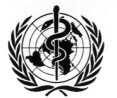

World Health Organization Classification of Tumours

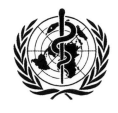

WHO   OMS

International Agency for Research on Cancer (IARC)

Pathology and Genetics of Tumours of Haematopoietic and Lymphoid Tissues

Edited by

Elaine S. Jaffe
Nancy Lee Harris
Harald Stein
James W. Vardiman

IARC*Press*
Lyon, 2001

World Health Organization Classification of Tumours

Series Editors   Paul Kleihues, M.D.
Leslie H. Sobin, M.D.

Pathology and Genetics of Tumours of Haematopoietic and Lymphoid Tissues

Editors   Elaine S. Jaffe, M.D.
Nancy Lee Harris, M.D.
Harald Stein, M.D.
James W. Vardiman, M.D.

Editorial Assistance   Wojciech Biernat, M.D.

Layout   Soyoung Lee
Sibylle Söring

Illustrations   Georges Mollon
Soyoung Lee

Printed by   Team Rush
69603 Villeurbanne, France

Publisher   IARC*Press*
International Agency for
Research on Cancer (IARC)
69008 Lyon, France

The WHO Classification of Tumours of
Haematopoietic and Lymphoid Tissues
was developed in collaboration with

Society for Hematopathology

European Association for Haematopathology

Steering Committee

Jacques Diebold

Georges Flandrin

Nancy Lee Harris

Elaine S. Jaffe

H. Konrad Müller-Hermelink

Harald Stein

James W. Vardiman

Emeritus Consultants

Costan W. Berard

Karl Lennert

Committee Chairs

Richard D. Brunning

Daniel Catovsky

Thomas M. Grogan

Nancy Lee Harris

Elisabeth Ralfkiaer

Martine Raphael

Harald Stein

Steven H. Swerdlow

James W. Vardiman

Roger A. Warnke

Lawrence M. Weiss

Members of the Clinical Advisory Committee are listed on page 310.

The Editorial and Consensus Meetings were supported by:

Cure for Lymphoma Foundation

Leukemia Clinical Research Foundation

Swiss Federal Office of Public Health

U.S. National Cancer Institute

University of Chicago Cancer Research Center

and

Frédérique Brupbacher
Charles Rodolphe Brupbacher Foundation for Cancer Research

Published by IARC Press, International Agency for Research on Cancer,
150 cours Albert Thomas, F-69008 Lyon, France

Format for bibliographic citations:
Jaffe E.S.,   Harris N.L., Stein H., Vardiman J.W. (Eds.): World Health Organization
Classification of Tumours. Pathology and Genetics of Tumours of Haematopoietic
and Lymphoid Tissues. IARC Press: Lyon 2001

IARC Library Cataloguing in Publication Data

Pathology and genetics of tumours of haematopoietic and lymphoid tissues/
        editors, E.S. Jaffe [et al.]

    (World Health Organization classification of tumours ; 3)

    1. Genetics 2. Hematopoietic System – pathology
    3. Lymphoid Tissue - pathology 4. Neoplasms I. Jaffe, Elaine Sarkin II.
    Series

    ISBN 92 832 2411 6   (NLM Classification: W1)

Contents

WHO Classification

The objective of the new WHO Classification of Tumours is to offer pathologists, oncologists and geneticists worldwide a system of classification for
human neoplasms that is based on their histopathological and genetic features. This is in accordance with the longstanding WHO principle that international agreement on criteria for the definition and classification of cancer types
and a standardized nomenclature are prerequisites for progress in clinical
oncology, multicentre therapy trials and comparative studies in different countries.

To ensure wide acceptance of the classification, great care is taken to select,
from different regions of the world, editors and contributors known for their scientific expertise and good judgment.

The present classification of tumours of haematopoietic and lymphatic tissues
is the result of several years of discussions and of consensus meetings aim-
ing at a nomenclature that is practical and which reflects the latest advances
in our understanding of the pathogenesis of these neoplasms.

Summary of the WHO classification of tumours of haematopoietic and lymphoid tissues

CHRONIC MYELOPROLIFERATIVE DISEASES

Chronic myelogenous leukaemia	9875/3*
Chronic neutrophilic leukaemia	9963/3
Chronic eosinophilic leukaemia/ hypereosinophilic syndrome	9964/3
Polycythaemia vera	9950/3
Chronic idiopathic myelofibrosis	9961/3
Essential thrombocythaemia	9962/3
Chronic myeloproliferative disease, unclassifiable	9975/3

MYELODYSPLASTIC / MYELOPROLIFERATIVE DISEASES

Chronic myelomonocytic leukaemia	9945/3
Atypical chronic myeloid leukaemia	9876/3
Juvenile myelomonocytic leukaemia	9946/3
Myelodysplastic/myeloproliferative diseases, unclassifiable	9975/3

MYELODYSPLASTIC SYNDROMES

Refractory anaemia	9980/3
Refractory anaemia with ringed sideroblasts	9982/3
Refractory cytopenia with multilineage dysplasia	9985/3
Refractory anaemia with excess blasts	9983/3
Myelodysplastic syndrome associated with isolated del(5q) chromosome abnormality	9986/3
Myelodysplastic syndrome, unclassifiable	9989/3

ACUTE MYELOID LEUKAEMIAS

Acute myeloid leukaemias with recurrent cytogenetic abnormalities

AML with t(8;21)(q22;q22), (AML1/ETO)	9896/3
AML with inv(16)(p13q22) or t(16;16)(p13;q22), (CBFβ/MYH11)	9871/3
Acute promyelocytic leukaemia (AML with t(15;17)(q22;q12), (PML/RARα) and variants)	9866/3
AML with 11q23 (MLL) abnormalities	9897/3

Acute myeloid leukaemia with multilineage dysplasia — 9895/3
with prior myelodysplastic syndrome
without prior myelodysplastic syndrome

Acute myeloid leukaemia and myelodysplastic syndrome, therapy related — 9920/3
Alkylating agent related
Topoisomerase II inhibitor-related

Acute myeloid leukaemia not otherwise categorised

Acute myeloid leukaemia, minimally differentiated	9872/3
Acute myeloid leukaemia without maturation	9873/3
Acute myeloid leukaemia with maturation	9874/3
Acute myelomonocytic leukaemia	9867/3
Acute monoblastic and monocytic leukaemia	9891/3
Acute erythroid leukaemia	9840/3
Acute megakaryoblastic leukaemia	9910/3
Acute basophilic leukaemia	9870/3
Acute panmyelosis with myelofibrosis	9931/3
Myeloid sarcoma	9930/3

Acute leukaemia of ambiguous lineage — 9805/3

B-CELL NEOPLASMS

Precursor B-cell neoplasm

Precursor B lymphoblastic leukaemia[1] / lymphoma[2]	9836/3[1] 9728/3[2]

Mature B-cell neoplasms

Chronic lymphocytic leukaemia[1] / small lymphocytic lymphoma[2]	9823/3[1] 9670/3[2]
B-cell prolymphocytic leukaemia	9833/3
Lymphoplasmacytic lymphoma	9671/3
Splenic marginal zone lymphoma	9689/3
Hairy cell leukaemia	9940/3
Plasma cell myeloma	9732/3
Solitary plasmacytoma of bone	9731/3
Extraosseous plasmacytoma	9734/3
Extranodal marginal zone B-cell lymphoma of mucosa-associated lymphoid tissue (MALT-lymphoma)	9699/3

Nodal marginal zone B-cell lymphoma	9699/3
Follicular lymphoma	9690/3
Mantle cell lymphoma	9673/3
Diffuse large B-cell lymphoma	9680/3
Mediastinal (thymic) large B-cell lymphoma	9679/3
Intravascular large B-cell lymphoma	9680/3
Primary effusion lymphoma	9678/3
Burkitt lymphoma[1] / leukaemia[2]	9687/3[1]
	9826/3[2]

B-cell proliferations of uncertain malignant potential

Lymphomatoid granulomatosis	9766/1
Post-transplant lymphoproliferative disorder, polymorphic	9970/1

T-CELL AND NK-CELL NEOPLASMS

Precursor T-cell neoplasms

Precursor T lymphoblastic leukaemia[1] / lymphoma[2]	9837/3[1]
	9729/3[2]
Blastic NK cell lymphoma**	9727/3

Mature T-cell and NK-cell neoplasms

T-cell prolymphocytic leukaemia	9834/3
T-cell large granular lymphocytic leukaemia	9831/3
Aggressive NK cell leukaemia	9948/3
Adult T-cell leukaemia/lymphoma	9827/3
Extranodal NK/T cell lymphoma, nasal type	9719/3
Enteropathy-type T-cell lymphoma	9717/3
Hepatosplenic T-cell lymphoma	9716/3
Subcutaneous panniculitis-like T-cell lymphoma	9708/3
Mycosis fungoides	9700/3
Sezary syndrome	9701/3
Primary cutaneous anaplastic large cell lymphoma	9718/3
Peripheral T-cell lymphoma, unspecified	9702/3
Angioimmunoblastic T-cell lymphoma	9705/3
Anaplastic large cell lymphoma	9714/3

T-cell proliferation of uncertain malignant potential

Lymphomatoid papulosis	9718/1

HODGKIN LYMPHOMA

Nodular lymphocyte predominant Hodgkin lymphoma	9659/3
Classical Hodgkin lymphoma	9650/3
Nodular sclerosis classical Hodgkin lymphoma	9663/3
Lymphocyte-rich classical Hodgkin lymphoma	9651/3
Mixed cellularity classical Hodgkin lymphoma	9652/3
Lymphocyte-depleted classical Hodgkin lymphoma	9653/3

HISTIOCYTIC AND DENDRITIC-CELL NEOPLASMS

Macrophage/histiocytic neoplasm

Histiocytic sarcoma	9755/3

Dendritic cell neoplasms

Langerhans cell histiocytosis	9751/1
Langerhans cell sarcoma	9756/3
Interdigitating dendritic cell sarcoma[1]/tumour[2]	9757/3[1]
	9757/1[2]
Follicular dendritic cell sarcoma[1]/tumour[2]	9758/3[1]
	9758/1[2]
Dendritic cell sarcoma, not otherwise specified	9757/3

MASTOCYTOSIS

Cutaneous mastocytosis	
Indolent systemic mastocytosis	9741/1
Systemic mastocytosis with associated clonal, haematological non-mast cell lineage disease	9741/3
Aggressive systemic mastocytosis	9741/3
Mast cell leukaemia	9742/3
Mast cell sarcoma	9740/3
Extracutaneous mastocytoma	9740/1

---

* Morphology code of the International Classification of Diseases (ICD-O), third edition. Behaviour is coded /3 for malignant tumours and /1 for lesions of low or uncertain malignant potential.

** Neoplasm of uncertain lineage and stage of differentiation.

WHO classification of tumours of haematopoietic and lymphoid tissues: Introduction

N.L. Harris
E.S. Jaffe
J.W. Vardiman
H. Stein
J. Diebold
H.K. Müller-Hermelink
G. Flandrin

The World Health Organization (WHO) Classification of Tumours of the Haematopoietic and Lymphoid Tissues was a collaborative project of the European Association for Haematopathology and the Society for Haematopathology. The project, which began in 1995, had a steering committee composed of members of both societies, and 10 disease-related committees that developed consensus lists of myeloid, lymphoid, and histiocytic neoplasms, with descriptions and criteria for diagnosis. The WHO classification is based on the principles defined in the "Revised European-American Classification of Lymphoid Neoplasms" (REAL) classification, originally published by the International Lymphoma Study Group (ILSG) in 1994 {496}. It incorporates input from additional experts in order to update and broaden the consensus on the lymphoid neoplasms, and extends the principles of disease definition and consensus-building to the classification of myeloid, mast cell and histiocytic neoplasms. Over 50 pathologists from around the world were involved in the project. Proponents of all major lymphoma and leukaemia classifications have agreed to accept the WHO as the standard classification of haematological malignancies. Thus, this classification represents the first true worldwide consensus classification of haematologic malignancies.

The REAL classification, published in 1994 by the ILSG, is a consensus list of lymphoid neoplasms that pathologists can recognise with available techniques, and that appear to be distinct clinical entities. This approach to lymphoma classification uses all available information – morphology, immunophenotype, genetic features, and clinical features – to define a disease entity. The relative importance of each of these features varies among diseases, and there is no one "gold standard." Morphology is always important, and some diseases are primarily defined by morphology, with immunophenotype as backup in difficult cases. Some diseases have a virtually specific immunophenotype, such that one would hesitate to make the diagnosis in the absence of the immunophenotype. In some lymphomas a specific genetic abnormality is an important defining criterion, while others lack specific known genetic abnormalities. Still others require knowledge of clinical features as well – nodal vs extranodal presentation, or specific anatomic site. Although its initial publication incited considerable controversy, experience over the last six years has shown that the REAL classification could be reproducibly used by expert haematopathologists, and that the entities it describes have distinctive clinical features, making it a useful and practical classification, despite its apparent complexity {8, 46}.

The REAL classification differed from prior lymphoma classifications in two ways. First, the emphasis on defining "real" disease entities, rather than focusing on subtleties of morphology or immunophenotype or primarily on patient survival, represented a new paradigm in lymphoma classification. Second, the ILSG recognised that the complexity of the field as the millennium approached made it impossible for a single person or small group to be completely authoritative, and also that broad agreement was necessary if the result were to be used by multiple pathologists, even if it required compromise. This consensus approach represented the second major departure from previous classifications, most of which represented the work of one or a few individuals

In order to ensure that the proposed WHO classification would be clinically useful, the Steering Committee invited expert haematologists and oncologists to form a Clinical Advisory Committee (CAC), with American and European co-chairs, to review the proposed classification and advise the pathologists on its clinical utility. Over 40 haematologists and oncologists from around the world participated. The proposed classification was circulated, and all participants were invited to submit topics and questions for discussion. The CAC and all pathologists involved in the WHO committees, as well as the Executive Committees of the two haematopathology societies, were invited to a meeting in 1997. The CAC meeting, which was organised around a series of clinical questions, was able to reach a consensus on most of the questions posed, and a number of modifications to the proposed classification were made {495}.

The WHO classification of haematological malignancies stratifies neoplasms primarily according to lineage: myeloid, lymphoid, histiocytic/dendritic cell and mast cell. Within each category, distinct diseases are defined according to a combination of morphology, immunophenotype, genetic features, and clinical syndromes. For each neoplasm, a cell of origin is postulated. For many of the lymphoid neoplasms, this "cell of origin" represents the stage of differentiation of the tumour cells that we see in the tissues, rather than the cell in which the initial transforming event occurs, since the latter is not known in many cases. Conversely, in some of the myeloid neoplasms, the "cell of origin" is known to be a pluripotential or multipotential stem cell, despite the fact that the majority of the tumour cells are at late stages of differentiation. It may well be that many haematologic malignancies originate in early precursor cells, and the specific genetic abnormality may determine what stage or stages the neoplastic cells differentiate to. Conversely, some neoplasms may truly arise in a later cell stage – such as a follicle centre cell – in which physiologic gene rearrangements and mutations create a substrate in which tumour-promoting genetic events can occur. The nomenclature for each entity reflects our best estimate of its lineage and stage of differentiation, recognising that our understanding is imperfect and that changes in lineage assignment and nomenclature may be necessary in the future as our understanding improves.

The classification recognises three major categories of lymphoid neoplasms: B cell neoplasms, T and NK cell neoplasms, and Hodgkin lymphoma (HL). Both lymphomas and lymphoid leukaemias are included in this classification, since both solid and circulating phases are present in many lymphoid neoplasms, and distinction between them is artificial. Thus, B-cell chronic lymphocytic leukaemia and B-cell small lymphocytic lymphoma are simply different manifestations of the same neoplasm, as are lymphoblastic lymphomas and lymphoblastic leukaemias and Burkitt lymphoma and Burkitt leukemia. Within the B and T/NK cell categories, two major categories are recognised – precursor neoplasms, corresponding to the earliest stages of differentiation, and peripheral or mature neoplasms, corresponding to more differentiated stages. Within the category of "non-Hodgkin" lymphomas, there are a large number of distinct diseases. These are associated with distinctive epidemiology, aetiology, clinical features and, often, distinctive responses to therapy. One of the corollaries of defining distinct entities is that it is neither possible nor helpful to sort them precisely according to histological grade or clinical aggressiveness. Histological grade is just one of many prognostic factors, which should be applied within a disease entity, not across the whole range of lymphoid neoplasms. Both the pathologist and the oncologist must "get to know" each disease entity and its spectrum of morphology and clinical behaviour. The lymphoid neoplasms can be sorted according to various principles, including their postulated normal counterpart in the immune system, their morphologic features, or their clinical features. The Clinical Advisory Committee considered the issue of clinical groupings and decided that sorting diseases according to prognosis was neither practical nor necessary, and could be misleading. Therefore, the WHO classification avoids such groupings. As the most practical approach, the peripheral T/NK-cell and B-cell neoplasms are grouped according to their most typical clinical presentations: predominantly disseminated, leukaemic, primary extranodal lymphomas, and predominantly nodal lymphomas.

A paradigm similar to that adopted for the REAL classification of lymphoid neoplasms has been applied to the myeloid disorders – namely, that a combination of morphology, immunophenotype, genetic features and clinical features is used to define distinct disease entities. The WHO Classification has four major groups of myeloid diseases. Chronic myeloproliferative diseases (CMPD) are clonal stem cell disorders characterised by effective haematopoiesis, resulting in elevated peripheral blood levels of one or more cell lines and, usually, hepatosplenomegaly; there is marrow hypercellularity with maturation and without dysplasia. Myelodysplastic/myeloproliferative diseases (MDS/MPD) are clonal stem cell disorders that have overlapping features between MDS and CMPD, with variably effective haematopoiesis and dysplastic features. Myelodysplastic syndromes (MDS) are clonal stem cell disorders characterised by ineffective haematopoiesis, resulting in cytopenias, and disordered (dysplastic) maturation of one or more cell lines. Acute myeloid leukaemias (AML) are clonal expansions of myeloid blasts. Although the French-American-British (FAB) morphologic classification of myeloid neoplasms has been accepted for many years, the discovery of a number of genetic lesions that predict clinical behaviour and outcome better than morphology alone necessitates the incorporation of specific genetic data into the classification scheme. In addition, acute leukaemias that arise in a background of myelodysplasia or from a previous MDS or MDS/MPD have sufficiently different biology from those lacking such features to warrant their own category. Finally, two distinctive categories of therapy-related AML have been recognised. Therefore, within the category of AML, four main groups are recognised: I. AML with recurrent cytogenetic abnormalities; II. AML with myelodysplasia-related features; III. Therapy-related AML and MDS; and IV. AML not otherwise categorised. Thus, the WHO classification not only incorporates specific genetic information as well as morphology into the classification of myeloid neoplasms, but also emphasises the relationships that exist between the four major categories of myeloid diseases. Because the technology of genetic analysis is moving rapidly, it is likely that advances in this field will necessitate revisions to any current classification in the near future.

Finally, a critical feature of any tumour classification is that it be periodically reviewed and updated to incorporate new information. Joint classification committees of the major societies of haematopathology will undertake this as an ongoing project. The experience of developing the WHO classification has produced a new and exciting degree of cooperation and communication among pathologists and oncologists from around the world, which should facilitate progress in the understanding and treatment of haematologic malignancies.

CHAPTER 1

Chronic Myeloproliferative Diseases

It is fitting that the Chronic Myeloproliferative Diseases (CMPDs) occupy the first chapter in this publication, because one of the members of this family of diseases, Chronic Myelogenous Leukaemia (CML), has a long tradition of being "first". CML was the first disorder for which the term leukaemia was used, the first malignancy associated with a recurring chromosomal abnormality (the Philadelphia chromosome), and the first disease in which the associated chromosomal abnormality was found to result from a translocation of genetic material from one chromosome to another to form a fusion gene (*BCR/ABL*). In addition, it was the first disease in which the fusion gene was recognised as giving rise to an abnormal fusion protein fundamental in the pathogenesis of the disease. Now, CML is the first disorder in which a therapeutic agent has been designed to specifically target the molecular defect.

Unfortunately, there is no specific genetic defect yet discovered for any of the remaining CMPD entities. For these, the diagnosis rests entirely upon the careful correlation of morphologic findings from blood and bone marrow specimens with laboratory and clinical observations. Only through consistency in classification of patients with these disorders will investigation into their underlying pathogenesis and the subsequent development of more effective therapies be successful.

WHO histological classification of chronic myeloproliferative diseases

Chronic myelogenous leukaemia (Philadelphia chromosome, t(9;22)(q34;q11), *BCR/ABL* positive)	9875/3
Chronic neutrophilic leukaemia	9963/3
Chronic eosinophilic leukaemia (and the hypereosinophilic syndrome)	9964/3
Polycythaemia vera	9950/3
Chronic idiopathic myelofibrosis (with extramedullary haematopoiesis)	9961/3
Essential thrombocythaemia	9962/3
Chronic myeloproliferative disease, unclassifiable	9975/3

Chronic myeloproliferative diseases: Introduction

J.W. Vardiman
R.D. Brunning
N.L. Harris

Definition and features

The Chronic Myeloproliferative Diseases (CMPDs) are clonal haematopoietic stem cell disorders characterised by proliferation in the bone marrow of one or more of the myeloid (i.e., granulocytic, erythroid and megakaryocytic) lineages. The proliferation is associated with relatively normal maturation that is effective, resulting in increased numbers of granulocytes, red blood cells and/or platelets in the peripheral blood, in contrast to the ineffective haematopoiesis observed in the myelodysplastic syndromes. Splenomegaly and hepatomegaly are commonly found, and are caused by sequestration of excess blood cells in the spleen or liver, extramedullary haematopoiesis, leukaemic infiltration, or any combination of these. The sum of these features distinguishes the CMPDs from the myelodysplastic syndromes, the myelodysplastic / myeloproliferative diseases, and from acute myeloid leukaemia.

Despite an often insidious clinical onset, all of the CMPDs have the potential to undergo clonal evolution and a stepwise progression that terminates in bone marrow failure due to myelofibrosis or ineffective haematopoiesis, or in transformation to an acute blast phase. Although the clinical, laboratory and morphologic changes associated with disease progression vary, cytogenetic or molecular evidence of clonal evolution is particularly noteworthy, and usually indicates the onset of an accelerated stage of the disease or of transformation to an acute process. An increase in the percentage of blasts in the blood or marrow, if persistent, is also an indication of worsening disease. The finding of 10-19% blasts in the blood or bone marrow generally signifies disease acceleration, and 20% or more is sufficient for a diagnosis of a blast phase.

A complicating feature of the myeloproliferative diseases is the frequent overlap of the clinical, laboratory and morphologic findings among the specific disease entities. Leukocytosis, thrombocytosis, excessive megakaryocytic proliferation, myelofibrosis and organomegaly are features that can occur in almost any of the individual diseases, and that sometimes blur the boundaries between them. For chronic myelogenous leukaemia (CML), the *BCR/ABL* fusion gene permits an unequivocal diagnosis when it is present in association with characteristic morphologic and clinical findings. Currently, however, no chromosomal or molecular markers specific for the other CMPD entities have been identified, although a number of recurring cytogenetic abnormalities have been reported. Still, most patients with CMPD have sufficiently characteristic clinical, laboratory and morphologic findings that, when considered together, allow them to be classified.

If the initial findings do not allow a specific classification, the designation as "unclassifiable" may be preferable until the process becomes more clearly defined.

Incidence / epidemiology

The CMPDs are primarily diseases of adults, and peak in frequency in the fifth to seventh decades of life. The incidence for all CMPDs combined is approximately 6-9/100,000 population annually. There appears to be no major difference in the geographical distribution of CML, but population and geographic-based data for the other CMPDs is limited. Data from Europe and North America suggest a similar incidence of polycythaemia vera (PV) and essential thrombocythaemia (ET) on the two continents, but they are much less common in Asia {1434, 355, 867, 1101}.

Table 1.01
Usual features of myeloid disorders at diagnosis.

Disease	BM cellularity	% Marrow Blasts	Maturation	Morphology	Haematopoiesis	Blood count(s)	Organomegaly
Myeloproliferative disorders	Usually increased	Normal or slightly increased (<10%)	Present	Relatively normal	Effective	One or more myeloid cell lines increased	Common
Myelodysplastic syndromes	Usually increased, occasionally decreased	Normal or increased (<20%)	Present	Dysplasia of one or more myeloid lineages	Ineffective	Cytopenia(s)	Uncommon
Myelodysplastic/ myeloproliferative diseases	Usually increased	Normal or increased (<20%)	Present	Dysplasia of one or more myeloid lineages frequent	Effective or ineffective; may vary among involved lineages	Variable	Common
Acute myeloid leukaemia	Usually increased, occasionally decreased	Increased (≥20%)	Varies, frequently minimal	May or may not be associated with dysplasia in one or more myeloid lines	Ineffective or effective	Variable	Uncommon

Introduction **17**

Pathogenesis

The major clinical and pathologic findings in the chronic myeloproliferative disorders are due to dysregulated proliferation and expansion of myeloid progenitors in the bone marrow, resulting in increased numbers of mature granulocytes, red blood cells and/or platelets in the peripheral blood. In most of the CMPDs, the genetic abnormality that initiates the myeloproliferative process occurs in a haematopoietic stem cell. This abnormality may bestow a proliferative advantage to only one or to all of the myeloid lineages, but regardless, all of the myeloid cells, and in some cases B and T lymphocytes, may be derived from the neoplastic clone.

Although no specific genetic abnormalities or disease-initiating events have yet been identified for most of the CMPDs, activation of tyrosine kinase signal transduction pathways are frequently implicated in their pathogenesis {15}. In CML, for example, the Philadelphia (Ph) chromosome results in the formation of a hybrid gene, the *BCR/ABL* fusion gene, that includes regions of the *ABL* gene translocated from chromosome 9 to chromosome 22, where they are juxtaposed with sequences of the *BCR* gene. The normal *ABL* gene encodes a nonreceptor tyrosine kinase important in signal transduction and regulation of cell growth. Juxtaposition of *ABL* with sequences of *BCR* results in enhanced tyrosine kinase activity and constitutive overactivity of tyrosine phosphokinase (reviewed in references {859, 1341}). Haematopoeitic cell lines transfected with BCR/ABL cDNA exhibit growth-factor independent proliferation in vitro, and tumourogenicity in vivo. Mice transplanted with stem cells transduced with BCR/ABL cDNA can develop a CML-like syndrome, with neutrophil proliferation and splenomegaly. Deletion of the tyrosine kinase or other key domains of the fusion protein abrogates these transforming effects. Thus, the BCR-ABL protein is necessary and sufficient for transformation. In addition, the protein leads to increased transcription of *MYC* and *BCL-2*, which may protect the leukaemic cells from apoptosis. Therefore the expansion of the neoplastic clone may be due not only to increased proliferation but also to prolonged survival.

Abnormal activation of tyrosine kinase-dependent signal transduction pathways have been implicated in the pathogenesis of other CMPDs as well. In PV, the erythroid progenitors are hypersensitive to a number of growth factors, including insulin-like growth factor-1 (IGF-1). The receptor for IGF-1, a member of the tyrosine kinase family of receptors, is hyperphosphorylated in the erythroid precursors in PV, and this could permit abnormal activation of a number of pathways such as RAS {249}. In addition, as in CML, there is increased transcription of genes that block apoptosis in PV {1055}. Whether similar molecular events will be found in the other CMPDs remain to be seen, but evidence for their presence is accumulating. The events that lead to disease progression in any of the CMPDs, including CML, are poorly understood at the current time.

One of the important bone marrow findings that overlaps the various CMPD entities is myelofibrosis. Although reticulin and/or collagen fibrosis is considered a hallmark of the fibrotic stage of CIMF, it can be associated with disease progression in the other entities as well, and sometimes creates diagnostic problems. The fibrosis is a secondary phenomenon in the CMPDs; the fibroblasts do not belong to the neoplastic clone. Instead, the fibrosis is most likely caused by the abnormal production and release of several cytokines and growth factors, such as platelet-derived growth factor and transforming growth factor-β (TFG-β), by megakaryocytes and other marrow cells {820}. These cytokines stimulate fibroblastic proliferation and the synthesis of fibronectin and collagen. The involvement of the megakaryocytes in eliciting the deposition of connective tissue is an attractive hypothesis to explain the often-observed relationship between atypical megakaryocytic proliferation and marrow fibrosis, not only in the CMPDs but also in acute megakaryoblastic leukaemia and the myelodysplastic syndromes.

Prognosis

If untreated, patients with a CMPDs may die within months after the onset of symp-

Table 1.02
Recurring genetic abnormalities and their frequency (%) in the myeloproliferative diseases at diagnosis {294, 740}.

Disease	Specific abnormalities	(%)	Recurring, nonspecific cytogenetic/genetic abnormalities	(%)
CML, CP	t(9;22)(q34;q11), *BCR/ABL*	100		
CML, AP/BP	t(9:22)(q34;q11), *BCR/ABL*	100	+8, +Ph, +19, i(17q), t(3;21)(q26;q22)(*EVI1/AML1*)	80
CNL	None		+8, +9, del (20q), del(11q14)	~10
CEL	None		+8, t(5;12)(q33;p13)(*TEL/PDGFβR*), dic(1;7), 8p11 (*FGFR1*)	?
PV	None		+8, +9, del(20q), del(13q), del(1p11)	~15
CIMF	None		+8, del(20q), -7/del(7q), del(11q), del(13q)	~35
ET	None		+8, del(13q)	~5

CML, CP = Chronic myelogenous leukaemia, chronic phase; CML, AP/BP = Chronic myelogenous leukaemia, accelerated or blast phase;
CNL = Chronic neutrophilic leukaemia; CEL = Chronic eosinophilic leukaemia; PV = Polycythaemia vera, proliferative phase;
CIMF = Chronic idiopathic myelofibrosis; ET = Essential thrombocythaemia' ?=insufficient data available

toms. However, when properly diagnosed and carefully managed, some patients may survive for many years, depending on the specific disease they have. Recent improvements in therapy, such as IFN alpha and bone marrow transplantation have substantially increased the life expectancy for patients with CML, so that median survival times of 5-7 years are commonly reported {355}. For PV and ET, median survival times longer than 10 years are not uncommon, and in view of the fact that they occur most frequently in older individuals, overall life expectancy may not be severely shortened {1434, 921, 909}. Perhaps the most exciting prospect for the future is therapy that targets specific molecular defects in the CMPDs, such as the recent development of an agent that inhibits the tyrosine kinase function of the BCR-ABL fusion protein in CML {321}. If similar mechanisms of pathogenesis do exist in the other CMPDs, tyrosine kinase inhibitors or similar agents may prove to be an important therapeutic tool that may significantly improve survival.

Rationale for classification

Although the ideal classification system for the CMPDs may ultimately be based on the underlying molecular pathogenesis, such knowledge is not yet available for each disorder. At the present time, therefore, the classification is based on the lineage of the predominant proliferating cells and the prominence of marrow fibrosis, together with a constellation of clinical and laboratory features. The classification of an individual patient's disease is based on the careful correlation of morphologic findings from well-prepared peripheral blood smears, bone marrow aspirate smears and bone marrow biopsy specimens with clinical and laboratory information, including cytogenetic and molecular genetic data. A bone marrow biopsy specimen is essential for diagnosis as well as for predicting prognosis, and should be stained with H&E, Giemsa or other appropriate stains that permit evaluation of histologic and cytologic features. The marrow biopsy specimen should also be stained for reticulin fibers to assess the marrow connective tissue. The blood and marrow specimens should be studied together as a unit in order to reach a diagnosis that has relevance for treatment and prognostic purposes.

Although the WHO classification for the CMPDs incorporates recent knowledge and techniques that aid in the recognition of the various entities, many of the guidelines proposed by the Polycythaemia Vera Study Group (PVSG) remain as integral components for the criteria for diagnosis of some of the entities. Perhaps the most important guideline established by the PVSG is that the proper management and understanding of the CMPDs are brought about by the interaction of the clinician, laboratorian and morphologist. This principal is endorsed in the WHO classification.

Chronic myelogenous leukaemia

J.W. Vardiman
R. Pierre
J. Thiele

M. Imbert
R.D. Brunning
G. Flandrin

Definition

Chronic myelogenous leukaemia (CML) is a myeloproliferative disease that originates in an abnormal pluripotent bone marrow stem cell and is consistently associated with the Philadelphia (Ph) chromosome and/or the *BCR/ABL* fusion gene. Although the initial major finding in CML is neutrophilic leukocytosis, the abnormal fusion gene is found in all myeloid lineages as well as in some lymphoid cells. The disease is bi- or triphasic: an initial indolent chronic phase (CML-CP) is followed by one or both of the aggressive transformed stages, accelerated phase (CML-AP) and blast phase (CML-BP).

ICD-O code   9875/3

Synonyms

Chronic granulocytic leukaemia
Chronic myeloid leukaemia

Epidemiology

CML is the most common of the myeloproliferative diseases. It accounts for 15-20% of all cases of leukaemia, and has a worldwide incidence of 1-1.5 cases per 100,000 population per year {1434, 473, 355}. The disease can occur at any age, but the median age at diagnosis is in the fifth and sixth decades of life. There is slight male predominance {1434, 473, 355}.

Site of involvement

In CML-CP, the leukaemic cells are minimally invasive, and the proliferation is largely confined to haematopoietic tissues, primarily the blood, bone marrow spleen and liver. During CML-BP, not only these sites but also a number of extramedullary tissues, including lymph nodes, skin, soft tissue and central nervous system, may show infiltration by blasts {900, 574}.

Clinical features

Most patients are diagnosed in the chronic phase, which usually has an insidious onset. Nearly 20-40% of patients are asymptomatic at diagnosis, and are discovered when a white blood cell (WBC) count performed at the time of a routine medical examination is found to be abnormal {355, 1147}.
Common findings at presentation include fatigue, weight loss, anaemia, night sweats and splenomegaly {355, 1147}. Atypical presentations, including initial presentation in CML-BP without a detectable chronic phase, may also occur {824, 25}. The transformed stages are generally accompanied by worsened performance status, and by symptoms related to severe anaemia, thrombocytopenia, or marked splenic enlargement {355}.

Aetiology

Factors predisposing to CML are unknown. Radiation exposure has been implicated in some cases {112, 250}. There does not appear to be an inherited disposition.

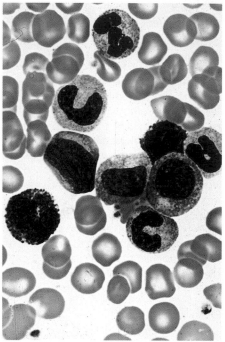

Fig. 1.01 CML, chronic phase. Peripheral blood smear shows leukocytosis and neutrophilic cells at varying stages of maturation. Basophilia is prominent. No dysplasia is present.

Morphology

Chronic phase (CML-CP)

In CML-CP, the peripheral blood smear shows leukocytosis (median WBC ~170 x 10^9/L) due mainly to neutrophils in different stages of maturation, with peaks in the percentages of myelocytes and of segmented neutrophils {1147, 1217}. Blasts

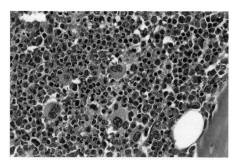

Fig. 1.02 CML, chronic phase. The bone marrow is nearly 100% cellular, due to granulocytic proliferation which shows maturation. There is concomitant megakaryocyte proliferation.

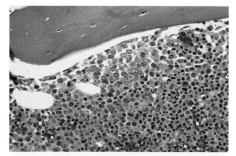

Fig. 1.03 CML, chronic phase. Often, a thickened layer of immature granulocytes, about 5-6 cells deep, surrounds the bony trabeculae. In normal marrow specimens, this layer is only 2-3 cells deep.

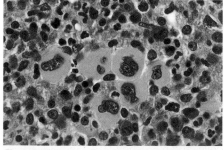

Fig. 1.04 CML, chronic phase. The megakaryocytes in CML are characteristically smaller than normal megakaryocytes.

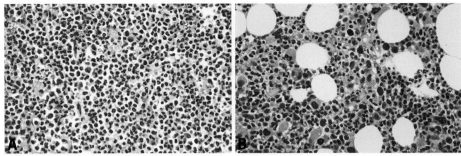

Fig. 1.05 CML. The number of megakaryocytes in CML is variable. **A** Marrow specimen in which the megakaryocytes are sparse, and the proliferation is mainly due to neutrophils. **B** A case of CML with numerous megakaryocytes. Some authorities {431} have used the variation in the numbers of megakaryocytes as the basis for a histologic subclassification scheme for CML.

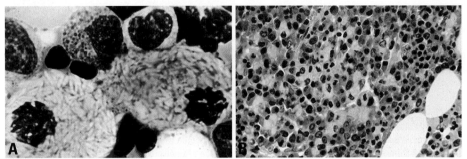

Fig. 1.06 CML, chronic phase. **A** The "pseudo-Gaucher cells" commonly observed in the marrow aspirates of patients with CML. **B** They may also be appreciated as foamy cells in bone marrow biopsy specimens. These histiocytes are secondary to increased cell turnover, although they are derived from the neoplastic clone of bone marrow cells.

usually account for <2% of the WBCs {1217, 91}. Absolute basophilia is invariably present, and many patients have eosinophilia as well {1217}. Significant dysgranulopoiesis is not observed {91}. Because the WBC count is increased, absolute monocytosis may be present, but the percent of monocytes is usually less than 3% {91}. The platelet count is normal or increased, and may exceed 1000 X 10^9/L; thrombocytopenia is very uncommon during the chronic phase {1147}. Most patients have mild anaemia. The bone marrow biopsy is hypercellular due to increased numbers of neutrophils and their precursors, which demonstrate a maturation pattern similar to that in the blood {928, 788}. In some cases, the paratrabecular cuff of immature neutrophils is thickened to 5-10 cells, in contrast to the 2-3 cell layer normally seen, and abundant segmented neutrophils are situated deeper in the intertrabecular regions of the marrow. Blasts usually account for fewer than 5% of the marrow cells, and more than 10% indicates transformation to the accelerated stage {194}. Megakaryocytes are characteristically smaller than normal and have hypolobated nuclei {431, 1290}. They may occur in normal or slightly decreased numbers, but in 40-50% of patients there is moderate to extensive proliferation of megakaryocytes {431, 1290}. Erythroid precursors vary in number, but are usually reduced in percentage. Up to 40% of patients display an increase in reticulin fibers in the initial marrow specimen, which can sometimes be marked {431, 1290, 277}. An increase in the amount of reticulin fibers in the bone marrow generally correlates with increased numbers of megakaryocytes, larger spleen size, and a more severe degree of anaemia {1290, 277}. Eosinophils may be substantially increased in some patients. Bone marrow aspirate smears generally reflect the changes described in the biopsy. Pseudo-Gaucher cells and sea-blue histiocytes are seen in about 30% of specimens. They are secondary to the increased bone marrow cell turnover, and are derived from the neoplastic clone {505, 26}.

In the chronic phase, the spleen is enlarged due to infiltration of the cords of the red pulp by granulocytes in different maturation stages, and a similar infiltrate may be seen in the hepatic sinusoids and portal areas.

Accelerated phase (CML-AP)

The accelerated phase of CML is characterised by one or more of the following changes: 1) Myeloblasts accounting for 10-19% of the peripheral blood white cells or of nucleated cells in the bone marrow, 2) peripheral blood basophils ≥20%, 3) persistent thrombocytopenia <100 X 10^9/L that is unrelated to therapy, 4) persistent thrombocytosis >1000 x 10^9/L despite adequate therapy, 5) increasing WBC count and increasing spleen size unresponsive to therapy,

Table 1.03
Chronic myelogenous leukaemia, accelerated phase.

The diagnosis of CML-AP may be made when one or more of the following are present:
- Blasts 10-19% of WBCs in peripheral blood and/or of nucleated bone marrow cells
- Peripheral blood basophils ≥20%
- Persistent thrombocytopenia (<100 x 10^9/L) unrelated to therapy, or persistent thrombocytosis (>1000 x 10^9/L) unresponsive to therapy
- Increasing spleen size and increasing WBC count unresponsive to therapy
- Cytogenetic evidence of clonal evolution
Megakaryocytic proliferation that occurs in sizeable sheets and clusters, associated with marked reticulin or collagen fibrosis, and/or severe granulocytic dysplasia, should be considered as suggestive of CML-AP. These latter findings, however, have not yet been analysed in large clinical studies to determine whether they are independent criteria for accelerated phase; they often occur simultaneously with one or more of the other features listed.

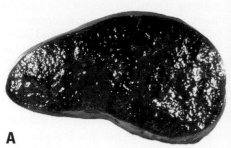 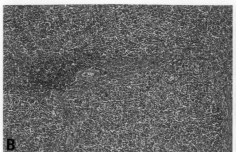 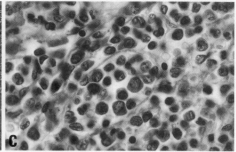

Fig. 1.07 CML. Splenomegaly is prominent in CML. **A** The gross appearance of the spleen in CML is solid and uniformly deep red, although areas of infarct may appear as lighter colored regions. **B** The red pulp distribution of the infiltrate usually compresses and obliterates the white pulp. **C** The leukaemic cells are present in the sinuses as well as in the splenic cords of the red pulp.

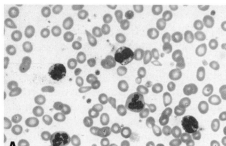 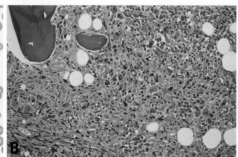 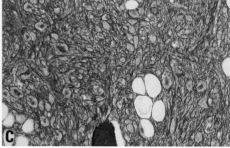

Fig. 1.08 CML, accelerated phase. **A** A peripheral blood smear from a patient in the accelerated phase. Basophils account for nearly 30% of the WBCs, and occasional blasts are also seen. **B** Bone marrow biopsy specimen, which shows areas of cellular depletion and prominence of small megakaryocytes. A marked increase in reticulin fibrosis is seen in **C**.

and/or 6) evidence of clonal evolution {355, 194, 628, 1146}. Marked dysplasia in the granulocytic lineage or prominent proliferation of small, dysplastic megakaryocytes in large clusters or sheets associated with marked reticulin or collagen fibrosis are suggestive of CML-AP {900, 154}, although the independent significance of these latter changes in defining this phase has not yet been well-tested in large clinical studies. Any lymphoblasts in the blood or marrow are always a cause for concern, and their number should be closely monitored, because they may indicate that a lymphoblastic transformation is imminent.

Blast phase (CML-BP)
The blast phase resembles acute leukaemia. The diagnosis of CML-BP can be made when 1) blasts ≥20% of the peripheral blood white cells or of the nucleated cells in the bone marrow, or 2) when there is an extramedullary proliferation of blasts, and/or 3) when there are large aggregates and clusters of blasts in the bone marrow biopsy specimen {574, 708, 251, 154}. In about 70% of cases, the blast lineage is myeloid, and may include neutrophilic, eosinophilic,

basophilic, monocytic, erythroid or megakaryocytic blasts, or any combination thereof. In approximately 20-30% of patients, the blast phase is due to proliferation of lymphoblasts. Rarely, patients

have separate populations of myeloid and lymphoid lineage blasts simultaneously {1130, 650, 917, 288}. The blast lineage may be obvious on morphologic grounds, but often the blasts are primi-

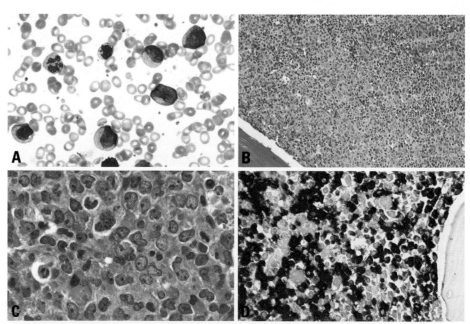

Fig. 1.09 CML, myeloid blast phase. **A** Peripheral blood of a patient with myeloid blast phase. The majority of the white blood cells are blasts. **B** and **C** illustrate sheets of myeloblasts in the bone marrow biopsy. **D** demonstrates myeloperoxidase detected immunohistochemically, proving the myeloid lineage of the blast proliferation.

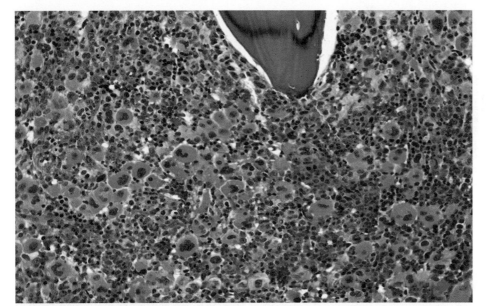

Fig. 1.10 CML, myeloid blast phase. Sheets of abnormal megakaryocytes, including micromegakaryocytes, are illustrated in the biopsy specimen. Blasts infiltrate between the abnormal megakaryocytes.

tive or heterogeneous, so immunophenotypic analysis is recommended.

Extramedullary blast proliferations most commonly present in the skin, lymph node, spleen, bone or central nervous system, but can occur anywhere, and may be of myeloid or lymphoid lineage {574}. If accumulations of blasts occupy focal but significant areas of the marrow, the diagnosis of CML-BP is warranted, even if the remainder of the marrow biopsy shows chronic phase {154}. However, foci of blasts that indicate BP must be distinguished from the foci of promyelo-

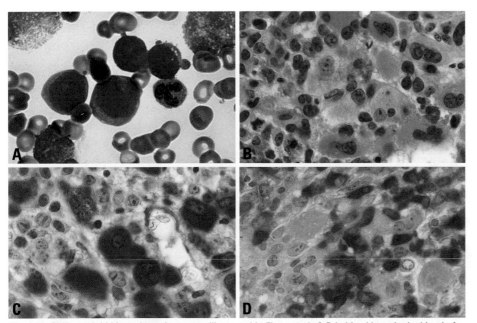

Fig. 1.11 CML, myeloid blast phase from case illustrated in Figure 1.10. **A** Primitive blasts in the blood of a patient who was diagnosed to have CML 5 years earlier. Flow cytometry demonstrated that the antigens CD13 and CD33 were expressed on most blasts, but a smaller number expressed the megakaryocyte-associated antigen, CD61. **B** There are numerous blasts between the abnormal megakaryocytes. **C** An immunohistochemical study for the megakaryocyte antigen, CD61, shows staining of occasional blasts as well as of the abnormal megakaryocytes. **D** More blasts were positive for myeloperoxidase than CD61. This myeloid blast phase is therefore mainly myeloblasts with a minor population of megakaryoblasts.

Table 1.04
Chronic myelogenous leukaemia, blast phase.

Blast phase may be diagnosed if one or more is present:
- Blasts ≥20% of peripheral blood white cells or of nucleated bone marrow cells
- Extramedullary blast proliferation
- Large foci or clusters of blasts in the bone marrow biopsy

cytes and myelocytes that often are prominent in paratrabecular and perivascular regions during chronic phase.

Cytochemistry / immunophenotype
The neutrophils in CML-CP have markedly decreased neutrophil alkaline phosphatase {976}, and may demonstrate delayed or weak expression of antigens normally found on neutrophils, such as CD15 and HLA-DR {460}. In BP of myeloid origin, the blasts may have strong, weak or no myeloperoxidase activity, but will have antigens associated with myeloid, monocytic (CD13, CD14, CD15, CD33, etc.), megakaryocytic (CDw41, CD61) and/or erythroid (glycophorin, haemoglobin A) differentiation. Not uncommonly, the myeloid blasts will express one or more lymphoid antigens as well {1130, 650, 917, 288}. Most cases of lymphoblastic BP are precursor B lymphoblasts (positive for CD10, CD19, CD34, and TdT but negative for sIg), but cases of precursor T cell origin (CD3, cCD3, CD7, TdT, etc.) also occur {251, 1130, 650, 917}. In many cases of lymphoid blast phase, one or more myeloid antigens is coexpressed on the blasts. Rarely, lymphoid and myeloid lineage blasts are present simultaneously {1130, 650, 917, 288}.

Genetics
At diagnosis, 90-95% of cases of CML have the characteristic t(9;22)(q34;q11) cytogenetic abnormality that results in the Philadelphia chromosome [der (22q)] {958, 1118}. This translocation fuses sequences of the *BCR* gene on chromosome 22 with regions of the *ABL* gene on chromosome 9 {79}. The remaining cases either have variant translocations that involve a third or even a fourth chromosome in addition to chromosomes 9 and 22, or have a cryptic translocation of 9q34

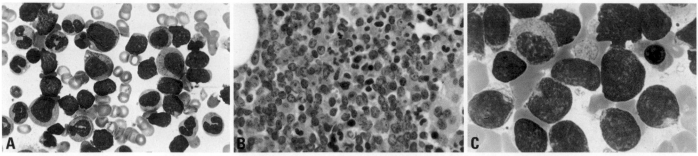

Fig. 1.12 CML, lymphoid blast phase. **A** Peripheral blood smear from a patient with lymphoid blast phase. Flow cytometry analysis of the blasts demonstrated a precursor B-cell phenotype: CD19, CD20, CD10, TdT and CD34 positive; a minor population of blasts co-expressed the myeloid-related antigen, CD33, with CD19. **B** Bone marrow biopsy and **C**, marrow aspirate smear from the same patient.

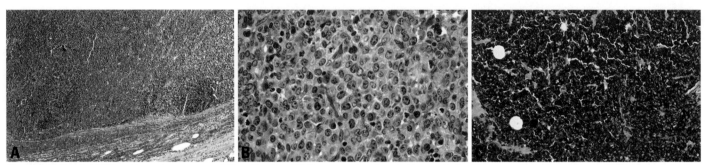

Fig. 1.13 CML, myeloid blast phase, in an extramedullary site. **A** and **B** illustrate a lymph node biopsy obtained from a patient with a history of CML for 3 years. The enlarged lymph node was the first evidence of blast phase. The lymph node architecture is largely effaced by a proliferation of medium to large sized cells. **C** an immunohistochemical study for lysozyme confirms the myeloid lineage of the blasts.

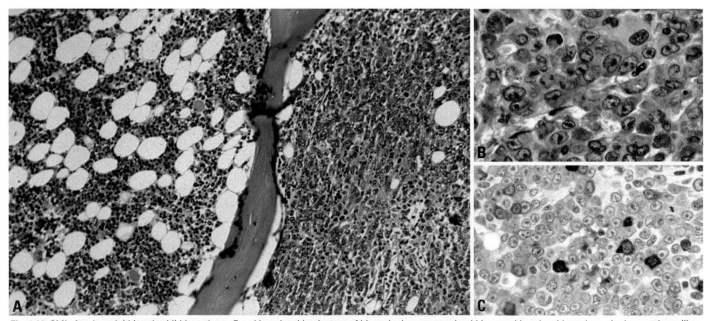

Fig. 1.14 CML, focal myeloid (erythroid) blast phase. Focal but sizeable clusters of blasts in the marrow should be considered as blast phase. In the specimen illustrated in **A**, much of the marrow biopsy shows chronic phase CML, but there is an adjacent, large sheet of blasts sufficient for a diagnosis of blast phase. **B** The blasts are large, with prominent nucleoli, and are demonstrated to be of erythroid lineage by immunostaining for haemoglobin A, which is shown in **C**.

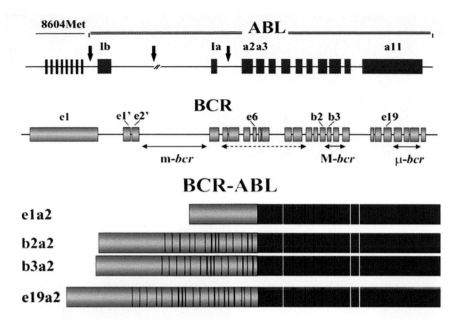

Fig. 1.15 Schematic representation of the *ABL* and the *BCR* genes disrupted in the t(9;22)(q34;q21) chromosomal abnormality. Exons are represented by boxes and introns by connecting horizontal lines. Breakpoints in *ABL*, illustrated as vertical arrows, almost invariably occur either upstream of exon Ib, between Ib and Ia, or between Ia and a2. The *BCR* gene contains 25 exons, including two putative alternative first (e1') and second (e2') exons. The breakpoints in *BCR* usually occur within one of three breakpoint cluster regions (bcr), the locations and probable extents of which are shown by the three double-headed horizontal arrows. In exceptional cases, the *BCR* breakpoints fall between m-bcr and M-bcr, within the region indicated by the double-headed dashed-line arrow. The lower half of the figure shows the structure of the various BCR-ABL m-RNA transcripts which are formed in accordance with the position of the breakpoint in *BCR*. Breaks in m-bcr give origin to BCR-ABL mRNA molecules with an e1a2 junction. The breaks in M-bcr occur either between exons b2 (e13) and b3 (e14) or between b3 (e14) and b4 (e15), generating fusion transcripts with a b2a2 or a b3a2 junction, respectively. Breakpoints in mu-bcr, the most 3' cluster region, result in BCR-ABL transcripts with an e19a2 junction, which was originally described as c3a2. Reproduced from Melo, J. {859}.

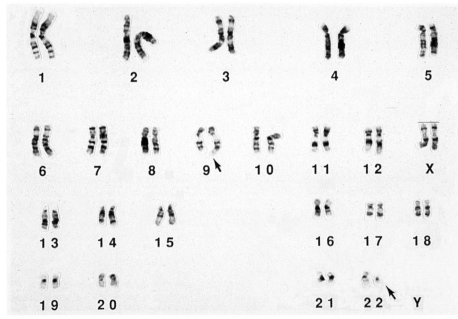

Fig. 1.16 CML. Karyotype from a patient with chronic phase CML. A reciprocal translocation involving chromosomes 9 and 22 has occurred. The der (22) chromosome is the Philadelphia chromosome.

and 22q11 that cannot be identified by routine cytogenetic analysis. In such cases, the *BCR/ABL* fusion gene is present, and can be detected by FISH analysis, RT-PCR or Southern blot techniques that detect the *BCR/ABL* fusion gene or the abnormal RNA fusion transcripts {859, 1380}.

The site of the breakpoint in the *BCR* gene may influence the phenotype of the disease {859}. In CML, the breakpoint on the *BCR* gene is almost always in the major breakpoint cluster region (M-BCR, *BCR* exons 12-16, also known as b1-b5) and an abnormal fusion protein, p210, is formed which has increased tyrosine kinase activity {859}. Rarely, the breakpoint in the *BCR* gene occurs in the mu region (μ–BCR, *BCR* exons 17-20, also known as c1-c4), and a larger fusion protein, p230, is encoded. Patients with this fusion may demonstrate prominent neutrophilic maturation {859, 998}. Although the minor breakpoint region, m-BCR, (*BCR* exons 1-2) leads to a shorter fusion protein (p190) and is most frequently associated with Ph positive ALL, small amounts of the p190 transcript can be detected in more than 90% of patients with CML as well, due to alternative splicing of the *BCR* gene {1127}. However, this breakpoint may also be seen in rare cases of CML that are distinctive for having increased numbers of monocytes, and thus can resemble chronic myelomonocytic leukemia {863}.

The significance of chromosomal abnormalities in addition to the Ph chromosome that are present at the time of diagnosis is not entirely clear. However, evidence of clonal evolution after the diagnostic specimen usually signifies transformation to more aggressive disease {355, 882, 881}. At the time of transformation to CML-AP or CML-BP, 80% of patients demonstrate cytogenetic changes in addition to the Ph chromosome, such as an extra Ph, +8, or i(17q). Genes shown to be altered in the transformed stages include *TP53*, *RB1*, *MYC*, *p16^{INK4a}*, *RAS*, and *AML1*, *EVI-1*, but their role in the transformation, if any, is currently unknown {881, 448}.

Postulated cell of origin
Pluripotent bone marrow stem cell.

Prognosis and predictive features
The natural history of CML is progression of disease from the chronic phase to CML-AP and/or CML-BP. Median survival

times have been prolonged through recent advances in therapy, such as interferon-alpha, so that median survival times of 5-7 years are now commonly reported {355}. Prognostic models have been proposed that consider a number of parameters at the time of initial diagnosis, such as patient age, spleen size, the numbers of blasts and of basophils in the marrow and blood and the amount of marrow fibrosis, that can, with varying degrees of success, stratify patients into low, intermediate and high risk groups {277, 1204, 629, 738, 1292}. Despite significant advances in therapy, including the recent development of agents that directly block the tyrosine kinase activity of the abnormal BCR/ABL fusion protein {321}, allogeneic bone marrow transplant is currently the only curative therapy.

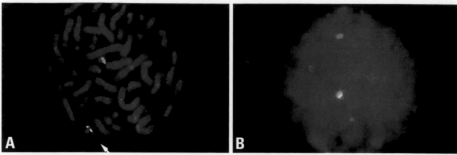

Fig. 1.17 CML. Fluorescent *in situ* hybridisation (FISH) depicting the *BCR/ABL* fusion gene. **A** depicts the fusion signal (arrow) in a metaphase preparation from a patient with CML, and **B** in an interphase cell.

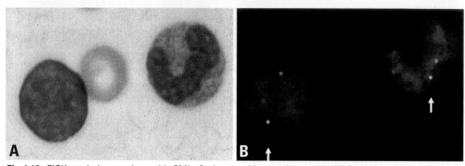

Fig 1.18 FISH study in a patient with CML. **A** shows a blast and a neutrophil from the peripheral blood. **B** After photography, FISH was performed on the Wright's stained slide (*BCR* probe, red signal, *ABL* probe, green signal, Ventana, Inc.), demonstrating the *BCR/ABL* fusion signals in the same cells.

Chronic neutrophilic leukaemia

M. Imbert
B. Bain
R. Pierre

J.W. Vardiman
R.D. Brunning
G. Flandrin

Definition

Chronic neutrophilic leukaemia (CNL) is a rare myeloproliferative disease, characterised by sustained peripheral blood neutrophilia, bone marrow hypercellularity due to neutrophilic granulocyte proliferation, and hepatosplenomegaly. There is no Philadelphia chromosome or BCR/ABL fusion gene. The diagnosis is one of exclusion of all causes of reactive neutrophilia and of all other myeloproliferative diseases.

ICD-O code   9963/3

Synonyms
None

Epidemiology

The true incidence of CNL is unknown, but fewer than 100 cases have been reported. In one study of 660 cases of chronic leukaemias of myeloid origin, not a single case of CNL was observed {1183}. CNL generally affects older adults, but has also been reported in adolescents {1443, 502, 1433}. The sex distribution is nearly equal {1443, 1433}.

Sites of involvement

The blood and bone marrow are always involved, and the spleen and liver usually show leukaemic infiltrates {1443, 1433, 1304}. However any tissue may be infiltrated by the neutrophils {1443, 1433, 1304}.

Clinical features

The most constant clinical feature reported is splenomegaly, which may be symptomatic. Hepatomegaly is usually present as well {1443, 1433}. A history of bleeding from mucocutaneous surfaces or from the gastrointestinal tract is reported in 25-30% of patients {1443, 502}. Gout and pruritus are other possible symptoms {1443}.

Aetiology

The cause of CNL is not known. In up to 20% of reported cases, the neutrophilia was associated with an underlying neoplasm, most usually multiple myeloma {1315, 1223, 190}. To date, no cases of CNL associated with myeloma have been reported in which a clonal chromosomal abnormality or evidence of clonality by molecular techniques has been convincingly demonstrated in the neutrophils {1224}. It is thus likely that most cases of "CNL" associated with myeloma are not autonomous proliferations of the neutrophils, but are secondary to abnormal cytokine release from the neoplastic plasma cells or other cells regulated by the plasma cell population.

Morphology

The peripheral blood smear shows neutrophilia $\geq 25 \times 10^9$/L. The neutrophils are usually segmented, but there may be a substantial increase in bands as well. In almost all cases, immature granulocytes (promyelocytes, myelocytes, metamyelocytes) account for fewer than 5% of the white cells, but occasionally, they may account for up to 10% {1443, 502, 1433}. Myeloblasts are almost never observed in the blood. The neutrophils often appear toxic, with abnormal, coarse granules, but they may also appear normal. Granulocytic dysplasia is not present. Red blood cell and platelet morphology is usually normal.

The bone marrow biopsy shows hypercellularity with neutrophilic proliferation. The myeloid-to-erythroid (M:E) ratio may reach 20:1 or greater. Blasts and promyelocytes are not increased in percentage at the time of diagnosis, but the

Table 1.05
Diagnostic criteria for chronic neutrophilic leukaemia.

1. Peripheral blood leukocytosis $\geq 25 \times 10^9$/L
   Segmented neutrophils and bands > 80% of white blood cells
   Immature granulocytes (promyelocytes, myelocytes, metamyelocyte) < 10% of white blood cells
   Myeloblasts <1% of white blood cells

2. Hypercellular bone marrow biopsy
   Neutrophilic granulocytes increased in percentage and number
   Myeloblasts < 5% of nucleated marrow cells
   Neutrophilic maturation pattern normal

3. Hepatosplenomegaly

4. No identifiable cause for physiologic neutrophilia
   No infectious or inflammatory process
   No underlying tumour, or if present, demonstration of clonality of myeloid cells by cytogenetic or molecular studies

5. No Philadelphia chromosome or BCR/ABL fusion gene

6. No evidence of another myeloproliferative disease
   No evidence of polycythaemia vera, i.e., normal red cell mass
   No evidence of chronic idiopathic myelofibrosis, i.e., no abnormal megakaryocytic proliferation, no reticulin or collagen fibrosis, no marked red blood cell poikilocytosis
   No evidence of essential thrombocythaemia, i.e., platelets < 600 x 10^9/L, no proliferation of mature, enlarged megakaryocytes

7. No evidence of a myelodysplastic syndrome or a myelodysplastic/myeloproliferative disorder
   No granulocytic dysplasia
   No myelodysplastic changes in other myeloid lineages
   Monocytes < 1 x 10^9/L

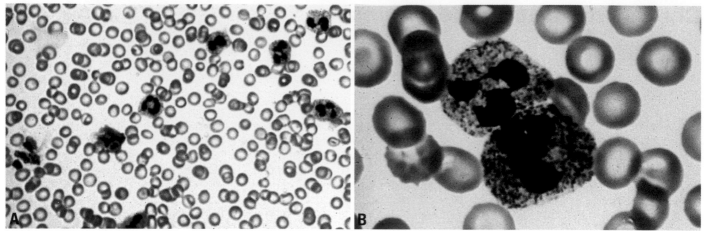

Fig. 1.19 Chronic neutrophilic leukaemia. **A** demonstrates the neutrophilia characteristic of the peripheral blood in CNL. **B** illustrates the toxic granulation commonly observed. Reproduced from Anastasi, J. and Vardiman, J.W. {669}.

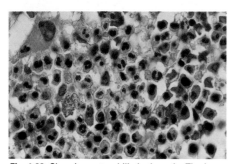

Fig. 1.20 Chronic neutrophilic leukaemia. The bone marrow biopsy specimen is hypercellular, and shows a markedly elevated M:E ratio with increased numbers of neutrophils, particularly mature segmented forms.

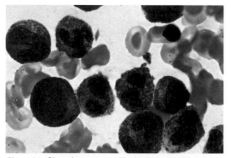

Fig. 1.21 Chronic neutrophilic leukaemia. The bone marrow aspirate smear demonstrates neutrophilic proliferation, with toxic granulation, but no other significant morphologic abnormalities.

percent of myelocytes and mature granulocytes is increased. Erythroid and megakaryocytic proliferation may also occur {1433}. Significant dysplasia is not present in any of the cell lineages, and if found, another diagnosis, such as atypical chronic myeloid leukemia, should be considered (see chapter 2). Reticulin fibrosis is uncommon {1443, 1433}.

In view of the reported frequency of CNL in association with multiple myeloma, the marrow should be examined for evidence of a plasma cell dyscrasia. If plasma cell abnormalities are present, clonality of the neutrophil lineage should be supported by cytogenetic or molecular techniques before making a diagnosis of CNL.

Splenomegaly and hepatomegaly result from tissue infiltration by the neutrophils. In the spleen, the infiltrate is mainly confined to the red pulp; in the liver, the sinusoids, portal areas or both, may be infiltrated {1443, 1433}.

Cytochemistry / immunophenotype

The neutrophil alkaline phosphatase score is increased, but no other cytochemical or immunophenotypic abnormality has been reported {1443, 502}.

Genetics

Cytogenetic studies are normal in nearly 90% of patients. In the remaining patients, clonal karyotypic abnormalities may include +8, +9, del (20q), and del (11q) {409, 1430, 295, 826}. There is no Ph chromosome or *BCR/ABL* fusion gene. A variant of Ph+, *BCR/ABL*+ chronic myelogenous leukemia (CML) has been reported that demonstrates peripheral blood neutrophilia similar to that seen in CNL {998}. In such cases, a variant BCR/ABL fusion protein, p230, is found. Cases with this molecular variant of the *BCR-ABL* fusion gene should be considered as CML, not CNL.

Postulated cell of origin

Unknown; most likely a bone marrow stem cell with limited lineage potential {409, 1430}.

Prognosis

Although generally regarded as a slowly progressive disorder, the survival of patients with CNL is variable, ranging from 6 months to more than 20 years. Usually the neutrophilia is progressive, and anaemia and thrombocytopenia may ensue. The development of myelodysplastic features may signal a transformation of the disease to acute leukaemia, which has been reported in some patients {1443, 502}. It is not clear whether the transformation was related to previous cytotoxic therapy in the cases reported.

Chronic eosinophilic leukaemia and the hypereosinophilic syndrome

B. Bain
R. Pierre
M. Imbert

J.W. Vardiman
R.D. Brunning
G. Flandrin

Definition
Chronic eosinophilic leukaemia (CEL) is a myeloproliferative disease in which an autonomous, clonal proliferation of eosinophilic precursors results in persistently increased numbers of eosinophils in the blood, bone marrow and peripheral tissues. Organ damage occurs as a result of leukaemic infiltration or the release of cytokines, enzymes or other proteins by the eosinophils.

In CEL, the eosinophil count is $\geq 1.5 \times 10^9$/L in the blood. There is no Ph chromosome or *BCR/ABL* fusion gene, and there are fewer than 20% blasts in the blood or bone marrow. To make a diagnosis of CEL, there should be evidence for clonality of the eosinophils or an increase in blasts in the blood or bone marrow. In many cases however, it is impossible to prove clonality of the eosinophils, in which case, if there is no increase in blast cells, the diagnosis of "idiopathic hypereosinophilic syndrome" is preferred. The idiopathic hypereosinophilic syndrome (HES) is defined as persistent eosinophilia ($\geq 1.5 \times 10^9$/L), for which no underlying cause can be found, and which is associated with signs of organ involvement and dysfunction {229, 1375}.

There is no evidence for eosinophil clonality. It is a diagnosis of exclusion, and may include some cases of true eosino-philic leukaemia as well as cases of cytokine-driven eosinophilia that are due to the abnormal release of eosinophil growth factors (e.g., interleukin-2, 3, and 5) for unknown reasons {229, 1375, 1163, 1222, 63}.

ICD-O code   9964/3

Synonyms
Chronic eosinophilic syndrome.

Epidemiology
Due to the difficulty in distinguishing CEL from HES, the true incidence of these diseases is unknown, although they are rare. HES is more common in men than women; the M:F ratio is ~9:1. Its peak incidence is in the fourth decade of life, although the disease may manifest at any age {229, 1375, 1163, 1222}. Eosinophilic leukaemia shows a marked male predominance.

Site of involvement
CEL and HES are multisystem disorders. The blood and bone marrow are always involved. Tissue infiltration by the eosinophils, and release of cytokines and humoral factors from the eosinophil granules lead to tissue damage in a number of organs, but the heart, lungs, central nervous system, skin and gastrointestinal tract are commonly involved. Evidence of splenic and hepatic involvement is present in 30-50% of patients {229, 1375, 1163, 1222}.

Clinical features
In about 10% of patients, eosinophilia is detected incidentally in patients who are otherwise asymptomatic. In others, constitutional symptoms, such as fever, fatigue, cough, angioedema, muscle pains, pruritus, and diarrhoea are found. The most serious clinical findings relate to endomyocardial fibrosis, with ensuing restrictive cardiomegaly. Scarring of the mitral / tricuspid valves leads to valvular regurgitation and formation of intracardiac thrombi, which may embolize to the brain. Peripheral neuropathy, central nervous system dysfunction, pulmonary symptoms due to lung infiltration, and rheumatologic findings are other frequent manifestations {229, 1375, 1163, 1222}.

Table 1.06
Diagnosis of chronic eosinophilic leukaemia and hypereosinophilic syndrome.

Required: Persistent eosinophilia $\geq 1.5 \times 10^9$/L in blood, increased numbers of bone marrow eosinophils, and myeloblasts <20% in blood or marrow
1. Exclude all causes of reactive eosinophilia secondary to: 　Allergy 　Parasitic disease 　Infectious disease 　Pulmonary diseases (hypersensitivity pneumonitis, Loeffler's, etc.) 　Collagen vascular diseases
2. Exclude all neoplastic disorders with secondary, reactive eosinophilia: 　T cell lymphomas, including mycosis fungoides, Sezary syndrome 　Hodgkin lymphoma 　Acute lymphoblastic leukaemia/lymphoma 　Mastocytosis
3. Exclude other neoplastic disorders in which eosinophils are part of the neoplastic clone: 　Chronic myelogenous leukaemia (Ph chromosome or *BCR/ABL* fusion gene positive) 　Acute myeloid leukaemia, including those with inv(16), t(16;16) (p13;q22) 　Other myeloproliferative diseases (PV, ET, CIMF) 　Myelodysplastic syndromes
4. Exclude T cell population with aberrant phenotype and abnormal cytokine production
5. If there is no demonstrable disease that could cause the eosinophilia, no abnormal T-cell population, and no evidence of a clonal myeloid disorder, diagnose HES
6. If all of the requirements, including conditions 1-4, have been met, and if the myeloid cells demonstrate a clonal chromosomal abnormality or are shown to be clonal by other means, or if blast cells are present in the peripheral blood (>2%) or are increased in the bone marrow (>5% but less than 19% of nucleated bone marrow cells), diagnose CEL.

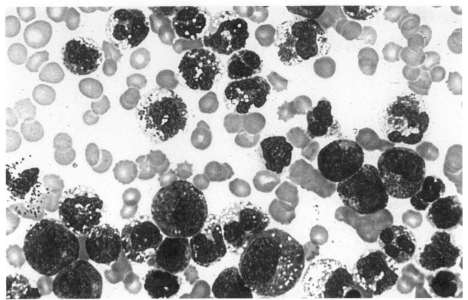

Fig. 1.22 Chronic eosinophilic leukaemia. Peripheral blood smear from a patient with a history of persistent eosinophilia. Immature as well as mature eosinophils are present. Cytogenetic analysis showed trisomy of chromosome 10.

Aetiology

The causes of CEL and of HES are unknown. It is important to exclude all causes of reactive eosinophilia, such as

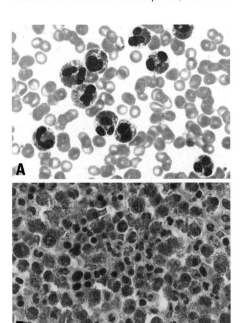

Fig. 1.23 Idiopathic HES. **A** Blood smear of a patient with cardiac failure, leukocytosis and hypereosinophilia. **B** Bone marrow of the same patient. Note the hypercellularity with markedly increased eosinophils and eosinophil precursors. Cytogenetic studies showed a normal karyotype. The patient succumbed to progressive cardiac failure, due to endomyocardial fibrosis, a complication of prolonged eosinophilia.

parasites and allergies, pulmonary diseases such as Loeffler's syndrome, collagen vascular disorders, skin diseases such as angiolymphoid hyperplasia, and Kimura's disease {63, 1142}. In addition, a number of neoplastic disorders such as T cell lymphoma, Hodgkin lymphoma, systemic mastocytosis, acute lymphoblastic leukaemia, and other myeloproliferative diseases may be associated with abnormal release of IL2, IL3, IL5 or GM-CSF and a secondary eosinophilia that mimics CEL or HES {63, 1142, 962, 1138, 1426, 856, 673, 677, 1217}. Some cases previously considered as HES have been shown to be due to the abnormal release of cytokines by T cells that are immunophenotypically aberrant and that may or may not be clonal {663, 152, 1197}. When such an aberrant T-cell population is present, the case should no longer be categorised as idiopathic HES.

Morphology

In CEL and HES, the most striking feature in the blood is eosinophilia, usually comprised mainly of mature eosinophils with only small numbers of eosinophilic myelocytes or promyelocytes {229, 1375, 1163, 1222, 387, 698}. There may be a range of eosinophil abnormalities, including sparse granulation with clear areas of cytoplasm, cytoplasmic vacuolisation, nuclear hypersegmentation or hyposegmentation, and enlarged size.

These changes may be seen in cases of reactive as well as of neoplastic eosinophilia, however, and are thus not very helpful in deciding whether a case should be considered as CEL or HES {63}. Neutrophilia often accompanies the eosinophilia, and some cases have monocytosis. Mild basophilia has been reported as well {387}. Blasts are infrequent if present at all, and >2% should prompt consideration of CEL.

The bone marrow is hypercellular due in part to eosinophilic proliferation {229, 1375, 387, 698, 154}. In most cases, eosinophil maturation is orderly, without a disproportionate increase in blasts. Charcot-Leyden crystals are often present. Erythropoiesis and megakaryocytopoiesis are usually normal. The finding of increased numbers of myeloblasts (5-19%) and of dysplastic features in the other cell lineages as well as in the eosinophils support the notion that the process is neoplastic, but does not necessarily prove the diagnosis of CEL unless the eosinophils are a predominant component and are proven to be part of the clonal process. Marrow fibrosis may be seen in some cases {387, 154}. The marrow should be carefully inspected for any process which might explain the eosinophilia as a secondary reaction, such as vasculitis, lymphoma, acute lymphoblastic leukaemia, or granulomatous disorders.

Any tissue may show eosinophilic infiltration, and Charcot-Leyden crystals are often present. Fibrosis is a common finding as well, and is caused by the degranulation of the eosinophils with the release of eosinophil basic protein and eosinophil cationic proteins {229, 1375, 1142}.

Cytochemistry / immunophenotype

Eosinophils exhibit cyanide-resistant myeloperoxidase activity. The peroxidase content of the eosinophils in CEL and HES is usually normal. Napthol ASD chloroacetate esterase is not normally detected in eosinophils, and when present has been regarded by some as evidence that the eosinophils are neoplastic {698, 776}.

However, it is not present in all neoplastic eosinophils, and has not been well studied in most cases of reactive eosinophilia, HES or CEL. No specific abnormality of the eosinophil immunophenotype has been reported in CEL or HES.

Genetics

No single or specific cytogenetic or molecular genetic abnormality has been identified in CEL. The detection of a Philadelphia chromosome or *BCR/ABL* fusion gene, even in cases in which eosinophilia is a predominant feature, indicates that the case is chronic myelogenous leukaemia, rather than CEL. Even when eosinophilia occurs in conjunction with a chromosomal abnormality that is usually myeloid-associated, it may be difficult to decide whether the eosinophils are part of the clonal process. However, the finding of a recurring karyotypic abnormality that is usually observed in myeloid disorders, such as +8 and i(17q), supports the diagnosis of CEL rather than HES {63, 1001}.

Haematological neoplasia associated with t(5;12)(q33;p13) is often associated with eosinophilia, and may be a discrete entity {100, 445, 71}. It usually has the features of chronic myelomonocytic leukaemia with eosinophilia (see section on chronic myelomonocytic leukaemia, chapter 2). Another cytogenetic/molecular genetic abnormality that may be associated with CEL is t(8;13)(p11;q12) and other 8p11 translocations, such as t(8;9)(p11;q32-34) and t(6;8)(q27;p11) {11}. The mechanism of leukemogenesis in the 8p11 syndromes is related to the *FGFR1* gene, which is fused with different partner genes in the variant translocations {1425}.

The 8p11 syndrome results from a mutation in a pluripotent lymphoid/myeloid stem cell. Although many patients present with eosinophilic leukaemia, the syndrome includes AML, precursor T lymphoblastic leukaemia/ lymphoma and occasionally, precursor B lymphoblastic leukaemia.

Postulated cell of origin

The cell of origin is a bone marrow stem cell, but the lineage potential of the affected cell may be variable. It may be a pluripotent stem cell [e.g., as in cases associated with the t(8;13) chromosomal abnormality], a multipotent stem cell, or possibly, a committed eosinophil precursor cell.

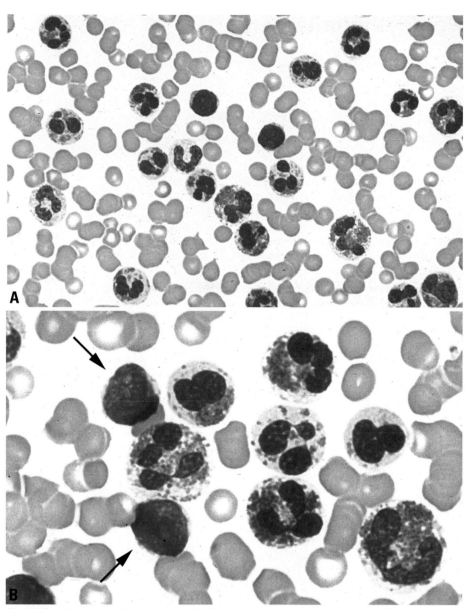

Fig. 1.24 Reactive eosinophilia in a patient with ALL. **A** Peripheral blood of a patient with ALL. The elevation of the white count in this case is due primarily to eosinophils, with only an occasional lymphoblast. **B** The lymphoblasts (arrows) are more clearly appreciated in the blood smear that is also illustrated in A. Eosinophilia is most frequently associated with cases of ALL that demonstrate the cytogenetic abnormality, t (5;14)(q31;q32).

Prognosis and predictive factors

Survival is quite variable. In some series in which patients with HES as well as those with probable eosinophilic leukaemia were included, 5 year survival rates approached 80% {229, 1375, 1163, 1222}. Marked splenomegaly, as well as the finding of blasts in the blood or increased blasts in the bone marrow, cytogenetic abnormalities, and dysplastic features in other myeloid lineages have been reported to be unfavourable prognostic findings {229, 1375, 1163, 1222}.

Polycythaemia vera

R. Pierre
M. Imbert
J. Thiele
J.W. Vardiman
R.D. Brunning
G. Flandrin

Definition
Polycythaemia vera (PV) is a myeloproliferative disease that arises in a clonal haematopoietic stem cell and is characterised by increased red blood cell production that is independent of the mechanisms that normally regulate erythropoiesis. Excessive proliferation of myeloid lineages in addition to the erythroid series is usually observed as well. Two phases of PV can be recognised: 1) an initial proliferative, polycythaemic phase, associated with an increased red cell mass, and 2) a "spent", or post-polycythaemic phase, in which cytopenias, including anaemia, are associated with ineffective haematopoiesis, bone marrow fibrosis, extramedullary haematopoiesis, and hypersplenism. The natural progression of PV also includes a low incidence of acute leukaemia. All causes of secondary erythrocytosis as well as inheritable polycythaemia must be excluded prior to making the diagnosis of PV.

ICD-O code   9950/3

Synonyms
Polycythaemia rubra vera

Epidemiology
The incidence of PV varies geographically, ranging from about 2 cases per million individuals per year in Japan, to about 13 per million per year in Australia. Europe and North America have a similar incidence of 8 - 10 cases per million population per year {884}. Most reports indicate a slight male predominance, with the M:F ratio ranging from 1-2:1 {884, 1196}. The

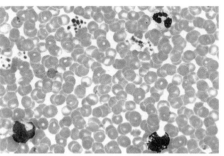

Fig. 1.25 Polycythaemia vera, polycythaemic phase. The peripheral blood smear from patients with PV demonstrates thick layering of red blood cells. In addition, thrombocytosis, neutrophilia and modest basophilia are commonly observed.

mean age at diagnosis is 60 years, and patients under 20 years old are rarely reported {264, 920}.

Sites of involvement
The blood and bone marrow are the major sites of involvement, but the spleen and liver are also affected, and are the major sites of extramedullary haematopoiesis in the later stages. However, any organ can be damaged as a result of the vascular consequences of the increased red cell mass.

Clinical features
The major symptoms are related to hypertension or to vascular abnormalities caused by the increased red cell mass. In nearly 25% of patients, an episode of venous or arterial thrombosis, such as deep vein thrombophlebitis, myocardial ischaemia or stroke, is the first manifestation {101, 980, 108}. Mesenteric and portal or splenic vein thrombosis should always lead to consideration of PV as a possible cause, and may even precede the onset of an overt polycythaemic stage {1323}. Headache, dizziness, visual disturbances, and paresthesias are also major complaints. Other findings may include pruritus, erythromelalgia (increased skin temperature, burning sensation, redness), and gout. Haemorrhage, particularly from the gastrointestinal tract, may also occur. Physical findings include

Table 1.07
WHO criteria for polycythaemia vera.

- A1 Elevated RBC mass > 25% above mean normal predicted value, or Hb > 18.5g/dl in men, 16.5 g/dl in women*

- A2 No cause of secondary erythrocytosis, including:
  - Absence of familial erythrocytosis
  - No elevation of erythropoietin (EPO) due to:
      hypoxia (arterial $pO_2 \leq 92$ %),
      high oxygen affinity haemoglobin,
      truncated EPO receptor
      inappropriate EPO production by tumour

- A3 Splenomegaly

- A4 Clonal genetic abnormality other than Ph chromosome or *BCR/ABL* fusion gene in marrow cells

- A5 Endogenous erythroid colony formation *in vitro*

- B1 Thrombocytosis >400 x 10^9/L

- B2 WBC > 12 x 10^9/L

- B3 Bone marrow biopsy showing panmyelosis with prominent erythroid and megakaryocytic proliferation

- B4 Low serum erythropoietin levels

Diagnose PV when A1 + A2 and any other category A are present, or when A1 + A2 and any two of category B are present.

* or > 99th percentile of method-specific reference range for age, sex, altitude of residence

plethora in 70% of patients, palpable splenomegaly in 70%, and hepatomegaly in 40% {101, 980, 108, 907}. Occasionally, patients may have clinical symptoms, peripheral blood abnormalities and bone marrow biopsy findings that are suggestive of PV, but the red cell mass and haemoglobin are not sufficiently elevated to make the diagnosis. The detection of endogenous erythroid colonies *in vitro* and of a low serum erythropoietin level in such cases may allow recognition of patients who are in an early "pre-polycythaemic" stage, and who may be expected to become polycythaemic at a later time {1323, 868}.

Aetiology

In most cases, the cause is unknown. A genetic predisposition has been reported in some families {150, 877}. Ionizing radiation, occupational exposure to toxins, and viruses have been suggested as possible causes in occasional patients {168, 132, 653}.

Morphology

The morphologic findings in bone marrow biopsy specimens of patients with polycythaemia vera, although characteristic, must be correlated with the clinical and laboratory findings in order to firmly establish the diagnosis.

Polycythaemic stage

In the polycythaemic stage, the major features of PV are normoblastic erythroid proliferation in the marrow, and an excess of normochromic, normocytic red cells in the peripheral blood. If iron deficiency due to bleeding is present, the red cells may be hypochromic and microcytic. Neutrophilia and basophilia are common in the blood smear. Occasional immature granulocytes may be seen, but circulating blasts are not generally observed. Thrombocytosis is found in more than 50% of patients {132, 906}.

Bone marrow cellularity has been reported to range from 35-100%, with a median cellularity of about 80%, but characteristically, the bone marrow biopsy is hypercellular for the patient's age {429, 342, 77, 1289}. Erythroid, mega-karyocytic and granulocytic proliferation (panmyelosis) account for the increased cellularity, but the increase in the numbers of erythroid precursors and of megakaryocytes is often most prominent

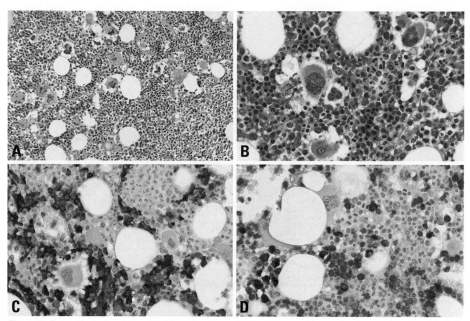

Fig. 1.26 Polycythaemia vera, polycythaemic phase. **A** Bone marrow biopsy specimens are characteristically hypercellular during the polycythaemic phase. **B** demonstrates the panmyelosis characteristic of PV. The megakaryocytic proliferation is easily appreciated in the H&E stained sections of the marrow biopsy. **C** An immunostain for haemoglobin A accentuates the erythroid proliferation. **D** An immunostain for myeloperoxidase, which demonstrates the granulocytic proliferation in the same case.

{429, 77, 1289}. Erythropoiesis is normoblastic, and granulopoiesis is morphologically normal. The percent of myeloblasts is not increased. Megakaryocytes are conspicuous, even when the marrow is normocellular. They tend to cluster around marrow sinusoids or to lie close to the bony trabeculae, and may show a pleomorphic aspect, i.e., often small to giant megakaryocytes are grouped together. They have deeply lobulated nuclei, and lack bizarre, dysplas-

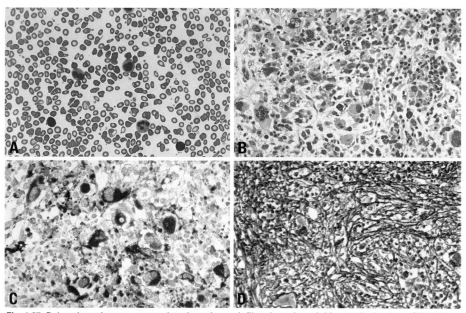

Fig. 1.27 Polycythaemia vera, post-polycythaemic myelofibrosis and myeloid metaplasia phase (PPMM). **A** Peripheral blood smear demonstrates leukoerythroblastosis with numerous teardrop shaped red blood cells (dacrocytes). **B** Bone marrow shows megakaryocytic proliferation and depletion of the erythroid and granulocytic cells. **C** An immunostain for CD61 illustrates the atypia in the megakaryocytic population, including a population of small megakaryocytes. **D** The reticulin fibrosis that is invariably present in PPMM.

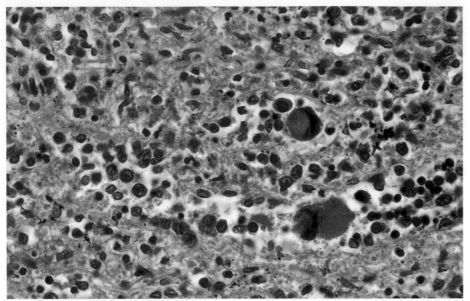

Fig. 1.28 Polycythaemia vera, post-polycythaemic myelofibrosis and myeloid metaplasia, splenectomy specimen. The splenic enlargement in the post-polycythaemic phase is due mainly to extramedullary haematopoiesis that occurs in the splenic sinuses, as well as fibrosis and entrapment of platelets and other haematopoietic cells in the splenic cords.

tic features. Silver stains will show a normal reticulin fiber network in about 70% of patients, but the remainder have reticulin fibrosis of variable degree {429, 342,

77, 1289}. Reactive nodular lymphoid aggregates may be found in up to 20% of cases {1295}. Stainable iron is lacking in the marrow aspirate in more than 95% of the cases {342}. The spleen and liver show mainly congestion; extramedullary haematopoiesis is minimal during the proliferative stage of PV {1401}.

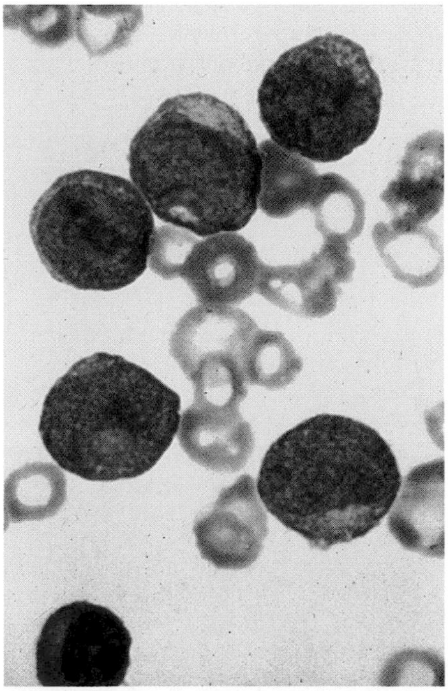

"Spent" phase and post-polycythaemic myelofibrosis and myeloid metaplasia (PPMM)
During the later stages of PV, the red cell mass normalises and then decreases, and the spleen further enlarges. Rarely, these findings occur in the face of a hypercellular marrow with minimal fibrosis {918}. The most common pattern of progression, however, is post-polycythaemic myelofibrosis and myeloid metaplasia (PPMM), which is characterised by a leukoerythroblastic blood smear, red blood cell poikilocytosis with teardrop-shaped red blood cells, and splenomegaly due to extramedullary haematopoiesis. The hallmark of this stage of the disease is reticulin and even collagen fibrosis of the marrow {429, 342}. The cellularity varies in PPMM, but hypocellular specimens are common. Clusters of megakaryocytes, often with hyperchromatic, dysmorphic nuclei are prominent. Erythropoiesis and granulopoiesis are decreased in amount, and are sometimes found, along with megakaryocytes, in

dilated marrow sinusoids. Osteosclerosis may also occur {429, 342, 77, 1289}. The splenic enlargement seen in PPMM is due to extramedullary haematopoiesis, with erythroid, granulocytic and megakaryocytic elements in the splenic sinuses. An increase in the number of immature cells may be observed at this time, but the finding of more than 10% blasts in the blood or marrow or the presence of significant myelodysplasia is unusual, and most likely signals transformation to a myelodysplastic syndrome or to acute leukaemia {871, 919}.

Immunophenotype
No unique immunophenotypic findings are reported for PV.

Genetics
No specific genetic defect has been identified. At diagnosis, cytogenetic abnormalities are found in only 10-20% of patients. The most common recurring abnormalities include +8, +9, del (20q), del (13q) and del (1p); sometimes +8 and +9 are found together. There is no Philadelphia chromosome or *BCR/ABL* fusion gene. These chromosomal abnormalities are seen with increasing frequency with disease progression and in nearly 80-90% of those with PPMM. Almost 100% of those who develop myelodysplastic syndrome or acute leukaemia have cytogenetic abnormalities, including those commonly observed in therapy-related MDS and AML {294, 1094, 1255} (see chapter 4).

Postulated cell of origin
Multipotent bone marrow stem cell.

Prognosis and predictive factors
Without therapy, the median survival of patients with PV is only a few months, but with currently available treatment, median survival times greater than 10 years are commonly reported {108, 907, 921}. Most patients die from thrombosis or haemorrhage, but up to 20% succumb to myelodysplasia or acute myeloid leukaemia {921}.
The factors that predict for thrombosis or haemorrhage are not well defined. The risk of MDS and acute leukaemia is only 2-3% in patients who have not been treated with cytotoxic agents, but increases to 10% or more following certain types of chemotherapy {108, 907, 921}.

Fig. 1.29 Acute leukaemia in polycythaemia vera. Blood smear from a patient with a long-standing history of PV. The patient had been treated with alkylating agents during the polycythaemic stage. The blasts expressed CD13, CD33, CD117 and CD34, and had a complex karyotype, consistent with therapy-related acute myeloid leukaemia.

Chronic idiopathic myelofibrosis

J. Thiele   J.W. Vardiman
R. Pierre   R.D. Brunning
M. Imbert   G. Flandrin

Definition
Chronic idiopathic myelofibrosis (CIMF) is a clonal myeloproliferative disease characterised by the proliferation of mainly megakaryocytic and granulocytic elements in the bone marrow, associated with reactive deposition of bone marrow connective tissue and with extra-medullary haematopoiesis (EMH). There is a stepwise evolution of the disease process with an initial prefibrotic stage that is characterised by a hypercellular bone marrow with minimal reticulin fibrosis that merges into a fibrotic stage, at which time the bone marrow demonstrates marked reticulin or collagen fibrosis, and often, osteomyelosclerosis. A leukoerythroblastic blood smear with tear-drop shaped red cells (dacrocytes) is a characteristic finding in the fibrotic stage. EMH contributes to the splenomegaly and hepatomegaly, which worsen throughout the disease course.

ICD-O code   9961/3

Synonyms
Agnogenic myeloid metaplasia
Myelosclerosis with myeloid metaplasia
Chronic granulocytic-megakaryocytic myelosis

Idiopathic myelofibrosis
Primary myelofibrosis

Epidemiology
The actual incidence of chronic idiopathic myelofibrosis is not known, but is estimated at 0.5-1.5 per 100,000 individuals per year {867, 1271}. It occurs most commonly in the seventh decade of life, and the two sexes are affected in nearly equal number {1271}. It rarely occurs in children {1171, 193}.

Site of involvement
The blood and bone marrow are always involved. The spleen and liver are the most common sites of extramedullary haematopoiesis, but lymph nodes, kidney, adrenal gland, dura mater, gastrointestinal tract, lung and pleura, breast and skin are other possible sites {1271, 1359, 1404, 363, 1285}. The EMH is largely responsible for the leukoerythroblastosis and abnormal red cell morphology.

Clinical features
Up to 30% of patients are asymptomatic at diagnosis, and are discovered by detection of splenomegaly during a routine physical examination or when a routine blood count discloses some abnor-

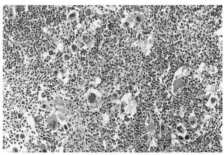

Fig. 1.30 Chronic idiopathic myelofibrosis, prefibrotic stage. The marrow is hypercellular and shows increased numbers of megakaryocytes that are atypical and that cluster together.

mality, such as anaemia or thrombocytosis {195, 298}. Symptoms may include fatigue, dyspnoea, weight loss, night sweats, low-grade fever, and bleeding. Gouty arthritis and renal stones occur due to hyperuricemia. Splenomegaly of varying degree is detected in up to 90% of patients and may be massive; nearly 50% have hepatomegaly {298, 1271, 193, 1359, 1294, 1349}.

Aetiology
The cause is unknown. Exposure to benzene and ionizing radiation have been documented in some cases, and rare examples of familial myelofibrosis have been reported {548, 29, 1006}.

Morphology
The classic picture of chronic idiopathic myelofibrosis is a blood smear that shows leukoerythroblastosis with poikilocytosis of red blood cells, particularly dacrocytes, a bone marrow biopsy specimen with marked fibrosis, and EMH that contributes to enlargement of the spleen and liver. But the morphologic findings at diagnosis vary considerably, depending on whether the patient is first encountered during the prefibrotic or the fibrotic stage.

Prefibrotic stage
Approximately 20-30% of patients are first detected in the prefibrotic stage (cellular phase) {157, 1287}. At this time, slight to

Table 1.08
Chronic idiopathic myelofibrosis: prefibrotic stage

Clinical findings	Morphological findings
Spleen and liver: No or mild splenomegaly or hepatomegaly	Blood: No or mild leukoerythroblastosis No or minimal red blood cell poikilocytosis; few if any dacrocytes

Haematology:
Haematologic parameters variable, but often:
  Mild anaemia
  Mild to moderate leukocytosis
  Mild to marked thrombocytosis
	Bone marrow:
	Hypercellularity
	Neutrophilic proliferation
	Megakaryocytic proliferation and atypia (clustering of megakaryocytes, abnormally lobulated megakaryocytic nuclei, naked megakaryocytic nuclei)
	Minimal or absent reticulin fibrosis

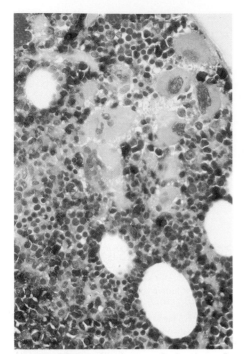

Fig. 1.31 CIMF, prefibrotic stage. During the prefibrotic stage, megakaryocytic and granulocytic proliferation are particularly conspicuous. This biopsy is stained with napthol ASD chloroacetate esterase (red reaction product) which enhances visualisation of the granulocytic component.

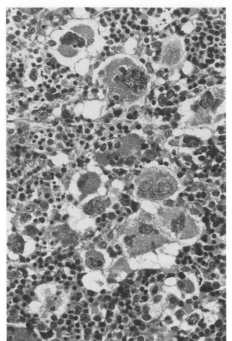

Fig. 1.32 CIMF, prefibrotic stage. Megakaryocytic abnormalities are a key to the diagnosis of CIMF. Note the abnormalities of megakaryopoiesis including anisocytosis, abnormal nuclear-cytoplasmic ratios, abnormal chromatin clumping with hyperchromatic nuclei, and plump lobulation of some nuclei.

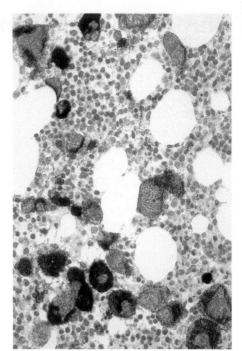

Fig. 1.33 CIMF, prefibrotic stage. This photograph demonstrates an immunostain with CD61 that highlights the megakaryocytic abnormalities described in Fig. 1.32, and also illustrates several small megakaryocytes that would not likely be appreciated on a routine H & E stain.

moderate anaemia is often present, and the blood smear typically shows mild leukocytosis and moderate to marked thrombocytosis {1288}. Nucleated red blood cells, dacrocytes, large atypical platelets, and immature granulocytes may be found in the blood during this stage, but usually in low numbers {1287}.

The bone marrow biopsy is hypercellular for the patient's age, with an increase in the number of neutrophils and of atypical megakaryocytes. There may be a "left shift" in granulopoiesis, but metamyelocytes, bands and segmented forms predominate. Clusters of myeloblasts are not observed, nor are they significantly increased in percentage (<10%) {157, 1287, 1288, 429}. Often, erythropoiesis is reduced in quantity, but early erythroid precursors may be prominent in some patients {1287}. Megakaryocytes are markedly abnormal, and their histotopography and morphology are key to recognising the prefibrotic stage. They often form clusters of variable size adjacent to sinuses and the bony trabeculae {157, 1287, 1288, 429}. Most megakaryocytes are enlarged, but small megakaryocytes may be seen, particularly with the aid of

immunohistochemical studies for platelet and megakaryocytic specific antigens {1287, 1288}. Deviations in the nuclear/cytoplasmic ratio, abnormal patterns of chromatin clumping associated with plump, "cloud-like" or "balloon-shaped" lobulation of megakaryocytic nuclei, as well as frequent naked megakaryocytic nuclei, are typical findings {1287}. Overall, the megakaryocytes are more atypical than in other chronic myeloproliferative diseases. Reticulin fibrosis is minimal or even absent during this stage, and when present, tends to be concentrated around

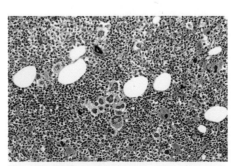

Fig. 1.34 CIMF, prefibrotic stage. This silver stain for bone marrow reticulin fibers shows only a minimal increase in reticulin fibers.

vessels. Vascular proliferation is usual in the marrow, and lymphoid nodules may be seen in up to 25% of specimens {1271, 1295}.

Fibrotic stage
Most patients with CIMF (70-80%) are initially diagnosed in the fibrotic stage. Splenomegaly and hepatomegaly due to EMH are invariably present at this time. Anaemia and a leukoerythroblastic blood smear with numerous dacrocytes are classic features of this stage {298, 193, 1359, 1404, 1294, 1349}. The white blood cell count may be normal, but severe leukopenia or marked leukocytosis are also possible. Dysgranulopoiesis is not common, and if present, suggests transformation to a more aggressive phase. A few myeloblasts are usual in blood smears during the fibrotic stage, but if they are 10% or more of the white blood cells they likely signify transformation to an accelerated or blast phase. Platelets may show a wide range of numerical values, but large, bizarre platelets and circulating megakaryocytic nuclei and fragments as well as micromegakaryocytes are frequent observations.

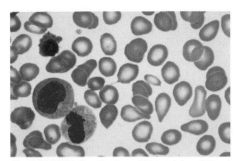

Fig. 1.35 CIMF, fibrotic stage. This peripheral blood smear shows dacrocytes, occasional nucleated red blood cells and immature granulocytes, and is typical of the changes observed in the fibrotic stage of CIMF.

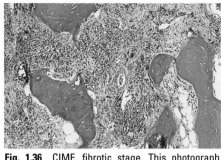

Fig. 1.36 CIMF, fibrotic stage. This photograph illustrates a bone marrow biopsy specimen showing cellular depletion and marrow fibrosis as well as osteosclerosis typical of the fibrotic stage of CIMF.

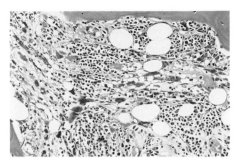

Fig. 1.37 CIMF, fibrotic stage. Megakaryocytes are often the most conspicuous haematopoietic element in the marrow in the fibrotic stage. Often the cells appear to "stream" through the marrow due to the underlying fibrosis.

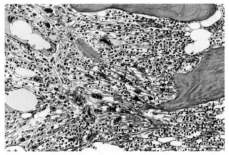

Fig. 1.38 CIMF, fibrotic stage. This silver stain for bone marrow reticulin fibers illustrates the marked reticulin fibrosis typical of this stage of CIMF.

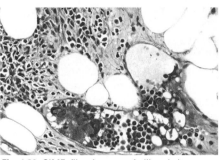

Fig. 1.39 CIMF, fibrotic stage. A dilated sinus contains immature haematopoietic elements, most notably megakaryocytes, which are well-stained with the PAS reaction. This "intrasinusoidal haematopoiesis" is characteristic but not diagnostic of CIMF.

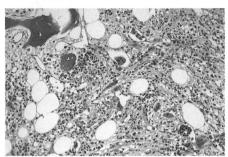

Fig. 1.40 CIMF, fibrotic stage. This photograph illustrates intrasinusoidal haematopoiesis. The cells are washed from the marrow sinuses into the blood, and may eventually lodge in tissues such as the spleen that permit their continued growth.

In the fibrotic stage, bone marrow biopsy specimens demonstrate reticulin or collagen fibrosis. The bone marrow may be hypercellular, but is more often normocellular or hypocellular, with patches of haematopoietic cells separated by regions of loose connective tissue or fat. Foci of immature cells may be prominent, although myeloblasts account for fewer than 10% of the marrow cells. Increased number and dilatation of marrow sinuses with intrasinusoidal haematopoiesis are characteristic {298, 1404, 1294}. Atypical megakaryocytes are often the most notable marrow elements, and occur in sizeable clusters or sheets {1287, 1286}, or within dilated sinuses {1404, 1294, 157, 1287}. Sometimes the bone marrow may be almost devoid of haematopoietic elements, and consists mainly of dense reticulin or collagen fibrosis, with small islands of haematopoietic precursors situated within the marrow sinuses. Osteoid or appositional new bone formation in bud-like endophytic plaques may be observed {1404, 157, 429}. The osteosclerotic tissue may form broad, irregular trabeculae that can occupy more than 50% of the marrow space.

In patients with a previously established diagnosis of CIMF, the finding of 10-19% blasts in the blood or marrow indicates an accelerated phase of the disease, and 20% or more signifies acute transfor-

Table 1.09
Chronic idiopathic myelofibrosis: fibrotic stage

Clinical findings	Morphological findings

Spleen and liver:
Moderate to marked splenomegaly and hepatomegaly
 	
Haematology:
  Moderate to marked anaemia
  Low, normal or elevated WBC
  Platelet count decreased, normal or elevated
	Blood:
	  Leukoerythroblastosis
	  Prominent red blood cell poikilocytosis with dacrocytes
	
	Bone marrow:
	  Reticulin and/or collagen fibrosis
	  Decreased cellularity
	  Dilated marrow sinuses with intraluminal haematopoiesis
	  Prominent megakaryocytic proliferation and atypia (clustering of megakaryocytes, abnormally lobulated megakaryocytic nuclei, naked nuclei)
	  New bone formation (osteosclerosis)

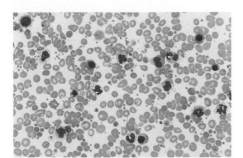

Fig. 1.41 CIMF, fibrotic stage. This peripheral blood smear is from the patient whose marrow is illustrated in Fig. 1.40. It shows marked leukoerythroblastosis, due largely to the abnormal release of cells from sites of EMH, including that within the bone marrow sinusoids.

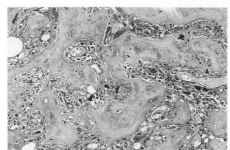

Fig. 1.42 CIMF with osteomyelosclerosis. Osteomyelosclerosis is characterised by broad, irregular bony trabeculae that can occupy up to 50% of the marrow space. Fibrosis, cellular depletion, sinusoidal dilatation and megakaryocytic proliferation are prominent in the intertrabecular areas.

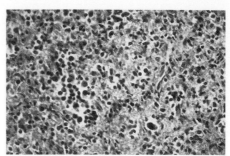

Fig. 1.43 CIMF with extramedullary haematopoiesis (EMH). In the spleen, EMH occurs mainly in the red pulp sinusoids. Megakaryocytes are prominent; erythroid and granulocytic proliferation are present as well. The splenic cords are often thickened due to fibrosis or to cellular sequestration.

mation. Occasionally, patients with CIMF can present in an accelerated phase. The differential diagnosis in such cases may include MDS with fibrosis (see chapter 3), MDS/MPD, unclassifiable (see chapter 2), or even acute panmyelosis with fibrosis (see chapter 4). These latter disorders usually lack the typical morphologic features and the marked hepatosplenomegaly that characterise CIMF. Patients with CIMF may also present initially in the acute phase with blasts accounting for 20% or more of the white blood cells or marrow cells. However, in these cases the diagnosis of acute leukaemia should be made outright, with only mention of the possible derivation from CIMF. Acute panmyelosis with myelofibrosis may also be considered, particularly if the patient lacks organomegaly.

Extramedullary haematopoiesis
The most common sites of EMH are the spleen and liver {1404, 363, 1285}.

Microscopic sections of the spleen show expansion of the red pulp by erythroid, granulocytic and megakaryocytic cells that are located mainly in the sinuses. Megakaryocytes are often the most conspicuous component of the EMH. The red pulp cords may show fibrosis as well as pooling of platelets. Hepatic sinuses also show EMH, but fibrosis and cirrhosis of the liver are also common. As noted above, a number of other sites may be involved by EMH {1359}.

Immunophenotype
No abnormal phenotypic features have been reported.

Genetics
No specific genetic defect has been identified. Cytogenetic abnormalities occur in about 60% of patients {328, 1096}. There is no Philadelphia chromosome or *BCR/ABL* fusion gene. The most common recurring abnormalities include del (13q), del (20q), and partial trisomy 1q, although

+8 and/or +9 are also reported {328, 1096}. Deletions affecting chromosomes 7 and 5 occur as well, but may be associated with prior cytotoxic therapy used to treat the myeloproliferative process. The genes associated with these abnormalities are currently unknown.

Postulated cell of origin
Bone marrow stem cell with multilineage potential.

Prognosis
Although survival times for patients with CIMF range from months to decades, the median survival time is approximately 3-5 years from diagnosis {1271, 193, 1349, 548, 328, 1096, 1124, 196, 707, 75}. Factors at presentation that adversely affect prognosis include age >70, severe anaemia (Hb <10g/dl), thrombocytopenia (<100 x 10^6/L), marked granulocytic immaturity in the blood, and an abnormal karyotype {1349, 548, 328, 1096, 1124, 196, 707, 75}. The major causes of morbidity and mortality are bone marrow failure (infection, haemorrhage), thromboembolic events, portal hypertension, cardiac failure, and acute leukaemia {1271}. The reported incidence of acute leukaemia ranges from 5-30% {1271, 328, 196}. Although some cases of acute leukaemia are related to prior cytotoxic therapy, many have been reported in patients who have never been treated, indicating that acute leukaemia is part of the natural history of CIMF. Any of the myeloid lineages may give rise to the acute leukaemia, and mixed-lineage phenotypes are also reported.

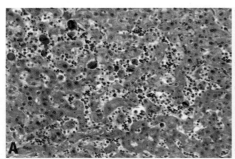 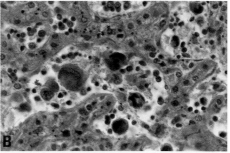

Fig. 1.44 CIMF, fibrotic stage, with EMH in liver. In the liver, the sinuoids are prominently involved by trilineage proliferation.

Essential thrombocythaemia

M. Imbert
R. Pierre
J. Thiele

J.W. Vardiman
R.D. Brunning
G. Flandrin

Definition
Essential thrombocythaemia (ET) is a clonal myeloproliferative disease that involves primarily the megakaryocytic lineage. It is characterised by sustained thrombocytosis in the blood and increased numbers of large, mature megakaryocytes in the bone marrow, and clinically, by episodes of thrombosis and/or haemorrhage. Currently there is no known genetic or biologic marker specific for ET, so other causes for thrombocytosis, including other myeloid disorders, underlying inflammatory and infectious diseases and solid tumours, must be excluded before making this diagnosis.

ICD-O code   9962/3

Synonyms
Primary thrombocytosis
Idiopathic thrombocytosis
Haemorrhagic thrombocythaemia

Epidemiology
The true incidence of ET is unknown, but is estimated to be 1-2.5 per 100,000 individuals annually {867}. Most cases are diagnosed in patients 50-60 years of age, with no major predilection for either sex. However, a second peak in frequency occurs at about 30 years of age, and then women are more often affected {867, 849, 908}. ET occurs in children, but is uncommon {1086}.

Sites of involvement
Bone marrow and blood are the prinicipal sites of involvement. The spleen shows minimal extramedullary haematopoiesis, but is a sequestration site for platelets {1405}.

Clinical features
More than one-half of patients are asymptomatic when a markedly elevated platelet count is discovered fortuitously on a routine complete blood count {908, 85, 909, 1015, 594}, but 20-50% of patients have some manifestation of vascular occlusion or of haemorrhage when they are first encountered. Microvascular occlusion may lead to transient cerebral ischaemia attacks or to digital ischaemia with parasthesias and gangrene. Thrombosis of major arteries and veins may also occur, and ET may be a cause of splenic or hepatic vein thrombosis. Bleeding occurs most commonly from mucosal surfaces, such as the gastrointestinal tract or upper airway passages {908, 85, 909, 1015, 594}. Modest splenomegaly is present in approximately 50% of patients at the time of diagnosis, and hepatomegaly is found in 15-20% {1405, 85, 909, 1015, 594}.

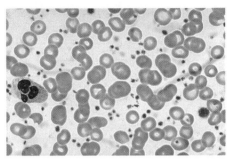

Fig. 1.45 Essential thrombocythaemia. The major abnormality in the peripheral blood smear is marked thrombocytosis. The platelets show anisocytosis, but are often not remarkably atypical.

Table 1.10
Diagnostic criteria for essential thrombocythaemia.

Positive criteria
1. Sustained platelet count ≥600 x 10⁹/L
2. Bone marrow biopsy specimen showing proliferation mainly of the megakaryocytic lineage with increased numbers of enlarged, mature megakaryocytes

Criteria of exclusion

1. No evidence of polycythaemia vera (PV)
   - Normal red cell mass or Hb <18.5 g/dl in men, 16.5g/dl in women
   - Stainable iron in marrow, normal serum ferritin or normal MCV
   - If the former condition is not met, failure of iron trial to increase red cell mass or Hgb levels to the PV range

2. No evidence of CML   - No Philadelphia chromosome and no *BCR/ABL* fusion gene

3. No evidence of chronic idiopathic myelofibrosis
   - Collagen fibrosis absent
   - Reticulin fibrosis minimal or absent

4. No evidence of myelodysplastic syndrome
   - No del(5q), t(3;3)(q21;q26), inv(3)(q21q26)
   - No significant granulocytic dysplasia, few if any micromegakaryocytes

5. No evidence that thrombocytosis is reactive due to:
   - Underlying inflammation or infection
   - Underlying neoplasm
   - Prior splenectomy

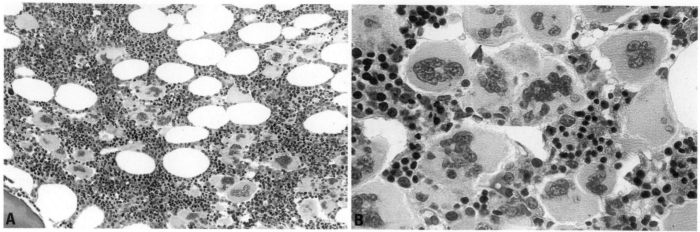

Fig. 1.46 Essential thrombocythaemia, bone marrow biopsy. **A** The bone marrow biopsy specimen may be normocellular, hypercellular or rarely, hypocellular. **B** The megakaryocytes are enlarged, show abundant amounts of mature cytoplasm and deeply lobulated and hyperlobated nuclei.

Aetiology

The cause of ET is unknown. Rare familial cases have been reported {351, 378}.

Morphology

The most striking abnormality on the blood smear is marked thrombocytosis. The platelets often display anisocytosis, and range from tiny forms to large, giant platelets. Bizarre shapes, pseudopods and agranular platelet cytoplasm may be seen, but are not common. The WBC count and leukocyte differential are usually normal, although mild elevations in the white count may occur {908, 909, 429, 510}. Basophilia is usually absent or minimal {908, 909}. The red blood cells are normocytic and normochromic, unless there has been previous haemor-

rhage, and then they may be hypochromic and microcytic due to iron deficiency. Leukoerythroblastosis and teardrop shaped red blood cells (dacrocytes) are not features of ET.

The bone marrow biopsy is normocellular or slightly to moderately hypercellular for the patient's age in most cases {1293, 158}, but hypocellularity has been reported {510}. The most striking abnormality is marked proliferation of large to giant megakaryocytes. They usually occur in loose clusters but may be dispersed in the marrow. The megakaryocytes have abundant, mature cytoplasm, and deeply lobulated and hyperlobulated nuclei, generally with smooth nuclear contours. Bizarre, highly atypical forms, such as those observed in chronic idiopathic

myelofibrosis, are not usually found in ET {429, 1291, 33}. Proliferation of erythroid precursors may be found in some cases, particularly if the patient has experienced previous haemorrhage. Granulocytic proliferation, if present, is usually mild. There is no increase in the percentage of myeloblasts, nor is there any granulocytic dysplasia. The network of reticulin fibers is normal or minimally increased, but significant reticulin fibrosis or any collagen fibrosis speaks strongly against a diagnosis of ET {429, 1293}. Bone marrow aspirate smears often show markedly increased numbers of large megakaryocytes, and large sheets of platelets. Emperipolesis of marrow elements in the cytoplasm of megakaryocytes is frequently observed

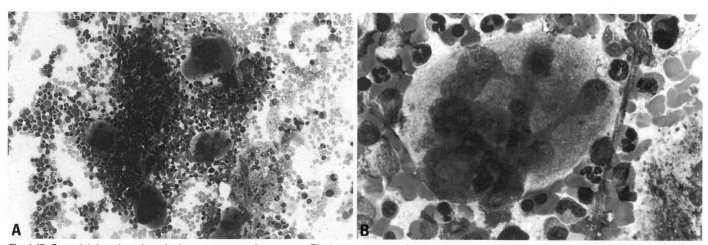

Fig. 1.47 Essential thrombocythaemia, bone marrow aspirate smear. The bone marrow aspirate smears generally mirror the changes seen in the biopsy. **A** An increase in the number and size of the megakaryocytes can be appreciated. **B** Note the deeply lobulated megakaryocytic nuclei, as well as sizeable pools of platelets. However, the aspirate smears fail to reveal the overall marrow architecture and distribution of the megakaryocytes that can be seen in the biopsy, and that is often necessary to establish the diagnosis of ET.

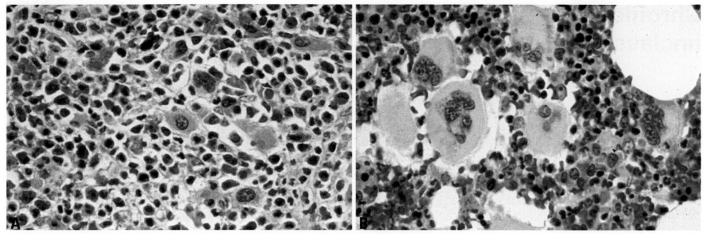

Fig. 1.48 Chronic myelogenous leukaemia **A** compared to essential thrombocythaemia **B**. CML often has an elevated platelet count, and may be confused with ET if the white blood cell count is not markedly elevated. Although cytogenetic and molecular genetic studies should always be performed if CML is suspected, the small size of the megakaryocytes in CML (**A**), will readily distinguish it from ET, in which the megakaryocytes are large (**B**).

in ET, but is not a specific finding {184}. Stainable iron is present in the marrow specimens of 40-70% of patients at diagnosis {908, 909}.

Extramedullary tissues are not significantly involved by the megakaryocytic proliferation. In the spleen and liver, some extramedullary haematopoiesis may be seen, but is scant if present. The splenic cords may be stuffed with platelets, and platelet aggregates may be seen in the splenic sinuses as well {1405}.

Immunophenotype

No aberrant phenotype has been described.

Genetics

No specific cytogenetic or molecular genetic abnormality is known at the current time. There is no Ph chromosome or *BCR/ABL* fusion gene; and cytogenetic and molecular genetic studies should always be done to exclude CML as a cause of the thrombocytosis. An abnormal karyotype is unusual in ET, and is found in only 5-10% of patients {2, 1179}. Recurring abnormalities reported include del (13q22), +8 and +9 {239}. Although the cytogenetic abnormalities, del (5q), t(3;3)(q21;q26.2) and inv (3)(q21q26.2)

are commonly associated with thrombocytosis, they are characteristic of MDS and AML rather than ET. The value of molecular techniques to determine clonality of the megakaryocytes or other myeloid lineages as a diagnostic procedure to establish the diagnosis of ET remains to be evaluated.

Postulated cell of origin

Bone marrow stem cell with variable lineage potential {382, 338}. Rare patients who meet the usual criteria for ET have been reported to have megakaryocytopoiesis that is nonclonal {498}. The relationship of such cases to the vast majority of cases of ET that have clonal haematopoiesis is not clear.

Prognosis and predictive factors

ET is an indolent disorder, characterised by long symptom-free intervals, interrupted by occasional life-threatening thromboembolic or haemorrhagic episodes. Median survival times of 10-15 years are commonly reported. Because ET usually occurs late in middle age, the life expectancy is near normal for many patients {908, 85, 909, 510}. The spleen serves as a site of sequestration of the platelets, thus splenectomy may result in a dramatic increase in the platelet count

and worse survival {1405}. Transformation of ET to acute myeloid leukaemia or a myelodysplastic syndrome occurs in fewer than 5% of patients, and when it does occur is likely related to previous cytotoxic therapy {909, 1184}. Although a few patients with ET develop marrow fibrosis after many years, such progression is uncommon {429}. The appearance of significant reticulin or any collagen fibrosis early in the disease process should prompt consideration of another diagnosis, such as chronic idiopathic myelofibrosis.

Provisional related entity

"Acquired sideroblastic anaemia associated with thrombocytosis".

Rarely, patients may present with diagnostic features of ET, but simultaneously have sideroblastic anaemia with many ringed sideroblasts in the marrow {6, 678, 474}. The classification and treatment of such patients is problematic. Because features of both a myelodysplastic and myeloproliferative process are present, it is best to consider this provisional entity as "Myelodysplastic/ Myeloproliferative disease, unclassifiable", until further studies determine the most appropriate category for such cases (see chapter 2).

Chronic myeloproliferative disease, unclassifiable

J. Thiele
M. Imbert
R. Pierre

J.W. Vardiman
R.D. Brunning
G. Flandrin

Definition

The designation, chronic myeloproliferative disease, unclassifiable (CMPD, U) should be applied only to cases that have definite clinical, laboratory and morphologic features of a myeloproliferative disease, but that fail to meet the criteria for any of the specific CMPD entities entities, or present with features that overlap two or more of the categories. There is no Philadelphia (Ph) chromosome or *BCR/ABL* fusion gene.

Most cases of CMPD, U, will fall into one of two groups: 1) Initial stages of PV, CIMF, or ET in which the characteristic features are not yet fully developed at the time of first presentation, or, 2) Late stage, advanced chronic myeloproliferative diseases, in which pronounced myelofibrosis, osteosclerosis, or transformation to a more aggressive stage obscures the underlying disorder {429, 1289, 1379}.

In patients with the initial stages of a CMPD that is unclassifiable, follow-up studies performed at intervals of 4-6 months will often provide sufficient information to permit a more precise designation. For patients with advanced disease in which the initial process is no longer recognisable, the designation of a late stage myeloproliferative disease that is otherwise unclassifiable may still provide useful prognostic information for therapeutic decisions.

The designation, CMPD, U, should not be used when the data necessary for proper classification are merely not available or have not been obtained, or when the bone marrow specimen is not of adequate quality or size for accurate evaluation {77, 1289}. These are the most frequent problems in routine practice, and account for the majority of the so-called unclassifiable cases. When these latter situations are encountered, it is preferable to describe the findings in the blood and marrow, and to suggest additional clinical and laboratory procedures that are needed to further classify the process, including adequate peripheral blood and bone marrow biopsy specimens.

If a case does not have the features of one of the well-defined entities, the possibility that it is not a myeloproliferative process must be strongly considered. A reactive marrow response to infection, chemotherapy, toxins, growth factors, cytokines and immunosuppresive agents may closely mimic a myeloproliferative disease. Furthermore, a number of other haematopoietic and non-haematopoietic neoplasms, such as lymphoma or metastatic carcinoma, may infiltrate the marrow and cause reactive changes, including dense fibrosis and osteosclerosis, that can be misconstrued as a CMPD.

Lastly, the defining characteristics of each myeloproliferative disease entity must be considered with the realisation that, as with any other biologic process, variations do occur. Furthermore, the CMPDs progress through different stages, so that with time the clinical and morphologic manifestations of the disease will change.

ICD-O code   9975/3

Synonyms
Undifferentiated myeloproliferative disease

Epidemiology
The exact incidence of CMPD, U is unknown, and varies according to the experience of the diagnostician as well as with the specific classification system and criteria utilised to classify myeloproliferative diseases. However, some reports indicate that the percentage of unclassifiable cases account for 10-20% of all cases of chronic myeloproliferative disease {429, 77, 1289, 1379, 161, 430}.

Sites of involvement
Similar to the other CMPDs.

Clinical features
The clinical features of CMPD, U are similar to those in the other myeloprolifera-

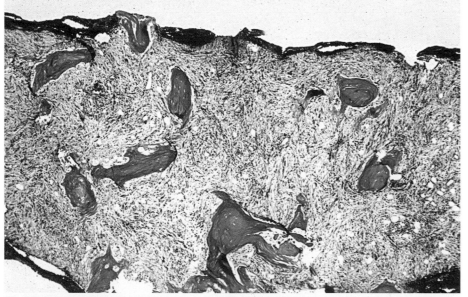

Fig. 1.49 Chronic myeloproliferative disease, unclassifiable, late fibrotic stage. A bone marrow biopsy specimen from a 75 year old man with pancytopenia, a leukoerythroblastic blood smear and marked splenomegaly. He had a history of haemotologic disease for 5 years but it had never been characterised. The biopsy shows cellular depletion and fibrosis, and distinction between post-polycythaemic myelofibrosis and myeloid metaplasia and CIMF is now impossible.

tive diseases. In patients with early, unclassifiable disease, organomegaly may be minimal or absent, but splenomegaly and hepatomegaly may be massive in those with advanced disease in whom bone marrow specimens are characterised by marked myelofibrosis or increased numbers of blasts. The haematologic values are also variable, and range from mild leukocytosis and moderate to marked thrombocytosis, with or without accompanying anaemia, to severe cytopenias due to bone marrow failure.

Aetiology
Unknown in most cases.

Morphology
Many cases that are diagnosed as CMPD, U are initial to very early stage disease in which the distinction between the pre-fibrotic stage of CIMF, the polycythaemic (or pre-polycythaemic) stage of PV, and ET is difficult. Often, the peripheral blood smear in such cases shows thrombocytosis and a variable degree of neutrophilia. The haemoglobin may be normal, mildly decreased or mildly increased. The bone marrow biopsy specimen shows hypercellularity and often prominent megakaryocytic proliferation, with variable amounts of granulocytic and erythoid proliferation. If the guidelines suggested in the previous sections on CMPD are carefully applied, most cases can be accurately assigned to a proper subtype, but if not, the designation of CMPD, U, is preferable until such time as careful follow-up data provides evidence of the correct diagnosis. In late stage disease, the bone marrow specimens show dense fibrosis and/or osteomyelosclerosis, indicating a terminal or burnt-out stage, and distinction between the post-polycythaemic stage of PV and the fibrotic stage of CIMF may be impossible if there is no previous history {77, 1359, 1404, 161, 430}. Although CML may also be accompanied by marked myelofibrosis, the small size of the megakaryocytes will alert the morphologist to the correct diagnosis, and cytogenetic and molecular genetic demonstration of the Ph chromosome and the *BCR/ABL* fusion gene will confirm the diagnosis of CML rather than of CMPD,U {429, 1289, 1379, 430}.

In patients with myeloproliferative diseases, more than 10% blasts in the blood

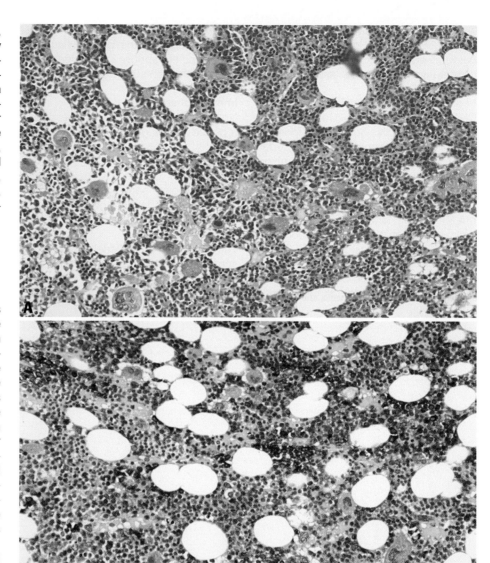

Fig. 1.50 Chronic myeloproliferative disease, unclassifiable, initial stage. **A** is an H&E stained section and **B** is a napthol ASD chloroacetate asterase reaction of the bone marrow biopsy specimen from a 46 year old man with a platelet count ranging from 500 to 1000 x 10⁹/L for several months. The bone marrow biopsy was obtained, and demonstrated hypercellularity with increased numbers of enlarged, mature megakaryocytes. The differential diagnosis was between essential thrombocythaemia and polycythaemia vera; over the next few months the haemoglobin level increased and a diagnosis of PV was established.

or marrow and/or the finding of significant myelodysplasia generally indicates transformation of the disease to a more aggressive, often terminal stage. If the initial diagnostic specimen has features of a myeloproliferative process that cannot be specifically categorised, but shows 10-19% blasts in the blood or bone marrow, diagnosis of the case as an accelerated stage of a myeloproliferative disease, unclassifiable, is appropriate. If blasts account for 20% or more of

the peripheral white blood cells or bone marrow cells in the initial specimen, then the diagnosis is acute leukaemia, and the suggestion that the case may be a blast transformation of a previous but unclassifiable myeloproliferative disease can be made. If the initial specimen shows changes suggestive of MDS as well as of CMPD, but there are insufficient criteria to diagnose a specific myelodysplastic or myeloproliferative disease, or if distinction between MDS with fibrosis and CMPD is impossible {992, 727, 822}, the case may be best categorised as myelodysplastic / myeloproliferative disease, unclassifiable (see chapter 2).

In summary, the morphologic findings in CMPD, U are variable. Care must be taken not to use this designation for reactive blood and bone marrow changes that may mimic myeloproliferative disorders, for well-defined myeloproliferative disorders in transformation to an accelerated or blast phase, or when an adequate clinical, laboratory and morphologic evaluation has not yet been performed. When the designation CMPD, U is used for cases that are most likely an initial, early stage of CIMF, PV or ET, every attempt must be made to provide a more specific diagnosis as soon as possible because of the prognostic differences and therapeutic implications associated with each subtype of CMPD.

Immunophenotype

No abnormal phenotype has been reported for this group of patients

Genetics

There is no cytogenetic or molecular genetic finding specific for this group. Abnormalities described in the other myeloproliferative diseases may also be seen in CMPD, U.

The finding of a Philadelphia chromosome or *BCR/ABL* fusion gene, however, indicates the diagnosis is CML and not CMPD, U.

Postulated cell of origin

Pluripotent or multipotent bone marrow stem cell.

Prognosis and predictive factors

There are no data available for this specific group. However, patients for whom this designation is used because their bone marrow specimens are markedly fibrotic or demonstrate blastic infiltration are likely to have advanced disease, and would be expected to have a poor prognosis. Patients who are in the early stages of disease will have a prognosis similar to those of the group into which their disease eventually evolves.

CHAPTER 2

Myelodysplastic /
Myeloproliferative Diseases

The MDS/MPD category includes myeloid disorders that have both dysplastic and proliferative features at the time of initial presentation. Such cases overlap the myelodysplastic syndromes (MDS) and chronic myeloproliferative disease (CMPD) groups, and are difficult to assign to either. It is not surprising that such diseases exist. Although the molecular abnormalities that lead to dysregulation of the pathways for myeloid proliferation, maturation and survival are likely different in most cases of MDS from those in CMPD, it is easy to envision that some genetic defects or combination of defects could lead to simultaneous proliferative and dysplastic features in the same patient.

Some of the disorders included in the WHO category of MDS/MPD, particularly chronic myelomonocytic leukaemia, have engendered considerable debate as to whether they should be classified as a myeloproliferative disorder or a myelodysplastic syndrome – a controversy that is not yet settled. The WHO classification provides a less restrictive view of these disorders, and creates a category which recognises the overlap that exists in some myeloid diseases. Classification of cases into this category may provide a focus for future studies of the molecular pathways involved in the control of proliferation, abnormal maturation, and dysplasia.

WHO histological classification of myelodysplastic / myeloproliferative diseases

Chronic myelomonocytic leukaemia	9945/3
Atypical chronic myeloid leukaemia	9876/3
Juvenile myelomonocytic leukaemia	9946/3
Myelodysplastic / myeloproliferative disease, unclassifiable	9975/3

Myelodysplastic / myeloproliferative diseases: Introduction

J.W. Vardiman

Definition and characteristic features

The myelodysplastic / myeloproliferative diseases (MDS/MPD) are clonal haematopoietic neoplasms that, at the time of initial presentation, have some clinical, laboratory or morphologic findings that might support a diagnosis of a myelodysplastic syndrome (MDS), and other findings that are more consistent with a chronic myeloproliferative disease (CMPD). They are characterised by hypercellularity of the bone marrow due to proliferation in one or more of the myeloid lineages. Frequently, the proliferation in one or more lineages is effective and results in increased numbers of circulating cells; however, they may be morphologically and functionally dysplastic. Simultaneously, one or more of the other lineages may exhibit ineffective proliferation, so that cytopenia(s) may be present as well. The blast percentage in the blood and marrow is always less than 20%. Although splenomegaly and hepatomegaly are commonly found, the clinical and laboratory findings vary, and can fall anywhere along a continuum between those usually associated with a myelodysplastic syndrome and a chronic myeloproliferative disease.

Patients with a history of a well-defined myeloproliferative disease who develop dysplasia and ineffective haematopoiesis should not be placed in this group. Such changes usually indicate progression of the initial myeloproliferative disease to a transformed phase. Rarely, however, some patients may present for the first time in a transformed stage of a CMPD that was not previously recognised, and they may have findings that suggest they belong to the MDS/MPD group. In such cases, if clinical and laboratory studies fail to reveal the nature of the underlying process, the designation of MDS/MPD, Unclassifiable, may be appropriate. Patients who have a Philadelphia chromosome or BCR/ABL fusion gene should not be placed in this category, but rather classified as chronic myelogenous leukaemia.

Incidence / epidemiology

The incidence of MDS/MPD varies widely, depending on the specific disease category. It may range from as many as 3/100,000 individuals over the age of 60 annually for the most common disorder, chronic myelomonocytic leukaemia (CMML), to as few as 0.13/100,000 children from 0-14 years of age annually for juvenile myelomonocytic leukaemia (JMML) {55, 501, 1393}. Atypical chronic myeloid leukaemia is a recently defined entity, and reliable data concerning its incidence are not available. In a series of over 500 patients with MDS classified according to the FAB criteria, 4.4% of cases (excluding cases diagnosed as CMML) had features of both MDS and CMPD, and could not be easily classified {945}.

Pathophysiology / pathogenesis

The major clinical and pathologic findings in MDS/MPD disorders are due to abnormalities in the regulation of the myeloid pathways for cellular proliferation, maturation, and cell survival. The clinical symptoms are due to the complications of cytopenia(s), production of dysplastic cells that do not function normally, leukaemic infiltration of various organ systems, or general constitutional symptoms such as fever and malaise {65}.

At the present time, there have been no genetic defects identified that are specific for any of the entities included in the MDS/MPD group, although there are some recurring chromosomal and molecular abnormalities that provide insight into possible mechanisms of their molecular pathogenesis. A relatively high frequency of mutations of N-RAS have been reported in each of the MDS/MPD disorders, suggesting that deregulation of the RAS pathway of signalling proteins may play some role in the abnormal proliferation {234}. Although they are rare, the t(5;12) (q31;p12) and t(5;10)(q33;q22) chromosomal aberrations that have been reported in CMML and aCML result in fusion proteins that apparently enhance the tyrosine kinase activity of the receptor, PDGFβR, and may lead to abnormal activation of the RAS pathway as well as abnormal regulation of other signal transduction pathways {445, 1195}. In addition, the increased incidence of JMML in patients with neurofibromatosis type-1 (NF1) has provided some clues that implicate abnormal RAS pathway regulation in the characteristic hypersensitivity of JMML leukaemic cells to GM-CSF. In children with JMML and NF1, there is loss of heterozygosity for the NF1 gene, so that the normal regulation of RAS by neurofibromin, the protein product of NF1, is lost, resulting in activation of the pathway {1180}. Thus, abnormalities in regulation of the RAS pathway appears to be a common finding in CMML, aCML and JMML, although individual patients may show different avenues in deregulating the RAS sequence. It is clear, however, that abnormalities in this pathway are not unique to MDS/MPD disorders, so that other mechanisms must interact with these molecular defects to produce the abnormal cellular kinetics observed in patients with MDS/MPD.

Prognosis / evolution

Survival times vary markedly for patients with MDS/MPD, and can range from months to years, depending on the individual disease. There is a tendency in each disorder for clonal evolution and disease progression. Patients may die of complications of cytopenia(s), leukaemic infiltration or a blast phase.

Rationale for classification

Although some authors believe that CMML, aCML and JMML are merely variations of the same disease process, there are sufficient clinical, morphologic and biological differences to warrant their separation in a classification scheme. There is also considerable controversy as to whether some entities included in this group should be classified as myeloproliferative or as myelodysplastic disorders {872}. The French-American-British group suggested that CMML could be divided into a myeloproliferative or a myelodysplastic type according to whether the WBC was greater or less than 13,000 x 10^9/L, respectively {91}. However, there is no convincing evidence that such a division of CMML is clinically or biologically relevant {432}. The WHO proposal to recognise the overlap that sometimes occurs between MDS and CMPD provides a less restrictive view of these disorders, and permits those who care for patients with these diseases to consider them in the context of which disease features predominate.

In addition to CMML, aCML and JMML, there are other disorders which may display proliferative and dysplastic features simultaneously, and could be included in a listing of MDS/MPD entities. One such disorder may be manifested as refractory anaemia with ringed sideroblasts (RARS) and marked thrombocytosis {474}. Patients with this disorder are not only a challenge to diagnose but also to treat effectively. Whether this disorder is merely a variant of RARS, the chance occurrence of two diseases in the same patient (RARS and essential thrombo-cythaemia), or a MDS/MPD will require further studies to determine. Until additional information is available, such cases are included in the MDS, Unclassifiable category.

The diseases that are included in the MDS/MPD category are instructive. They teach us that disorders of the marrow stem cell do not always readily fit into single diagnostic slots, and that an ideal classification will only come about as we learn more about the defects in the pathways that control cell proliferation, maturation and survival.

Chronic myelomonocytic leukaemia

J.W. Vardiman
R. Pierre
B. Bain
J.M. Bennett

M. Imbert
R.D. Brunning
G. Flandrin

Definition

Chronic myelomonocytic leukaemia (CMML) is a clonal disorder of a bone marrow stem cell, in which monocytosis is a major defining feature. It is characterised by: 1) persistent monocytosis >1 x 10^9/L in the peripheral blood, 2) absence of a Philadelphia chromosome and *BCR/ABL* fusion gene, 3) fewer than 20% blasts in the blood or bone marrow, and 4) dysplasia involving one or more myeloid lineages. However, if convincing myelodysplasia is not present, the diagnosis of CMML can still be made if the other requirements are met, and an acquired, clonal cytogenetic or molecular genetic abnormality is present in the marrow cells, or if the monocytosis has persisted for at least 3 months and all other causes of monocytosis, such as a tumour, infection or inflammation, have been excluded. The clinical, haematologic and morphologic features of CMML are heterogeneous, and vary along a spectrum from predominantly myelodysplastic to mainly myeloproliferative in nature.

ICD-O code   9945/3

Synonyms

Subacute myelomonocytic leukaemia
Chronic myelomonocytic syndrome

Epidemiology

There are no reliable incidence data for CMML, because in some epidemiologic surveys, CMML is grouped with chronic myeloid leukaemia and in others, as a myelodysplastic syndrome (MDS) {55}. In one study in which CMML accounted for 31% of the cases of MDS, the incidence of MDS was estimated to be approximately 12.8 cases per 100,000 individuals per year {1393}. The median age at diagnosis is 65-75 years, with a male predominance of 1.5-3:1 {1205, 374, 5, 1239, 432}.

Sites of involvement

The blood and bone marrow are always involved. The spleen, liver, skin, and lymph nodes are the most common sites of extramedullary leukaemic infiltration {374, 5, 432}.

Clinical features

In approximately 50% of patients, the white blood cell (WBC) count is normal or slightly decreased. Although monocytosis is present in such cases, there may be neutropenia, and the clinical and other haematologic findings may be identical to those of a myelodysplastic disorder. In the remaining patients, the WBC count is increased at the time of diagnosis, and the disease has features that are more myeloproliferative in nature. However, the incidence of the most common presenting complaints of fatigue, weight loss, fever, and night sweats are similar in both groups of patients, as is the rate of infection and of bleeding due to thrombocytopenia {1205, 374, 5, 1239, 432}.

Although splenomegaly and hepatomegaly may be present in either group, they are more frequent (up to 50% of patients) when the WBC count is increased above normal {432}.

Aetiology

The specific aetiology of CMML is unknown. Occupational and environmental carcinogens, ionizing irradiation and cytotoxic agents may be possible causes in some cases {55}.

Morphology

Peripheral blood monocytosis is the hallmark of CMML. By definition, monocytes are always >1 x 10^9/L and usually range from 2 to 5 x 10^9/L, but may exceed 80 x 10^9/L {374, 5, 816, 872}. The percentage of monocytes is almost always >10% of the WBCs {1183, 91}. The monocytes generally are mature, with unremarkable morphology, but can exhibit abnormal granulation, unusual nuclear lobation, or finely dispersed nuclear chromatin {687}. Blasts and promonocytes may be seen, but if they account for ≥20% of the WBC, the diagnosis is AML rather than CMML (see below). Other changes in the blood are variable. The WBC may be normal or slightly decreased, with neutropenia, but in nearly one-half of patients it is increased due not only to monocytosis but also to neutrophilia {432, 816, 872, 1183}. Neutrophil precursors (promyelocytes, myelocytes) usually account for fewer than 10% of the WBCs {1183, 91}. Mild basophilia is sometimes present. Eosinophils are usually normal or slightly increased in number, but in some cases, eosinophilia may be striking. Because cases of CMML with eosinophilia may be associated with specific cytogenetic/

Table 2.01
Diagnostic criteria for chronic myelomonocytic leukaemia.

1. Persistent peripheral blood monocytosis >1 x 10^9/L
2. No Philadelphia chromosome or *BCR/ABL* fusion gene
3. Fewer than 20% blasts* in the blood or bone marrow

4. Dysplasia in one or more myeloid lineages. If myelodysplasia is absent or minimal, the diagnosis of CMML may still be made if the other requirements are met, and:
   - an acquired, clonal cytogenetic abnormality is present in the marrow cells, *or*
   - the monocytosis has been persistent for at least 3 months *and*
   - all other causes of monocytosis have been excluded.

* Blasts include myeloblasts, monoblasts and promonocytes. Promonocytes are monocytic precursors with abundant light gray or slightly basophilic cytoplasm with a few scattered, fine lilac-coloured granules, finely-distributed, stippled nuclear chromatin, variably prominent nucleoli, and delicate nuclear folding or creasing, and in this classification are equivalent to blasts.

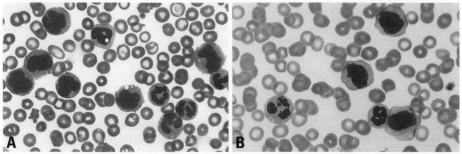

Fig. 2.01 Chronic myelomonocytic leukaemia-1. The degree of leukocytosis, neutrophilia and dysplasia is variable in CMML. **A** The white blood count is elevated with minimal dysplasia in the neutrophil series. **B** A normal white blood cell count with absolute monocytosis, neutropenia and dysgranulopoiesis.

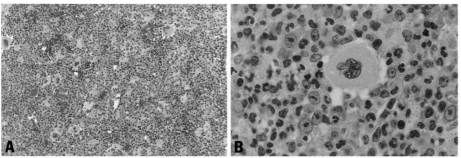

Fig. 2.02 Chronic myelomonocytic leukaemia-1. **A** A bone marrow biopsy specimen from a patient with CMML-1. Often, the granulocytic component is most obvious in the biopsy specimen, and monocytes may not be readily appreciated. **B** The folded nuclei and delicate nuclear chromatin characteristic of monocytes can be appreciated among the granulocytes.

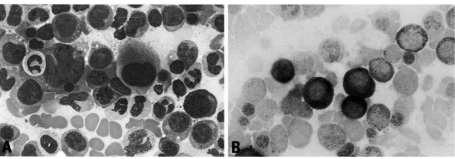

Fig. 2.03 Chronic myelomonocytic leukaemia-1. **A** In the Wright-Giemsa stained preparation, the dysplastic granulocytic component is obvious. **B** The monocytic component is appreciated with the special stains, napthol ASD chloroacetate esterase reaction combined with alpha naphthyl butyrate esterase (monocytes brown, neutrophils blue, dual staining cells have mixture of blue and brown).

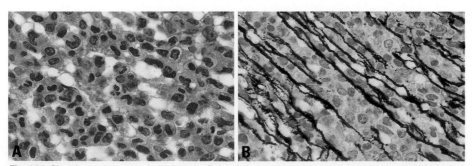

Fig. 2.04 Chronic myelomonocytic leukaemia. Some degree of fibrosis may be seen in up to 30% of cases. **A** and **B** This composite slide illustrates increased reticulin fibrosis in a marrow biopsy specimen of a patient with CMML.

molecular genetic abnormalities, and because the persistently elevated eosinophil count may be associated with severe tissue damage, such cases should be specifically identified (see below). Dysgranulopoiesis, including neutrophils with hypolobated or abnormally lobated nuclei or abnormal cytoplasmic granulation, is present in most cases, but may be less prominent in patients with leukocytosis than those with a normal or low WBC count {816, 687}. Mild anaemia, often normocytic but sometimes macrocytic, is common. Platelet counts vary, but moderate thrombocytopenia is often present. Atypical, large platelets may be observed {5, 816}. The bone marrow is hypercellular in over 75% of cases, but normocellular and even hypocellular specimens may occur {1239, 872}. Granulocytic proliferation is often the most striking finding in the bone marrow biopsy, but an increase in erythroid precursors may be seen as well {872, 91}. Monocytic proliferation is invariably present, but can be difficult to appreciate in the biopsy or on marrow aspirate smears. Cytochemical studies that aid in the identification of monocytes, such as alpha naphthyl acetate esterase or alpha naphthyl butyrate esterase, used alone or in combination with naphthol ASD chloroacetate esterase, are strongly recommended when the diagnosis of CMML is suspected {1272}. Dysgranulopoiesis, similar to that found in the blood, is present in the marrow of most patients with CMML, and dyserythropoiesis (megaloblastic changes, abnormal nuclear contours, ringed sideroblasts, etc.) is observed in over one-half of patients {432, 816, 872}. Micromegakaryocytes and/or megakaryocytes with abnormally lobated nuclei are found in up to 80% of patients {816, 872}. Fibrosis of variable degree is seen in the bone marrow specimens of nearly 30% of patients with CMML {822}.

The splenic enlargement in CMLL is usually due to infiltration of the red pulp by the leukemia cells. Lymphadenopathy is uncommon, but when it occurs, it may signal transformation to a more acute phase, and the lymph node may show diffuse infiltration by myeloid blasts. Sometimes, there is lymph node and less commonly splenic involvement by a diffuse infiltration of plasmacytoid monocytes. In some patients generalised lymphadenopathy due to tumoural prolifera-

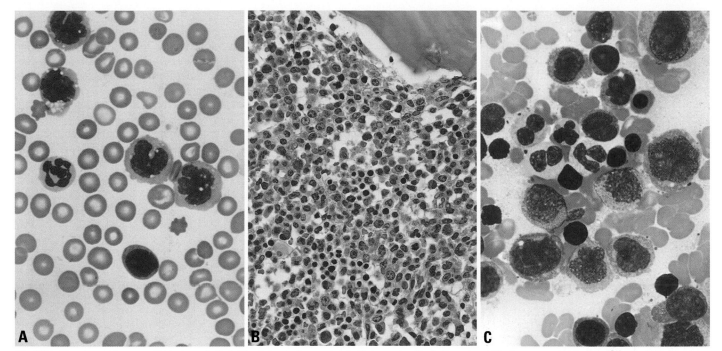

Fig. 2.05 Chronic myelomonocytic leukaemia-2. **A** Blood smear from a newly diagnosed patient. Occasional blasts were noted in the peripheral blood smear. **B** Biopsy from the same patient. The immaturity of the bone marrow elements can be readily appreciated. **C** In the aspirate smear, blasts and promonocytes account for 12% of the marrow cells.

tions of plasmacytoid monocytes may be the presenting manifestation of CMML. These cells have round nuclei, finely dispersed chromatin, inconspicuous nucleoli, and a rim of eosinophilic cytoplasm. The cytoplasmic membrane is usually distinct, with well-defined cytoplasmic borders. This imparts a cohesive appearance to the infiltrating cells. Apoptotic bodies, often within starry sky histiocytes, are frequently present. The relationship of the plasmacytoid monocyte proliferation to the leukemic myelomonocytic cells is uncertain. While plasmacytoid monocytes are proposed to be of monocytic lineage, it is not proven that the plasmacytoid monocytes are clonally related to the neoplastic cells of CMML {59, 536, 353, 493}.

The number of blasts, including promonocytes (in this classification, promonocytes are equivalent to blasts), usually account for fewer than 5% of the peripheral blood WBCs and less than 10% of the nucleated marrow cells at the time of diagnosis. A higher blast count than this may identify patients who are at risk of having a poor prognosis or a rapid transformation to acute leukaemia {374, 5, 1239, 1272, 1414, 372, 451}.

It is recommended that CMML be further divided into two subcategories, depending on the number of blasts found in the peripheral blood and bone marrow, as follows:

CMML-1
Blasts <5% in the blood, <10% in the bone marrow.

CMML-2
Blasts 5-19% in the blood or 10-19% in the bone marrow, or when Auer rods are present and the blast count is less than 20% in blood or marrow.

The finding of >20% blasts in the blood and/or the bone marrow indicates AML rather than CMML.

CMML with eosinophilia
An additional subset, CMML with eosinophilia, may be diagnosed when the criteria for CMML are present, but in addition, the eosinophil count in the peripheral blood is >1.5 x 10⁹/L. Patients in this category may have complications related to the degranulation of the eosinophils (see chapter 1). This subset should be designated as CMML-1 or CMML-2 with eosinophilia according to the above guidelines.

Immunophenotype
The blood and marrow cells usually express the expected myelomonocytic antigens, such as CD33 and CD13, with variable expression of CD14, CD68 and CD64 {810, 119, 1411}. Few cases of CMML have been reported with detailed immunophenotypic data, but rare cases with unexpected phenotypes have been reported {1411}. An increased percentage of CD34+ cells may be associated with early transformation to acute leukaemia {1411}.

The plasmacytoid monocytes associated with CMML have a characteristic immunophenotype. They are positive for CD14, CD43, CD56, CD68, and CD4. T-cell associated antigens such as CD2 and CD5 are often present. Based on these features, in the past these cells had been interpreted as "plasmacytoid T-cells". However, a T-cell derivation has been disproved.

Genetics
Clonal cytogenetic abnormalities are found in 20-40% of patients with CMML, but none are specific {374, 5, 1239, 432, 1272, 1306, 476, 375}. The most frequent recurring abnormalities include +8, -7/del (7q) and structural abnormalities of 12p. Abnormalities of 11q23 are uncommon in CMML, and suggest instead the diagnosis of acute leukaemia. Some authors have suggested that patients with isolated i(17q) are a unique group within the myelodysplastic/myelo-

proliferative category, but many patients with this abnormality can be classified as CMML; whether they should be placed in a special category awaits further study {847, 385}. As many as 40% of patients exhibit point mutations of *RAS* genes at diagnosis or during the disease course {1246, 999, 1394}.

The myelodysplastic/myeloproliferative disorder associated with t(5;12)(q31;p12), which results in the formation of an abnormal fusion gene, *TEL/PDGFβR*, has been recognised by some as a unique entity, although most patients are reported to have CMML {445, 71}. It occurs in fewer than 1-2% of patients with CMML, and is usually accompanied by marked eosinophilia. Cases of CMML with eosinophilia associated with other rearrangements of the *TEL* gene have also been reported {1399}.

Postulated cell of origin
Bone marrow stem cell.

Prognosis and predictive factors
Survival of patients with CMML is reported to vary from 1 to more than 100 months, but the median survival time in most series is 20-40 months {1205, 374, 5, 1239, 432, 1272, 1414, 372, 451}. Progression to acute leukaemia occurs in approximately 15-30% of cases. A number of clinical and haematologic parameters, including splenomegaly, severity of anaemia and degree of leukocytosis, have been reported to be important factors in predicting the course of the disease. However, in virtually all studies, the percentage of blood and bone marrow blasts is the most important factor in determining survival {1205, 374, 5, 1239, 432, 1272, 1414, 372, 451}.

Atypical chronic myeloid leukaemia

J.W. Vardiman   B. Bain
M. Imbert   R.D. Brunning
R. Pierre   G. Flandrin

Definition
Atypical chronic myeloid leukaemia (aCML) is a leukaemic disorder that demonstrates myelodysplastic as well as myeloproliferative features at the time of initial diagnosis. It is characterised by principal involvement of the neutrophil series with leukocytosis comprised of immature and mature neutrophils that are dysplastic. Multilineage dysplasia is common, however, and reflects the stem cell origin of aCML. The neoplastic cells do not have a Philadelphia chromosome or the *BCR/ABL* fusion gene.

ICD-O code   9876/3

Synonyms
Subacute myeloid leukaemia

Epidemiology
The exact incidence of aCML is not known, but is reported to be only 1-2 cases for every 100 cases of Ph+, *BCR/ABL+* CML {1183}. Patients with aCML tend to be elderly; in the few series reported to date the median age at diagnosis is in the seventh or eighth decade of life {1183, 514, 816, 252}. The reported M:F ratio varies from 1:1 to 2.5:1 {514, 816, 252}.

Sites of involvement
The peripheral blood and bone marrow are always involved; splenic and hepatic involvement is also common.

Clinical features
There are few reports of the clinical features of patients with aCML. Most patients have symptoms related to anaemia or sometimes to thrombocytopenia, whereas in others, the chief complaint may be related to splenomegaly {1183, 514, 816, 252}.

Aetiology
The cause of aCML is unknown.

Morphology
In the peripheral blood, the white blood cell (WBC) count is variable; median val-

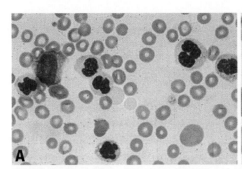
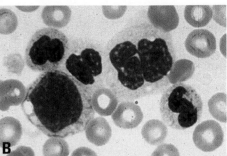

Fig. 2.06 Atypical chronic myeloid leukaemia. **A** shows an elevated WBC in the peripheral blood. **B** illustrates marked dysplasia and immature granulocytes. Cytogenetic studies revealed a +8, but no Ph-chromosome, and no *BCR/ABL* fusion gene was detected by FISH.

ues ranging from 35-96 x 10^9/L have been reported, and some patients may have WBC counts in excess of 300 x 10^9/L {1183, 514, 816, 252, 1190, 91}. Blasts usually account for fewer than 5% and always for less than 20% of the peripheral blood white cells. Immature granulocytes (promyelocytes, myelocytes and metamyelocytes) usually total

Table 2.02
Diagnostic criteria of atypical chronic myeloid leukaemia (aCML).

- Peripheral blood leukocytosis due to increased numbers of mature and immature neutrophils

- Prominent dysgranulopoiesis

- No Ph chromosome or *BCR/ABL* fusion gene

- Neutrophil precursors (promyelocytes, myelocytes, metamyelocytes) ≥10% of WBCs

- No or minimal absolute basophilia; basophils <2% of WBCs

- No or minimal absolute monocytosis; monocytes <10% of WBCs

- Hypercellular bone marrow biopsy with granulocytic proliferation and granulocytic dysplasia, with or without dysplasia in the erythroid and megakaryocytic lineages.

- Fewer than 20% blasts in the blood or bone marrow

10-20% or more. Although the absolute monocyte count may be increased, the percentage of monocytes rarely exceeds 10%. Basophilia may be observed, but is not prominent {1183, 514, 816, 252, 91}. The major characteristic that distinguishes aCML is dysgranulopoiesis, which is often pronounced. Acquired Pelger-Huet or other nuclear abnormalities, such as abnormally condensed nuclear chromatin or bizarrely segmented nuclei, and abnormal cytoplasmic granularity, are abnormalities that may be seen in the neutrophils. Moderate anaemia is frequent, and the red cells may show changes indicative of dyserythropoiesis, including macro-ovalocytosis. The platelet count is variable, but thrombocytopenia is common {1183, 514, 816, 252, 91}.

The bone marrow biopsy demonstrates hypercellularity because of granulocytic proliferation. Blasts may be modestly increased in number, but large sheets or clusters of blasts are not present, and blasts account for fewer than 20% of the marrow cells. Dysgranulopoiesis is a constant finding in aCML, and the changes in the neutrophilic series in the marrow are similar to those described for the blood. Megakaryocytes may be decreased, normal or increased in number, but in most cases some megakaryocytes are dysplastic. Erythropoiesis is variable in quantity. Usually the M:E ratio is greater than 10:1, but in some cases erythroid precursors may account for

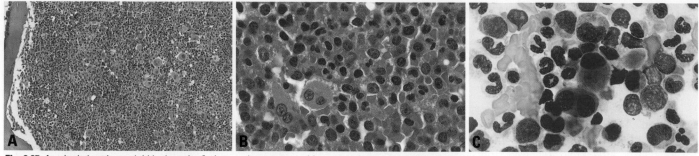

Fig. 2.07 Atypical chronic myeloid leukaemia. **A** shows a bone marrow biopsy specimen from the same case illustrated in fig. 2.06. It shows hypercellularity, due to granulocytic proliferation. **B** Note an increase in the number of megakaryocytes, with small, abnormal forms. From the biopsy alone, the morphology would be difficult to differentiate from Ph chromosome positive chronic myelogenous leukaemia. **C** Bone marrow aspirate smear. Dysplasia in the granulocytic and the megakaryocytic cells is evident.

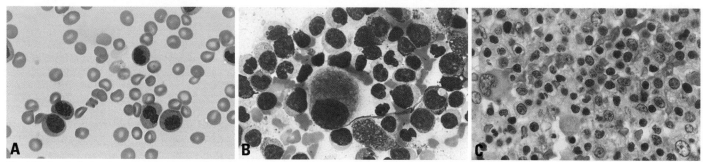

Fig. 2.08 Atypical chronic myeloid leukaemia. These microphotographs illustrate the blood smear and bone marrow aspirate and biopsy of a patient with aCML and the cytogenetic abnormality, i(17q). **A** Cells in the blood are dysplastic, with hypercondensed nuclear chromatin. Note also the thrombocytopenia. **B** In the bone marrow aspirate the neutrophil nuclei are condensed. **C** In the biopsy the nuclei of the neutrophils are so condensed, they appear as mononuclear cells.

over 30% of the marrow cells, and dyserythropoiesis may be present {1183, 514, 816, 252, 91, 1190}. Increased reticulin fibers are seen in some cases at the time of diagnosis, or may appear later in the course of the disease.

Cytochemistry / immunophenotype
No specific immunophenotypic or cytochemical abnormality has been reported to date. Leukocyte alkaline phosphatase scores may be low, normal or elevated, and thus are not useful for diagnosis {816, 252}.

Genetics
Cytogenetic abnormalities, including +8, +13, del(20q), i(17q) and del(12p), are found in up to 80% of patients with aCML, but none are specific {514, 816, 252, 1190}. There is no Philadelphia chromosome or *BCR/ABL* fusion gene. A single case of aCML with t(5;10)

(q33;q22), which results in the abnormal fusion gene, *PDGFβR/H4/D10S170*, has been reported {1195, 699}.

Postulated cell of origin
Bone marrow myeloid stem cell.

Clinical course and prognosis
Patients with aCML fare poorly. The data reported to the present time include small numbers of patients, but median survival times reported are less than 20 months {1183, 514, 1190}. Thrombocytopenia and marked anaemia are poor prognostic factors {514}. In approximately 25-40% of patients, aCML evolves to acute leukaemia, whereas the remainder die of marrow failure {252, 1190}.

Variant
Syndrome of abnormal chromatin clumping
The "syndrome of abnormal chromatin clumping" can be considered as a vari-

ant of aCML {369, 143, 561}. It is characterised in the peripheral blood by a high percentage of immature and mature neutrophils that exhibit exaggerated clumping of the nuclear chromatin. Nuclear hypolobation and cytoplasmic hypogranularity are also commonly found. In most patients, the white blood cell count is increased, but occasional patients may have normal values {369}. Anaemia and thrombocytopenia are often severe. The bone marrow is hypercellular, and shows granulocytic proliferation and the same nuclear abnormalities as in the blood. Moderate dysplastic changes in the erythroblastic and megakaryocytic lineages are often present as well. Survival times are similar to those reported in aCML {369, 143, 561}.

Juvenile myelomonocytic leukaemia

J.W. Vardiman
R. Pierre
M. Imbert

B. Bain
R.D. Brunning
G. Flandrin

Definition

Juvenile myelomonocytic leukaemia (JMML) is a clonal haematopoietic disorder of childhood that is characterised by proliferation principally of the granulocytic and monocytic lineages. Erythroid and megakaryocytic abnormalities are frequently present as well, which is in keeping with evidence that JMML arises from a bone marrow stem cell with multilineage potential in the myeloid series {22, 164, 876}. Recently, diagnostic criteria for JMML have been proposed {953} and are outlined in Table 2.03.

ICD-O code   9946/3

Synonyms

Juvenile chronic myelomonocytic leukaemia

Epidemiology

The incidence of JMML is estimated to be approximately 1.3 per million children 0 - 14 years of age per year. It accounts for less than 2-3% of all leukaemia in children, but for 20-30% of all cases of myelodysplastic and myeloproliferative disease in patients less than 14 years old {501, 43, 795, 186}. The age at diagnosis ranges from 1 month to early adolescence, but 75% of cases occur in children less than 3 years of age {795, 186, 952, 1245}. Boys are affected nearly twice as frequently as girls {795}. Approximately 10% of cases occur in children with the clinical diagnosis of neurofibromatosis type 1 (NF-1) {795, 186}.

Sites of involvement

The blood and bone marrow always show evidence of myelomonocytic proliferation. Leukaemic infiltration of the liver and spleen is found in virtually all cases. Although any tissue may be infiltrated, lymph node, skin and the respiratory

The authors wish to thank Dr. C. Niemeyer and Dr. H. Hasle for their review and comments regarding the manuscript.

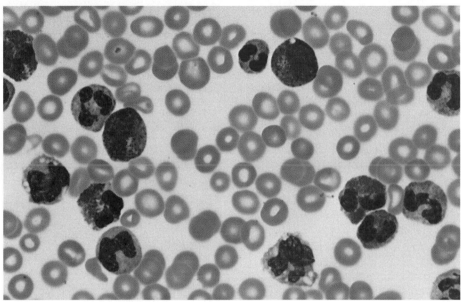

Fig. 2.09 Juvenile myelomonocytic leukaemia. The peripheral blood smear demonstrates leukocytosis comprised of neutrophils, including immature forms, and increased numbers of monocytes. Thrombocytopenia is also present.

tract are other common sites of involvement {953, 795, 186}.

Clinical features

Most patients present with constitutional symptoms, including malaise, pallor and fever, or evidence of an infection {795, 186, 952, 1245}. Symptoms of bronchitis or tonsillitis are observed in nearly one-half of cases at the time of initial presentation, and nearly as many have evidence of bleeding {795, 186, 952}.

Table 2.03
Diagnostic criteria of juvenile myelomonocytic leukaemia*.

1. Peripheral blood monocytosis > 1 x 10^9/L

2. Blasts (including promonocytes)** are <20% of the WBCs in the blood and of the nucleated bone marrow cells

3. No Ph chromosome or *BCR/ABL* fusion gene

4. Plus two or more of the following:
    Haemoglobin F increased for age
    Immature granulocytes in the peripheral blood
    WBC count >10 x 10^9/L
    Clonal chromosomal abnormality (e.g. may be monosomy 7)
    GM-CSF hypersensitivity of myeloid progenitors *in vitro*

 *Modified from {953}
**In this classification, promonocytes are equivalent to blasts. Promonocytes are monocytic precursors with abundant light grey or slightly basophilic cytoplasm with a few scattered, fine lilac-coloured granules, finely-distributed, stippled nuclear chromatin, variably prominent nucleoli, and delicate nuclear folding or creasing.

Maculopapular skin rashes occur in 40-50%, and café-au-lait spots may be seen in patients with NF-1. Hepatospleno-megaly is present in almost all cases {795, 186, 952, 1245}.

The laboratory tests that aid in the diagnosis of JMML are outlined in Table 2.03. Important abnormalities of the myeloid progenitor cells in JMML include their ability to form spontaneous granulocyte-macrophage colonies *in vitro* and their marked hypersensitivity to GM-CSF {344, 404, 1038}. These studies are strongly recommended to confirm the diagnosis of JMML. Additional laboratory features include polyclonal hypergammaglobu-linemia in the majority of patients, and increased serum lysozyme levels {795}.

The clinical and laboratory features of JMML sometimes closely mimic infectious diseases, including those due to Epstein-Barr virus, cytomegalovirus, human herpesvirus 6, histoplasma, mycobacteria and toxoplasma. Infections due to these agents must be excluded as a cause for the clinical and haematologic findings by appropriate laboratory testing {796}.

Aetiology

The cause of JMML is not known. In some cases, there is a genetic predisposition. Rare cases have been reported in identical twins {795}. In addition, there is an important association between neurofibromatosis type 1 (NF-1) and JMML. In contrast to adults who have NF-1, children with the clinical diagnosis of NF-1 are reported to have a 200- to 500-fold increased risk of developing a myeloid malignancy, mainly JMML {1245, 21}.

Morphology

The peripheral blood is often the most important specimen in proving the diagnosis. It shows leukocytosis, anaemia, and often, thrombocytopenia {795, 186, 952, 1245, 1004, 519}. The median reported WBC count varies from 25-35 x 10^9/L, but is > 100 x 10^9/L in 5-10% of children. The leukocytosis is comprised mainly of neutrophils, including immature forms such as promyelocytes and myelocytes, as well as of monocytes. Blasts (including promonocytes) usually account for fewer than 5% of the white cells, and always for less than 20%. Eosinophilia and basophilia are observed in a minority of patients. Nucleated red blood cells are often seen.

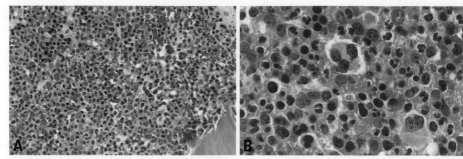

Fig. 2.10 Juvenile myelomonocytic leukaemia. **A** Bone marrow biopsy specimen from a patient with JMML. The marrow is hypercellular with granulocytic proliferation. **B** The megakaryocytes are reduced in number, but appear morphologically normal in the biopsy. Blasts are not substantially increased in number as judged from the biopsy.

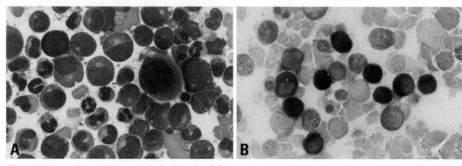

Fig. 2.11 Juvenile myelomonocytic leukaemia. **A** Bone marrow aspirate smear from a patient with JMML. The aspirate usually reflects the changes noted in the blood, but the monocyte component is difficult to appreciate. **B** A combined alpha napthyl acetate esterase and napthol ASD chloroacetate esterase reaction identifies the granulocytic (blue reaction product) and the monocytic component (brown reaction product). A few cells contain both products.

Red blood cell changes may include macrocytosis, particularly in patients with monosomy 7, but normocytic red cells are more common, and microcytosis may be seen as well {1245}. Although platelet counts are variable, thrombocytopenia is usual and may be severe {795, 186, 952, 1245, 1004, 519}.

The bone marrow aspirate and biopsy are hypercellular with granulocytic proliferation, although in some patients erythroid precursors may comprise nearly one-half of the bone marrow cells {1245, 1004, 519}. Monocytes generally account for 5-10% of the marrow cells, but 30% or more may be present. Blasts (including promonocytes) account for fewer than 20% of the marrow cells, and Auer rods are never seen. Dyspoiesis, including pseudo-Pelger-Huet neutrophils, hypogranularity of neutrophil cytoplasm, or megaloblastic changes in the erythroid precursors, may be noted in some cases, but most often dysplasia is minimal if present at all. Megakaryocytes are often reduced in number, but marked megakaryocytic dysplasia is unusual {186, 952, 1245, 1004, 519}.

Leukaemic infiltrates are common in the skin, where myelomonocytic cells infiltrate the superficial and deep dermis. In the lung, leukaemic cells spread from the peribronchial lymphatics into adjacent alveolar septae, and in the spleen, they infiltrate the red pulp, and have a predilection for trabecular and central arteries. In the liver, the sinusoids and the portal tracts are infiltrated {519}.

Cytochemistry / immunophenotype

No specific cytochemical or immunophenotypic abnormalities have been reported in JMML.

In extramedullary tissues, the monocytic component is best detected by immunohistochemical techniques that detect lysozyme, because myelo-peroxidase may be weakly expressed. In bone marrow aspirate smears, cytochemical stains for alpha naphthyl acetate esterase or butyrate esterase, alone or in combination with napthol ASD chloroacetate esterase, may be helpful in detection of the monocytic component. Although leukocyte alkaline phosphatase scores are reported to be decreased in about

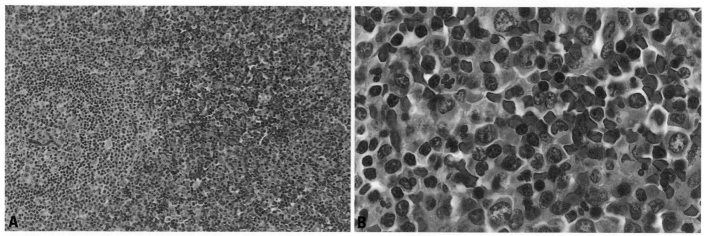

Fig. 2.12 Juvenile myelomonocytic leukaemia. **A** The leukaemic infiltrate is seen in the red pulp region of the spleen, and spares the germinal center. **B** shows that the infiltrate is comprised mainly of immature and mature neutrophils and monocytes.

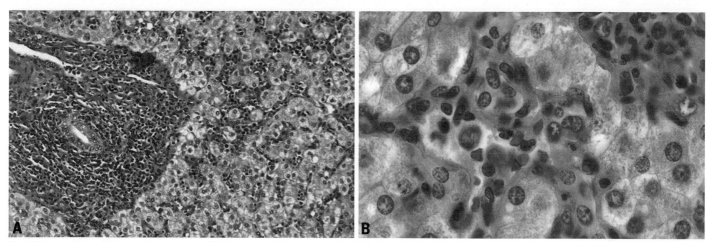

Fig. 2.13 Juvenile myelomonocytic leukaemia. The leukaemic infiltrate in the liver is in the portal regions **(A)** as well as in the hepatic sinusoids **(B)**.

50% of patients, it is not helpful in establishing the diagnosis {795}.

Genetics
There is no Philadelphia chromosome or *BCR/ABL* fusion gene. Cytogenetic abnormalities, including monosomy 7, occur in 30-40% of patients, but none are specific for JMML {186, 1245, 519, 1192}.
Point mutations of *RAS* are reported in the leukaemic cells of 20% of patients {389}. Loss of the normal *NF1* allele is common in those patients with JMML associated with NF-1, and loss of heterozygosity for *NF1* has also been reported in some patients with JMML who lack the NF-1 phenotype {1192}. This genetic alteration leads to loss of neurofibromin, a protein which is important in the regu-

lation of the RAS family of oncogenes {1192, 186}.

Postulated cell of origin
Multipotent or pluripotent bone marrow stem cell.

Prognosis and predictive factors
The course of JMML is quite variable, but overall the prognosis is poor. If untreated, approximately 30% of patients have rapid progression, and die within a year of diagnosis {795, 186, 1245}. However, some children may experience a longer course characterised by clinical improvement even without therapy. Median survival times of 5 months to more than 4 years have been reported, depending on the type of therapy chosen. The prognosis is better when the

disease appears in children less than 1 year of age, and children more than 2 years old at the time of diagnosis have a decidedly worse prognosis {795, 186, 1245}. Platelet counts <33 x 10^9/L or haemoglobin F levels >15% at the time of diagnosis are poor prognostic findings {1245}. Most children die from organ failure, such as respiratory failure due to leukaemic infiltration. Relatively few patients, perhaps 10-20%, evolve to acute leukaemia {795, 186, 952}. Although chemotherapy may benefit some patients, the overall response is usually poor, and currently, bone marrow transplant is the only therapy that has been demonstrated to clearly improve survival time {43, 795, 186, 1245}.

Myelodysplastic / myeloproliferative disease, unclassifiable

B. Bain
J.W. Vardiman
M. Imbert
R. Pierre

Definition

The designation, myelodysplastic/myeloproliferative disorder, unclassifiable (MDS/MPD, U) may be applied to cases that have clinical, laboratory and morphologic features that support a diagnosis of a myelodysplastic syndrome (MDS), as well as clinical, laboratory and morphologic features that support a diagnosis of a myeloproliferative disorder (MPD), but that do not meet the criteria for any of the other entities included in the MDS/MPD category.

These disorders are characterised by proliferation of one or more of the myeloid lineages that is ineffective, dysplastic, or both, and simultaneously, effective proliferation, with or without dysplasia, in one or more of the other myeloid lineages {945, 65, 292}. The identification of such cases can be of clinical importance because both the myelodysplastic and the myeloproliferative features may have to be considered in choice of therapy {474}.

It is important that the designation, MDS/MPD, U not be used for patients with a previous, well-defined myeloproliferative disease who develop dysplastic features in association with transformation to a more aggressive phase. Genetic studies for the Philadelphia chromosome and *BCR/ABL* fusion gene should always be done before assigning a patient to this category, because a positive result would indicate that the diagnosis is CML (most likely in an accelerated phase) and not MDS/MPD. On the other hand, MDS/MPD, U may indeed include some patients in whom the chronic phase of a CMPD was not previously detected, and who initially present in transformation with myelodysplastic features. If the underlying myeloproliferative process cannot be identified, the designation of MDS/MPD, U is appropriate.

Effects of any previous cytotoxic or growth factor therapy on an underlying, previously unrecognised myelodysplastic or myeloproliferative disorder should be considered before making a diagnosis of MDS/MPD, U. If therapy has been admin-istered recently, follow-up clinical and laboratory observations to demonstrate that the blood and marrow changes are not due to the treatment would be prudent.

ICD-O code   9975/3

Synonym

Mixed myeloproliferative/myelodysplastic syndrome, unclassifiable
"Overlap" syndrome, unclassifiable

Epidemiology

The incidence of MDS/MPD, U is unknown. Among patients meeting the criteria for the myelodysplastic syndrome, refractory anaemia with ringed sideroblasts (RARS), as many as 15% have a platelet count >500 x 10^9/l {706, 1242, 611}. If, as in this classification (see below) patients with RARS and platelet counts >600 x 10^9/L are placed in the category, MDS/MPD, U, the percentage of patients with overlapping features will be slightly lower.

Sites of involvement

The bone marrow and peripheral blood are always involved; spleen, liver, and other extramedullary tissues may be involved as well.

Clinical findings

The clinical features of MDS/MPD, U overlap those found in the MDS and MPD categories. Some patients have splenomegaly and hepatomegaly.

Aetiology

Unknown

Morphology

Laboratory features usually include anaemia, with or without macrocytosis, and dimorphic red blood cells on the peripheral smear. In addition, there is evidence of effective proliferation in one or more lineages, either as thrombocytosis (platelet count > 600 x 10^9/L) or leukocytosis (WBC count >13 x 10^9/L). Neutrophils may show dysplastic features and there may be giant or hypogranular platelets. Blasts account for fewer than 20% of the WBCs and of the nucleated cells of the bone marrow, and a finding of more than 10% likely indicates transformation to a more aggressive stage. The bone marrow biopsy specimen is hyper-

Table 2.04
Diagnostic criteria for myelodysplastic/myeloproliferative disease, unclassifiable.

- The case has clinical, laboratory and morphologic features of one of the categories of MDS (refractory anaemia, refractory anaemia with ringed sideroblasts, refractory cytopenia with multilineage dysplasia, refractory anaemia with excess of blasts), with <20% blasts in the blood and bone marrow

AND

- Has prominent myeloproliferative features, e.g., platelet count equal to or greater than 600 x 10^9/L associated with megakaryocytic proliferation, or WBC equal to or greater than 13.0 x 10^9/L, with or without prominent splenomegaly,

AND

- Has no preceding history of an underlying CMPD or of MDS, no history of recent cytotoxic or growth factor therapy that could explain the myelodysplastic or myeloproliferative features, and no Philadelphia chromosome or *BCR/ABL* fusion gene, del (5q), t(3;3)(q21;q26) or inv(3)(q21q26)

OR

- The patients has mixed myeloproliferative and myelodysplastic features and cannot be assigned to any other category of MDS, CMPD or of MDS/MPD.

cellular and may show proliferation in any or all of the myeloid lineages. However, dysplastic features are simultaneously present in at least one cell line.

Provisional entity: MDS/MPD, U - Refractory anaemia with ringed sideroblasts (RARS) associated with marked thrombocytosis.

A number of patients have been described with the clinical and morphologic features of the myelodysplastic syndrome, RARS (see chapter 3) but who also have a markedly elevated platelet count (> 600 x 10⁹/L) {474, 1242, 611}. The bone marrow specimens in these cases demonstrate that more than 15% of the erythroid precursors are ringed sideroblasts. In addition, there is megakaryocytic proliferation. The megakaryocytes are reported to have variable morphology, but are often normal or enlarged in size, and may resemble those seen in essential thrombocythemia (see chapter 1). Whether this is a distinct entity, one end of the spectrum of RARS, or the simultaneous occurrence of two separate disorders (RARS and essential thrombocythaemia) is not yet clear, so that the designation of MDS/MPD, U is appropriate until future studies indicate a more exact classification. Some patients with del (5q) may have similar findings {678}, but should be assigned to the MDS category of the "5q- syndrome" if they meet the criteria for that diagnosis {292}. Patients with MDS or AML and abnormalities of chromosome 3q21q26 may also show thrombocytosis which is associated with micromegakaryocytes {955, 183, 1168}. Such patients usually have a poor prognosis, and should be classified in the appropriate MDS category if the blast count is less than 20% in the blood or marrow, or as AML if 20% or more blasts are present.

Genetics

There is no cytogenetic or molecular genetic finding specific for this group. A Philadelphia chromosome and *BCR/ABL* fusion gene should always be excluded prior to making the diagnosis of MDS/MPD, U.

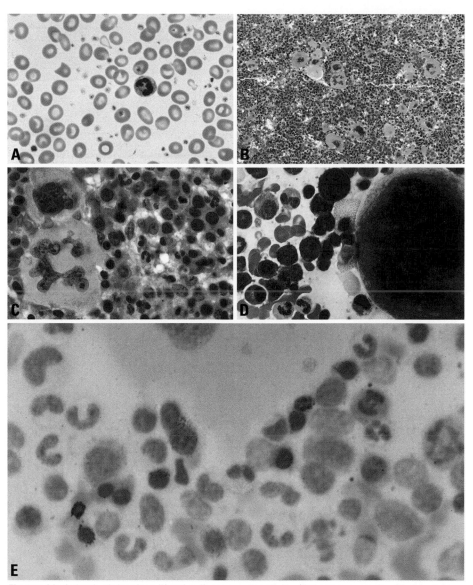

Fig. 2.14 Myelodysplastic/myeloproliferative disease, unclassifiable. (Refractory anaemia with ringed sideroblasts and marked thrombocytosis). This sequence of microphotographs illustrate blood and bone marrow changes of a 58 year old man with severe anaemia and a platelet count of 950 x 10⁹/L. **A** illustrates marked thrombocytosis in the peripheral blood and red blood cell abnormalities, including hypochromia. **B** demonstrates that the bone marrow biopsy specimen is hypercellular with marked erythroid and megakaryocytic proliferation. **C** and **D** show enlarged megakaryocytes similar to those observed in essential thrombocythemia. **E** shows nearly 30% of the erythroid precursors are ringed sideroblasts.

Postulated cell of origin

Pluripotent or multipotent haematopoietic stem cell.

Prognosis and predictive factors

Not known.

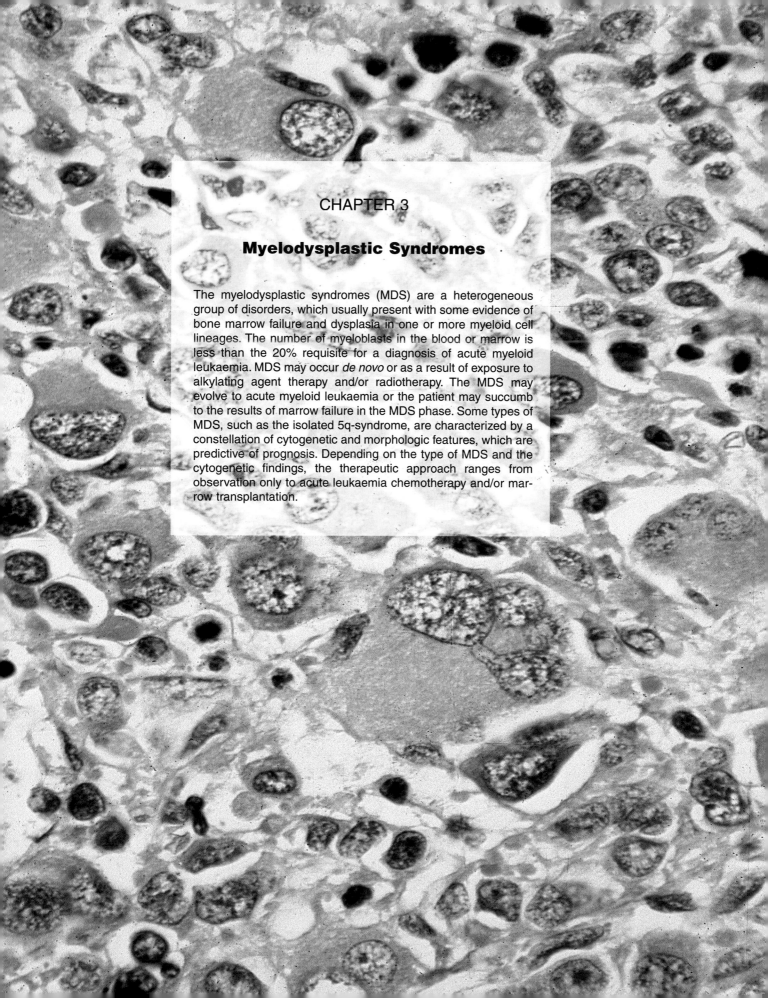

CHAPTER 3

Myelodysplastic Syndromes

The myelodysplastic syndromes (MDS) are a heterogeneous group of disorders, which usually present with some evidence of bone marrow failure and dysplasia in one or more myeloid cell lineages. The number of myeloblasts in the blood or marrow is less than the 20% requisite for a diagnosis of acute myeloid leukaemia. MDS may occur *de novo* or as a result of exposure to alkylating agent therapy and/or radiotherapy. The MDS may evolve to acute myeloid leukaemia or the patient may succumb to the results of marrow failure in the MDS phase. Some types of MDS, such as the isolated 5q-syndrome, are characterized by a constellation of cytogenetic and morphologic features, which are predictive of prognosis. Depending on the type of MDS and the cytogenetic findings, the therapeutic approach ranges from observation only to acute leukaemia chemotherapy and/or marrow transplantation.

WHO histological classification of myelodysplastic syndromes

Refractory anaemia	9980/3
Refractory anaemia with ringed sideroblasts	9982/3
Refractory cytopenia with multilineage dysplasia	9985/3
Refractory anaemia with excess blasts	9983/3
Myelodysplastic syndrome, unclassifiable	9989/3
Myelodysplastic syndrome associated with isolated del(5q) chromosome abnormality	9986/3

Myelodysplastic syndromes: Introduction

R.D. Brunning
J.M. Bennett
G. Flandrin
E. Matutes

D. Head
J.W. Vardiman
N.L. Harris

Definition

The myelodysplastic syndromes (MDS) are a group of clonal haematopoietic stem cell diseases characterised by dysplasia and ineffective haematopoiesis in one or more of the major myeloid cell lines {92, 508, 4}. The dysplasia may be accompanied by an increase in myeloblasts but the number is less than 20%, which is the requisite threshold recommended for the diagnosis of acute myeloid leukaemia. It is important to recognise that the threshold of 20% blasts in the blood or marrow for the distinction of acute leukaemia from MDS does not represent a therapeutic mandate for treating patients with $\geq$ 20% blasts as acute leukaemia. A treatment decision to manage the patient as AML or MDS must be based on several factors including age, prior history of a myelodysplastic syndrome, overall clinical findings and evolution, which are the same determinant factors for patients with $\geq$30% blasts. Although progression to acute myeloid leukaemia is the natural course in many cases of MDS, the percentage varies substantially in the various subtypes; a higher percentage of MDS with increased myeloblasts transforms to acute leukaemia. Although the majority of MDS are characterised by progressive marrow failure, the biologic course in some patients is relatively indolent.

Chronic myelomonocytic leukaemia (CMML), which heretofore has been categorised with the myelodysplastic syndromes, is frequently difficult to classify specifically as a myelodysplastic syndrome or a myeloproliferative disorder because of variability in the leukocyte count, and presence or absence of myelodysplasia. As a result, in this classification of haematopoietic tumours, chronic myelomonocytic leukaemia is placed in a new category of diseases, "myelodysplastic / myeloproliferative disorders" (see chapter 2) which includes diseases which may share features of both of these two groups of disorders.

Synonyms

Dysmyelopoietic syndromes
Preleukaemic syndromes
Oligoblastic leukaemia

Epidemiology

MDS occurs predominantly in older adults (median age: 70 years), with a non-age corrected incidence of 3/100,000 but rising to 20/100,000 over age 70 years. An increasing number of secondary MDS /

Table 3.01
Peripheral blood and bone marrow findings in myelodysplastic syndromes.

Disease	Blood findings	Bone marrow findings
Refractory anaemia (RA)	Anaemia No or rare blasts	Erythroid dysplasia only <5% blasts <15% ringed sideroblasts
Refractory anaemia with ringed sideroblasts (RARS)	Anaemia No blasts	$\geq$15% ringed sideroblasts Erythroid dysplasia only <5% blasts
Refractory cytopenia with multilineage dysplasia (RCMD)	Cytopenias (bicytopenia or pancytopenia) No or rare blasts No Auer rods <1x10^9/L monocytes	Dysplasia in $\geq$10% of the cells of two or more myeloid cell lines <5% blasts in marrow No Auer rods <15% ringed sideroblasts
Refractory cytopenia with multilineage dysplasia and ringed sideroblasts (RCMD-RS)	Cytopenias (bicytopenia or pancytopenia) No or rare blasts No Auer rods <1x10^9/L monocytes	Dysplasia in $\geq$10% of the cells in two or more myeloid cell lines $\geq$15% ringed sideroblasts <5% blasts No Auer rods
Refractory anaemia with excess blasts –1 (RAEB-1)	Cytopenias <5% blasts No Auer rods <1x10^9/L monocytes	Unilineage or multilineage dysplasia 5-9% blasts No Auer rods
Refractory anaemia with excess blasts –2 (RAEB-2)	Cytopenias 5-19% blasts Auer rods ± <1x10^9/L monocytes	Unilineage or multilineage dysplasia 10%-19% blasts Auer rods ±
Myelodysplastic syndrome – unclassified (MDS-U)	Cytopenias No or rare blasts No Auer rods	Unilineage dysplasia: one myeloid cell line <5% blasts No Auer Rods
MDS associated with isolated del(5q)	Anaemia Usually normal or increased platelet count <5% blasts	Normal to increased megakaryocytes with hypolobated nuclei <5% blasts Isolated del(5q) cytogenetic abnormality No Auer rods

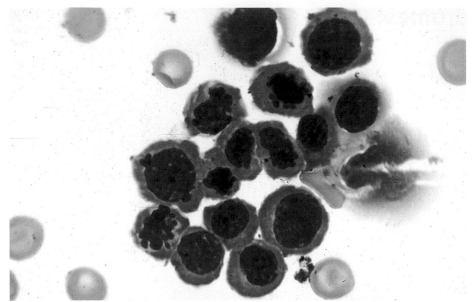

Fig. 3.01 Arsenic intoxication. Bone marrow smear from a 47 year-old male with pancytopenia and obtunded mental status being chronically poisoned with arsenic by his wife. There is marked dyserythropoiesis. The patient received Dimercaprol and rapidly recovered.

AML have been recognised as a result of chemotherapy/radiation therapy for other malignant disorders. The incidence is not known but may represent as many as 10-15% of all the AML's and MDS's diagnosed each year {56, 1393}.

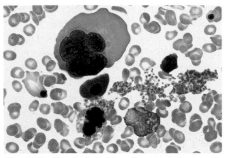

Fig. 3.02 Congenital dyserythropoietic anaemia. Marked dyserythropoiesis in a marrow smear from a patient with congenital dyserythropoiesis, type III.

Fig. 3.03 Parvovirus B19 infection. Bone marrow smear from a patient with parvovirus B19 infection showing marked erythroid hypoplasia with occasional giant erythroblasts with dispersed chromatin and fine cytoplasmic vacuoles.

Clinical features
The majority of patients present with symptoms related to cytopenia(s), most frequently anaemia, and less commonly neutropenia and/or thrombocytopenia. Organomegaly is infrequently observed.

Aetiology
The MDS occur as primary or *de novo* disorders and as therapy-related diseases. The primary *(de novo)* myelodysplastic syndromes occur without a known history of toxic exposure. The therapy related MDS occur in patients who have a known history of exposure to chemotherapeutic agents and/or radiation therapy; the chemotherapeutic agents are usually alkylating agent type.

In "*de novo*" MDS possible aetiologies include viruses and benzene exposure. Benzene exposure has been implicated in the aetiology of both AML and MDS in exposed petrochemical employees at levels well above the minimal requirements allowed by most government agencies. Cigarette smoking increases the risk by about two-fold. Some inherited haematological disorders, such as Fanconi's anaemia, are also associated with an increased incidence of MDS.

Morphology
The morphological classification of the myelodysplastic syndromes is principally based on the percent of blasts in the marrow and blood, the type and degree of dysplasia and the presence of ringed sideroblasts {92}. In determining the blast percentage in the marrow, a 500 cell differential should be performed and in the blood, a 200 leukocyte differential. The characteristics of the dysplasia are relevant when distinguishing between the various types of MDS and may be important in predicting biology. In addition, some cytogenetic abnormalities are associated with characteristic morphologic findings, e.g. isolated del(5q) and hypolobated megakaryocytes and del(17p) with hypolobated neutrophils.

A major problem in the differential diagnosis and classification of the myelodysplastic syndromes is the determination whether the presence of myelodysplasia is due to a clonal disorder or is the result of some other factor. The presence of dysplasia is not in itself evidence of a clonal disorder. There are several nutritional and toxic factors which may cause myelodysplastic changes including vitamin B12 and folic acid deficiency, and exposure to heavy metals, particularly arsenic {1381}. Congenital haematological disorders such as congenital dyserythropoietic anaemia must also be considered as a cause of dysplasia when it is confined to the erythroid cells {154}. Parvovirus B19 infection may cause erythroblastopenia with giant megaloblastoid erythroblasts. Chemotherapeutical agents may result in marked dysplasia. Granulocyte colony stimulating factor may cause marked dysplasia of the neutrophil series with marked hypergranularity, Dohle bodies and striking nuclear hypolobulation. Blasts may be observed in the blood and may reach levels of 9-10% {1161}. As a result it is extremely important to be aware of the clinical history and consider non-clonal disorders as possible aetiologies when evaluating cases with myelodysplasia, particularly those cases with no increase in blasts. Paroxysmal nocturnal haemoglobinuria may present with features similar to a myelodysplastic syndrome.

In an attempt to more accurately predict clinical behaviour, cases of MDS without an increase in blasts are recognised as manifesting either unilineage or multilineage dysplasia. In refractory anaemia and refractory anaemia with ringed sideroblasts with unilineage dysplasia the dysplasia is confined to the erythroid lineage. Unilineage dysplasia may also occur in the granulocytes and megakaryocytes but these processes are less frequent than unilineage dysplasia involving the erythroid cells, and such cases may be categorized as MDS, unclassifiable. In refractory cytopenia with multilineage dysplasia and refractory cytopenia with multilineage dysplasia and ringed sideroblasts, "significant" dysplastic features are recognised in two or more of the major myeloid cell lineages. The recommended requisite percentage of cells manifesting dysplasia to qualify as "significant" is ten percent {433}. This admittedly is an arbitrary threshold and will result in some cases being misclassified. Future studies may result in this number being adjusted.

Assessment of the degree of dysplasia may be problematic depending on the quality of the smear preparations and the stain. Poor quality smears may result in misinterpretation of the presence or absence of dysplasia. Because of the critical importance of recognition of dysplasia to the diagnosis of an MDS, the necessity of high quality slide preparation cannot be overemphasised. Slides for the assessment of dysplasia should be made from freshly obtained specimens; specimens exposed to anticoagulants for more than two hours are unsatisfactory.

Dyserythropoiesis is manifested principally by alterations in the nucleus including budding, internuclear bridging, and karyorrhexis, multinuclearity, and megaloblas-

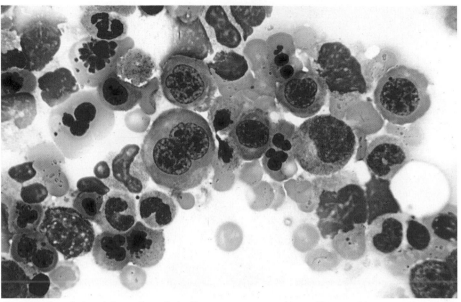

Fig. 3.04 Drug induced dyserythropoiesis. Bone marrow smear from a 57 year-old woman who shortly before this bone marrow examination received several chemotherapeutic agents for breast carcinoma including folic acid antagonists. The cytogenetics were normal and the megaloblastic changes were no longer present three weeks following this biopsy.

toid changes; cytoplasmic features include ring sideroblasts, vacuolisation, and periodic acid-Schiff positivity, either diffuse or granular. Dysgranulopoiesis is characterised primarily by small size, nuclear hypolobation (pseudo Pelger-Huet), and hypersegmentation, hypogranularity and pseudo Chediak-Higashi granules {433}. Megakaryocyte dysplasia may be characterised by hypolobulated micromegakaryocyte, non-lobulated nuclei in megakaryocytes of all sizes, and multiple, widely-separated nuclei.

The characteristics of the dysplasia may be relevant in predicting biology of a myelodysplastic disorder and the relationship to specific cytogenetic abnormalities. Unilineage dysplasia involving the erythroid cells is commonly observed in refractory anaemia and ringed sideroblastic anaemia. Multilineage dysplasia involving two or three of the myeloid cell lines is more frequently observed in the high-grade myelodysplastic syndromes and is used to distinguish refractory cytopenia with multilineage dysplasia from refractory anaemia {1110}. Similarly, the presence of multilineage dysplasia is used to separate refractory anaemia with ringed sideroblasts into two categories,

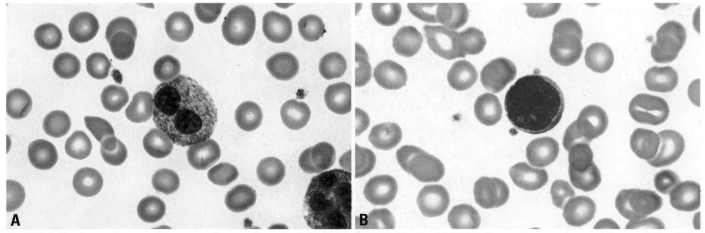

Fig. 3.05 A Blood smear from a patient on granulocyte colony stimulating factor. A neutrophil with a bilobed nucleus and increased azurophilic granulation. **B** The same specimen as A showing a myeloblast.

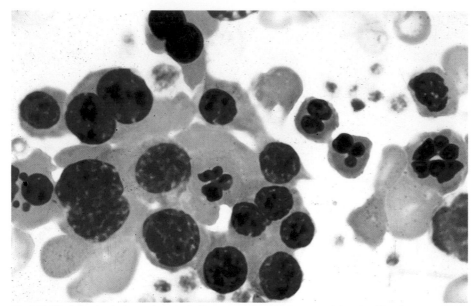

Fig. 3.06 Myelodysplastic dyserythropoiesis. Bone marrow smear from an adult male with refractory cytopenia with multilineage dysplasia (RCMD) and complex cytogenetic abnormalities including del(17p) and del(5q).

refractory anaemia with ringed sideroblasts with unilineage dysplasia (RARS) and refractory cytopenia with multilineage dysplasia with ringed sideroblasts (RCMD-RS). An increased number of ringed sideroblasts, occasionally >15% of the erythroid precursors, may be observed in other types of myelodysplastic syndromes, including RAEB. If the defining criteria for these forms of MDS are present, they dictate the classification.

The marrow is usually hypercellular or normocellular; the cytopenias result from ineffective haematopoiesis. A minority of the cases have a hypocellular marrow.

The presence of small clusters or aggregates of myeloblasts and promyelocytes (5-8 cells) in marrow trephine biopsies localised in the central portion of the marrow away from the vascular structures and endosteal surface of the bone trabeculae in the MDS is referred to as abnormal localisation of immature precursors (ALIP) {154, 84}. The presence of three or more of these foci in a section is considered as ALIP positive, and is frequently present in cases of RAEB. The occurrence of ALIP in the other MDS subtypes has been reported to be associated with a more rapid evolution to acute leukaemia. If increased ALIP is noted in a case of RA, RARS with unilineage dysplasia, or RCMD, the peripheral blood and bone marrow aspirate smears should be carefully re-evaluated to exclude a higher-grade lesion. The presence of ALIP should be noted in the histopathology report.

Genetics

Cytogenetic and molecular studies have a major role in the evaluation of patients with myelodysplastic syndromes in regard to prognosis, the recognition of morphological cytogenetical correlates, and determination of clonality {451, 4, 1394}. The *de novo* "5q- syndrome," which occurs primarily in women, is characterised by megakaryocytes with hypolobated nuclei, refractory macrocytic anaemia, normal or increased platelet count, a favourable clinical course and an isolated del(5q) chromosome abnormality, and is recognised as a specific type of MDS in this classification. The occurrence of a del(17p) deletion is associated with MDS or AML with pseudo Pelger-Huet anomaly, small vacuolated neutrophils, *TP53* mutation and unfavourable clinical course; it is most common in therapy related MDS {595, 719}. Complex cytogenetical abnormalities, usually including chromosomes 5 and/or 7, are generally associated with an unfavourable clinical course. Several other cytogenetic findings appear to be associated with characteristic morphologic abnormalities such as isolated del(20q) with involvement of erythroid cells and megakaryocytes and abnormalities of chromosome 3, which are associated with MDS and AML with increased abnormal megakaryocytes. New cytogenetic, morphological, clinical correlations are anticipated.

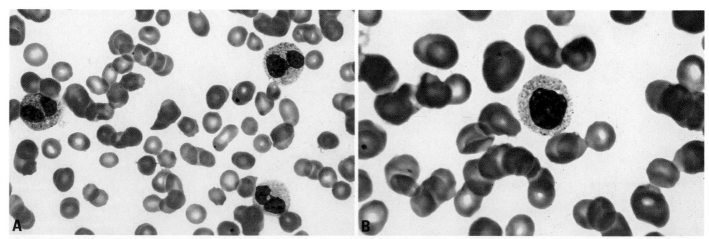

Fig. 3.07 A Dysgranulopoiesis. Blood smear. This blood smear from a patient with refractory cytopenia with multilineage dysplasia (RCMD) and a complex karyotype including del(17p) shows three neutrophils with bilobed nuclei. **B** Higher magnification of the same smear showing a neutrophil with a non-lobulated nucleus.

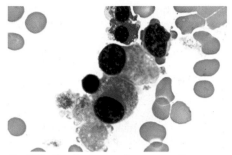

Fig. 3.08 Dysplastic megakaryocytes. Bone marrow section from a 37 year-old male with pancytopenia showing a markedly hypercellular marrow with markedly increased megakaryocytes, many with dysplastic features.

Postulated cell of origin
Haematopoietic stem cell.

Prognosis and predictive factors
The morphological subtypes of the myelodysplastic syndromes can be generally categorised into two risk groups based on duration of survival and incidence of evolution to acute leukaemia. The low risk groups are refractory anaemia (RA) and refractory anaemia with ringed sideroblasts (RARS). The high-risk groups are refractory anaemia with excess blasts (RAEB) and refractory cytopenia with multilineage dysplasia with or without ringed sideroblasts.

The importance of cytogenetic studies as a prognostic indicator in MDS has been recognised and codified by an international study group {451}. Three major risk categories of cytogenetic findings have

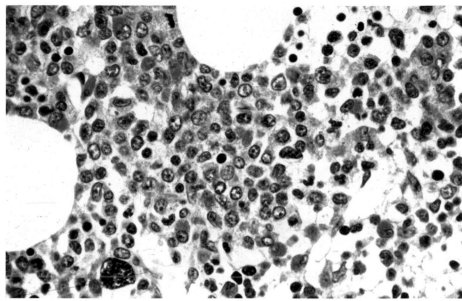

Fig. 3.09 Abnormal localisation of immature precursors. Bone marrow section. This section from a case of RAEB-1 contains a focus of immature myeloid precursors.

been defined: i) good risk - normal cytogenetics, isolated del(5q), isolated del (20q), and -Y; ii) poor risk – complex abnormalities, i.e. >3 recurring abnormalities, or abnormalities of chromosome 7; and iii) intermediate risk - all other abnormalities.

A scoring system for predicting survival and evolution to acute leukaemia based on percent marrow blasts, type of cytogenetic abnormalities, and degree and number of cytopenias has been proposed by the International Myelo-dysplastic Syndrome Working Group {451}.

Four risk groups based on this scoring system are recognised: low 0; INT (intermediate)-1, 0.5-1.0; INT-2, 1.5-2.0; and high, ≥2.5. In general, the higher risk groups are related to higher marrow blast percentage, more unfavourable cytogenetic findings and more severe degree of cytopenia.

Consideration of age improves predictability of survival; patients younger than 60 years of age have improved survival in the individual risk categories compared to patients older than 60 years.

Table 3.02
International prognostic scoring system for MDS {451}.

Score	0	0.5	1.0	1.5	2.0
Prognostic variables					
% blasts	<5	5-10	–	11-20	20-30*
Karyotype**	Good	Intermediate	Poor		
Cytopenias***	0-1	2-3			

*This group is recognized as AML in this propsed classification
**Karyotype: Good = normal, -Y, del(5q), del(20q);
       Poor = complex (≥3 abnormalities) or chromosome 7 anomalies;
       intermediate = other abnormalities
***Cytopenias = Hb <10 gm/dL
       Neutrophils <1500/µL
       Platelets <100k/µL

Refractory anaemia

R.D. Brunning
J.M. Bennett
G. Flandrin
E. Matutes

D. Head
J.W. Vardiman
N.L. Harris

Definition
Refractory anaemia (RA) is a myelodysplastic syndrome characterised mainly by unilineage dysplasia affecting the erythroid series. Ineffective dyserythropoiesis leads to anaemia refractory to haematinic therapy. The degree of dysplasia varies and may be minimal, but the detection of unequivocal dyserythropoiesis is essential. All other aetiological possibilities for the erythroid abnormalities must be excluded, including drug and toxin exposure, viral illness, immunologic disorders, congenital abnormalities, and vitamin deficiencies. If a clonal cytogenetic abnormality is not present, there should be a period of observation of six months and reevaluation, before a definitive diagnosis of RA is established. Myeloblasts are <1% in the blood and account for less than 5% of marrow cells. The process should be reclassified in the appropriate classification if evidence of dysplasia in other myeloid cell lines evolves or if the blasts increase in number.

ICD-O code   9980/3

Synonyms
Aregenerative anaemia

Epidemiology
Refractory anaemia is uncommon, comprising approximately 5-10% of all cases of MDS. It is primarily a disease of older adults.

Sites of involvement
The blood and bone marrow are the principal sites of involvement.

Clinical features
The presenting symptoms are related to anaemia, which is refractory to haematinic therapy.

Aetiology
Unknown.

Morphology
In the peripheral blood, the red blood cells are usually normochromic, and normocytic or normochromic and macrocytic. Unusually, cases have a hypochromic population of red blood cells. The anisocytosis and poikilocytosis vary from none to marked abnormalities. Blasts are rarely seen, and if present account for <1% of the white blood cells. The neutrophils and platelets are usually normal in number and morphology. The erythroid precursors in the marrow vary from decreased to markedly increased; dys-erythropoiesis varies from slight to moderate. Dyserythropoiesis is manifested principally by alterations in the nucleus including budding, internuclear bridging, and karyorrhexis, multinuclearity, and megaloblastoid changes; cytoplasmic features include vacuolisation and periodic acid-Schiff positivity, either diffuse or granular {612}.
Ringed sideroblasts may be present but are less than 15% of erythroid precursors. Myeloblasts account for <5% of the marrow cells. Auer rods are not seen. The neutrophils and megakaryocytes are normal or may show minimal dysplasia. The bone marrow biopsy is generally hypercellular due to erythroid hyperplasia, but may be normocellular or even hypocellular.

Immunophenotype
Immunophenotyping is not relevant in the diagnosis of refractory anaemia.

Genetics
Cytogenetic abnormalities may be observed in up to 25% of cases. Several different acquired clonal chromosomal abnormalities may be identified, and although useful for establishing a diagnosis of RA, they are not specific. The abnormalities generally associated with myelodysplastic syndromes include del(20q), +8, and abnormalities of 5 and/or 7.

Postulated cell of origin
Bone marrow stem cell.

Prognosis and predictive factors
The clinical course is protracted; the median survival of RA is approximately 66 months and the rate of progression to acute leukaemia is approximately 6% {433}.

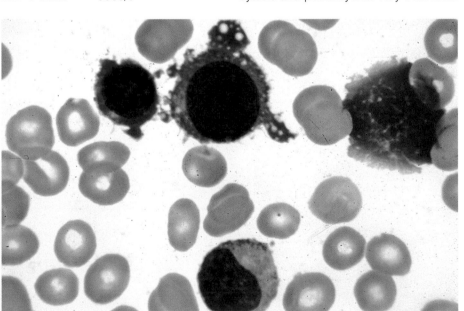

Fig. 3.10 Myelodysplastic syndrome; refractory anemia. Bone marrow smear. This specimen showed dysplastic features only in the erythroid precursors; occasional erythroblasts showed vacuolated cytoplasm and slightly megaloblastoid nuclei.

Refractory anaemia with ringed sideroblasts

R.D. Brunning
J.M. Bennett
G. Flandrin
E. Matutes

D. Head
J.W. Vardiman
N.L. Harris

Definition

Refractory anaemia with ringed sideroblasts (RARS) is a myelodysplastic syndrome characterised by an anaemia in which 15% or more of the erythroid precursors in the marrow smears are ringed sideroblasts. The ringed sideroblast is defined as an erythroid precursor in which one third or more of the nucleus is encircled by ten or more siderotic granules as demonstrated in an iron stained smear. Myeloblasts are less than 5% in the marrow and are not present in the blood. Secondary causes of ringed sideroblasts, such as anti-tuberculosis drugs and alcoholism, must be excluded.

ICD-O code   9982/3

Synonyms

Pure sideroblastic anaemia
Acquired idiopathic sideroblastic anaemia
Sideroblastic anaemia

Epidemiology

RARS accounts for approximately 10-12% of cases of MDS. It occurs primarily in older individuals, and more frequently in males than females.

Sites of involvement

The blood and bone marrow are the principal sites of involvement. The liver and spleen may show evidence of iron overload.

Clinical features

The presenting symptoms are related to anaemia, which is usually of moderate degree. There may be symptoms related to progressive iron overload. Uncommonly, patients present with the findings of sideroblastic anaemia and marked thrombocytosis. This combination of findings is discussed in the section on myelodysplastic/myeloproliferative diseases.

Aetiology

Unknown.

Morphology

The red cells in the blood smear may manifest anisochromasia (dimorphic pattern) with a major population of normochromic red blood cells and a minor population of hypochromic cells; some cases present with normochromic macrocytic or normocytic anaemia. Blasts are not present in the blood.

The bone marrow shows erythroid hyperplasia. Fifteen percent or more of the red cell precursors are ringed sideroblasts, as defined by 10 or more iron granules encircling one third or more of the nucleus in an iron-stained smear. Dysplasia is restricted to the erythroid lineage; in addition to the 15% ringed sideroblasts, there may be other evidence of dyserythropoiesis, including nuclear lobation and megaloblastoid features. The bone marrow biopsy is normocellular to markedly hypercellular, usually with marked erythroid hyperplasia. Myeloblasts number fewer than 5% of the marrow cells. Neutrophils and megakaryocytes are normal in number and they show no evidence of dysplasia. Hemosiderin-laden macrophages are often abundant.

An increased number of ringed sideroblasts, occasionally >15%, may be observed in other types of myelodysplastic syndromes, including RAEB. If the defining criteria for these forms of MDS are present, they dictate the classification.

Immunophenotype

Not relevant.

Genetics

Clonal chromosomal abnormalities are seen in fewer than 10% of cases of RARS. If a clonal cytogenetic abnormality develops in the course of the disease, the case should be re-evaluated and appropriately reclassified if evidence of another form of MDS or AML develops.

Postulated cell of origin

Bone marrow stem cell.

Prognosis and predictive factors

Approximately 1-2% of cases of RARS with unilineage dysplasia evolve to acute myeloid leukaemia. The overall median survival is approximately 6 years {433}.

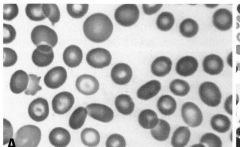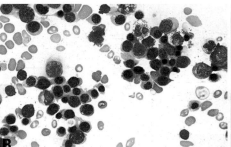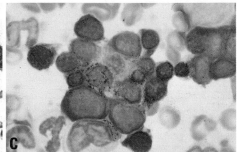

Fig. 3.11 Refractory anaemia with ringed sideroblasts; unilineage dysplasia. **A** Blood smear with dimorphic red blood cells and macrocytes (Wright-Giemsa). **B** Bone marrow smear from the case illustrated in A showing marked erythroid hyperplasia (Wright-Giemsa). **C** Iron stain of bone marrow smear from case illustrated in A and B showing numerous ringed sideroblasts.

Refractory cytopenia with multilineage dysplasia

R.D. Brunning
J.M. Bennett
G. Flandrin
E. Matutes
D. Head
J.W. Vardiman
N.L. Harris

Definition
Refractory cytopenia with multilineage dysplasia (RCMD) is a myelodysplastic syndrome with bi-cytopenia or pancytopenia, and dysplastic changes in 10% or more of the cells in two or more of the myeloid cell lines. There are less than 1% blasts in the blood and less than 5% in the marrow. Auer rods are not present and the monocytes in the blood are less than 1×10^9/L.

ICD-O code   9985/3

Synonym
Myelodysplastic syndrome, unclassified

Epidemiology
Occurs in older individuals. Refractory cytopenia with multilineage dysplasia accounts for approximately 24% of cases of MDS {433}. RCMD-RS accounts for approximately 15% of cases of MDS.

Clinical features
Most patients present with evidence of bone marrow failure, with cytopenia in two or more myeloid lineages.

Morphology
Dysplastic changes are present in ≥10% of the cells in two or more myeloid cell lines; the dysplasia may be marked {1110}. Neutrophils may manifest hypogranulation and/or nuclear hyposegmentation (pseudo Pelger-Huet nuclei). Myeloblasts account for fewer than 5% of the marrow cells. In some cases there is marked erythroid hyperplasia. Erythroid precursors may show cytoplasmic vacuoles and marked nuclear irregularity including multilobation, multinucleation and megaloblastoid nuclei. Erythroid precursors may be periodic acid-Schiff positive. In RCMD, ringed sideroblasts may be identified, but are less than 15% of nucleated red blood cells. If ringed sideroblasts are more than 15% of the erythroid precursors, the case should be classified as the subtype, Refractory cytopenia with multilineage dysplasia and ringed sideroblasts (RCMD-RS). Megakaryocyte abnormalities which may be observed include hypolobulated nuclei and/or micromegakaryocytes.

Immunophenotype
Not relevant.

Genetics
Clonal chromosome abnormalities including trisomy 8, monosomy 7, del(7q), monosomy 5, del(5q), and del(20q), as well as complex karyotypes, may be found in up to 50% of patients with RCMD and RCMD-RS.

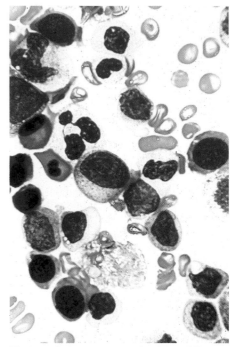

Fig. 3.12 Refractory cytopenia with multilineage dysplasia. Bone marrow smear. This bone marrow specimen from a patient with a therapy related myelodysplastic syndrome shows evidence of dysplasia in both the erythroid precursors and the neutrophils. The mature neutrophils are small and have hypolobulated nuclei. Cytogenetic studies showed a very complex karyotype including del(5q)(q13q33) and del(17p).

Postulated cell of origin
Bone marrow myeloid stem cell.

Prognosis and predictive factors
The clinical course varies. Prognostic factors relate to the degree of cytopenia and dysplasia. The frequency of acute leukaemia evolution is approximately 11% {433}. The overall median survival is approximately 33 months. RCMD and RCMD-RS have similar survivals. Patients with complex karyotypes have survivals similar to patients with refractory anaemia with excess of blasts (RAEB).

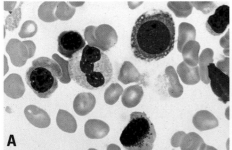
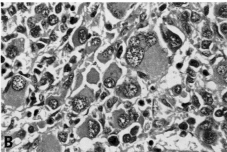

Fig. 3.13 Myelodysplastic syndrome: refractory cytopenia with multilineage dysplasia and complex cytogenetic abnormalities. **A** Bone marrow smear from a 37 year-old male with pancytopenia. This smear shows erythroid precursors with megaloblastoid nuclei and a red cell precursor with the nucleus encircled by Pappenheimer bodies (iron granules); ringed sideroblasts were present in an iron stained smear. **B** Bone marrow section from the specimen in A. Megakaryocytes are markedly increased and many have dysplastic features.

Refractory anaemia with excess blasts

R.D. Brunning
J.M. Bennett
G. Flandrin
E. Matutes

D. Head
J.W. Vardiman
N.L. Harris

Definition

Refractory anaemia with excess blasts (RAEB) is a myelodysplastic syndrome with 5-19% myeloblasts in the bone marrow. Because of a well documented difference in survival and incidence of evolution to acute myeloid leukaemia between patients with RAEB with bone marrow blast percentage of 5-10%, and those with 10-20% blasts, two categories of RAEB are recognised: RAEB-1, defined by 5-9% blasts in the bone marrow and <5% blasts in the blood, and RAEB-2, defined by 10-19% blasts in the bone marrow {451}. Patients with 5-19% blasts in the blood and <10% blasts in the bone marrow are also placed in the RAEB-2 group. The significance of the detection of Auer rods with a blast percentage less than 20% in the bone marrow or blood is not completely clear; it is recommended that cases of RAEB with Auer rods be classified as RAEB-2.

ICD-O code   9983/3

Synonyms
None

Epidemiology
This disease affects primarily individuals over 50 years of age. It accounts for approximately 40% of all patient with MDS.

Clinical features
Most patients initially present with symptoms related to bone marrow failure, including anaemia and/or thrombocytopenia and/or neutropenia.

Morphology
The blood smear frequently shows abnormalities in all three myeloid cell lines: anisopoikilocytosis with macrocytes, atypical platelets, hypogranulation and nuclear hyposegmentation (pseudo Pelger-Huet nuclei) in neutrophils. In the blood myeloblasts range from 0–19%. In the marrow, blasts range from 5-19% of the cells, and there is usually neutrophil hyperplasia with variable degrees of dysplasia. Dysgranulopoiesis is characterised primarily by small size, nuclear hypolobation (pseudo Pelger-Huet), and hypersegmentation, cytoplasmic hypo-granularity and pseudo Chediak-Higashi granules {433}. Erythroid precursors may show dyserythropoiesis including abnormally lobulated nuclei, multinucleated cells, and megaloblastoid nuclei; mega-karyocyte dysplasia may be characterised by hypolobulated micromegakaryocytes, non-lobulated nuclei in megakaryocytes of all sizes and multiple widely-separated nuclei.

The bone marrow biopsy is hypercellular in the majority of cases; a minority of cases are normocellular or hypocellular. Foci of immature neutrophils and blasts unrelated to bone trabeculae and vascular structures, referred to as abnormal localisation of immature precursors (ALIP), may be present. The marrow biopsy is hypocellular in approximately 10-15% of patients.

Genetics
A variable percentage of cases (30%-50%) have clonal cytogenetic abnormalities including +8, -5, del(5q), -7, del(7q), and del(20q). Complex karyotypes may also be observed.

Postulated cell of origin
Bone marrow myeloid stem cell.

Immunophenotype
The blasts express one or more myeloid antigens, including CD13, CD33 and CD117.

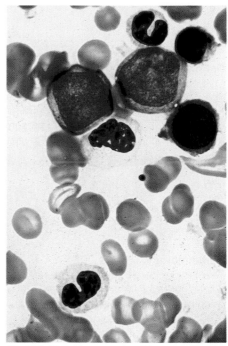

Fig. 3.14 Refractory anemia with excess blasts-1 (RAEB-1). Bone marrow smear. The mature neutrophils in this case show nuclear hypolobulation (pseudo Pelger-Huet nuclei) and cytoplasmic hypogranularity.

Prognosis and predictive factors
Refractory anaemia with excess blasts is usually marked by progressive marrow failure with increasing cytopenias. Approximately 25% of cases of RAEB-1 and 33% of patient's with RAEB-2 progress to a frank acute myeloid leukaemia; the remainder succumb to the effects of marrow failure. The median survival is approximately 18 months for RAEB-1 and 10 months for RAEB-2 {433}.

Myelodysplastic syndrome, unclassifiable

R.D. Brunning
J.M. Bennett
G. Flandrin
E. Matutes

D. Head
J.W. Vardiman
N.L. Harris

Definition
Myelodysplastic syndrome, unclassifiable (MDS-U) is a myelodysplastic syndrome which lacks findings appropriate for classification as RA, RARS, RCMD, RAEB. The blasts in the blood and bone marrow are not increased.

ICD-O code   9989/3

Synonyms
None

Epidemiology
The incidence of myelodysplastic syndrome, unclassifiable, is unknown. It is principally a disease of older individuals but occasional cases may occur in younger individuals, including children. A history of exposure to cytotoxic or radiation therapy may be present.

Clinical features
Patients present with symptoms similar to those seen in the other myelodysplastic syndromes.

Morphology
There are no specific morphological findings. There is a neutropenia or thrombocytopenia. Dysplasia is restricted to either the neutrophil or megakaryocytic cell lines and may be marked.
The bone marrow biopsy is usually hypercellular but may be normocellular and less commonly hypocellular. Dysplastic megakaryocytes may be prominent.

Genetics
There are no specific cytogenetic findings. Chromosome studies may be normal, or clonal cytogenetic findings similar to those in the other subtypes of MDS may be present.

Postulated cell of origin
Myeloid stem cell.

Immunophenotype
Not relevant

Prognosis and predictive factors
The survival or percent of cases evolving to acute leukaemia or higher grade myelodysplastic syndrome are unknown. If defining characteristics of a specific form of myelodysplastic syndrome develop, the process should be reclassified.

Myelodysplastic syndrome associated with isolated del(5q) chromosome abnormality ("5q- syndrome")

R.D. Brunning
J.M. Bennett
G. Flandrin
E. Matutes

D. Head
J.W. Vardiman
N.L. Harris

Definition
A myelodysplastic syndrome associated with an isolated del(5q) cytogenetic abnormality. The number of blasts in the bone marrow and blood is <5% {127, 829}.

ICD-O code
9986/3

Synonyms
None

Epidemiology
The "5q-syndrome" occurs predominantly but not exclusively in middle age to older women.

Clinical features
The most common symptoms are usually related to refractory anaemia, which is often severe. Occasional patients may have significantly elevated platelet counts.

Morphology
There is usually marked macrocytic anaemia. There may be slight leukopenia. The platelet count is generally normal to elevated. Occasional blasts (but always <5%) may be observed in the blood. The marrow is usually hypercellular or normocellular with normal to increased megakaryocytes, many of which may have hypolobated nuclei. The number of blasts in the marrow is <5% {127}. Dysplastic features of variable degree are present in the erythroid precursors.
The marrow biopsy usually shows a hypercellular marrow. The megakaryocytes are usually normal to increased in number and normal to slightly decreased in size; many megakaryocytes have hypolobated nuclei. There frequently are scattered aggregates of small lymphocytes.

Genetics
The sole cytogenetic abnormality involves a deletion between bands q31 and 33 on chromosome 5; the size of the deletion and the break points are variable. If any additional cytogenic abnormality is present, the case should not be placed in this category.

Postulated cell of origin
Bone marrow stem cell.

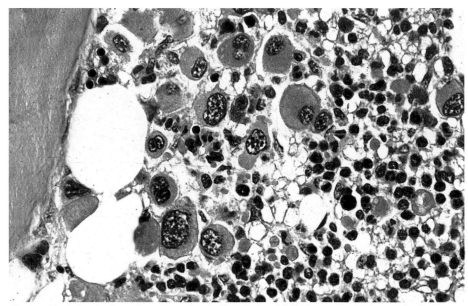

Fig. 3.15 Myelodysplastic syndrome associated with an isolated del(5q) cytogenetic abnormality. Bone marrow section. Numerous megakaryocytes of various size are present. Several have hypolobulated nuclei.

Prognosis and predictive factors
These findings are associated with long survival. Karyotypic evolution is uncommon. Additional cytogenetic abnormalities are usually associated with evolution to acute myeloid leukaemia or a higher grade myelodysplastic process. The significance of more than 5% marrow blasts in a patient with an isolated del(5q) is not clear, although some reports indicate they have a worse prognosis than those with less than 5% blasts {127, 829}.

CHAPTER 4

Acute Myeloid Leukaemias

There is increasing recognition of the importance of genetic events in the classification and therapy of the acute myeloid leukaemias. As a result, the WHO classification of the acute myeloid leukaemias incorporates and interrelates morphology, cytogenetics, molecular genetics and immunologic markers in an attempt to structure a classification that is universally applicable and prognostically relevant. The prognostic importance of genetic events is most clearly demonstrated in the acute myeloid leukaemias characterised by recurrent chromosome translocations: t(15;17)(q22;q12); t(8;21)q22;q22) and inv 16(p13q22) which generally have a favourable prognosis when treated with appropriate therapeutic agents. In contrast, leukaemias with complex karyotypes, partial deletions or loss of chromosome 5 and/or 7 are frequently characterised by multi-lineage dysplasia, a high incidence of multi-drug resistant glycoprotein positivity and an unfavourable response to therapy. It is anticipated that advances in molecular technology will reveal additional markers that will result in more effective and less toxic therapeutic regimens.

WHO histological classification of acute myeloid leukaemias

Acute myeloid leukaemia with recurrent genetic abnormalities

Acute myeloid leukaemia with t(8;21)(q22;q22); *(AML1(CBFa)/ETO)*	9896/3
Acute myeloid leukaemia with abnormal bone marrow eosinophils inv(16)(p13q22) or t(16;16)(p13;q22); *(CBFb/MYH11)*	9871/3
Acute promyelocytic leukaemia (AML with t(15;17)(q22;q12) *(PML/RARa)* and variants	9866/3
Acute myeloid leukaemia with 11q23 (*MLL*) abnormalities	9897/3

Acute myeloid leukaemia with multilineage dysplasia	9895/3
Acute myeloid leukaemia and myelodysplastic syndromes, therapy-related	9920/3

Acute myeloid leukaemia not otherwise categorised

Acute myeloid leukaemia minimally differentiated	9872/3
Acute myeloid leukaemia without maturation	9873/3
Acute myeloid leukaemia with maturation	9874/3
Acute myelomonocytic leukaemia	9867/3
Acute monoblastic and monocytic leukaemia	9891/3
Acute erythroid leukaemias	9840/3
Acute megakaryoblastic leukaemia	9910/3
Acute basophilic leukaemia	9870/3
Acute panmyelosis with myelofibrosis	9931/3
Myeloid sarcoma	9930/3

Acute leukaemia of ambiguous lineage	9805/3
Undifferentiated acute leukaemia	9801/3
Bilineal acute leukaemia	9805/3
Biphenotypic acute leukaemia	9805/3

Acute myeloid leukaemia: Introduction

R.D. Brunning
E. Matutes
N.L. Harris
G. Flandrin

J. Vardiman
J. Bennett
D. Head

Definition

Acute myeloid leukaemia (AML) is a clonal expansion of myeloid blasts in bone marrow, blood or other tissue.

ICD-O code   9861/3

Rationale for classification

The WHO classification of the acute leukaemias incorporates morphologic, immunophenotypic, genetic, and clinical features in an attempt to define entities that are biologically homogenous and that have clinical relevance. The acute leukaemias are classified as myeloid or lymphoid based on the lineage of the blast cells.

The classification of the acute myeloid leukaemias (AML) encompasses four major categories:

(1) Acute myeloid leukaemia with recurrent genetic abnormalities
(2) Acute myeloid leukaemia with multilineage dysplasia
(3) Acute myeloid leukaemia, therapy related
(4) Acute myeloid leukaemia not otherwise categorised.

The first three categories recognise the importance of several factors in predicting the biology of the leukaemic process. Some cytogenetic profiles that reflect specific molecular events are highly correlated with response to therapy and survival {114, 461, 1060, 1200}. Acute myeloid leukaemia associated with certain recurrent translocations such as t(8;21)(q22;q22) and inv(16)(p13q22) or t(16;16)(p13;q22) occur predominantly in younger individuals and generally are accompanied by a relatively favourable response to therapy and clinical behaviour. In contrast, acute myeloid leukaemia with multilineage dysplasia occurs most frequently in older individuals, is often associated with an unfavourable cytogenetic profile, e.g. –7/del(7q), –5/del(5q), a higher incidence of multidrug resistance glycoprotein (MDR-1) positivity and unfavourable response to therapy. The therapy related acute myeloid leukaemias occurring after alkylating agent chemotherapy closely resemble *de novo* acute myeloid leukaemia with multilineage dysplasia both morphologically and cytogenetically.

The last category of acute myeloid leukaemia, those cases not otherwise categorised, is morphology based and reflects the French-American-British (FAB) classification with some significant modifications {93, 220}. The most significant change from the FAB classification is the recommendation that the requisite blast percentage for a diagnosis of acute myeloid leukaemia be ≥20 myeloblasts in the blood or marrow. This is admittedly an arbitrary threshold but is supported by

Table 4.01
Classification of acute myeloid leukemia (AML).

Acute myeloid leukaemia with recurrent genetic abnormalities
– Acute myeloid leukaemia with t(8;21)(q22;q22); (*AML1/ETO*) – Acute myeloid leukaemia with abnormal bone marrow eosinophils inv(16)(p13q22) or t(16;16)(p13;q22); (*CBFβ/MYH11*) – Acute promyelocytic leukaemia (AML with t(15;17)(q22;q12) (*PML/RARα*) and variants – Acute myeloid leukaemia with 11q23 (*MLL*) abnormalities
Acute myeloid leukaemia with multilineage dysplasia
– Following a myelodysplastic syndrome or myelodysplastic syndrome/myeloproliferative disorder – Without antecedent myelodysplastic syndrome
Acute myeloid leukaemia and myelodysplastic syndromes, therapy-related
– Alkylating agent-related – Topoisomerase type II inhibitor-related (some may be lymphoid) – Other types
Acute myeloid leukaemia not otherwise categorised
– Acute myeloid leukaemia minimally differentiated – Acute myeloid leukaemia without maturation – Acute myeloid leukaemia with maturation – Acute myelomonocytic leukaemia – Acute monoblastic and monocytic leukaemia – Acute erythroid leukaemia – Acute megakaryoblastic leukaemia – Acute basophilic leukaemia – Acute panmyelosis with myelofibrosis – Myeloid sarcoma

The authors gratefully acknowledge the Clinical Cytometry Society, meeting in Montpellier, France, in May 2000, for providing commentary on the use of flow cytometry in the classification of acute leukaemia.

studies that demonstrate a survival pattern for cases with 20-30% blasts that is similar to cases with ≥30% myeloblasts in the bone marrow {349, 350, 451}. However, it must be emphasised that the diagnosis of acute leukaemia is not in itself a therapeutic mandate; clinical factors must be taken into consideration when a therapeutic decision to treat for acute myeloid leukaemia is made. In certain instances the diagnosis of acute myeloid leukaemia can be established when the blast percentage in the marrow is less than 20, e.g. cases with an associated t(8;21)(q22;q22) and inv(16)(p13q22) or t(16;16)(p13;q22). It is anticipated that this classification will evolve as additional discoveries with clinical relevance are made.

Epidemiology

Worldwide, the overall incidence of acute leukaemia is approximately 4/100,000 population per year, with 70% of these cases being acute myeloid leukaemia (AML). Acute lymphoblastic leukaemia (ALL) is predominantly a disease of children, 75% of cases usually under 6 years of age. The vast majority of cases of AML occur in adults, median age 60 years with an incidence of 10/100,000 population per year in individuals 60 years and older.

Acute leukaemia comprises approximately one-third of cases of childhood cancer. The estimated number of new cases of acute leukaemia in adults in the United States in 2000 is approximately 13,000, 3200 cases of acute lymphoblastic leukaemia and 9700 cases of acute myeloid leukaemia. In adults, the male to female ratio for ALL is approximately 1.2:1 and that for AML is 1:1. Approximately 2600 cases of acute leukaemia are predicted in children (<15 years of age); the number is slightly higher in males and Whites. The incidence of AML in children is higher in the first years of life {1143, 1202}.

Aetiology

The possible aetiologic factors associated with the leukaemias and myelodysplastic syndromes (MDS) include viruses; ionizing radiation, cytotoxic chemotherapy and benzene {1143}. Exposure to the atomic bomb detonations in Hiroshima and Nagasaki increased the incidence of both AML, ALL, and CML in the survivors. Benzene has been implicated in the aetiology of both AML and MDS. Cigarette smoking increases the risk by about two-fold. Despite these associations, at the present time, only 1-2% of the diagnosed leukaemias can be attributed to these genotoxic agents.

Morphology

The primary specimens for classification of acute myeloid leukaemia are blood, bone marrow and particle crush smears. In cases with marked marrow fibrosis, the marrow trephine biopsy may be the only specimen available; subclassification in these cases may not be possible. The standard bone marrow Romanowsky stains such as Wright-Giemsa or May-Grünwald-Giemsa should be used. The Wright stain is unsuitable, as it stains granules suboptimally and does not allow discrimination of immature cell types.

Myeloblasts vary in size from slightly larger than mature lymphocytes to the size of monocytes or larger with moderate to abundant basophilic to blue-grey cytoplasm; the nuclei are round to oval with fine granular chromatin and usually several nucleoli. They may contain a few azurophilic granules. Auer rods are myeloid lineage specific. In contrast, lymphoblasts vary from the size of mature lymphocytes to larger than neutrophils; there is scant to moderate amounts of light to basophilic or blue-grey cytoplasm which may contain amphophilic granules; the nuclear chromatin varies from finely granular to slightly clumped with inconspicuous to prominent nucleoli. The abnormal promyelocytes in acute promyelocytic leukaemia, monoblasts and promonocytes in acute monocytic leukaemia and megakaryoblasts in acute megakaryocytic leukaemia are considered blast equivalents for the purposes of establishing a diagnosis of acute leukaemia. Erythroblasts are not included in the blast count.

Bone Marrow Biopsy

The bone marrow biopsy is necessary for evaluation of cellularity and recognition of marrow fibrosis. In addition, in cases in which inadequate smear specimens are obtained because of fibrosis or other factors, immunohistochemistry with a variety of antibodies may be the primary methodology for determining cell lineage. Antibodies to haemoglobin A and glycophorin A are useful for erythroid precursors and detection of CD61, CD41, and factor VIII expression is useful for recognition of cells of megakaryocytic lineage. CD34 is expressed by haematopoietic stem cells but is not lineage specific. Antibody to TdT recognises blast populations but is more frequently positive in ALL than AML.

Hypocellular acute myeloid leukaemia:

In some cases of acute myeloid leukaemia the marrow cellularity is less than 20%, so called "hypocellular" or "hypoplastic" acute myeloid leukaemia. This is not a specific diagnostic category. Hypocellular AML must be differentiated from aplastic anaemia. Bone marrow hypocellularity in aplastic anaemia is

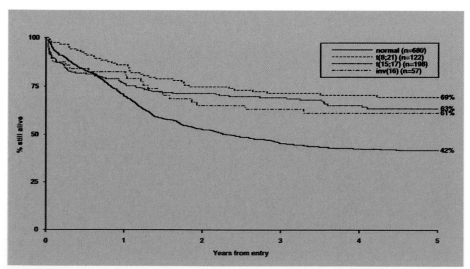

Fig. 4.01 Survival curves from the MRC AML 10 trial for patients with acute myeloid leukaemia associated with recurrent cytogenetic translocation. Reproduced from Grimwade D, et al {461}.

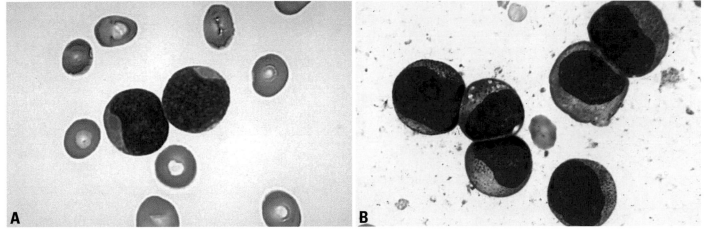

Fig. 4.02 Acute myeloid leukaemia. **A** Agranular myeloblasts. **B** Granulated myeloblasts.

usually more pronounced without evidence of increased blasts; the interstitial cells are well differentiated lymphocytes, plasma cells, mast cells, and scattered maturing haemopoietic cells. The distinction from hypocellular myelodysplastic syndrome may be difficult. For a diagnosis of hypocellular AML the blasts should be ≥ 20%. Immunohistochemical reaction with antibody to CD34 will usually show a significant positive population in hypoplastic acute leukaemia; in aplastic anaemia the reaction is negative or only a rare cell may be positive.

Cytochemistry
Myeloperoxidase (MPO)
Myeloperoxidase activity is specific for myeloid differentiation. Methods using 0-Tolidine or amino ethyl carbazole as substrate have counterstains that allow ready identification of cell types and are less carcinogenic than substrates using benzidine. Myeloperoxidase activity is stable for approximately four weeks in unstained smears kept at cool room temperature and protected from light. Myeloperoxidase activity in myeloblasts is granular and often concentrated in the Golgi zone. Monoblasts may be negative or positive with scattered fine granules. Lymphoblasts and megakaryoblasts are MPO negative.

Sudan Black B (SBB)
SBB reactivity is similar to MPO in myeloblasts and monoblasts, and is stable for months in unstained slides. The intensity of SBB staining varies with methodology and its specificity for the myeloid lineage is less than MPO. Positive cells usually stain more intensely with SBB than MPO. Lymphoblasts are usually negative; in rare cases, lymphoblasts contain granules which may stain light gray, contrasting to the black granules in neutrophils and myeloblasts.

Non-Specific Esterase (NSE)
Alpha Naphthyl Butyrate (ANB): Reactivity in monoblasts with most methodologies is diffuse cytoplasmic. Lymphoblasts, especially granular lymphoblasts, may show multifocal punctate or Golgi zone cytoplasmic positivity. Neutrophils are negative or only weakly positive.

Alpha Naphthyl Acetate (ANA): Reactivity in monoblasts and lymphoblasts is similar to ANB. Megakaryoblasts and erythroblasts may contain multifocal punctate cytoplasmic positivity that is partially resistant to NaF inhibition. The ANA positivity in monoblasts is totally inhibited by NaF; lymphoblast positivity is variably inhibited. Neutrophils are negative or only weakly positive.

Immunophenotype
Immunophenotypic analysis has a central role in distinguishing between minimally differentiated acute myeloid leukaemia and acute lymphoblastic leukaemia, in the recognition of acute megakaryoblastic leukaemia, and in the separation of B and T cell ALL. In addition, there are subcategories in this classification that have characteristic immunophenotypic features, and in many cases particular diagnoses can be suggested or excluded based on immunophenotypic results. Immunophenotyping may be performed by flow cytometry or by immunohistochemistry on slides. However, the value of particular markers may differ depend-ing on the technique used. In particular, many of the most specific cytoplasmic markers (see below) have been reported to be less specific when tested using slide-based immunocytochemical stains when compared to flow cytometry {39}. A detailed discussion of immunophenotyping and in particular of flow cytometry are outside of the scope of this document. Because of this, the immunophenotypic information described here should only be viewed as general guidelines for interpretation. Particularly for flow cytometry, a detailed knowledge of technical issues, including choice of fluorochrome, details of gating, and relative patterns and intensities of many antigens, often in combination, can provide important information relative to the diagnosis and classification of acute leukaemias beyond what is outlined here. Where possible, we have emphasised those disease categories in which these issues are of critical importance.

Antigens most frequently used for assignment of particular lineages are

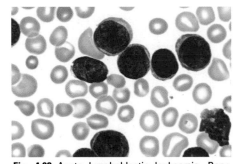

Fig. 4.03 Acute lymphoblastic leukaemia. Bone marrow smear. Several lymphoblasts from a case of precursor lymphoblastic leukaemia. Compare with appearance of blasts in Figure 4.02.

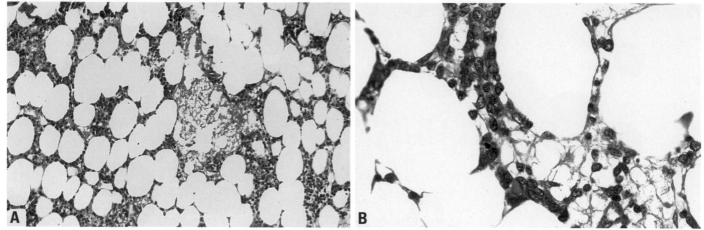

Fig. 4.04 Hypoplastic acute myeloid leukaemia. Bone marrow section. **A** This marrow trephine biopsy from a 64 year-old patient with acute myeloid leukaemia is markedly hypocellular. **B** High magnification of the same biopsy. The predominant cells are blasts which were slightly myeloperoxidase positive on a smear preparation.

lineage specific, although the majority are only lineage-associated. Some antigens tend to be expressed in the cytoplasm rather than on the surface: when several surface markers of a given lineage are studied, accurate lineage assignment can be achieved. The use of multiple markers helps to recognise cases of bilineal or biphenotypic leukaemias. Moreover, multiple markers may help to identify phenotypes associated with particular cytogenetic abnormalities, or may help to identify phenotypic aberrancies that may be useful in patient monitoring for detecting minimal residual disease {662, 978}.

In addition to the considerations used in this classification in an attempt to predict biologic behaviour, identification of other factors may also be relevant. The expression on the leukaemic blasts of the multidrug resistance glycoprotein (MDR-1) which is a transmembrane efflux pump that actively extrudes chemotherapeutic agents from leukaemic cells is more frequently observed in the blasts of acute myeloid leukaemia occurring in older individuals and is a predictor of decreased complete response rate. In elderly patients with AML, the expression of MDR-1 is associated with a higher frequency of unfavourable cytogenetic profiles than cases of elderly patients with AML in which the blasts are MDR-1 negative and in whom there is a higher complete response rate {745, 746}. These findings occur in both *de novo* and secondary acute myeloid leukaemias. The occurrence of these unfavourable factors increases with age; they are present in 17% of patients less than 35 years of age and 71% of patients over the age of 55 {745, 746}.

Genetics

Cytogenetic and genotypic studies are important for the subclassification of haematopoietic malignancies {171, 316, 899, 461, 1076}. T and B-cell precursor lymphoblastic proliferations may demonstrate clonal rearrangement of T-cell receptor and immunoglobulin genes respectively, but these changes are not lineage restricted and are not helpful in lineage assignment. T cell receptor gene rearrangement may occasionally be seen in myeloid leukaemias. Specific details of genetic studies are discussed in the following sections by disease entities.

Table 4.02
Panel of monoclonal antibodies for the classification of acute leukaemias.

Haematopoietic precursors: CD34, HLA-Dr, TdT, CD45[2]
B-lineage: CD19, CD20, CD22[1], CD79a[1,3]
T-lineage: CD2, CD3[1], CD5, CD7
Myeloid: CD13, CD33, CD15, MPO[1], CD117
Megakaryoblastic: CD41, CD61

Antigens identified with an asterisk are considered lineage specific when detected in the cytoplasm by flow cytometry.
[1] Cytoplasmic expression
[2] CD45 is generally more dimly expressed than on normal lymphocytes and it may be negative in some cases of ALL or megakaryoblastic leukaemia
[3] CD79a has also been reported in some cases of precursor T-ALL

Acute myeloid leukaemia with recurrent genetic abnormalities

R.D. Brunning
E. Matutes
G. Flandrin
J. Vardiman

J. Bennett
D. Head
N.L. Harris

This group is characterised by recurrent genetic abnormalities, mainly balanced translocations, and often a high rate of complete remission, and favourable prognosis.

The most commonly identified abnormalities are reciprocal translocations: t(8;21), inv(16) or t(16;16), t(15;17) and various translocation involving the 11q23 breakpoint {171}. Molecular studies have shown that these structural chromosome rearrangements create a fusion gene encoding a chimeric protein. All of these categories have some degree of correlation with morphology.

Many of the translocations are detected by reverse transcriptase-polymerase chain reaction (RT-PCR) which has a higher sensitivity (1×10^{-5}) than cytogenetics (1×10^{-2}). The altered expression and/or structure of cellular gene products results in functional activation that may contribute to the initiation or progression of leukaemogenesis.

Other recurring cytogenetic abnormalities in AML are significantly less frequent and described in AML not otherwise categorised.

cases of acute myeloblastic leukaemia with maturation {171}. It occurs predominantly in younger patients.

Clinical features

Tumour manifestations, such as myeloid sarcomas (granulocytic sarcomas), may be present at presentation. In such cases the initial bone marrow aspiration may show a misleading low number of blast cells, but should be diagnosed as AML despite a blast percentage in the bone marrow of <20.

Morphology and cytochemistry

The common morphological features include the presence of large blasts with abundant basophilic cytoplasm, often containing numerous azurophilic granulation; a few blasts in some cases show very large granules (pseudo Chediak-Higashi granules), suggesting abnormal fusion. Auer rods are frequently found and appear as a single long and sharp rod with tapered ends; they may be detected in mature neutrophils. In addition to the large blast cells, some smaller blasts, predominantly in the peripheral

blood, may be found. Promyelocytes, myelocytes, and mature neutrophils with variable dysplasia are present in the bone marrow. These cells may show abnormal nuclear segmentation (e.g. pseudo Pelger-Huet nuclei) and/or cytoplasmic staining abnormalities, including homogenous pink coloured cytoplasm in neutrophils.

Eosinophil precursors are frequently increased but they do not exhibit the cytological or cytochemical abnormalities characteristic of acute myelomonocytic leukaemia associated with abnormalities of chromosome 16; basophils and/or mast cells are sometimes present in excess. The monocytic component is usually reduced or absent. Erythroblasts and megakaryocytes are morphologically normal.

Acute myeloblastic leukaemia with maturation is the predominant morphologic type correlating with the t(8;21), but some cases without maturation or with monocytic differentiation have also been reported. Rare cases with a bone marrow blast percentage <20 occur. These should be classified as AML and not as RAEB.

*Acute myeloid leukaemia with t(8;21)(q22;q22);(AML1/ETO)**

Definition

Acute myeloid leukaemia (AML) with t(8;21)(q22;q22); (*AML1 / ETO*) is an acute myeloid leukaemia generally showing maturation in the neutrophil lineage.

ICD-O code   9896/3

Epidemiology

The translocation t(8;21)(q22;q22) is one of the most common structural aberrations in acute myeloid leukaemia and is found in 5-12% of cases of AML and in one-third of karyotypically abnormal

* Editor's note: The AML1 gene is also referred to as the RUNX1 gene.

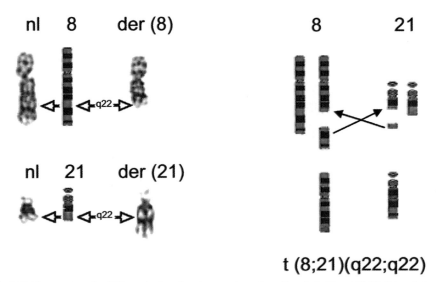

Fig. 4.05 The translocation 8;21 results from breakage and reunion of bands 8q22 and 21q22. G-banded normal (nl) 8 and 21 chromosomes (left) and the derivative (der) 8 and 21 chromosomes resulting from the translocation are shown on the right.

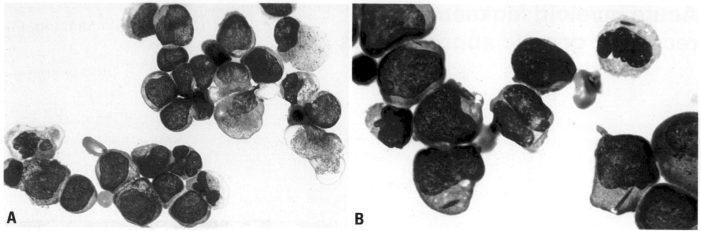

Fig. 4.06 Acute myeloblastic leukaemia with maturation and an associated t(8;21)(q22;q22). **A** Bone marrow smear. Note myeloblasts and more mature stages of neutrophil maturation; one blast contains a prominent slender Auer rod. **B** Bone marrow smear showing several blasts and a dysplastic segmented neutrophil with prominent Auer rods.

Immunophenotype

In addition to the expression of myeloid markers (CD13, CD33, MPO), AML with the t(8;21) frequently shows coexpression of the lymphoid marker CD19; in contrast to ALL it is generally present only on a subset of the blasts {551, 662}. CD34 is characteristically present, and CD56 is often expressed, although not as consistently as CD19. CD56 expression is not

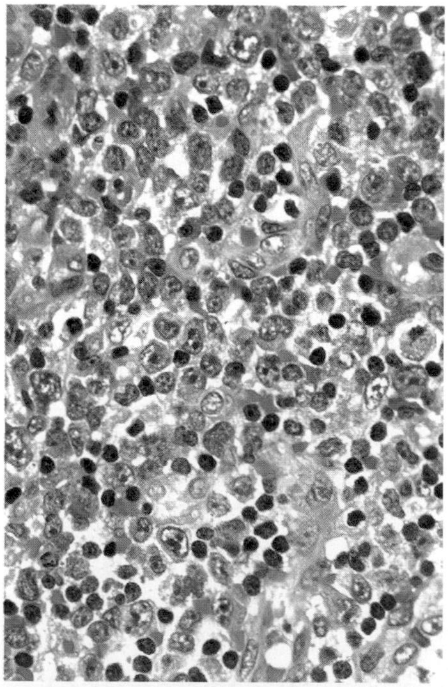

Fig. 4.07 Myeloid sarcoma. Biopsy of an orbital mass from a child with AML with a t(8;21)(q22;q22). There are eosinophil precursors scattered in the predominant blast population.

specific but may have adverse prognostic significance {61}. Some cases are TdT positive; however, its expression is generally dim.

Genetics

The genes for both heterodimeric components of core binding factor (CBF), CBFα and CBFβ are known to be involved in translocations associated with acute leukaemias. The translocation t(8;21)(q22;q22) involves the *AML1* gene, also known as *RUNX1,* which encodes CBFα, and the *ETO* (eight-twenty-one) gene {171, 316, 317}. The AML1/ETO fusion transcript is consistently detected in patients with t(8;21) AML. The disruption of *AML1* gene has been reported to occur within a single intron; AML1/ETO transcripts have similarities to the Drosophila segmentation gene called RUNT. It has been reported that some patients having the morphologic findings typical of the t(8;21) described above, may have rearrangement of *AML1* and *ETO* genes, but are cytogenetically negative for the t(8;21) translocation.

Postulated cell of origin

Myeloid stem cell with predominant neutrophil differentiation.

Prognosis and predictive factors

Acute myeloid leukaemia with the t(8;21) is usually associated with good response to chemotherapy and high complete remission rate with long-term disease-free survival when treated with high dose

cytarabine in the consolidation phase {114, 461}. A large number of patients show additional chromosome abnormalities: e.g., loss of a sex chromosome and del(9)(q22). Some factors appear to adversely affect survival including CD56 expression and secondary karyotypic abnormalities {61, 1095, 1162}.

Acute myeloid leukaemia with inv(16)(p13q22) or t(16;16)(p13;q22); (CBFβ/MYH11)

Definition

Acute myeloid leukaemia with inv(16)(p13q22) or t(16;16)(p13;q22); *(CBFβ/MYH11)* is an acute myeloid leukaemia that usually shows monocytic and granulocytic differentiation and the presence of a characteristically abnormal eosinophil component in the marrow {741, 815}. The combination of acute myelomonocytic leukaemia with abnormal eosinophils is referred to as AMML Eo.

ICD-O code   9871/3

Epidemiology

The inv(16)(p13q22) is found in approximately 10-12% of all cases of AML. It can occur in all age groups but predominantly in younger patients.

Clinical features

Myeloid sarcomas may be present at initial diagnosis or at relapse and may constitute the only evidence of relapse in some patients.

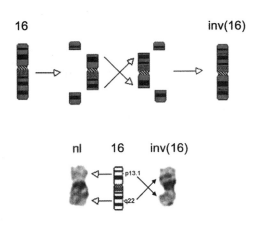

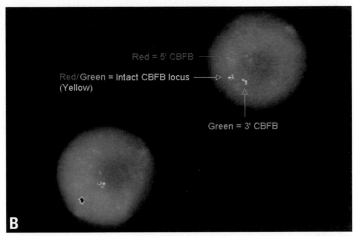

A

B

Fig. 4.08 Acute myelomonocytic leukaemia with associated inv(16)(p13q22). **A** The inversion 16 results from breakage and rejoining of bands 16p13.1 and 16q22. G-banded normal (nl) 16 and inv(16) are shown. **B** Dual color fluorescence-in-situ-hybridization: the 5′ region of *CBFβ* is labeled in red; the 3′ region in green. A normal chromosome 16 has the 5′ and 3′ regions contiguous to each other resulting in a single yellow or overlapping red/green signals. The inversion 16 splits the *CBFβ* locus resulting in separate red and green signals. Both °interphase cells shown have one normal 16 chromosome and one inv(16).

Morphology and cytochemistry

In these cases, in addition to the morphological features of acute myelomonocytic leukaemia, the bone marrow shows a variable number of eosinophils (sometimes <5%) at all stages of maturation without significant maturation arrest. The most striking abnormalities involve the immature eosinophilic granules, mainly evident at the promyelocyte and myelocyte stages. The abnormalities are usually not present at later stages of eosinophil maturation. The eosinophilic granules are often larger than those normally present in immature eosinophils, purple-violet in colour, and in some cells are so dense that they obscure the cell morphology. The mature eosinophils may occasionally show nuclear hyposegmentation. The naphthol ASD chloroacetate esterase reaction, which is normally negative in eosinophils, is characteristically faintly positive in these abnormal eosinophils. Such a reaction is not seen in eosinophils of AML with the t(8;21). Auer rods may be observed in myeloblasts. At least 3% of the blasts show MPO reactivity. The monoblasts and promonocytes usually show non-specific esterase reactivity, although it may be weaker than expected in some cases.

In addition to the predominant monocytic and eosinophil components, the neutrophils in the bone marrow are usually sparse, with a decreased number of mature neutrophils. The peripheral blood is not different from other cases of AMML; eosinophils are not usually increased but an occasional case has been reported

with abnormal and increased eosinophils in the blood.

While the majority of cases of inv(16)(p13q22) have been identified as AMML Eo, occasional cases with this genetic abnormality have been reported to lack the eosinophilia, to show only myeloid maturation without a monocytic component or only monocytic differentiation. Not infrequently, the blast percentage is only at the threshold level of 20% or occasionally lower. Similar to cases with the t(8;21) with less than 20% bone marrow blasts, cases with this characteristic genetic abnormality should be diag-

nosed as acute myeloid leukaemia. The marrow trephine biopsy is usually hypercellular but may occasionally be normocellular.

Immunophenotype

In addition to myeloid antigens (CD13, CD33, MPO) the blasts in this type of leukaemia may frequently show markers characteristic of monocytic differentiation including some or all of the following: CD14, CD4, CD11b, CD11c, CD64, CD36 and lysozyme; none of these is specific for the inv(16). In AMML with inv(16), coexpression of CD2 with

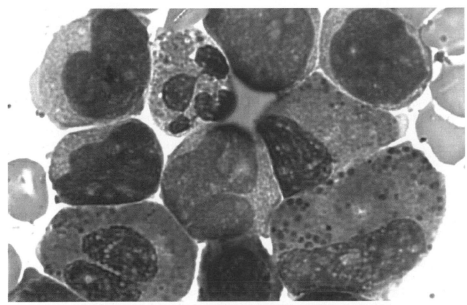

Fig. 4.09 Acute myelomonocytic leukaemia with associated inv(16)(p13q22). Increased abnormal eosinophils, one with large basophilic colored granules, are present.

myeloid markers has been frequently documented but it is not specific for this diagnosis.

Genetics

Inv(16)(p13q22) and t(16;16)(p13;q22) both result in the fusion of the *CBFβ* gene at 16q22 to the smooth muscle myosin heavy chain (MYH11) at 16p13. MYH11, located at 16p13, codes for a smooth muscle myosin heavy chain gene {171}. The *CBFβ* gene is located at 16q22 and codes for the Core Binding Factor (CBF) β subunit, a heterodimeric transcription factor known to bind the enhancers of various murine leukaemia viruses and similar motifs in the enhancers of T cell receptor (TCR) genes. The CBFβ subunit heterodimerises with CBFα, the gene product of *AML1*, one of the genes involved in the t(8;21) translocation usually associated with AML with maturation. Occasionally cytological features of AMML Eo may be present without karyotypic evidence of a chromosome 16 abnormality, the *CBFβ/MYH11* being nevertheless demonstrated by molecular studies. By conventional cytogenetics, the inv(16) is a subtle rearrangement that may be overlooked when metaphase preparations are suboptimal. Thus, at diagnosis, the use of FISH and RT-PCR methods may be necessary to document the genetic alteration.

Postulated cell of origin

Haematopoietic stem cell with potential to differentiate into granulocytic and monocytic lineages.

Prognosis and predictive factors

Clinical studies have shown that patients with AMML with inv(16) and t(16;16) achieve higher complete remission (CR) rates when treated with high dose cytarabine in the consolidation phase {461, 899}.

Acute promyelocytic leukaemia (AML with t(15;17)(q22;q12); (PML/RARα) and variants)

Definition

Acute promyelocytic leukaemia (AML with t(15;17)(q22;q12)* is an acute myeloid leukaemia in which abnormal promyelocytes predominate. Both hyper-

granular or "typical" APL and microgranular (hypogranular) types exist.

ICD-O code   9866/3

Epidemiology

APL comprises 5-8% of AML {1225}. The disease can occur at any age but patients are predominantly adults in mid-life.

Clinical features of APL

Typical and microgranular APL are frequently associated with disseminated intravascular coagulation (DIC). In microgranular APL, unlike typical APL, the leukocyte count is very high, with a rapid doubling time.

Morphology and cytochemistry

The nuclear size and shape in the abnormal promyelocytes of hypergranular APL are irregular and greatly variable; they are often kidney-shaped or bilobed. The cytoplasm is marked by densely packed or even coalescent large granules, staining bright pink, red or purple in Roma-nowsky stains. The cytoplasmic granules may be so large and/or numerous that they totally obscure the nuclear cytoplasmic margin. In some cells the cytoplasm is filled with fine dust-like granules. Characteristic cells containing bundles of Auer rods ("faggot cells") randomly distributed in the cytoplasm are present in most cases. Myeloblasts with single Auer rods may also be observed. Auer rods in hypergranular APL are usually larger than in other types of AML and they may have a characteristic morphology at ultrastructural level with a hexagonal arrangement of tubular structures with a specific periodicity of approximately 250 mμ in contrast to the 6-20 laminar periodicity of Auer rods in other types of AML. The myeloperoxidase reaction is always strongly positive in all the leukaemic promyelocytes, with the reaction product covering the entire cytoplasm and often the nucleus. The nonspecific esterase reaction may be weakly positive in approximately 25% of cases. Only occasional obvious leukaemic promyelocytes may be observed in the blood.

Cases of microgranular (hypogranular) APL are characterised by distinct morphological features such as apparent paucity or absence of granules, and predominantly bilobed nuclear shape {444}. The apparent hypogranular cytoplasm relates to the submicroscopic size of the

azurophilic granules. This may cause confusion with acute monocytic leukaemia on Romanowsky stained smears; however, a small number of the abnormal promyelocytes show clearly visible granules and/or bundles of Auer rods (faggot cells). The leukocyte count is frequently markedly elevated in the microgranular variant of APL with numerous abnormal microgranular promyelocytes in contrast to typical APL. The MPO reaction is strongly positive contrasting with the weak or negative reaction in monocytes. Abnormal promyelocytes with deeply basophilic cytoplasm have been described mainly in the relapse phase in patients who have been previously treated with all trans-retinoic acid.

The marrow biopsy is usually hypercellular. The abnormal promyelocytes have relatively abundant cytoplasm with numerous granules; occasionally Auer rods may be identified in well-prepared specimens. The nuclei are frequently convoluted.

Immunophenotype

Acute promyelocytic leukaemia with the t(15;17) has a characteristic but not diagnostic myeloid phenotype. By flow cytometry, CD33 is usually homogeneously positive and bright, while CD13 is heterogeneous. HLA-DR and CD34 are generally absent; if they are expressed, they are only found on a subset of the leukaemic cells. The more mature marker CD15 is negative or only dimly expressed and is never coexpressed with CD34 {978}. There is frequent coexpression of CD2 and CD9. By immunocytochemistry, antibodies against the PML gene product show a characteristic nuclear multigranular pattern with nucleolar exclusion in contrast to the speckled pattern seen in normal promyelocytes or blasts from other types of AML {358}.

Genetics

In addition to its therapeutic impact, the sensitivity of APL cells to all trans-retinoic acid has led to the discovery that the retinoic acid receptor alpha (*RARα*) gene

---

*Editor's note: the precise location of the *RARa* breakpoint on chromosome 17 has been variably reported in the literature. Although it was originally described to be 17q21, most authorities now agree its location is 17q11.2-12, and generally denoted as 17q12.

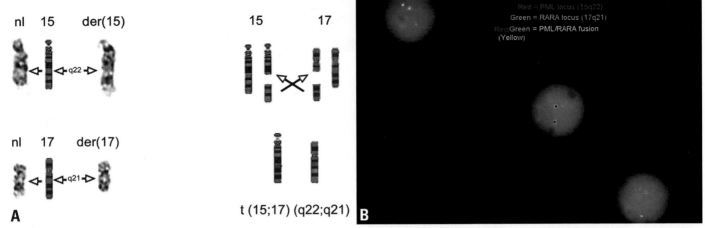

Fig. 4.10 Acute promyelocytic leukaemia with t(15;17)(q22;q12). A The translocation 15;17 results from breakage and reunion of bands 15q22 and 17q12. G-banded normal (nl) 15 and 17 chromosomes (left) and the derivative (der) 15 and 17 resulting from the translocation are shown on the right. B Dual color fluorescence-in-situ-hybridisation with probes PML (15q22) and RARa(17q21)* demonstrate the presence of a PML/RARa fusion resulting from the 15;17 translocation. Each of the three interphase cells has one separate red (PML) signal, one separate green (RARa) signal, and one yellow or overlapping red/green signal consistent with the presence of a PML/RARa gene fusion.

on 17q12 fuses with a nuclear regulatory factor on 15q22 (promyelocytic leukaemia or *PML* gene) giving rise to a PML-RARα gene fusion product {171, 272, 857}.

Rare cases of APL lacking the classic t(15;17) (q22;q12) on routine cytogenetic studies have been described either as cases having complex variant translocations involving both chromosomes 15 and 17 with additional chromosome abnormalities and expressing PML/RARα transcript, or cases where neither chromosome 15 nor chromosome 17 apparently is involved, but with submicroscopic insertion of *RARα* into *PML* leading to the expression of the PML/RARα transcript; these latter cases are considered as cryptic or masked t(15;17). Morphologic

analysis shows no major differences between the t(15;17) positive group and the *PML/RARα* positive patients without t(15;17).

Postulated cell of origin
Myeloid stem cell with potential to differentiate to granulocytic lineage.

Prognosis
Acute promyelocytic leukaemia has a particular sensitivity to treatment with all trans-retinoic acid, which acts as a differentiating agent {185, 1261}. The prognosis in APL, treated optimally with all trans-retinoic acid and an anthracycline is relatively favourable similar to AML with t(8;21) or inv(16) {373}.

Variants
APL with variant translocations:
t(11;17)(q23;q21), t(5;17)(q32;q12);
t(11;17)(q13;q21)

Genetics
There are three variant translocations involving *RARα*: t(11;17)(q23;q21) in which *RARα* on chromosome 17 fuses with promyelocytic leukaemia zinc finger gene (*PLZF*) on chromosome 11, t(5;17)(q23;q12) in which the nucleophosmin gene on chromosome 5 (*NPM*) fuses with *RARα*, and t(11;17)(q13;q21) in which the nuclear matrix associated gene (*NuMA*) on chromosome 11 fuses with *RARα* {857}.

There have been several reported cases

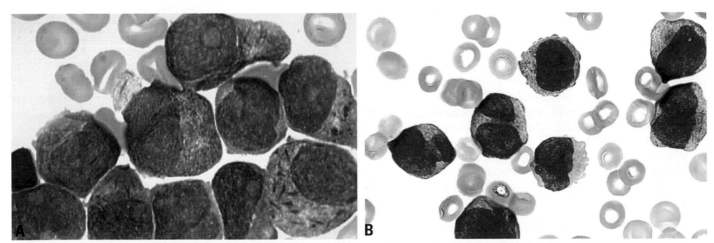

Fig. 4.11 Acute promyelocytic leukaemia. **A** Hypergranular type in bone marrow smear. There are several abnormal promyelocytes with intense azurophilic granulation. Several of the promyelocytes contain numerous Auer rods (Faggot cells). **B** Microgranular variant, in blood smear. There are several abnormal promyelocytes with lobulated, almost cerebriform nuclei. The cytoplasm contains numerous small azurophilic granules; other cells appear sparsely granular.

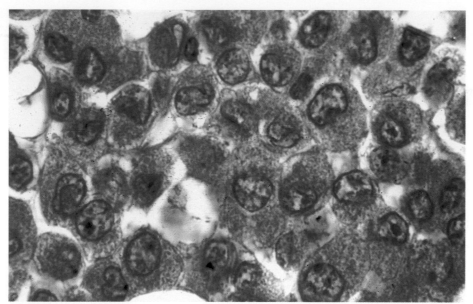

Fig. 4.12 Acute promyelocytic leukaemia. Bone marrow biopsy. Abnormal promyelocytes with abundant hypergranulated cytoplasm. The nuclei are generally round to oval. Several of the nuclei are irregular and invaginated.

of the AML with translocation t(11;17) (q23;q21), in which the *PLZF* gene on chromosome 11 is fused with the *RARα* gene on 17q21 {218, 857, 1132}. The variant translocation t(5;17)(q32;q12) in which the *NPM* gene on chromosome 5, fuses with the retinoic acid receptor (*RARα*) gene on chromosome 17 is rare and is usually classified as atypical APL. Two alternative spliced transcripts are expressed which differ in 129 bases immediately upstream of the *RARα* sequence {103, 272, 857, 1092}. The *RARα* sequences are the same as the sequence found in the *PML/RARα* and *PLZF/RARα* fusion in the t(15;17) and t(11;17) respectively.

Morphology and cytochemistry

The cases with variant translocations have initially been reported as having APL morphology {1132}. However, the t(11;17)(q23;q21) *PLZF/RARα* subgroup shows some morphological differences with a predominance of cells with regular nuclei, many granules, usually absence of Auer rods, an increased number of pseudo Pelger-Huet cells and strong MPO activity {1132}. These particular characteristics could allow the definition of a separate morphological entity among APL. The initial cases of APL associated with the t(5;17)(q32;q12) had a predominant population of hypergranular promyelocytes and a minor population of hypo-

granular promyelocytes; Auer rods were not identified by light microscopy {248}.

Clinical features

Acute promyelocytic leukaemia variant with t(11;17)(q23;q21) is resistant to ATRA, both *in vivo* and *in vitro* {857}. APL with the t(5;17)(q23;q12) appears to respond to ATRA {857}.

Acute myeloid leukaemia with 11q23 (MLL) abnormalities

Definition

Acute myeloid leukaemia with 11q23 abnormalities, is usually associated with monocytic features.

ICD-O code   9897/3

Epidemiology

Abnormalities of 11q23 are found in 5-6% of cases of AML. These abnormalities can occur at any age but are more common in children. Two clinical subgroups of patients have a high frequency of 11q23 aberration and AML: one is AML in infants and the other group is therapy-related leukaemia usually occurring after treatment with DNA topoisomerase II inhibitors. In general, the translocations in therapy related leu-

kaemias are the same as those occurring in "*de novo*" leukaemia, i.e. t(9;11), t(11;19), t(4;11) {1016, 1061, 1169}.

Clinical features

Patients may present with disseminated intravascular coagulation. They may have extramedullary monocytic sarcomas and/or tissue infiltration (gingiva, skin).

Morphology and cytochemistry

There is a strong association between acute monocytic and myelomonocytic leukaemias and deletions/translocations involving 11q23, mainly with acute monoblastic leukaemia, although occasionally it is detected in AML with and without maturation. Monoblasts and promonocytes typically predominate. Monoblasts are large cells, with abundant cytoplasm which can be moderately to intensely basophilic and may show pseudopod formation. Scattered fine azurophilic granules and vacuoles may be present. The monoblasts usually have round nuclei with delicate lacy chromatin, and one or more large prominent nucleoli.

Promonocytes have a more irregular and delicately convoluted nuclear configuration; the cytoplasm is usually less

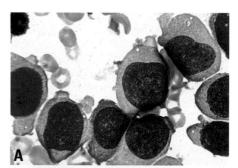

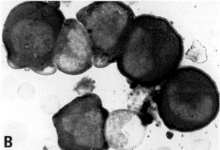

Fig. 4.13 Acute monoblastic leukaemia. Bone marrow smears. **A** Several monoblasts, some with very abundant cytoplasm and fine myeloperoxidase negative azurophilic granules are present. **B** Nonspecific esterase reaction showing intensely positive monoblasts.

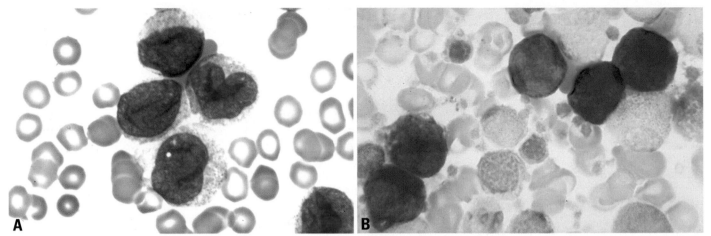

Fig. 4.14 Acute monocytic leukaemia, differentiated. Bone marrow smears. **A** There are several monoblasts and promonocytes with very pale cytoplasm containing numerous fine azurophilic granules. The promonocytes have delicate nuclear folds. **B** Non-specific esterase stain. The promonocytes are intensely reactive.

basophilic and sometimes more obviously granulated, with occasional large azurophilic granules and vacuoles. Monoblasts and promonocytes usually show strong positive non-specific esterase reactions. The monoblasts often lack MPO reactivity.

Immunophenotype
Cases of AML variably express myeloid associated antigens (CD13, CD33). There are no immunophenotypic features that are specific for AMLs with 11q23 translocations; those showing monoblastic morphology will generally be CD34 negative and express markers of monocytic differentiation including CD14, CD4, CD11b, CD11c, CD64, CD36 and lysozyme.

Genetics
Molecular studies have identified a human homolog of the Drosophila trithorax gene designated *HRX* or *MLL*, which is a developmental regulator and is structurally altered in leukaemia associated translocations that show an abnormality at band 11q23. The *MLL* gene on 11q23 is involved in a number of translocations with different partner chromosomes {171}.

The most common translocations observed in childhood AML are the t(9;11)(p21;q23) and the t(11;19)(q23;p13.1)/t(11;19)(q23;p13.3); other

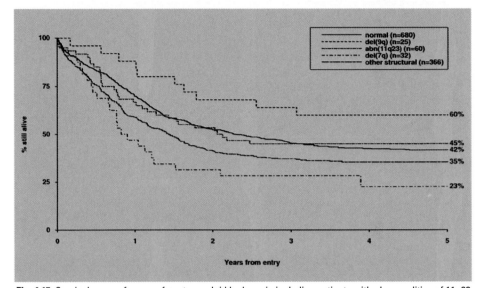

Fig. 4.15 Survival curve of cases of acute myeloid leukaemia including patients with abnormalities of 11q23 with intermediate prognosis. Reproduced from Grimwade D, et al {461}.

observed translocations of 11q23 involve approximately 20 different partner chromosomes. Molecular studies have shown that the *MLL* gene is rearranged more frequently than is revealed by conventional cytogenetic studies {171}.

A partial tandem duplication of *MLL* gene has been reported in a few adult patients whose leukaemic blast cells have a +11 and in some with normal karyotype.

Postulated cell of origin
Haematopoietic stem cell with multilineage potential.

Prognosis and predictive factors
Acute myeloid leukaemia with associated abnormalities of chromosome 11q23 have an intermediate survival.

Acute myeloid leukaemia with multilineage dysplasia

R.D. Brunning
E. Matutes
N.L. Harris
G. Flandrin

J. Vardiman
J. Bennett
D. Head

Definition

Acute myeloid leukaemia (AML) with multilineage dysplasia is an acute leukaemia with ≥20% blasts in blood or marrow, and dysplasia in 2 or more myeloid cell lines, generally including megakaryocytes. Dysplasia must be present in ≥50% of the cells of at least 2 lines {410}. These features must be present in a pre-treatment specimen. This entity may occur *de novo* or following MDS or a myelodysplastic/myeloproliferative disorder (MDS/MPD).

When a myelodysplastic syndrome precedes acute myeloid leukaemia, the diagnostic terminology should reflect the evolution, i.e. acute myeloid leukaemia evolving from a myelodysplastic syndrome.

ICD-O code   9895/3

Epidemiology

This category of AML occurs mainly in elderly patients and is rare in children {506, 746}.

Clinical features

Patients with AML and multilineage dysplasia often present with severe pancytopenia.

Precursor lesions

AML with multilineage dysplasia may follow a myelodysplastic syndrome.

Morphology and cytochemistry

This category of AML is morphologically defined by the presence of multilineage dysplasia. These features must be assessed on well-stained, pre-treatment smears of blood or bone marrow. Dysplasia must be present in ≥50% of two cell lines. Dysgranulopoiesis is characterised by neutrophils with hypogranular cytoplasm, hyposegmented nuclei (pseudo Pelger-Huet anomaly) or bizarrely segmented nuclei. In some cases, these features may be more readily identified on peripheral blood than bone marrow smears. Dyserythropoiesis is characterised by megaloblastic nuclei, karyorrhexis, nuclear fragments or multinucleation. Ringed sideroblasts, cytoplasmic vacuoles, and PAS positivity are additional features of dyserythropoiesis. Dysmegakaryopoiesis is characterised by micromegakaryocytes and normal size or large megakaryocytes with monolobed or multiple separated nuclei. It is important to distinguish the various abnormal megakaryocytes: normal sized megakaryocytes with non-lobed ("monol-obed") nuclei and small ("micro") megakaryocytes with hypolobated nuclei {410}. Dysplastic megakaryocytes may be more readily appreciated in sections than smears.

Differential diagnosis

The principal differential diagnoses are acute erythroid-myeloid leukaemia and acute myeloblastic leukaemia with maturation. Adherence to the diagnostic criteria for each of these entities should resolve the problem in the majority of cases. Some cases may overlap two morphologic types. It is appropriate to focus on one classification and note the difficulty in the exact definition in the report.

Immunophenotype

Immunophenotyping studies reflect the heterogeneity of the underlying morphology. Blasts frequently constitute only a subpopulation of the cell population and these are generally CD34+ and express pan-myeloid markers (CD13, CD33). There is frequent aberrant expression of CD56 and/or the lymphoid-associated marker CD7. The maturing myeloid cells may show patterns of antigen expression that differ from that seen in normal

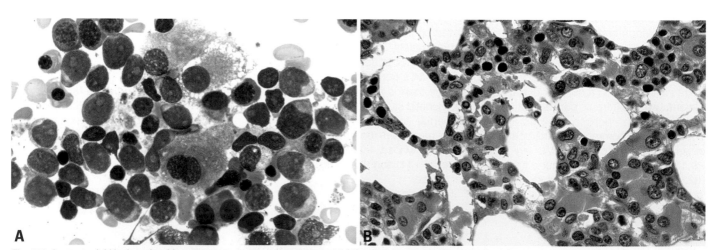

Fig. 4.16 Acute myeloid leukaemia with multilineage dysplasia associated with (A) inv(3)(q21q26) and (B) t(3;3)(q21;q26). **A** Bone marrow smear shows several blasts and a binucleated megakaryocyte and a megakaryocyte with a hypolobulated nucleus. Some of the erythroid precursors show dysplastic features. **B** Bone marrow section shows numerous megakaryocytes with hypolobated nuclei.

myeloid development, and there may be alterations in the light scatter properties of maturing cells, particularly granulocytes. There is an increased incidence of multidrug resistance glycoprotein (MDR-1) expression on the blast cells {745, 746}.

Genetics
Chromosome abnormalities are similar to those found in myelodysplastic syndromes and often involve gain or loss of major segments of certain chromosomes: -7/del(7q), -5/del(5q), +8, +9, +11, del(11q), del(12p), -18, +19, del(20q), +21 and less often specific translocations (t(2;11), t(1;7)) and translocations involving 3q21 and 3q26 {506, 745, 746, 899}. Abnormalities in the 3q26 region such as inv(3)(q21q26), t(3;3)(q21;q26) or ins(3;3), are associated with multilineage AML and MDS with increased platelet production; inv(3)(q21q26) is also seen in other types of AML and myeloproliferative syndromes associated with thrombocytosis and increased bone marrow mega-karyocytes. The t(3;21)(q21;q26) is usually therapy related, or associated with chronic myeloid leukaemia as a second event at

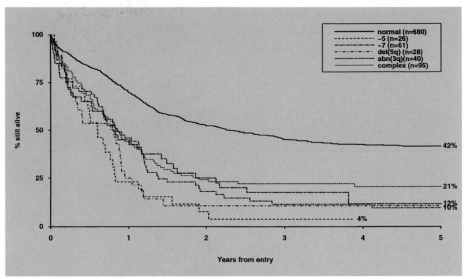

Fig. 4.17 Survival curve for cases of acute myeloid leukaemia with adverse cytogenetic findings in the MRC-AML 10 trial. Reproduced from Grimwade D, et al {461}.

blastic crisis while the t(3;5)(q25;q34) is associated with multilineage dysplasia but has no thrombocytosis.

Postulated cell of origin
Haematopoietic stem cell.

Prognosis and predictive factors
Multilineage dysplasia in AML has an adverse effect on the probability of achieving complete remission {506, 745, 746}.

Acute myeloid leukaemias and myelodysplastic syndromes, therapy related

R.D. Brunning
E. Matutes
G. Flandrin
J. Vardiman

J. Bennett
D. Head
N.L. Harris

Definition
Acute myeloid leukaemias (AML) and myelodysplastic syndromes (MDS), therapy related arise as a result of cytotoxic chemotherapy and/or radiation therapy. Two major types are recognised based on the causative agents: alkylating agent/radiation related and topoisomerase II inhibitor related {343, 1016, 1061, 1067}. These types of AML and MDS may be classified if appropriate in a specific morphologic or genetic category with the qualifying term "therapy related".

ICD-O code   9920/3

Alkylating agent related acute myeloid leukaemia and myelodysplastic syndrome

Epidemiology
The alkylating agent/radiation related disorders usually occur 5-6 years following exposure to the mutagenic agent; the reported range is approximately 10–192 months {343, 873}. The risk for occurrence is related to the total cumulative

dose of the alkylating agent and the age of the patient.

Aetiology
This disorder arises as a result of the mutagenic effect of alkylating agents and/or ionizing radiation.

Clinical features
The process frequently presents initially as a myelodysplastic syndrome with evidence of bone marrow failure: isolated cytopenias or pancytopenia with associ-

ated myelodysplastic changes. This stage is followed by frank dysplastic features in multiple cell lineages; the blast percentage in the marrow is usually less than 5%. Approximately two-thirds of cases in the MDS phase satisfy the criteria for refractory cytopenia with multilineage dysplasia; approximately a third of these cases have ringed sideroblasts in excess of 15%. About 25% of cases satisfy the criteria for refractory anaemia with excess blasts 1 or 2. The MDS phase may evolve to acute myeloid leukaemia or a higher grade MDS; a substantial number of patients succumbs to the disease in the myelodysplastic phase. A minority of patients may present with overt acute leukaemia.

Morphology

This type of therapy-related AML, either presenting as AML or evolving from MDS, usually involves all myeloid cell lines, i.e., a panmyelosis. Dysplastic changes characterised by nuclear hypolobation and cytoplasmic hypogranulation in the neutrophils and dyserythropoiesis are present in virtually all patients. Ringed sideroblasts are present in up to 60% of cases and exceed 15% in approximately one third of cases. Increased marrow basophils are present in 25% of cases and increased dysplastic megakaryocytes are present in approximately one fourth of the cases. Auer rods occur in a minority of cases. Some cases correspond to acute myeloid leukaemia with maturation; lesser numbers of cases are acute myelomonocytic leukaemia, acute monocytic leukaemia, erythroleukaemia, or acute megakaryocytic leukaemia; acute promyelocytic leukaemia is rare.

The marrow biopsy is hypercellular in 50% of cases and normocellular or hypocellular in 25% of cases respectively. Slight to marked marrow fibrosis occurs in approximately 15% of cases.

Immunophenotype

Immunophenotyping studies reflect the heterogeneity of the underlying morphology. Blasts frequently constitute only a subpopulation of the cell population and these are generally CD34+ and express pan-myeloid markers (CD13, CD33). There is frequent aberrant expression of CD56 and/or the lymphoid-associated marker CD7. The maturing myeloid cells may show patterns of antigen expression that differ from that seen in normal

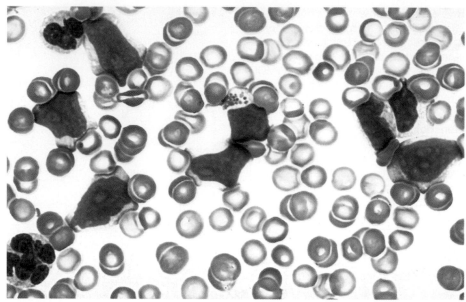

Fig. 4.18 Acute myeloid leukaemia, therapy related. Bone marrow smear from a case of acute myeloid leukaemia with increased basophils from a patient with alkylating agent related acute myeloid leukaemia.

myeloid development, and there may be alterations in the light scatter properties of maturing cells, particularly neutrophils. There is an increased incidence of multidrug resistance glycoprotein (MDR-1) expression on the blast cells {745, 746}.

Genetics

Alkylating agent/radiation therapy-related AML or MDS have a high incidence of clonal cytogenetic abnormalities. These are similar to those seen in AML with multilineage dysplasia and *de novo* MDS, refractory cytopenia with multilineage dysplasia (RCMD) or refractory anaemia with excess blasts (RAEB). They are primarily unbalanced translocations or deletions involving chromosomes 5 and/or 7 consisting of loss of all or part of the long arm of the chromosome; the deletion of the long arm of chromosome 5 usually includes bands q23 to q32 {1016}.
Other chromosomes frequently involved in a non-random manner include 1, 4, 12, 14, and 18; complex chromosomal abnormalities are the most common finding.

Postulated cell of origin

Haematopoietic stem cell.

Prognosis and predictive factors

This type of therapy-related acute myeloid leukaemia is generally refractory to anti leukaemia therapy and is associated with short survival {873}.

Topoisomerase II inhibitor related acute myeloid leukaemia

Epidemiology

This type of leukaemia occurs in patients of all ages treated with topoisomerase II inhibitors. Topoisomerase II related AML generally has a shorter latency period from the time of institution of the causative therapy to the development of leukaemia than the alkylating agent/radiation related type; the reported interval is approximately 12-130 months with a median of 33-34 months.

Aetiology

This type of therapy related acute myeloid leukaemia occurs in patients treated with drugs targeting DNA-topoisomerase II; the major agents implicated are the epipodophyllotoxins, etoposide and teniposide. The anthracyclines, doxorubicin and 4-epi-doxorubicin, have also been implicated {1016, 1061, 1067}.

Clinical features

This type of therapy related leukaemia usually, but not invariably, presents without a preceding myelodysplastic phase.

Morphology

Topoisomerase II inhibitor-related AML characteristically has a significant monocytic component. Most cases fall in the categories of acute monoblastic or myelomonocytic leukaemia. Cases with granulocyte differentiation have been observed. Acute promyelocytic leukaemia has been reported in some series {636}. Occasionally the presenting features are those of a myelodysplastic syndrome or megakaryoblastic leukaemia {1169}.

Cases of acute lymphoblastic leukaemia (ALL) also occur following topoisomerase II inhibitors and are usually associated with a t(4;11)(q21;q23) chromosomal abnormality {1169}.

Genetics
The predominant cytogenetic finding is a balanced translocation involving 11q23 (the *MLL* gene) primarily t(9;11), t(11;19) and t(6;11) {1169}. Other observed abnormalities include t(8;21) and t(3;21) involving band 21q22, inv(16), t(8;16), and t(6;9) {636, 1016, 1061, 1067}. Cases of APL with a typical t(15;17)(q22;p21) may also be observed. Acute lymphoblastic leukaemia may also be observed and is usually associated with a t(4;11)(q21;q23) {1169}.

Prognosis and predictive factors
Preliminary data suggest that most cases respond to initial therapy in a manner similar to that of patients with *de novo* acute leukaemia of the corresponding type. Insufficient long-term follow-up exists to predict the ultimate survival of these patients {1061, 1067}.

Acute myeloid leukaemia not otherwise categorised

R.D. Brunning
E. Matutes
G. Flandrin
J. Vardiman

J. Bennett
D. Head
N.L. Harris

This category of the classification of the acute myeloid leukaemias encompasses those cases that do not fulfill criteria for inclusion in one of the previously described groups. The primary basis for subclassification within this category is the morphologic and cytochemical features of the leukaemia cells and the degree of maturation.

The defining criterion for acute myeloid leukaemia is twenty percent (20%) or more myeloblasts in the blood or marrow; the abnormal promyelocytes in APL and the promonocytes in AML with monocytic differentiation are considered blast equivalents. The classification or pure erythroid leukaemia is unique and is based on the percent of abnormal erythroblasts. It is recommended that the blast percentage in the marrow be determined from a 500 cell differential count using an acceptable Romanowsky stain. In the blood the differential should include 200 leukocytes; if there is a marked leukopenia, buffy coat smears should be used.

The major criteria required for this category are based on examination of bone marrow aspirates and blood smears. Bone marrow biopsy is necessary to assess marrow cellularity prior to and fol-

lowing therapy and for diagnosis of cases of hypocellular acute leukaemia, and for leukaemias associated with myelofibrosis. The recommendations for classification are applicable only to specimens obtained prior to chemotherapy.

Acute myeloblastic leukaemia, minimally differentiated

Definition
Acute myeloblastic leukaemia, minimally differentiated is an acute leukaemia with no evidence of myeloid differentiation by morphology and light microscopy cytochemistry {1339}. The myeloid nature of the blasts is demonstrated by immunological markers and/or ultrastructural studies including ultrastructural cytochemistry. Immunophenotyping studies are essential in all cases to distinguish this disease from acute lymphoblastic leukaemia.

ICD-O code   9872/3

Synonym
FAB: Acute myeloid leukaemia, M0

Epidemiology
These cases comprise approximately 5% of cases of AML. Most patients are adults.

Clinical features
Patients with AML, minimally differentiated usually present with evidence of marrow failure with anaemia, thrombocytopenia and neutropenia. There may be leukocytosis with markedly increased number of blasts.

Morphology and cytochemistry
The blasts are usually of medium size with dispersed nuclear chromatin, round

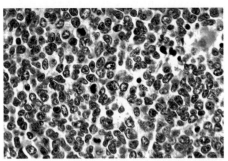

Fig. 4.19 Acute myeloblastic leukaemia, minimally differentiated. Bone marrow section. This marrow is completely replaced by blasts without differentiating features. There are numerous mitotic figures.

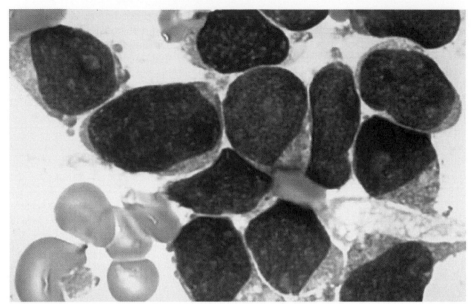

Fig. 4.20 Acute myeloblastic leukaemia, minimally differentiated. Bone marrow smear. The blasts vary in size, amount of cytoplasm and prominence of nucleoli. There are no differentiating features.

or slightly indented nuclei with one or two nucleoli. The cytoplasm is agranular with a varying degree of basophilia. Less frequently the blasts are small with more condensed chromatin, inconspicuous nucleoli and scanty cytoplasm resembling lymphoblasts. The cytochemical reactions for myeloperoxidase (MPO), Sudan Black B (SBB) and naphthol ASD chloroacetate esterase are negative (less than 3% positive blasts); alpha naphthyl acetate and butyrate esterases are negative or may show a nonspecific weak reaction distinct from that of monocytic cells.

In some unusual cases of acute myeloblastic leukaemia, minimally differentiated, there may be a residual normal population of maturing neutrophils. These cases may resemble acute myeloblastic leukaemia with maturation, but are distinguished by the absence of MPO or SBB positivity in the blasts and the absence of Auer Rods.

The marrow sections are usually markedly hypercellular with poorly differentiated blasts.

With sensitive ultrastructural studies, MPO activity may be demonstrated in small granules, endoplasmic reticulum, Golgi area and/or nuclear membranes.

Differential diagnosis

The differential diagnosis includes ALL, acute megakaryoblastic leukaemia, biphenotypic/mixed lineage acute leu-

kaemia and more rarely, the leukaemic phase of large cell lymphoma. Immunophenotyping studies are essential to distinguish these conditions.

Immunophenotype

Blast cells express one and usually more pan-myeloid antigens including CD13, CD33, and CD117 and are negative with B and T lymphoid restricted antibodies: cCD3, cCD79a, and cCD22. Anti-MPO may be positive in a few blasts, but is often negative. Most cases express primitive haematopoietic associated antigens such as CD34, CD38, and HLA-DR and generally lack antigens associated with myelomonocytic maturation such as CD11b, CD15, CD14, and CD65. TdT may be positive in one third or more of cases. Frequently, there may be expression of some antigens associated with but not specific for lymphoid differentiation including CD7, CD2, or CD19, but these are generally expressed at lower intensity than in lymphoid leukaemias.

Genetics

No unique chromosome abnormality has been identified in AML minimally differentiated. The most common abnormalities are complex karyotypes, trisomy 13, trisomy 8, trisomy 4 and monosomy 7 {1339}. The immunoglobulin heavy chain gene and T-cell receptor chain genes, in most cases, are in germline configuration.

Postulated cell of origin

Haematopoietic stem cell at the earliest stage of myeloid differentiation/maturation.

Prognosis and predictive factors

Minimally differentiated acute myeloid leukaemia appears to have a poor prognosis with a lower remission rate and more frequent early relapse and shorter survival compared to other AML types.

Acute myeloblastic leukaemia without maturation

Definition

Acute myeloblastic leukaemia without maturation is characterised by a high percentage of bone marrow blasts without significant evidence of maturation to more mature neutrophils. Blasts constitute ≥90% of the non-erythroid cells. The myeloid nature of the blasts is demonstrated by MPO or SBB (>3% of blasts) positivity and/or Auer rods.

ICD-O code   9873/3

Synonym

FAB: Acute myeloid leukaemia, M1

Epidemiology

AML without maturation comprises approximately 10% of cases of AML. It may occur at any age but the majority of patients are adults; the median age is approximately 46 years {1095}.

Clinical features

The patients usually present with evidence of marrow failure with anaemia, thrombocytopenia and neutropenia. There may be a leukocytosis with markedly increased blasts.

Morphology

Some cases of AML without maturation are characterised by obvious myeloblasts, some of which have azurophilic granulation and/or unequivocal Auer rods. In other cases, the blasts resemble lymphoblasts and lack azurophilic granules: MPO and SBB positivity is present in a variable number of blasts, but always ≥3%.

The bone marrow biopsy sections are usually markedly hypercellular. Normocellular or hypocellular cases may occur.

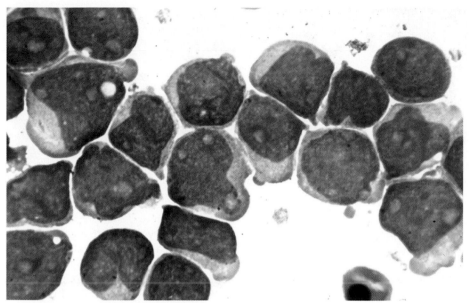

Fig. 4.21 Acute myeloblastic leukaemia without maturation. Bone marrow smear. The cells are predominantly myeloblasts; occasional myeloblasts contain azurophilic granules or Auer rods. There is no evidence of maturation beyond the myeloblast stage.

The blasts in sections may react with antibodies to MPO, lysozyme and CD34.

Differential diagnosis
The differential diagnosis includes acute lymphoblastic leukaemia in cases of AML without maturation with no granules and low percentage of MPO positive blasts, or AML with maturation when the latter shows a high percentage of blasts.

Immunophenotype
The blasts in AML without maturation express at least two myelomonocytic antigens including CD13, CD33, CD117 and/or MPO. CD34 is often positive. There is generally no expression of markers associated with monocytic matura-

tion such as CD11b or CD14. Immunohistochemistry in biopsy specimens may show reactivity of the blasts with antibodies to MPO, Lysozyme, CD117 and/or CD34. Lymphoid antigens such as CD3, CD20 and CD79a are typically absent.

Genetics
There is no demonstrated association between AML without maturation and specific recurrent chromosomal abnormalities. The immunoglobulin heavy chain gene and T-cell receptor chain genes, in most cases, are in germline configuration.

Postulated cell of origin
Precursor haematopoietic cell at the earliest stage of myeloid differentiation.

Prognosis and predictive factors
This type of acute myeloid leukaemia usually follows an aggressive course particularly in patients presenting with hyperleukocytosis.

Acute myeloblastic leukaemia with maturation

Definition
Acute myeloblastic leukaemia with maturation is characterised by the presence

of ≥20% blasts in the bone marrow or blood and evidence of maturation to more mature neutrophils (≥10% neutrophils at different stages of maturation); monocytes comprise <20% of bone marrow cells.

ICD-O code   9874/3

Synonym
FAB: Acute myeloid leukaemia, M2

Epidemiology
Acute myeloblastic leukaemia with maturation comprises approximately 30-45% of cases of AML {1225}. It occurs in all age groups; twenty percent of patients are less than 25 years of age and forty percent are ≥60 years of age {1225}.

Clinical features
Patients often present with symptoms related to anaemia, thrombocytopenia and neutropenia. The white blood cell count is variable as is the number of blasts.

Morphology
Blasts with and without azurophilic granulation are present. Auer rods are frequently present. Promyelocytes, myelocytes and mature neutrophils comprise ≥10% of the marrow cells; variable degrees of dysplasia are frequently present. The neutrophils may show abnormal nuclear segmentation, including hyper- and hypo-segmentation (pseudo Pelger-Huet nuclei), and/or hypogranulation. Eosinophil precursors are frequently increased but do not exhibit the cytological or cytochemical abnormalities characteristic of the eosinophils in acute myelomonocytic leukaemia (AMML), associated with inv(16). Basophils and/or

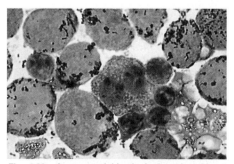

Fig. 4.22 Acute myeloblastic leukaemia without maturation. Bone marrow smear. Myeloperoxidase reaction showing numerous myeloblasts with strong peroxidase reactivity. There are several peroxidase negative erythroid precursors in the center.

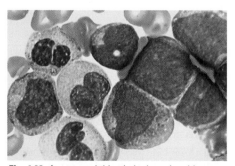

Fig. 4.23 Acute myeloblastic leukaemia with maturation. Bone marrow smear. In addition to the myeloblasts, there are several more mature neutrophils; one neutrophil has a pseudo Pelger-Huet nucleus.

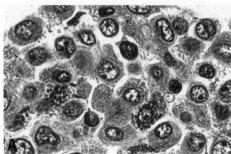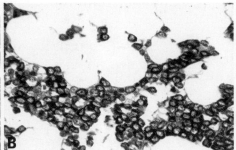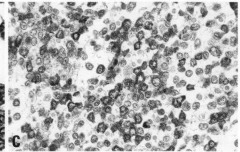

Fig. 4.24 Acute myeloid leukaemia with maturation. **A** Bone marrow biopsy presents the myeloblasts with abundant cytoplasm and azurophilic granules. Occasional blasts contain an Auer rod. Scattered eosinophils are present. **B, C** In these bone marrow biopsies numerous blasts show intense myeloperoxidase activity **(B)** and lysozyme positivity **(C)**.

mast cells are sometimes increased. Cases with increased marrow basophils may have recurrent cytogenetic abnormalities, including deletions and translocations at 12p (11-13) and t(6;9) (p23;q34). AML with the t(8;21)(q22:q22) is usually AML with maturation, and is described under AML with recurrent genetic abnormalities.

The marrow biopsy is usually hypercellular. The blasts and maturing neutrophils show reactivity with antibodies to MPO and lysozyme.

Differential diagnosis
The differential diagnosis includes refractory anaemia with excess blasts in cases with a low blast percentage, acute myeloid leukaemia without maturation when the percentage of blasts is high, and acute myelomonocytic leukaemia in cases with increased monocytes.

Immunophenotype
The blasts in AML with maturation usually express one or more of the myeloid-associated antigens, CD13, CD33, and CD15. They may express CD117, CD34, and HLA-DR.

Genetics
Deletion and translocations involving chromosome 12p band 11-13, such as del(12)(p11-p13) are associated with increased bone marrow basophils. The translocation t(6;9)(p23;q34) results in the formation of a chimeric fusion gene: *DEK/CAN*. Rare cases have t(8;16) (p11;p13); these are often associated with haemophagocytosis, particularly erythrophagocytosis {899, 1226}.

Postulated cell of origin
Haematopoietic precursor cell at the earliest stage of myeloid development.

Prognosis and predictive factors
AML with maturation responds frequently to aggressive therapy. Survival rates vary. Cases with a t(8;21) have a favourable prognosis. Cases with t(6;9)(p23;q34) have an overall poor prognosis.

Acute myelomonocytic leukaemia

Definition
Acute myelomonocytic leukaemia (AMML) is an acute leukaemia characterised by the proliferation of both neutrophil and monocyte precursors. The bone marrow has ≥20% blasts; neutrophils and their precursors and monocytes and their precursors each comprise ≥20% of marrow cells. This arbitrary minimal limit of 20% monocytes and precursors distinguishes AMML from cases of AML with or without maturation in which some monocytes may be present. A high number (usually ≥ 5x10⁹/l) of circulating blood monocytic cells may be present.

ICD-O code   9867/3

Synonym
FAB: Acute myeloid leukaemia, M4

Clinical features
Patients typically present with anaemia and thrombocytopenia, fever and fatigue. The white blood cell count may be high with numerous blasts.

Epidemiology
Acute myelomonocytic leukaemia comprises approximately 15-25% of cases of AML {1225}. Some patients have a pre-

ceding history of chronic myelomonocytic leukaemia. It occurs in all age groups but is more common in older individuals; the median age is 50 years. There is a male to female ratio of 1.4 to 1.0.

Morphology and cytochemistry
The monoblasts are large cells, with abundant cytoplasm which can be moderately to intensely basophilic and may show pseudopod formation. Scattered fine azurophilic granules and vacuoles may be present. The monoblasts usually have round nuclei with delicate lacy chromatin, and one or more large prominent nucleoli. Promonocytes have a more irregular and delicately convoluted nuclear configuration; the cytoplasm is usually less basophilic and sometimes more obviously granulated, with occasional large azurophilic granules and vacuoles. Monocytes and promonocytes may not always be readily distinguishable in routinely stained bone marrow smears. The peripheral blood typically shows an increase in monocytes, which are often more mature than those in the marrow. The monocytic component may be more evident in the blood than in the marrow.

At least 3% of the blasts should show myeloperoxidase (MPO) positivity. The monoblasts, promonocytes, and monocytes are typically non-specific esterase positive, although in some cases reactivity may be weak or absent. If the cells meet morphologic criteria for monocytes, absence of NSE does not exclude the diagnosis. Double staining for NSE and naphthol ASD chloroacetate esterase or MPO may show dual positive cells.

Differential diagnosis
The major differential diagnoses include AML with maturation and acute monocyt-

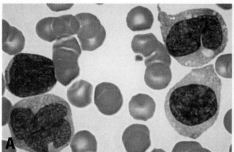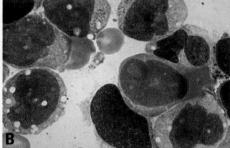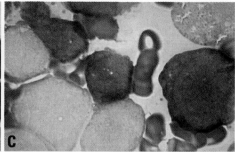

Fig. 4.25 Acute myelomonocytic leukaemia. **A** Blood smear, myeloblast, monoblast, and promonocytes. **B** Bone marrow smear. Myeloblasts and several more mature monocytes including promonocytes. **C** Non-specific esterase reaction on a bone marrow smear. Several NSE positive cells are present. The non-reacting cells are predominantly myeloblasts and neutrophil precursors.

ic leukaemia. The distinction from both of these types is based on the cytochemical findings and percent of monocytic cells.

Immunophenotype

These leukaemias variably express myeloid antigens (CD13, CD33) and generally show some markers characteristic of monocytic differentiation such as CD14, CD4, CD11b, CD11c, CD64, CD36 and lysozyme. Intensity of expression of many of these markers, or patterns of coexpression of some of these in combination may be particularly helpful in the recognition of monocytic differentiation. There is often a residual population of less-differentiated myeloblasts that expresses CD34 and pan-myeloid markers.

Genetics

Nonspecific cytogenetic abnormalities are present in the majority of the cases. Cases with inv(16) are described under AML with recurrent genetic abnormalities. Some cases may have abnormalities of 11q23 (see AML with recurrent genetic abnormalities).

Postulated cell of origin

Haematopoietic precursor cell with potential to differentiate into neutrophil and monocytic lineages.

Prognosis and predictive factors

Acute myelomonocytic leukaemia frequently responds to aggressive therapy. Survival rates vary. Patients with increased and abnormal marrow eosinophils with associated abnormality involving chromosome 16 have a favourable prognosis (see section on AML with recurrent translocations). Other cases have a survival similar to other types of AML.

Acute monoblastic leukaemia and acute monocytic leukaemia

Definition

Acute monoblastic leukaemia and acute monocytic leukaemia are myeloid leukaemias in which 80% or more of the leukaemic cells are of monocytic lineage including monoblasts, promonocytes, and monocytes; a minor neutrophil component, less than 20%, may be present. Acute monoblastic leukaemia and acute monocytic leukaemia are distinguished by the relative proportions of monoblasts and promonocytes. In acute monoblastic leukaemia, the majority of the monocytic cells are monoblasts (typically ≥80%). In acute monocytic leukaemia, the majority of the monocytic cells are promonocytes.

ICD-O code   9891/3

Synonym

FAB: Acute monoblastic leukaemia, M5a; Acute monocytic leukaemia, M5b.

Epidemiology

Acute monoblastic leukaemia comprises 5-8% of cases of AML {1225}. It may occur at any age but is most common in young individuals.
In infancy it is frequently associated with abnormalities of 11q23. Extramedullary lesions may occur. Acute monocytic leukaemia comprises 3-6% of cases of AML; the male to female ratio is 1.8 to 1.0. It is more common in adults; the median age is 49 years {1225}.

Clinical features

Bleeding disorders are common presenting features. Extramedullary masses and cutaneous and gingival infiltration and CNS involvement are common.

Morphology and cytochemistry

Monoblasts are large cells, with abundant cytoplasm which can be moderately to intensely basophilic and may show pseudopod formation. Scattered fine azurophilic granules and vacuoles may be present. The monoblasts usually have round nuclei with delicate lacy chromatin, and one or more large prominent nucleoli. Promonocytes have a more irregular and delicately convoluted nuclear configuration; the cytoplasm is usually less basophilic and sometimes more obviously granulated, with occasional large azurophilic granules and vacuoles.
Auer rods are rare in acute monoblastic leukaemia and, when present, are usually in cells identifiable as myeloblasts. Haemophagocytosis (erythrophagocytosis) may be observed and suggests an associated t(8;16)(p11;p13) {1226}.
The monoblasts and promonocytes usually show intense non-specific esterase activity in most cases. In up to 10-20% of cases of acute monoblastic leukaemia, the non-specific esterase reaction is negative or very weakly positive. In some of these, immunophenotyping may be necessary to establish monocytic differentiation. Monoblasts are typically myeloperoxidase (MPO) negative; promonocytes may show some scattered MPO positivity.
The marrow biopsy in acute monoblastic leukaemia is usually hypercellular with a predominant population of large, poorly differentiated blasts with abundant cytoplasm. Nucleoli may be prominent. The monoblast typically reacts with antibody to lysozyme and usually is non-reactive with antibody to MPO. The promonocytes in acute monocytic leukaemia, show marked nuclear lobulation and react with antibodies to lysozyme and CD68 (PG-M1). Similar patterns of reactivity are

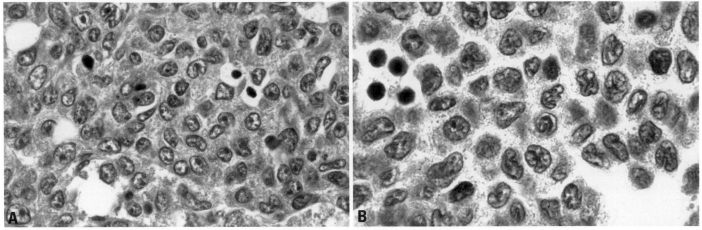

Fig. 4.26 Acute monoblastic leukaemia. **A** Bone marrow biopsy showing complete replacement by a population of large blasts with abundant cytoplasm. The nuclei are generally round to oval; occasional nuclei are distorted. **B** Acute monocytic leukaemia. Bone marrow section. The nuclear folds in the promonocytes are prominent.

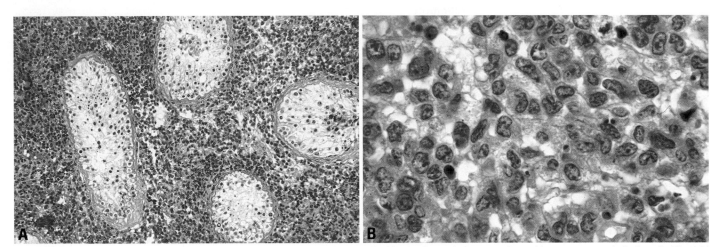

Fig. 4.27 Acute monocytic leukaemia, testicular infiltration. **A** Low magnification of a biopsy of a testis from a patient with acute monocytic leukaemia. There is extensive expansion and infiltration of the space between the seminiferous tubules. **B** The monocytic cells have relatively abundant cytoplasm and very dispersed chromatin; nucleoli are not prominent.

present in extramedullary lesions. The extramedullary lesion may be predominantly of monoblasts or promonocytes or an admixture of two cell types.

Differential diagnosis

The major differential diagnosis of acute monoblastic leukaemia includes AML without maturation, AML minimally differentiated, and acute megakaryoblastic leukaemia. Extramedullary monoblastic sarcomas may be confused with malignant lymphoma or soft tissue sarcomas; they are distinguished from non-Hodgkin lymphomas by reactivity with antibodies to CD68 and/or lysozyme and lack of expression of lymphoid antigens. Occasional cases resemble prolymphocytic leukaemia; they are readily distinguished by immunophenotypic analysis and cytochemistry. The major differential diagno-

sis of acute monocytic leukaemia includes AMML and microgranular APL. These can be distinguished with well stained smears. The abnormal promyelocytes in APL are intensely MPO positive whereas the monocytes are weakly reactive or negative.

Immunophenotype

These leukaemias variably express myeloid antigens CD13, CD33, CD117 and generally show some markers characteristic of monocytic differentiation including CD14, CD4, CD11b, CD11c, CD64, CD68, CD36, and lysozyme. CD34 is frequently negative, and CD33 is often very brightly expressed. Many cases will not express more mature markers of monocytic differentiation such as CD14, while CD36, CD64, CD4, and CD11c are more frequently expressed.

Intensity of many of these markers, or patterns of coexpression of some of these in combination may be particularly helpful in the recognition of monocytic differentiation. By flow cytometry, MPO antigen may be expressed in acute monocytic leukaemia and less often in monoblastic leukaemia. By immunohistochemistry in paraffin-embedded marrow biopsy specimens and in extramedullary monocytic sarcomas, lysozyme is typically expressed, while myeloperoxidase is typically negative or weakly positive in some cases; CD68 (PG-M1) may be positive.

Genetics

There is a strong association between acute monoblastic leukaemia and deletions and translocations involving chromosome 11 band q23; these cases are included with AML with recurrent genetic abnormalities. Occasional cases of acute monocytic leukaemia and acute myelomonocytic leukaemia (AMML), and occasionally AML with or without maturation may manifest a similar abnormality. Translocation t(8;16)(p11;p13) may be associated with acute monocytic leukaemia or AMML and, in the majority of cases, is associated with haemo-phago-cytosis by leukaemic cells, particularly erythrophagocytosis and coagulopathy. These findings may also be observed in AML with maturation.

Postulated cell of origin
Bone marrow stem cell with some commitment to monocytic differentiation.

Prognosis and predictive factors
Both acute monoblastic leukaemia and acute monocytic leukaemia differentiated may follow an aggressive clinical course.

Acute erythroid leukaemias

Definition
Acute erythroid leukaemias are acute leukaemias that are characterised by a predominant erythroid population. Two subtypes are recognised based on the presence or absence of a significant myeloid component.

Erythroleukaemia (erythroid/myeloid)
This subtype is defined by the presence in the bone marrow of ≥50% erythroid precursors in the entire nucleated cell population and ≥20% myeloblasts in the non-erythroid cell population, i.e. the myeloblasts are calculated as a percent of the non-erythroid bone marrow cells.

Pure erythroid leukaemia
This represents a neoplastic proliferation of immature cells committed exclusively to the erythroid lineage (>80% of marrow cells) with no evidence of a significant myeloblastic component {419}.

ICD-O code   9840/3

Synonyms
FAB: Acute myeloid leukaemia M6a (erythroid/myeloid)
Acute myeloid leukaemia, M6b (pure erythroid leukaemia)
Erythremic myelosis (pure erythroid)

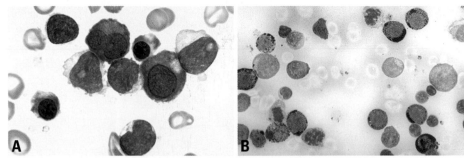

Fig. 4.28 Acute erythroleukaemia, erythroid/myeloid. **A** Bone marrow smear. Myeloblasts and several erythroid precursors showing dyserythropoietic changes are present. **B** Bone marrow smear. Periodic acid-Schiff reaction. There are several erythroid precursors at varying stages of maturation with PAS positive cytoplasm. The more immature precursors have a coarsely granular-globular reaction; the later stage precursors have a diffuse cytoplasmic positivity.

Epidemiology
Erythroleukaemia (erythroid/myeloid) is predominantly a disease of adults. It comprises approximately 5-6% of cases of AML {1225}. Pure erythroid leukaemia is extremely rare and can occur at any age, including childhood. Occasional cases of chronic myeloid leukaemia undergo erythroblastic transformation and show features similar to erythroleukaemia or more rarely, pure erythroid leukaemia.

Clinical features
The clinical features of the erythroid leukaemias are not unique but profound anaemia and normoblastemia are common. Erythroleukaemia (erythroid/myeloid) may present *de novo* or evolve from a myelodysplastic syndrome, either refractory anaemia with excess of blasts (RAEB) or refractory anaemia with multilineage dysplasia with or without ringed sideroblasts.

Morphology and cytochemistry
Erythroleukaemia (erythroid/myeloid): All maturation stages of the erythroid precursors may be present, frequently with a shift to immaturity. The erythroid precursors are dysplastic with megaloblastoid nuclei and/or bi or multinucleated forms; the cytoplasm in the more immature cells frequently contains poorly demarcated vacuoles, which may coalesce. Large multinucleated erythroid cells may be

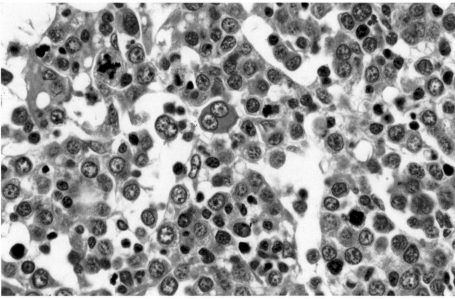

Fig. 4.29 Acute erythroid leukaemia; erythroid myeloid leukaemia. Bone marrow biopsy. There is a population of erythroid precursors and myeloblasts reflecting the dual lineage hyperplasia. A binucleate megakaryocyte is present.

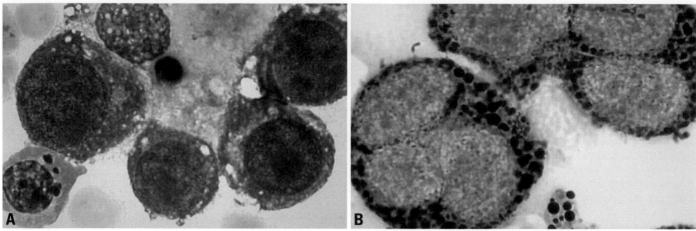

Fig. 4.30 Pure erythroid leukaemia. **A** Bone marrow smear shows four abnormal proerythroblasts. The erythroblasts are large with finely dispersed chromatin, prominent nucleoli and cytoplasmic vacuoles, some of which are coalescent. **B** Periodic acid-Schiff stain. The cytoplasm of the proerythroblasts shows intense globular PAS positivity.

present. The myeloblasts are of medium size, often containing a few cytoplasmic granules and occasionally Auer rods and are similar to the myeloblasts in AML with and without maturation. The iron stain may show ringed sideroblasts and the PAS stain may be positive in the erythroid precursors either in a globular or diffuse pattern. The myeloperoxidase (MPO) and Sudan Black B (SBB) stains may be positive in the myeloblasts.

The marrow biopsy in erythroid myeloid leukaemia is usually hypercellular. There may be prominent megakaryocytic dysplasia.

Pure erythroid leukaemia: The undifferentiated form of pure erythroid leukaemia is usually characterised by the presence of medium to large size erythroblasts usually with round nuclei, fine chromatin and one or more nucleoli; the cytoplasm is deeply basophilic, often agranular and frequently contains poorly demarcated vacuoles which are often PAS positive. More rarely the blasts may be smaller and resemble the lymphoblasts of ALL. Transmission electron microscopy demonstrates features characteristic of the erythroid cells such as free ferritin particles or siderosomes in the cytoplasm and rhopheocytosis. A platelet peroxidase like reaction has also been described. The blasts are negative for MPO and SBB; they show reactivity with alpha-naphthyl acetate esterase, acid phosphatase and PAS, the latter usually in a block-like staining pattern.

In the marrow biopsies of pure acute erythroid leukaemia the cells appear undifferentiated. Reactivity with antibody to

haemoglobin A varies from a few scattered positive cells to numerous positive cells.

Differential diagnosis

Erythroleukaemia (erythroid/myeloid) should be distinguished from RAEB and acute myeloid leukaemia with maturation with increased erythroid precursors. A bone marrow differential count of all nucleated cells should be performed. If the erythroid precursors are ≥50% of all cells, the differential count of non-erythroid cells should be calculated. If blasts are ≥20% of non-erythroid cells, the diagnosis is erythroleukaemia (erythroid/myeloid); if <20%, the diagnosis is RAEB.

The differential diagnosis also includes AML with multilineage dysplasia. If there is dysplasia involving ≥50% of myeloid or megakaryocyte-lineage cells, the case should be classified as AML with multilineage dysplasia.

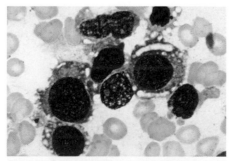

Fig. 4.31 Pure erythroid leukaemia. Bone marrow smear with numerous very immature erythroid precursors; these cells have cytoplasmic vacuoles which occasionally coalesce.

The differential diagnosis of pure erythroid leukaemia includes megaloblastic anaemia due to vitamin B12 or folate deficiency. Patients with vitamin B12 and/or folate deficiency respond to these vitamins and the dysplastic changes are not generally as marked as in pure erythroid leukaemia. Neutrophil precursors with premature nuclear segmentation are an additional hallmark of B12 and folate deficiency.

Pure erythroid leukaemia without morphologic evidence of erythroid maturation may be difficult to distinguish from other types of AML, particularly megakaryoblastic, and also from ALL or lymphoma. Lack of expression of lymphoid antigens will exclude the latter diagnoses.* Distinction from megakaryoblastic leukaemia is the most difficult; if the immunophenotype is characteristic of erythroid precursors, a diagnosis can be established, however some cases are ambiguous and there may be cases with concurrent erythroid-megakaryocytic involvement. If these cases satisfy the criteria for multilineage involvement, they should be classified as acute myeloid leukaemia with multilineage involvement.

Immunophenotype

Erythroleukaemia (erythroid/myeloid)

The erythroblasts in erythroleukaemia generally lack myeloid-associated markers and are negative with anti-MPO; they react with antibodies to glycophorin A and haemoglobin A. The myeloblasts express a variety of myeloid associated antigens including CD13, CD33, CD117

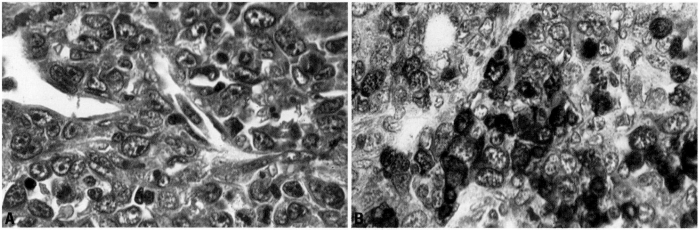

Fig. 4.32 Pure erythroid leukaemia. Bone marrow section. Composite figure of pure acute erythroid leukaemia showing a predominant population of very immature erythroid precursors in **A** routinely stained section and **B** section stained for haemoglobin A. Many of the erythroid precursors including the very immature ones are reactive.

(c-kit) and MPO with or without expression of precursor-cell markers; e.g., CD34 and class-II HLA-DR determinants similar to the blasts in other AML subtypes.

Pure erythroid leukaemia
The more differentiated forms can be detected by the expression of glycophorin A and haemoglobin A and absence of MPO and other myeloid markers; the blasts are often negative with monoclonal antibodies to class II HLA-DR determinants and CD34. The more immature forms are usually negative for glycophorin A or this is only weakly expressed in a minority of blasts; other markers such as carbonic anhydrase 1, Gero antibody against the Gerbich blood group or CD36 are usually positive as they detect erythroid progenitors at earlier stages of differentiation. CD36 is not specific for erythroblasts and may be expressed by monocytes and megakaryocytes. Antigens associated with mega-karyocytes (CD41 and CD61) are typically negative but may be partially expressed in some cases.
Immunohistochemical reactivity with antibody to haemoglobin A may be helpful in establishing cell origin in biopsy specimens.

Genetics
There is no specific chromosome abnormality described in this type of AML. Complex karyotypes with multiple structural abnormalities are common, with chromosomes 5 and 7 the most frequently affected.

Postulated cell of origin
Erythroleukaemia (erythroid/myeloid)
Multipotent stem-cell with wide myeloid potential.

Pure erythroid leukaemia
Primitive (BFU-E/CFU-E) stem cell with some degree of commitment to the erythroid lineage.

Prognosis and predictive factors
Erythromyeloid leukaemia is generally associated with an aggressive clinical course. The morphologic findings may evolve to a more predominant myeloblast picture. Pure erythroid leukaemia is usually associated with a rapid clinical course.

Acute megakaryoblastic leukaemia

Definition
Acute megakaryoblastic leukaemia is an acute leukaemia in which ≥50% of the blasts are of megakaryocyte lineage.

ICD-O code   9910/3

Synonym
FAB: Acute myeloid leukaemia, M7

Epidemiology
Acute megakaryoblastic leukaemia occurs in both adults and children. This is an uncommon disease comprising approximately 3-5% of cases of AML.

Clinical features
Patients present with cytopenias, often thrombocytopenia although some may have thrombocytosis. Dysplastic features in the neutrophils and platelets may be present. Organomegaly, e.g., hepatosplenomegaly is infrequent except in children with acute megakaryoblastic leukaemia associated with the t(1;22) who often present with prominent abdominal masses {103}. Radiographic evidence of bone lytic lesions has been observed in children. An association of acute megakaryoblastic leukaemia and mediastinal germ cell tumours has been observed in young adult males {950}. The leukaemic process presents 0-122 months following the diagnosis of the germ cell tumour. Other types of AML and histiocytosis have also been reported.

Morphology and cytochemistry
The megakaryoblasts are usually of medium to large size (12-18 μ) with a round, slightly irregular or indented nucleus with fine reticular chromatin and one to three nucleoli. The cytoplasm is basophilic, often agranular, and may show distinct blebs or pseudopod formation. In some cases the blasts are predominantly small with a high nuclear-cytoplasmic ratio resembling lymphoblasts; large and small blasts may be present in the same patients. Occasionally, the blasts occur in small clusters. Circulating micromega-karyocytes, megakaryoblastic fragments, dysplastic large platelets and hypogranular neutrophils may be present. Micro-megakaryocytes are small cells with 1 or 2 round nuclei with condensed chromatin

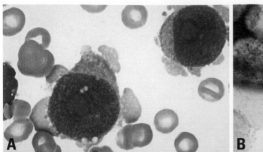

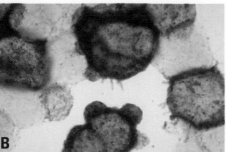

Fig. 4.33 Acute megakaryoblastic leukaemia. **A** Bone marrow smear. The two megakaryoblasts are large cells with cytoplasmic pseudopod formation; portions of the cytoplasm are "zoned" with granular basophilic areas and clear cytoplasm. Nucleoli are unusually prominent. **B** Bone marrow smear reacted with antibody to CD61 (platelet glycoprotein IIIa). The cytoplasm of the megakaryoblasts is intensely reactive (APAAP).

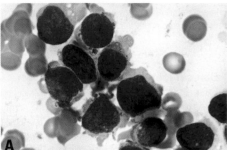

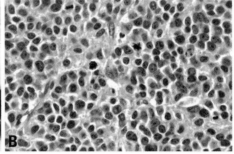

Fig. 4.34 Acute megakaryoblastic leukaemia, poorly differentiated. **A** This marrow smear from a 22 month-old child is completely replaced by poorly differentiated blasts which by flow cytometry expressed CD61 (platelet glycoprotein IIIa) and CD41 (platelet glycoprotein IIb/IIIa). **B** Bone marrow section.

and mature cytoplasm; these should not be counted as blasts. In some patients, because of extensive marrow fibrosis resulting in a "dry tap", the percent of marrow blasts is estimated from the marrow biopsy. Imprints of the biopsy may also be useful. Although acute megakaryoblastic leukaemia may be associated with extensive fibrosis, this is not an invariant finding.

The histopathology of the biopsy varies from cases with a uniform population of poorly differentiated blasts to a mixture of poorly differentiated blasts and maturing dysplastic megakaryocytes; varying degrees of reticulin fibrosis may be present. The megakaryoblasts in megakaryoblastic leukaemia associated with a t(1;22)(p13;q13) in infants may show a stromal pattern of marrow infiltration mimicking a metastatic tumour {103, 182}. Cytochemical stains for SBB and MPO are consistently negative in the megakaryoblasts; the blasts may show reactivity with PAS and acid phosphatase and a punctuate non-specific esterase reactivity. Electron microscopy cytochemistry shows the blasts to contain peroxidase activity confined to the

nuclear membranes and endoplasmic reticulum with the platelet peroxidase (PPO) reaction; this is not demonstrable by the myeloperoxidase (MPO) reaction on fixed cells.

Differential diagnosis

The differential diagnosis includes minimally differentiated AML, acute panmyelosis with myelofibrosis, ALL, pure erythroid leukaemia, and blastic transformation of chronic myeloid leukaemia or idiopathic myelofibrosis. In both of the latter two conditions there is usually a history of a chronic phase and splenomegaly is an almost constant finding. In addition, in idiopathic myelofibrosis there are marked changes in the red cell morphology; in chronic myeloid leukaemia a Philadelphia chromosome or BCR/ABL fusion protein is always documented. Some metastatic tumours in the bone marrow, particularly in children, e.g. alveolar rhabdomyosarcoma, may resemble acute megakaryoblastic leukaemia. Acute megakaryoblastic leukaemia with t(1,22) in infants may mimic metastatic neuroblastoma, particularly in sections. The distinction between acute megakary-

oblastic leukaemia and acute panmyelosis with fibrosis is not always completely clear. In general, acute megakaryoblastic leukaemia represents a proliferation predominantly of megakaryoblasts. Acute panmyelosis is characterised by a trilineage proliferation, i.e. granulocytes, megakaryocytes and erythroid precursors. In some instances a clear distinction cannot be made.

Immunophenotype

The megakaryoblasts express one or more of the platelet glycoproteins: CD41 glycoprotein (IIb/IIIa), and/or CD61 (glycoprotein IIIa). The more mature platelet-associated marker CD42 (glycoprotein Ib) is less frequently present. The myeloid markers CD13 and CD33 may be positive although CD34, the panleukocyte marker CD45, and class II HLA-DR are often negative, especially in children; CD36 is characteristically positive.

Blasts are negative with the anti-MPO antibody and with other markers of myeloid differentiation. Lymphoid markers and TdT are not expressed, but there may be aberrant expression of CD7. Cytoplasmic expression of CD41 or CD61 are more specific and sensitive than surface staining, particularly by flow cytometry, because of possible adherence of platelets to blast cells.

In the bone marrow trephine biopsies abnormal megakaryocytes and in some cases megakaryoblasts can be recognised by a positive reaction with antibodies to factor VIII or the platelet glycoproteins (CD61); the detection of the latter marker is highly dependent on proce-

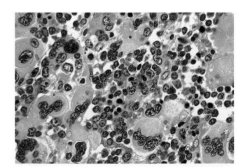

Fig. 4.35 Acute megakaryoblastic leukaemia. This bone marrow biopsy from an adult with acute megakaryoblastic leukaemia shows virtually complete replacement by a population of blasts and well differentiated megakaryocytes. There is a minor population of erythroid precursors. The blasts expressed CD61 (platelet glycoprotein IIIa).

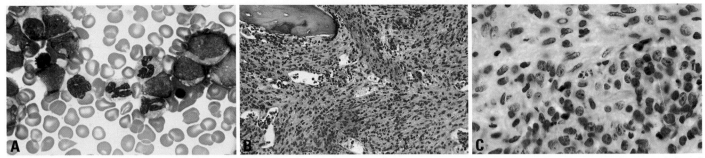

Fig. 4.36 Acute myeloid leukaemia with associated t(1;22)(p13;q13). **A** Bone marrow smear from a 3.5 month-old child contains a heteromorphous population of blasts. **B** Bone marrow section shows extensive replacement of marrow by intertwining bundles of blast cells. **C** High magnification of the specimen shows blasts without differentiating features.

dures used for fixation and decalcification.

Genetics

There is no unique chromosomal abnormality associated with acute megakaryoblastic leukaemia in adults; some cases show inv(3)(q21;q26) but this abnormality is also found in other types of acute myeloid leukaemia, e.g., AML without maturation, or AML with maturation often in association with thrombocytosis.

In children and particularly infants under 1 year of age, there may be an association with a t(1;22)(p13;q13), with distinct clinical features {103, 182}.

In young males with mediastinal germ cell tumours and acute megakaryoblastic leukaemia, several cytogenetic abnormalities have been observed including i(12p).

Postulated cell of origin

Haemopoietic precursor cell committed to the megakaryocytic lineage and possibly erythroid lineage and/or able to differentiate into these lineages.

Prognosis and predictive factors

Prognosis is usually poor, particularly in infants with the t(1;22).

Variant: Acute myeloid leukaemia / transient myeloproliferative disorder in Down syndrome

Definition

Individuals with Down syndrome have an increased predisposition to acute leukaemia, predominantly myeloid type {1442, 1441}. The major morphologic subtype appears to be acute megakaryoblastic leukaemia. In some patients the leukaemia undergoes spontaneous remission; this latter process has been referred to as transient myeloproliferative disorder or transient leukaemia.

Clinical features

This disorder usually manifests in the neonatal period frequently with marked leukocytosis. The blast percentage in the blood is usually in excess of thirty and frequently exceeds fifty percent. The magnitude of the leukocyte count or the degree of thrombocytopenia are not reliable distinguishing features between acute leukaemia and the transient disease. There may be prominent extramedullary involvement.

Morphology and cytochemistry

The morphology of the leukaemic cells in the major type of AML in Down syndrome patients is somewhat unusual. The blasts are 12-15 υm with round to slightly irregular nuclei and a moderate amount of basophilic cytoplasm; cytoplasmic blebs may be present. The cytoplasm of a variable number of blasts contains coarse azurophilic granules resembling basophil granules. Promegakaryocytes and micromegakaryocytes are frequently present. Dyserythropoiesis is common; dys-granulopoiesis is usually minimal. The blasts in the "transient" myeloproliferative disorder are morphologically indistinguishable from the blasts in the cases of persistent leukaemia. Increased basophils may be observed in the blood {1442}.

The blasts are MPO and SBB and TdT negative. Some blasts contain scattered granular PAS positivity. A variable percentage of blasts manifests platelet peroxidase reactivity by ultrastructural cytochemistry.

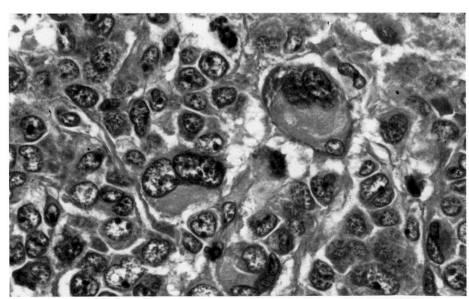

Fig. 4.37 Acute megakaryoblastic leukaemia in a patient with Down syndrome. Lymph node. Abdominal lymph node from an infant with Down syndrome and acute megakaryoblastic leukaemia. There is extensive nodal replacement by megakaryoblasts and occasional mature megakaryocytes.

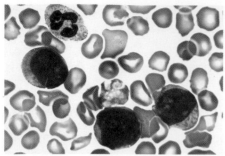

Fig. 4.38 Transient myeloproliferative disorder in Down syndrome. Blood smear. Three blasts. This process underwent spontaneous remission in eight weeks with no evidence of recurrence eighteen years later.

Immunophenotype

The markers expressed are generally similar to those of other cases of megakaryoblastic leukaemia in childhood; the blasts may also express CD7.

Genetics

In addition to trisomy 21, some cases show additional clonal abnormalities; the most frequent is trisomy 8 {1442, 688}. The t(1;22) is not found. Studies with fluorescent *in situ* hybridisation have shown that the additional cytogenetic abnormalities are present in erythroid precursors as well as in the megakaryoblasts.

Molecular studies in a few cases with the transient myeloproliferative disorder have shown clonality by X-chromosome linked polymorphism analysis.

Postulated cell of origin

Myeloid precursor cell with potential for megakaryocytic and erythroid differentiation.

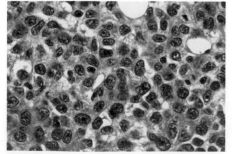

Fig. 4.39 Acute basophilic leukaemia. Bone marrow trephine biopsy. The blasts are poorly differentiated.

Prognosis

In the transient cases the process remits spontaneously in one to three months. Recurrence followed by second remission or persistent disease may occur. Cases with persistent disease typically respond well to a modified therapeutic regimen for childhood AML but most ultimately relapse and die of their disease.

Acute basophilic leukaemia

Definition

Acute basophilic leukaemia is an acute myeloid leukaemia in which the primary differentiation is to basophils. Some cases may represent blast transformation of a clinically and haematologically undetected Philadelphia chromosome, *BCR/ABL* positive CML {1030}.

ICD-O code   9870/3

Epidemiology

This is a very rare disease with a relatively small number of reported cases, comprising <1% of all cases of AML.

Clinical features

As in other acute leukaemias, patients present with features related to bone marrow failure and may or may not have circulating blasts. In addition, cutaneous involvement, organomegaly, some lytic lesions and symptoms related to hyper-histaminemia may be present.

Morphology and cytochemistry

The circulating blood and bone marrow blasts are medium size with a high nuclear-cytoplasmic ratio, an oval, round or bilobed nucleus characterised by dispersed chromatin and one to three prominent nucleoli. The cytoplasm is moderately basophilic and contains a variable number of coarse basophilic granules which may stain positive in metachromatic stains; vacuolation of the cytoplasm may be present. Mature basophils are usually sparse. Dysplastic features in the erythroid precursors may be present. Electron microscopy shows that the granules contain structures characteristic of either basophil precursors or mast cells; they contain an electron-dense particulate substance, are internally bisected, e.g. have a theta character, or contain crystalline material arranged in a pattern of scrolls or lamellae, the latter finding is more typical of mast cells. Coexistence of basophil and mast cell granules may be identified in the same immature cells {1030}.

The most characteristic cytochemical reaction is metachromatic positivity with toluidine blue. In addition, the blasts usually show a diffuse pattern of staining with acid phosphatase and, in some cases, PAS positivity in blocks; the blasts are often negative by light microscopy for SBB, MPO and non-specific esterase; however, with electron microscopy peroxidase activity may be detected in the nuclear membrane, endoplasmic reticulum and granules.

The bone marrow trephine biopsy shows diffuse replacement by blasts cells, sometimes with an increased number of basophil precursors. In cases with mast cell differentiation, differentiated mast cells having a distinct morphology with an oval nucleus and elongated cytoplasm, may be identified close to the trabeculi. Reticulin fibrosis is often prominent in the latter cases.

Differential diagnosis

The differential diagnosis includes blast crisis of CML, other AML subtypes with basophilia such as AML with maturation (M2) associated with abnormalities of 12p or t(6;9), acute eosinophilic leukaemia and, more rarely, a rare subtype of acute lymphoblastic leukaemia with prominent coarse granules.

The clinical features, cytogenetics and blast cell morphology will distinguish between cases presenting "*de novo*" from those resulting from transformation of a chronic myeloid leukaemia and from AML with basophilia. Immunological markers will distinguish between granulated acute lymphoblastic leukaemia and acute basophilic leukaemia and light microscopic cytochemistry for myeloperoxidase and electron microscopy will distinguish acute basophilic leukaemia from eosinophilic leukaemia.

Immunophenotype

The blasts express myeloid markers such as CD13 and CD33 and early haematopoietic markers, CD34 and class-II HLA-DR.

Usually the blasts show a positive reaction with CD9 and some cases may be TdT+ but are, as a rule, negative for specific lymphoid markers.

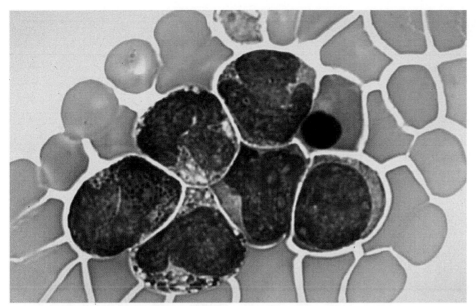

Fig. 4.40 Acute basophilic leukaemia. Bone marrow smear. Blasts and immature basophils. The basophil granules vary from large coarse granules to smaller granules.

Genetics
There is no consistent chromosome abnormality identified in these cases. Involvement of 12p or t(6;9), which may occur in some AML cases with increased basophils, have not been identified. A few cases may present as *de novo* Philadelphia chromosome positive acute leukaemia, with a t(9;22)(q34;q11).

Postulated cell of origin
Early myeloid cell committed to the basophil lineage.

Prognosis and predictive factors
Since this is a rare type of acute leukaemia, there is little information on survival. The cases observed have generally been associated with a poor prognosis.

Acute panmyelosis with myelofibrosis

Definition
Acute panmyelosis with myelofibrosis is an acute panmyeloid proliferation with accompanying fibrosis of the bone marrow {1248}.

Synonyms
Acute myelofibrosis
Acute myelosclerosis
Acute myelodysplasia with myelofibrosis

ICD-O code   9931/3

Epidemiology
Acute panmyelosis with myelofibrosis is a very rare form of AML. It is primarily a disease of adults but has also been reported in children. This process may occur either *de novo* or in patients who have been treated with alkylating-agent chemotherapy and/or radiation (see AML and MDS, therapy-related).

Clinical features
Patients present with constitutional symptoms including weakness and fatigue. Marked pancytopenia is common. There is no or minimal splenomegaly. The clinical evolution is usually rapidly progressive.

Morphology and cytochemistry
The blood usually shows marked pancytopenia. The red blood cells show no or minimal poikilocytosis; some degree of anisocytosis with a variable number of macrocytes and rare normoblasts are frequent. Occasional immature neutrophils including blasts may be identified. Dysplastic changes in myeloid cells are frequent. Atypical platelets may be noted.
Bone marrow aspiration is frequently unsuccessful; either no fluid marrow or a suboptimal specimen is obtained. The marrow biopsy is hypercellular with variable degrees of hyperplasia of the erythroid precursors, granulocytes and megakaryocytes. Foci of immature cells, including blasts, are scattered throughout the marrow; clusters of late stage erythroid precursors may be prominent. Megakaryocytes may be particularly conspicuous; an increased number of small to large megakaryocytes with dysplastic features is virtually always present; the nuclei are frequently non-lobated with dispersed chromatin. The cytoplasm is uniformly eosinophilic and may be accentuated with the periodic acid-Schiff stain and antibodies to factor VIII-associated antigen and CD61.
The degree of fibrosis is variable. In most patients there is a marked increase in reticulin fibers; frank collagenous fibrosis is uncommon.

Differential diagnosis
The major differential diagnosis of acute panmyelosis with myelofibrosis includes acute megakaryoblastic leukaemia, other types of acute leukaemia with associated marrow fibrosis, metastatic tumour with a desmoplastic reaction, and chronic idiopathic myelofibrosis (CIMF). The distinction between AML, particularly acute megakaryoblastic leukaemia with myelofibrosis and AML with multilineage dysplasia with fibrosis, and acute panmyelosis with myelofibrosis may be arbitrary and whether it is clinically relevant is not clear. In general, if the proliferative process is predominantly one cell type, i.e. the myeloblasts, and there is an associated fibrosis, the case should be classified as AML with a specific subtype designated with the qualifying phase "with myelofibrosis". If the proliferative process involves all of the major myeloid cell lines, i.e. the granulocytes, erythroid cells and megakaryocytes, the term acute panmyelosis with myelofibrosis is more appropriate. This may be a variant of AML with multilineage dysplasia in some cases. Immunohistochemistry is necessary to identify involvement of multiple cell lines.
Acute panmyelosis with myelofibrosis is distinguished from CIMF by the predominance of more immature cells in the acute process and the characteristics of the megakaryocytes. In CIMF the majority of the megakaryocytes have markedly contorted nuclei with condensed nuclear chromatin; in the acute process the chromatin is dispersed in many cells and non-lobated or hypolobated nuclei are

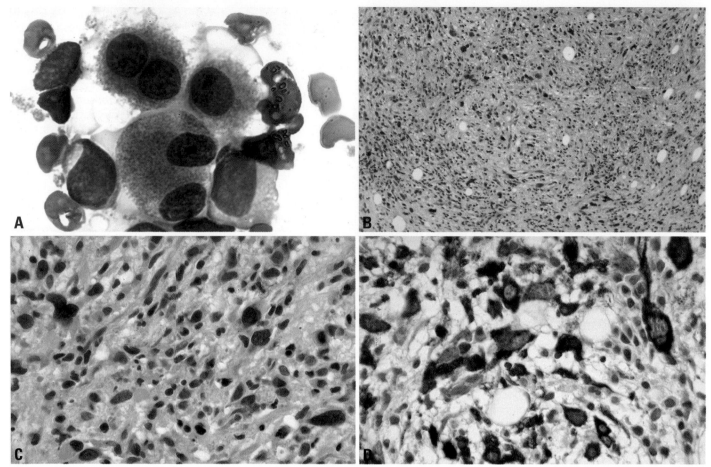

Fig. 4.41 Acute myelofibrosis. **A** A marrow trephine imprint from a patient with acute panmyelosis. There are several megakaryocytes with hypolobulated nuclei and blast forms. **B** Bone marrow biopsy from a 75 year-old woman with severe pancytopenia, no evidence of splenomegaly and a complex karyotype including del(5q), del(7q), and del(12p). The marrow is markedly hypercellular with a marked increase in reticulin fibers. Numerous megakaryocytes can be identified. **C** High magnification of the specimen illustrated in B. Many cells are distorted. Several megakaryocytes with hypolobulated nuclei are present. **D** Immunoperoxidase reaction with antibody to factor VIII. Numerous megakaryocytes, many with hypolobulated nuclei, are positive. A substantial number of non-reacting cells is present.

usually frequent. Physical findings in the chronic disorder invariably include splenomegaly, which may be marked. Splenomegaly is absent or minimal in the acute process.

Metastatic tumour is excluded by studies with appropriate antibodies to both haematopoietic and non-haematopoietic cells.

Immunophenotype
If sufficient specimen is obtained for immunologic markers, the cells show phenotypic heterogeneity, and express varying degrees of expression of myeloid associated antigens. The blasts may express one or more myeloid-associated antigens: CD13, CD33, CD117 and MPO. In some cases a proportion of immature cells express erythroid or megakaryocytic antigens as discussed

under those subtypes of leukaemia. Immunohistochemistry on the biopsy specimen using antibodies to myeloperoxidase, lysozyme, the megakaryocyte markers, CD41, CD61 and factor VIII, and erythroid markers such as glycophorin A and haemoglobin A identify the relative proportions of the various myeloid components.

Genetics
If sufficient specimen for cytogenetics is obtained, the results are usually abnormal. Complex abnormalities may be present and frequently involve chromosomes 5 and/or 7.

Postulated cell of origin
Myeloid haematopoietic stem cell. The fibroblastic proliferation is an epiphenomenon.

Prognosis and predictive factors
The disease is usually associated with poor response to chemotherapy and short survival.

Myeloid sarcoma

Definition
Myeloid sarcoma is a tumour mass of myeloblasts or immature myeloid cells occurring in an extramedullary site or in bone. The tumour mass may precede or occur concurrently with acute or chronic myeloid leukaemia or with other types of myeloproliferative disorders or myelodysplastic syndromes. A myeloid sarcoma may also be the initial manifestation of relapse in a previously treated AML in remission.

Synonyms
Extramedullary myeloid tumour
Granulocytic sarcoma
Chloroma

ICD-O code   9930/3

Sites of involvement
The most common sites of occurrence are subperiosteal bone structures of the skull, paranasal sinuses, sternum, ribs, vertebrae, and pelvis; lymph nodes and skin are also common sites.

Clinical features
Myeloid sarcomas may occur *de novo* or concurrently with acute myeloid leukaemia, or a myeloproliferative disorder; a myeloid sarcoma may be the first evidence of AML.
There may occasionally be a long interval (months or years) between the occurrence of myeloid sarcoma and AML.

Morphology and cytochemistry
The most common type of myeloid sarcoma is the granulocytic sarcoma, which is composed of myeloblasts and neutrophils and neutrophil precursors (see figure 4.07). There are three major types based on degree of maturation: 1) blastic; 2) immature; and 3) differentiated. The blastic type is composed primarily of myeloblasts, the immature type of myeloblasts and promyelocytes and the differentiated type of promyelocytes and more mature neutrophils.
A less common form of myeloid sarcoma is the monoblastic sarcoma, which may precede or occur simultaneously with acute monoblastic leukaemia. This type is usually composed of a population of monoblasts.

Tumours with trilineage haematopoiesis or predominantly erythroid precursors or megakaryocytes may occur in conjunction with transformation of chronic myeloproliferative disorders.
The definitive diagnosis of a myeloid sarcoma is based on reactivity of the blasts in cytochemical reactions or by immunophenotypic analysis. On imprints the myeloblasts and neutrophils are positive for myeloperoxidase. The neutrophils are also naphthol ASD chloroacetate esterase positive. The monoblastic tumours may be positive for non-specific esterase. Naphthol ASD chloroacetate esterase is an excellent histochemical stain for neutrophils but may be ablated by fixation and decalcifying agents.

Differential diagnosis
The major differential diagnoses are non-Hodgkin lymphoma of the lymphoblastic type, Burkitt lymphoma, large-cell lymphoma, and small round cell tumours, particularly in children (neuroblastoma, rhabdomyosarcoma, Ewing's/PNET and medulloblastoma). Immunophenotyping by flow cytometry or immunohistochemistry for expression of myelomonocytic antigens and the myeloid associated enzymes myeloperoxidase and chloroacetate esterase are essential. A high index of suspicion for myeloid sarcoma when confronted with poorly differentiated lesions is necessary to avoid missing this lesion.

Immunophenotype
Staining of sections with antibody to MPO, lysozyme and chloroacetate esterase are critical to the recognition of these lesions. The myeloblasts in the granulocytic sarcomas have antigenic

profiles similar to the blasts and precursor cells in AML with and without maturation, expressing myeloid-associated antigens: CD13, CD33, CD117, MPO. The monoblasts in the monoblastic sarcomas have surface antigens similar to that of monoblasts in acute monoblastic leukaemia, CD14, CD116, CD11c, and usually react with antibodies to lysozyme and CD68 by immunohistochemistry. Most myeloid sarcomas will express CD43. Reactivity of tumour cells with CD43 but not with CD3 in a neoplasm of uncertain origin should prompt consideration of a myeloid tumour, and more specific studies for MPO, lysozyme, CD61 should be performed.

Genetics
An association between myeloid sarcoma and AML with maturation and t(8;21)(q22;q22) and AMML Eo with inv (16)(p13q22) or t(16;16) (p13;q22) may be observed. The monoblastic sarcoma may be associated with translocations involving 11q23.

Postulated cell of origin
Primitive myeloid haematopoietic cell.

Prognosis and predictive factors
If a myeloid sarcoma occurs in a setting of MDS or MPD, it is equivalent to blast transformation. In a setting of AML, the prognosis is that of the underlying leukaemia. When a myeloid sarcoma occurs as isolated lesion without any evidence of leukaemia, curative radiotherapy to the lesion may result in a very prolonged survival.

Acute leukaemias of ambiguous lineage

R.D. Brunning
E. Matutes
M. Borowitz
G. Flandrin
D. Head
J. Vardiman
J. Bennett

Definition

Acute leukaemias of ambiguous lineage are forms of acute leukaemia in which the morphologic, cytochemical and immuno-phenotypic features of the proliferating blasts lack sufficient evidence to classify as myeloid or lymphoid origin (acute undifferentiated leukaemia) or which have morphologic and/or immunophenotypic characteristics of both myeloid and lymphoid cells or both B and T lineages (acute bilineal leukaemia and acute biphenotypic leukaemia) {485, 744, 837, 1247}.

Synonyms

Acute leukaemia of indeterminate lineage
Mixed phenotype acute leukaemia
Mixed lineage acute leukaemia
Hybrid acute leukaemia

ICD-O code

Undifferentiated acute leukaemia
9801/3
Bilineal acute leukaemia   9805/3
Biphenotypic acute leukaemia
9805/3

Epidemiology

These are rare leukaemias and account for less than 4% of all cases of acute leukaemia. They occur both in children and adults but are more frequent in adults.

Aetiology

Similar to other forms of acute leukaemia the aetiology is unknown. Environmental toxins and radiation exposure are possible causes.

Clinical features

The clinical features relate to bone marrow failure and include fatigue, infections and bleeding disorders related to anaemia, neutropenia and thrombocytopenia.

Morphology

In acute undifferentiated leukaemia, the leukaemic cells lack any differentiating features.

Acute biphenotypic leukaemia and acute bilineal leukaemia may present either as one of the subtypes of AML, namely monoblastic or poorly differentiated myeloid, or with features of acute lymphoblastic leukaemia. It is not unusual to identify in the same case populations of small blasts resembling lymphoblasts and larger blasts; in some cases the blasts are morphologically undifferentiated {837, 1247}.

Immunophenotype

Undifferentiated acute leukaemia

These leukaemias lack markers considered specific for a given lineage including cCD79a*, cCD22, CD3 and MPO. They also will not generally express more than one lineage-associated marker. The blasts in these leukaemias often express HLA-DR, CD34, CD38 and may express TdT and CD7.

Bilineal acute leukaemia

These cases are defined by the detection of a dual population of blasts with each population expressing markers of a distinct lineage, i.e. myeloid and lymphoid or B and T. These cases may evolve into biphenotypic acute leu-

kaemia and the relationship between these two entities is not completely clear {485, 837}.

Biphenotypic acute leukaemia

This category of acute leukaemias is characterised by blasts which coexpress myeloid and T or B lineage specific antigens or concurrent B and T lineage antigens. Rarely the blasts in a case coexpress markers for all three lineages, i.e. myeloid, B and T {654, 744, 837}.

Many markers are only lineage-associated and not specific particularly in early haematopoietic cell development. Thus the coexpression of one or two cross lineage antigens is not a sufficient criterion to diagnose biphenotypic leukaemia. Myeloid-antigen positive ALL, or lymphoid antigen-positive AML are often seen and should not be equated with biphenotypic acute leukaemia. Rather, the diagnosis should be reserved for cases in which there is ambiguity of lineage assignment because of the presence of multiple antigens associated with more than one lineage. In some cases there is immunophenotypic evidence of "lineage switch"; this may occur after a relatively short period of time and

Table 4.03
Scoring system for markers proposed by the European Group for the Immunologic Classification of Leukaemia (EGIL). Biphenotypic leukaemia is diagnosed when the score is 2 or more for the myeloid lineage, and 2 or more for one of the lymphoid lineages.

Score	B-lymphoid	T-lymphoid	Myeloid
2	CytCD79a* Cyt IgM CytCD22	CD3(m/cyt) anti-TCR	MPO
1	CD19 CD20 CD10	CD2 CD5 CD8 CD10	CD117 CD13 CD33 CD65
0.5	TdT CD24	TdT CD7 CD1a	CD14 CD15 CD64

*CD79a may also be expressed in some cases of precursor T lymphoblastic leukaemia/lymphoma.

therapeutic intervention {997, 1022, 1091}. In many cases "lineage switch" probably represents the expansion of a pre-existent minor population of blasts of a different lineage following the therapeutic suppression of the major population of cells, i.e. there was a pretherapy bilineal blast population of different magnitudes. In addition, in some cases there appears to be lineage instability.

In the classification of a case of acute leukaemia, antigenic determinants may be assigned different degrees of specificity. Table 4.03 is a scoring system for markers proposed by the European Group for the Immunologic Classification of Leukaemia {10}.

Differential diagnosis

As noted, biphenotypic acute leukaemia must be distinguished from myeloid antigen positive ALL or lymphoid antigen positive AML. Undifferentiated acute leukaemia must be distinguished from minimally differentiated myeloid leukaemia, and rarely from unusual precursor-B-cell or T-cell ALL. The distinction is based on immunological markers.

Genetics

A high percentage of cases of bilineal and biphenotypic acute leukaemia present with cytogenetic abnormalities {180, 485, 744, 997, 1247}. About a third of cases have the Philadelphia chromosome; these usually have a CD10+ precursor B lymphoid component. Some cases are associated with the t(4;11)(q21;q23) or other 11q23 abnormalities and often manifest a CD10-negative precursor B population with a separate recognisable component of monocytic leukaemia.

Cases of T/myeloid biphenotypic or bilinial leukaemia do not have these cytogenetic findings but may have other complex karyotypic abnormalities.

DNA analysis of the Ig and TCR chain genes show that a substantial proportion of cases have rearrangement or deletions of the Ig-heavy chain gene or TCR chain genes, including those which apparently present as "AML".

Postulated cell of origin

Multipotent progenitor stem cell.

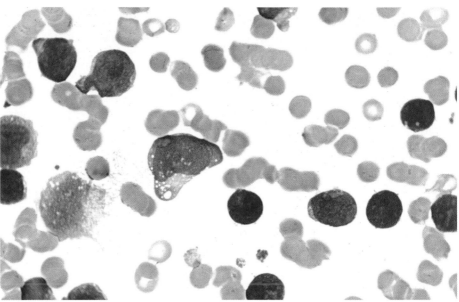

Fig. 4.42 Biphenotypic acute leukemia. Bone marrow smear from a case of acute leukemia with an associated t(9;22)(q34;q11.2). The blasts vary from small lymphoid appearing blasts to large blasts with dispersed chromatin, prominent nucleoli and a moderate amount of pale cytoplasm.

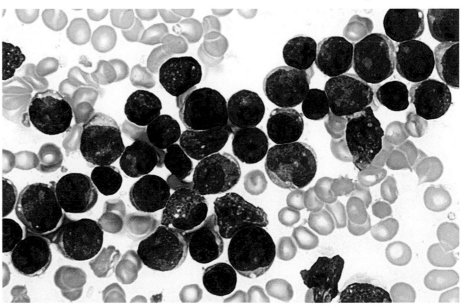

Fig. 4.43 Acute biphenotypic leukemia. Bone marrow smear from a case of acute leukemia with morphologic features of acute lymphoblastic leukemia in which the blasts expressed lymphoid and myeloid antigens.

Prognostic and predictive factors

The prognosis appears to be unfavourable, particularly in adults; the occurrence of the t(4;11) or the Philadelphia chromosome are particularly unfavourable prognostic findings {654, 744}. The optimal approach for therapy is unknown but probably includes aggressive chemotherapy and allogenic or autologous stem cell transplantation.

CHAPTER 5

Precursor B-Cell and
T-Cell Neoplasms

Some of the most significant advances in the therapy of leukaemias and lymphomas in the last two decades has occurred with the precursor B and T lymphoblastic leukaemias and lymphomas. The "cure rate" in some types of precursor B lymphoblastic leukaemia approaches 80%. Some types however are still associated with low rates of remission. The cyto-genetic profiles, genotype and immunophenotype of the malig-nant cell have had considerable impact on prognostic stratifi-cations with recognition of low and high risk groups. These stratifications have resulted in more specific therapeutic regi-mens with higher remission rates for unfavourable prognostic groups.

WHO histological classification of precursor B-cell and T-cell neoplasms

Precursor B lymphoblastic leukaemia[1]/lymphoblastic lymphoma[2]   9835/3[1]
(precursor B-cell acute lymphoblastic leukaemia)   9728/3[2]

Precursor T lymphoblastic leukaemia[1]/lymphoblastic lymphoma[2]   9837/3[1]
(precursor T-cell acute lymphoblastic leukaemia)   9729/3[2]

Precursor B lymphoblastic leukaemia / lymphoblastic lymphoma
(Precursor B-cell acute lymphoblastic leukaemia)

R.D. Brunning*
M. Borowitz
E. Matutes
D. Head

G. Flandrin
S.H. Swerdlow
J.M. Bennett

Definition

Precursor B lymphoblastic leukaemia (B-ALL)/lymphoblastic lymphoma (B-LBL) is a neoplasm of lymphoblasts committed to the B-cell lineage, typically composed of small to medium-sized blast cells with scant cytoplasm, moderately condensed to dispersed chromatin and inconspicuous nucleoli, involving bone marrow and blood (B lymphoblastic leukaemia) and occasionally presenting with primary involvement of nodal or extranodal sites (B lymphoblastic lymphoma).

Because of the biologic unity of B-ALL and B-LBL, the use of one or the other term in some patients is arbitrary. When the process is confined to a mass lesion without any or minimal evidence of blood and marrow involvement, the diagnosis is lymphoma. With extensive marrow and blood involvement, lymphoblastic leukaemia is the appropriate term. If the patient presents with a mass lesion and 25% or fewer lymphoblasts in the marrow, the designation lymphoma is preferred. This is an arbitrary distinction and exceptions may apply {910}.

ICD-O code

Precursor B lymphoblastic leukaemia
9836/3
Precursor B lymphoblastic lymphoma
9728/3

Synonyms

Acute lymphoblastic leukaemias
FAB: L1 and L2

Epidemiology

Acute lymphoblastic leukaemia is primarily a disease of children; 75% of cases occur in children under six years of age. The estimated number of new cases in the United States in the year 2000 is approximately 3200: approximately 80-85% are of precursor B-cell phenotype {1103, 1143, 1202}.

Precursor B lymphoblastic lymphoma is an uncommon type of lymphoma and constitutes approximately 10% of cases of lymphoblastic lymphoma {118}. Approximately 75% of cases reported in a literature review were less than 18 years of age; 88% of patients in a series of 25 cases were under 35 years of age and the median age was 20 years {806}. One report indicated a male predominance {769}.

Aetiology

The aetiology of B-ALL/LBL is unknown. There is evidence to suggest a genetic factor in some cases.

Sites of involvement

The marrow and blood are involved in all cases of precursor B ALL. Extramedullary involvement is frequent with particular predilection for the central nervous system, lymph nodes, spleen, liver, and gonads.

The most frequent sites of involvement in B-LBL are the skin, bone, soft tissue, and lymph nodes {102, 769, 806}. Mediastinal masses are infrequent {102, 1139}.

Clinical features

Most patients with B-ALL present with evidence and consequences of bone marrow failure: thrombocytopenia and/or anaemia and/or neutropenia. The leukocyte count may be decreased, normal or markedly elevated. Lymphadenopathy, hepatomegaly and splenomegaly are frequent. Bone pain and arthralgias may be prominent symptoms.

A small number of patients with a precursor B lymphoblastic neoplasm present primarily as lymphomas with or without blood and bone marrow involvement {769, 806, 1361}. The B-LBL most frequently present in the skin, bone and lymph nodes; the cutaneous involvement may manifest as multiple nodules. Marrow and blood involvement may be pres-

* The authors acknowledge the Clinical Cytometry Society, meeting in Montpellier, France in May, 2000, for providing commentary on the use of flow cytometry in the classification of acute leukaemia.

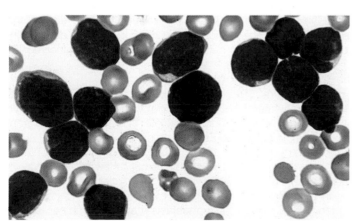

Fig. 5.01 Precursor B lymphoblastic leukaemia. Bone marrow smear with several lymphoblasts with a high nuclear cytoplasmic ratio and variably condensed nuclear chromatin.

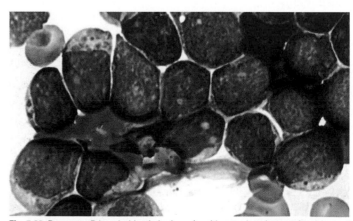

Fig. 5.02 Precursor B lymphoblastic leukaemia with cytoplasmic granules. Many of the lymphoblasts in this bone marrow smear contained numerous coarse azurophilic granules.

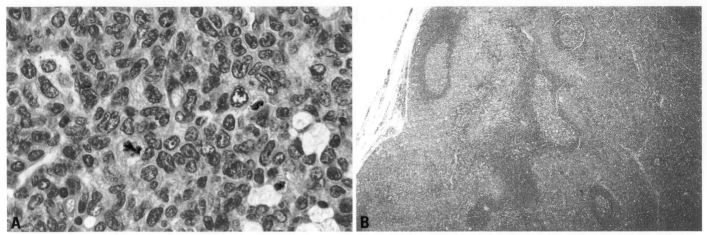

Fig. 5.03 Precursor B lymphoblastic leukaemia. **A** This bone marrow from an adult with t(9;22) positive B-ALL is completely replaced by lymphoblasts. Mitotic figures are numerous. **B** Lymph node. The neoplastic cells infiltrate diffusely sparing normal follicles.

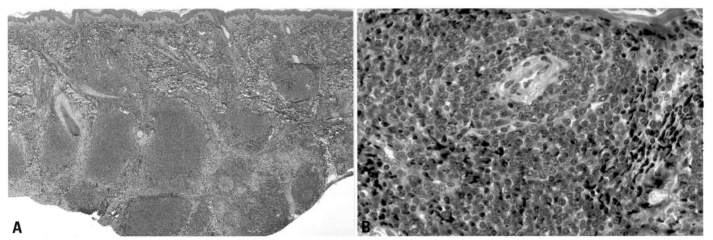

Fig. 5. 04 Precursor B lymphoblastic lymphoma. **A** Skin. The neoplastic cells diffusely infiltrate the dermis with sparing of the epidermis. **B** Same case at higher magnification shows lymphoblasts surrounding blood vessel.

ent, but the percentage of lymphoblasts in the marrow is less than 25.

Morphology
The lymphoblasts in B-ALL/LBL in smear and imprint preparations vary from small blasts with scant cytoplasm, condensed nuclear chromatin and indistinct nucleoli to larger cells with moderate amounts of light blue to blue-grey cytoplasm, occasionally vacuolated, dispersed nuclear chromatin and multiple variably prominent nucleoli. Coarse azurophilic granules are present in some lymphoblasts in approximately 10% of cases. This finding may be associated with a t(9;22)(q34;q11.2) cytogenetic abnormality. In some cases the lymphoblasts have cytoplasmic pseudopods (hand mirror cells).

In marrow biopsies, the lymphoblasts in B-ALL are relatively uniform in appearance with round to oval to indented, sometimes convoluted nuclei. Nucleoli are variably prominent and are usually inconspicuous or indistinct. The chromatin is finely dispersed. The number of mitotic figures usually varies; mitotic figures are less numerous in marrow biopsies of B-ALL than in T-ALL {850}.

Lymphoblastic lymphoma is generally characterised by a diffuse pattern of lymph node or other tissue involvement; in some cases with partial node involvement the lymphoblasts infiltrate the paracortical area with sparing of germinal centres.

The lymphoblasts are somewhat homogeneous in appearance with round to oval nuclei which may manifest varying degrees of convolution of the nuclear membrane. The nuclear chromatin is finely stippled; nucleoli are generally incon-

spicuous. In most cases, mitotic figures are numerous and in some cases there may be a focal "starry sky" pattern. The morphologic features of B and T lymphoblastic proliferations are similar and morphology cannot be used as a distinguishing feature of immunophenotype.

Cytochemistry
Lymphoblasts are negative for myeloperoxidase and myeloid type reactivity with Sudan Black-B (SBB). Lymphoblast granules may stain light grey with SBB staining but less intensely than myeloblasts. Lymphoblasts may show PAS positivity; in some cases the nuclei may be partially encircled by a rim of PAS reactivity. Lymphoblasts may react with non-specific esterase with a multifocal punctate or Golgi zone pattern with variable inhibition with sodium fluoride.

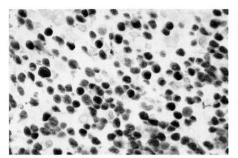

Fig. 5.05 Precursor B lymphoblastic leukaemia, TdT. Immunohistochemical demonstration of nuclear TdT in a bone marrow biopsy.

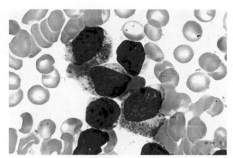

Fig. 5.06 Precursor B lymphoblastic leukaemia with a t(9;22) chromosomal abnormality. Bone marrow smear from a 24 year-old male. Several of the lymphoblasts have abundant cytoplasm with numerous coarse azurophilic granules.

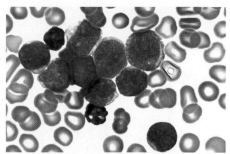

Fig. 5.07 Precursor B lymphoblastic leukaemia with a t(4;11) chromosomal abnormality. Several lymphoblasts in the marrow of an eight month-old child.

Immunophenotype

The lymphoblasts in B-ALL/LBL are terminal deoxynucleotidyl tranferase (TdT)-positive, HLAT-DR positive and are almost always positive for CD19 and cytoplasmic CD79a. The lymphoblasts are positive for CD10 and CD24 in most cases; the lymphoblasts in t(4;11) (q21;q23) ALL are usually CD10 negative and frequently CD24 negative {120, 274, 1000}. There is variable expression of CD22 and CD20. CD45 may be absent. Cytoplasmic CD22 is considered lineage-specific. The myeloid–associated antigens CD13 and CD33 may be expressed but the presence of these myeloid markers does not exclude the diagnosis of precursor B-ALL. The degree of differentiation of precursor B lineage lymphoblasts has clinical and genetic correlates. In the earliest stage, so called early precursor B-ALL, the blasts express CD19, cytoplasmic CD79a, cytoplasmic CD22 and nuclear TdT. In the intermediate stage, so called common ALL, the blasts express CD10. In the most mature precursor B differentiation stage, so called pre-B-ALL,

the blasts express cytoplasmic mu chains (cyt-mu). Surface immunoglobulin is characteristically absent although if present does not exclude a diagnosis of precursor B-ALL/LBL {939}.

Genetics

The cytogenetic abnormalities in precursor B ALL/lymphoma are considered in several groups: hypodiploid, hyperdiploid <50, hyperdiploid >50, translocations and pseudodiploid {974, 1060, 1075}.

ALL - t(9;22) (q34;q11.2); *BCR/ABL*
ALL - (v; 11q 23); *MLL* Rearranged
ALL - t(12;21) (p13;q22); *TEL/AML1* *
ALL - t(1;19) (q23;p13.3); *PBX/E2A*
ALL - hypodiploid
ALL - hyperdiploid >50

These findings are prognostically important, and are used to modify treatment in paediatric disease. With current treatment good prognostic groups are: i) hyperdiploidy between 51 and 65 chromosomes, corresponding to a flow cytometric DI (DNA content) of 1.16 to 1.6; and ii)

t(12;21)(p12;q22). The t(12;21)(p13;q22) is the result of fusion of the *TEL* gene at 12p13 with the transcription factor-encoding *AML1* gene at 21q22; molecular techniques are required for recognition as it is not detected by standard cytogenetics. Several cytogenetic findings are associated with a poor prognosis with current treatment; i) The t(9;22), which results from fusion of *BCR* at 22q11.2 and the cytoplasmic tyrosine kinase gene *ABL* at 9q34 is more frequent in adults. In most childhood cases of ALL with the t(9;22), a p190 kd BCR/ABL fusion protein is produced. In adults about one-half of cases of ALL with the t(9,22) produce the p210 kd fusion protein that is present in CML, and the remainder produce the p190. No definite clinical differences have been attributed to these two different gene products. ii) B-precursor ALL in early stages of differentiation (early precursor B ALL) may have a t(4;11), with fusion of the *MLL* gene at 11q23 encoding a putative DNA-binding protein and *AF4* at 4q21. Other translocations at 11q23 result from fusion of the *MLL* locus with other partner genes. ALL with 11q23 abnormalities may also occur as therapy related leukaemia secondary to etoposide {1169}. iii) The t(1;19), found in the 25% of childhood B-ALL with cytoplasmic mu expression, fuses the transcription factor-encoding gene *E2A* at 19p13.3 with *PBX* at 1q23; this is associated with a poor prognosis with some treatment regimens. iv) Hypodiploidy is associated with a poor prognosis. Other abnormalities (del(6q), del(9p), del(12p), hyperdiploidy less than 51, near triploidy,

Table 5.01
Prognostic implications of genetic alterations in childhood precursor B lymphoblastic leukaemia.

Cytogenetic findings	Genetic alteration	Frequency	Prognosis
t(9;22)(q34;q11.2)	*BCR/ABL*	3 - 4%	Unfavourable
t(4;11)(q21;q23)[1]	*AF4/MLL*	2 - 3%	Unfavourable
t(1;19)(q23;p13.3)	*PBX/E2A*	6% (25% of pre-B-ALL)	Unfavourable[2]
t(12;21)(p13;q22)[3]	*TEL/AML1*	16 - 29%	Favourable
Hyperdiploid >50		20 - 25%	Favourable
Hypodiploidy		5%	Unfavourable

[1] Prototype 11q23 translocation in precursor B ALL; other translocations may involve the MLL gene
[2] Not uniformly Unfavourable with all therapeutic regimens
[3] Detected by molecular studies

* Editor's note: The *AML1* gene is also known as *RUNX1*.

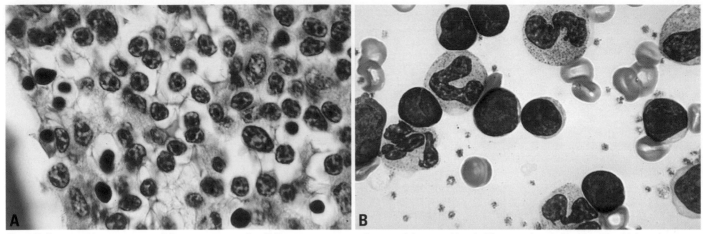

Fig. 5.08 Increased haematogones. **A** Bone marrow section. **B** Bone marrow smear from an eight year-old male. There are lymphoid cells with a high nuclear cytoplasmic ratio and very homogeneous nuclear chromatin; nucleoli not observed or are indistinct. These cells resemble the lymphoblasts in ALL of childhood.

and near tetraploidy) are associated with an intermediate prognosis.

Some of the genetically defined entities described above have characteristic immunophenotypes. *MLL* rearranged leukaemias are characteristically CD10-, and also frequently CD24- and CD15+ {1000}. B-ALL t(1;19) is CD10+, CD34- and CD20- or dim and usually cytoplasmic mu positive. B-ALL with t(12;21) shows high density expression of CD10 and HLA-DR while CD9 and CD20 are usually negative.

Postulated cell of origin
Precursor B-lymphoblast.

Differential diagnosis
The differential diagnosis of B-ALL includes T-ALL, acute myeloid leukaemia (AML) minimally differentiated and reactive bone marrow with increased haematogones. T-ALL, B-ALL, and AML, minimally differentiated can be distinguished from each other only by immunophenotype.

Haematogones may be increased in the marrows of very young children and in the marrows from older individuals with a variety of disorders, including iron deficiency anaemia, neuroblastoma and idiopathic thrombocytopenic purpura as well as following cytotoxic therapy {174}. These cells have a very high nuclear cytoplasmic ratio and a homogeneous nuclear chromatin; the nuclei may show indentations or clefts. Nucleoli are not usually identified; if present they are indistinct. Haematogones are not generally found in the peripheral blood. In marrow biopsies, the haematogones are distributed uniformly in the interstitium. The

nuclear chromatin is very clumped. Nucleoli and mitotic figures are rarely identified.

Haematogones may be difficult to distinguish immunophenotypically from leukaemic B lymphoblasts. Both the haematogones and lymphoblasts are TdT positive and may express CD10. However, in multiparameter flow cytometry, the immunophenotype of haematogones is characteristic in that they lack aberrant antigen expression and show a reproducible pattern of coexpression of markers associated with B-cell lymphoid differentiation including CD10, CD19, CD20, CD34 and CD45. There is a continuum of expression of these antigens in haematogones, indicating maturation. There is a predominance of intermediate (CD10+, CD19+, TdT negative, SIg-) and late immunophenotypic stage (CD19+, CD20+, SIg+). In contrast, the lymphoblasts in almost all cases of B-cell precursor ALL show patterns that differ from normal with a predominance of immature cells (TdT+, CD19+, SIg-, CD20-) and a paucity of mature cells {1106, 1362}.

In lymph nodes and extranodal tissues, the major differential diagnosis of lymphoblastic lymphoma in children is Burkitt lymphoma; in adults the differential diagnosis also includes the blastoid variant of mantle cell lymphoma. These lymphomas are readily distinguished with TdT determination.

Lymphoblastic lymphoma is the only lymphoma that shows nuclear TdT positivity. Myeloblastic infiltration may be distinguished by chloroacetate esterase or antibodies to myeloperoxidase and lysozyme.

Prognosis and predictive factors
Precursor B-ALL is generally a good prognosis leukaemia. In the paediatric age group overall the complete remission rate is approximately 95%, in adults 60-85%. The disease free survival rate in children is 70%. Approximately 80% of children with B-ALL appear to be cured. Paediatric risk groups in B-ALL are based on cytogenetic profile, age, leukocyte count, sex, and response to initial therapy {367, 492, 649, 730, 819, 1075, 1095}. There is a high association in infancy with translocations involving the *MLL* gene at 11q23, which conveys a poor prognosis regardless of age. In childhood, over 50% of patients have good prognostic hyperdiploid karyotype or t(12;21) genetic changes with 85-90% long-term survival. Predictive factors for durable remission and prolonged survival in children are age 4-10, hyperdiploid chromosomes, particularly 54-62 with trisomy 4 and/or 10 and/or 17, t(12;21)(p13;q22), and low or normal leukocyte count at diagnosis {509, 819, 1077}. Adverse factors include very young age, <1 year, the t(9;22) (q34;q11.2) and t(4;11)(q21;q23) cytogenetic abnormalities.

In adult precursor B-ALL, cases have not been as well characterised genetically; the poor prognosis t(9;22)(q34;q11.2) (Ph[1]) cytogenetic abnormality is found in 25% of cases; translocations at 11q23 are more frequent than in children, and the good risk features, hyperdiploidy with 51-65 chromosomes and t(12;21), are infrequent.

Precursor B lymphoblastic lymphoma has a high remission rate with a median survival of approximately 60 months {769}.

Precursor T lymphoblastic leukaemia / lymphoblastic lymphoma
(Precursor T-cell acute lymphoblastic leukaemia)

R.D. Brunning
M. Borowitz
E. Matutes
D. Head

G. Flandrin
S.H. Swerdlow
J.M. Bennett

Definition
Precursor T lymphoblastic leukaemia (T-ALL)/lymphoblastic lymphoma (T-LBL) is a neoplasm of lymphoblasts committed to the T-cell lineage, typically composed of small to medium-sized blast cells with scant cytoplasm, moderately condensed to dispersed chromatin and inconspicuous nucleoli, involving bone marrow and blood (T-ALL) and sometimes presenting with primary involvement of nodal or extranodal sites (T-LBL).

Because of the biologic unity of precursor T lymphoblastic leukaemia and T lymphoblastic lymphoma, the use of one or the other term in some patients is arbitrary. When the process is confined to a mass lesion without any or minimal evidence of blood and marrow involvement, the diagnosis is lymphoma. With extensive marrow and blood involvement, acute lymphoblastic leukaemia is the appropriate term. If the patient presents with a mass lesion and 25% or fewer lymphoblasts in the marrow, the designation lymphoma is preferred. This is an arbitrary distinction and exceptions may apply {910}.

ICD-O code
Precursor T acute lymphoblastic leukaemia
9837/3
Precursor T lymphoblastic lymphoma
9729/3

Synonyms
Acute lymphoblastic leukaemia
FAB: L1 and L2
Lukes and Collins: Convoluted T cell lymphoma

Epidemiology
Precursor T-ALL comprises about 15% of childhood ALL; it is more common in adolescents than younger children and more common in males than females. T-ALL comprises approximately 25% of cases of adult ALL.

Precursor T lymphoblastic lymphoma comprises approximately 85-90% of lymphoblastic lymphomas; similar to its leukaemic counterpart, it is most frequent in adolescent males {1361}.

Aetiology
The aetiology of these tumours is basically unknown.

Clinical features
Precursor T-ALL typically presents with a high leukocyte count, and often a large mediastinal mass or other tissue mass. For a given leukocyte count and tumour burden, precursor T-ALL patients may

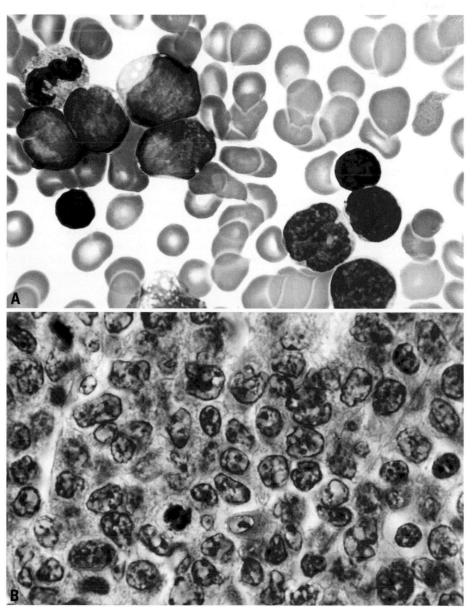

Fig. 5.09 Precursor T lymphoblastic leukaemia. **A** Blood smear. The lymphoblasts vary in size from large cells to small cells with a very high nuclear cytoplasmic ratio. **B** Bone marrow section.

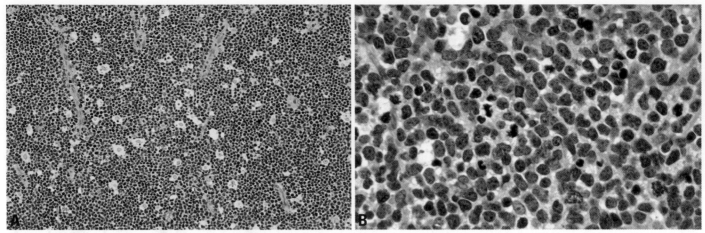

Fig. 5.10 Precursor T lymphoblastic lymphoma. **A** Low magnification of a lymph node showing complete replacement by lymphoblastic lymphoma. Numerous tingible body macrophages are scattered throughout the node. **B** High magnification of the specimen in **A** showing lymphoblasts with round to oval to irregularly shaped nuclei with dispersed chromatin and distinct but not unusually prominent nucleoli. Several mitotic figures are present.

have relative sparing of normal marrow haematopoiesis compared to other subtypes of ALL.

T lymphoblastic lymphoma frequently presents with a mass lesion in the mediastinum often exhibiting rapid growth. Pleural effusions are common.

Sites of involvement

The blood and marrow are involved in all cases of T-ALL. Approximately 50% of T lymphoblastic lymphomas present as a mediastinal mass; other possible sites include peripheral lymph nodes, skin, liver, spleen, Waldeyer's ring, central nervous system and gonads.

Morphology

The lymphoblasts in T-ALL/LBL are similar to precursor B lymphoblasts. In smears the cells are of medium size with a high nuclear cytoplasmic ratio; there may be a considerable size range from small lymphoblasts with very condensed nuclear chromatin and no evident nucleoli to larger blasts with finely dispersed chromatin and relatively prominent nucleoli. Cytoplasmic vacuoles may be present.

In marrow sections the lymphoblasts have a high nuclear-cytoplasmic ratio, finely stippled chromatin and inconspicuous nucleoli. The number of mitotic figures is reported to be higher in T-ALL than B-ALL.

In T-LBL the lymph node generally shows complete effacement, with involvement of the capsule. A "starry-sky" effect may be present. Partial involvement in a paracortical location with sparing of germinal centres may occur. In some cases, the predominant population of blasts has convoluted nuclei; mitotic figures may be numerous.

A small number of patients with T-LBL, eosinophilia and myeloid hyperplasia has been observed {11} (see also chapter 1). In some cases there has been an associated t(8;13) (p11.2;q11-22) cytogenetic abnormality observed in bone marrow cells {560}. The lymphoblastic lymphoma is usually infiltrated by eosinophils. Several of these cases have developed a myeloid malignancy, either acute myeloid leukaemia, myelodysplastic syndrome or myeloid sarcoma. This constellation of findings is more frequent in males than females.

Cytochemistry

T-lymphoblasts frequently show focal acid phosphatase activity in smear and imprint preparations.

Immunophenotype

The lymphoblasts in T-ALL/LBL are TdT positive and variably express CD1a, CD2, CD3, CD4, CD5, CD7 and CD8. Of these, CD7 and cytoplasmic CD3 are most often positive, and only CD3 is considered lineage specific. CD4 and CD8 are frequently co-expressed on the blasts, and CD10 may be positive. CD79a positivity has been observed in some cases. One or both of the myeloid associated antigens CD13 and CD33 are often present and, rarely, CD117 (c-kit). The presence of the myeloid markers by themselves does not exclude the diagnosis of T-ALL/LBL. T lymphoblasts may demonstrate clonal rearrangement of the T-cell receptor genes (TCR), but this is not lineage specific {1037}. T-ALL/LBL can be stratified into different stages of intrathymic differentiation according to the number and sequence of antigens expressed (cytoplasmic CD3, CD2 and CD7 expressed early, followed by CD5, CD1a, followed by membrane CD3). Some studies have shown a correlation between the stages of T-cell differentiation and survival {259} but no definite genetic correlation has been found. T-ALL may be less differentiated than T-LBL, but the groups overlap.

Genetics

In about one third of T-ALL/LBL translocations have been detected involving the alpha and delta T-cell receptor loci at 14q11.2, the beta locus at 7q35, and the gamma locus at 7p14-15, with a variety of partner genes {974}. Genes include the transcription factors *MYC* (8q24.1), *TAL1* (1p32), *RBTN1* (11p15), *RBTN2* (11p13), and *HOX11* (10q24), and the cytoplasmic tyrosine kinase *LCK* (1p34.3-35). In most cases, these translocations lead to a dysregulation of transcription of the partner gene by juxtaposition with the regulatory region of one of the T-cell receptor loci.

In about 25% of cases of T-ALL the *TAL1* locus is dysregulated by a microscopic deletion in its 5' regulatory region, rather than by translocation. The deletion del(9p), resulting in loss of the tumour suppressor gene *CDKN2A* (an inhibitor of the cyclin-dependent kinase CDK4), occurs more frequently in T-ALL, (about 30% of cases by cytogenetics, a higher percentage by molecular testing) than in other immunologic subsets. These genetic features are identical to those in T-LBL, and have no evident specific clinical significance.

Postulated cell of origin
Precursor T lymphoblast.

Differential diagnosis
The differential diagnosis of T-ALL includes B-ALL, acute myeloid leukaemia (AML) minimally differentiated and reactive bone marrow with increased haematogones. T-ALL, B-ALL, and AML, minimally differentiated can be distinguished from each other only by immunophenotype.

Haematogones may be increased in the marrows of very young children and in the marrows from older individuals with a variety of disorders, including iron deficiency anaemia, neuroblastoma and idiopathic thrombocytopenic purpura as well as following cytotoxic therapy {154}. These cells have a very high nuclear cytoplasmic ratio and a homogeneous nuclear chromatin; the nuclei may show indentations or clefts. Nucleoli are not usually identified; if present they are indistinct. Haematogones are not generally found in the peripheral blood. In marrow biopsies, the haematogones are distributed uniformly in the interstitium. The nuclear chromatin is very clumped. Nucleoli and mitotic figures are rarely identified.

Haematogones may be difficult to distinguish immunophenotypically from leukaemic T lymphoblasts. Both the haematogones and lymphoblasts are TdT positive and may express CD10. However, in multiparameter flow cytometry, the immunophenotype of haematogones is characteristic in that they lack aberrant antigen expression and show a reproducible pattern of coexpression of markers associated with B-cell lymphoid differentiation including CD10, CD19, CD20, CD34 and CD45. There is a continuum of expression of these antigens in haematogones, indicating maturation. There is a predominance of intermediate (CD10+, CD19+, TdT negative, SIg-) and late immunophenotypic stage (CD19+, CD20+, SIg+). In contrast, the lymphoblasts in all cases of T-ALL show T-cell antigen expression.

In lymph nodes and extranodal tissues, the major differential diagnosis of lymphoblastic lymphoma in children is Burkitt lymphoma; in adults the differen-

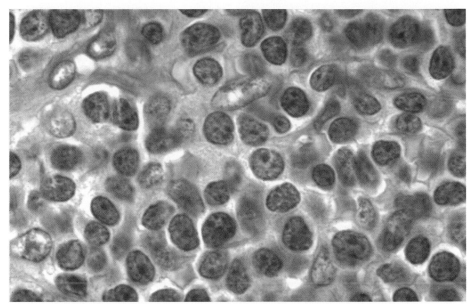

Fig. 5.11 Precursor T lymphoblastic leukaemia. In this example, the lymphoblasts lack nuclear convolutions. The chromatin is finely stippled.

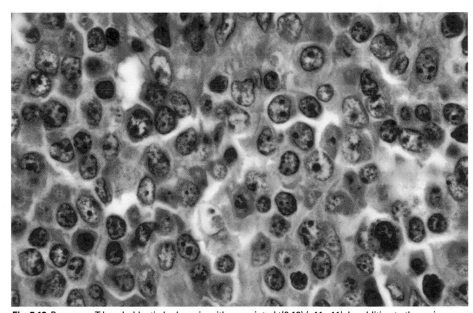

Fig. 5.12 Precursor T lymphoblastic leukaemia with associated t(8;13) (p11;q11). In addition to the major population of lymphoblasts there are eosinophils at different stages of maturation.

tial diagnosis also includes the blastoid variant of mantle cell lymphoma. These lymphomas are readily distinguished with TdT determination. Lymphoblastic lymphoma is the only lymphoma that shows nuclear TdT positivity. Myeloblastic infiltration may be distinguished by chloroacetate esterase or antibodies to myeloperoxidase and lysozyme.

Prognosis and predictive factors
In paediatric protocols T-ALL is usually treated as high risk disease, similar to

T-LBL. In adult protocols, T-ALL is treated similarly to other types of ALL. Prior to the advent of current therapeutic protocols, the prognosis for childhood T-ALL was unfavourable; with current treatment regimens, survival is comparable to B-ALL.

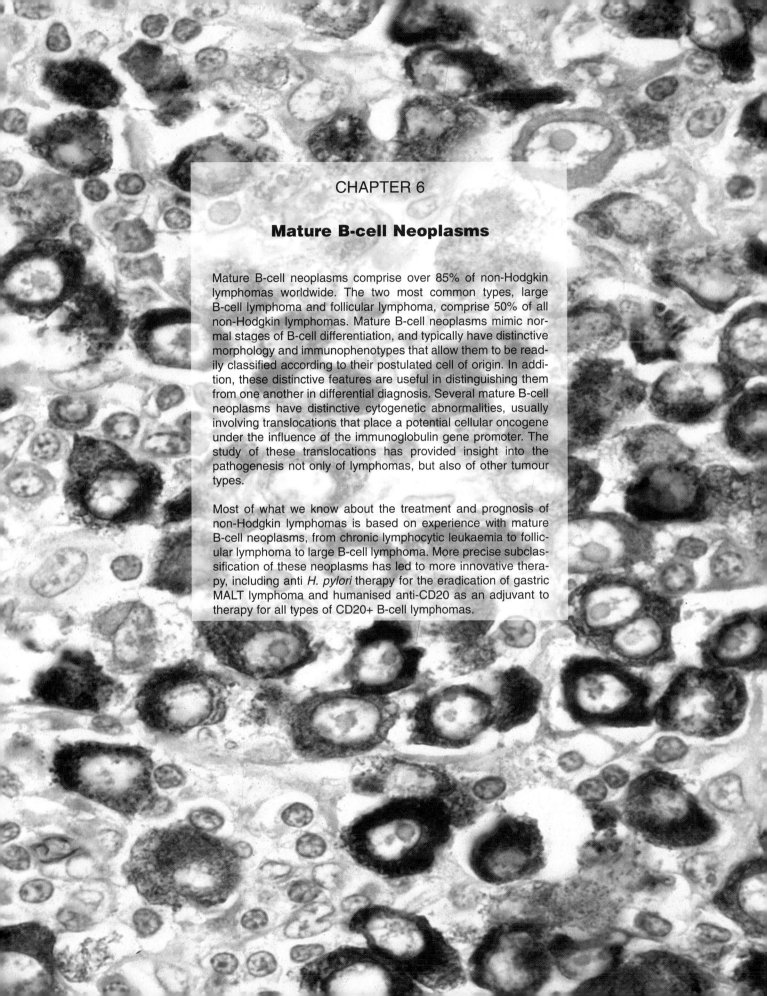

CHAPTER 6

Mature B-cell Neoplasms

Mature B-cell neoplasms comprise over 85% of non-Hodgkin lymphomas worldwide. The two most common types, large B-cell lymphoma and follicular lymphoma, comprise 50% of all non-Hodgkin lymphomas. Mature B-cell neoplasms mimic normal stages of B-cell differentiation, and typically have distinctive morphology and immunophenotypes that allow them to be readily classified according to their postulated cell of origin. In addition, these distinctive features are useful in distinguishing them from one another in differential diagnosis. Several mature B-cell neoplasms have distinctive cytogenetic abnormalities, usually involving translocations that place a potential cellular oncogene under the influence of the immunoglobulin gene promoter. The study of these translocations has provided insight into the pathogenesis not only of lymphomas, but also of other tumour types.

Most of what we know about the treatment and prognosis of non-Hodgkin lymphomas is based on experience with mature B-cell neoplasms, from chronic lymphocytic leukaemia to follicular lymphoma to large B-cell lymphoma. More precise subclassification of these neoplasms has led to more innovative therapy, including anti *H. pylori* therapy for the eradication of gastric MALT lymphoma and humanised anti-CD20 as an adjuvant to therapy for all types of CD20+ B-cell lymphomas.

WHO histological classification of mature B-cell neoplasms

B-cell neoplasms

Precursor B-cell neoplasm

Precursor B lymphoblastic leukaemia[1] / lymphoma[2]	9835/3[1] 9728/3[2]

Mature B-cell neoplasms

Chronic lymphocytic leukaemia[1] / small lymphocytic lymphoma[2]	9823/3[1] 9670/3[2]
B-cell prolymphocytic leukaemia	9833/3
Lymphoplasmacytic lymphoma	9671/3
Splenic marginal zone lymphoma	9689/3
Hairy cell leukaemia	9940/3
Plasma cell myeloma	9732/3
Monoclonal gammopathy of undetermined significance (MGUS)	9765/1
Solitary plasmacytoma of bone	9731/3
Extraosseous plasmacytoma	9734/3
Primary amyloidosis	9769/1c
Heavy chain diseases	9762/3

Extranodal marginal zone B-cell lymphoma of mucosa-associated lymphoid tissue (MALT-lymphoma)	9699/3
Nodal marginal zone B-cell lymphoma	9699/3
Follicular lymphoma	9690/3
Mantle cell lymphoma	9673/3
Diffuse large B-cell lymphoma	9680/3
Mediastinal (thymic) large B-cell lymphoma	9679/3
Intravascular large B-cell lymphoma	9680/3
Primary effusion lymphoma	9678/3
Burkitt lymphoma[1] / leukaemia[2]	9687/3[1] 9826/3[2]

B-cell proliferations of uncertain malignant potential

Lymphomatoid granulomatosis	9766/1
Post-transplant lymphoproliferative disorder, polymorphic	9970/1

Mature B-cell neoplasms: Introduction

N.L. Harris

Definition

Mature B-cell neoplasms are clonal proliferations of B cells at various stages of differentiation, ranging from naïve B cells to mature plasma cells. B-cell neoplasms in many respects appear to recapitulate stages of normal B-cell differentiation, so that they can be to some extent classified according to the corresponding normal B-cell stage. However, some common B-cell neoplasms – for example, hairy cell leukaemia – do not clearly correspond to a normal B-cell differentiation stage, while others – for example, chronic lymphocytic leukaemia – appear to be of heterogeneous origin. Thus, the normal counterpart of the neoplastic cell cannot at this time be the sole basis for the classification.

Epidemiology

Mature B-cell neoplasms comprise over 90% of lymphoid neoplasms worldwide {8, 46}. They comprise approximately 4% of new cancers each year around the world. They are more common in developed countries, particularly the United States, Australia and New Zealand, and Europe. The annual incidence ranges from over 15/100,000 in the United States to only 1.2/100,00 in China, with intermediate rates in South America, Africa and Japan {999a}. The most common types are follicular lymphoma and diffuse large B-cell lymphoma, which together make up 50% of all non-Hodgkin lymphomas {8, 46}, and plasma cell myeloma. In the United States, B-cell neoplasms, including non-Hodgkin lymphoma (50,000), chronic lymphocytic leukaemia (CLL) (7800) and plasma cell myeloma (13,700), account for over 70,000 new cases/year, or 6% of all cancers {729a}. The individual B-cell neoplasms vary in their relative frequency in different parts of the world. Follicular lymphoma is more common in developed countries, particularly in the United States (10% of non-Hodgkin lymphomas) and Western Europe, and is uncommon in South America, Eastern Europe, Africa and Asia. Burkitt lymphoma is endemic in equatorial Africa, where it is the most

common childhood malignancy, but it comprises only 1-2% of lymphomas in the United States and Western Europe. The median age for all types of mature B-cell neoplasms is in the 6th and 7th decades, but mediastinal large B-cell lymphoma has a median age of 37 years, and Burkitt lymphoma has a median age in adults of 30 years. Of the mature B-cell lymphomas, only Burkitt lymphoma and large B-cell lymphoma occur with any significant frequency in children. Most types have a slight male predominance (52-55%), but mantle cell lymphoma has a striking male predominance (74%), while females predominate in follicular lymphoma (58%) and most particularly in mediastinal large B-cell lymphoma (66%).

The major known risk factor for mature B-cell neoplasia appears to be an abnormality of the immune system, either immunodeficiency or autoimmune disease. Although evidence of immune system abnormalities are lacking in most patients with mature B-cell neoplasms, immunodeficient patients have a markedly increased incidence of B-cell neoplasia, particularly large B-cell lymphoma and Burkitt lymphoma {96, 931, 176}.

Major forms of immunodeficiency currently include infection with the human immunodeficiency virus (HIV), iatrogenic immunosuppression to prevent allograft rejection or graft vs host disease (GVHD), and primary immune deficiencies. Some autoimmune diseases are also associated with an increased risk of lymphoma, particularly extranodal marginal zone /

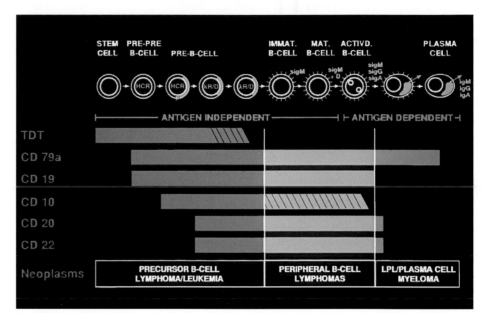

Fig. 6.01 B-cell differentiation showing sequence of antigen expression during B-cell differentiation.

Table 6.01
Frequency of B and T/NK cell lymphomas {8}.

Diagnosis	% of total cases
Diffuse large B-cell lymphoma	30.6%
Follicular lymphoma	22.1%
MALT lymphoma	7.6%
Mature T-cell lymphomas (except ALCL)	7.6%
Chronic lymphocytic leukaemia/ small lymphocytic lymphoma	6.7%
Mantle cell lymphoma	6.0%
Mediastinal large B-cell lymphoma	2.4%
Anaplastic large cell lymphoma	2.4%
Burkitt lymphoma	2.50%
Nodal marginal zone lymphoma	1.8%
Precursor T lymphoblastic	1.7%
Lymphoplasmacytic lymphoma	1.2%
Other types	7.4%

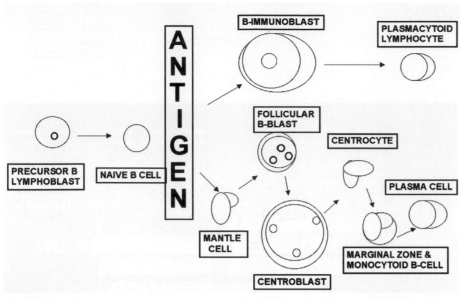

Fig. 6.02 Scheme of B-cell differentiation, showing maturation from the precursor B lymphoblast to the mature plasma cell. There is some evidence that in the early immune response, naive B cells may transform directly to immunoblasts and mature to IgM-producing plasma cells. In the late primary and secondary responses, the germinal centre recation gives rise to immunoglobulin variable region gene mutations, heavy chain class switch, and generation of IgG and IgA-producing plasma cells and memory B cells.

mucosa-associated lymphoid tissue (MALT) lymphoma in patients with lymphoepithelial sialadenitis or Hashimoto thyroiditis {637, 638}.

Aetiology

Infectious agents have been shown to contribute to the development of several types of mature B-cell lymphomas. Epstein-Barr virus (EBV) is present in nearly 100% of endemic Burkitt lymphoma and in 40% of sporadic and HIV-associated cases {1058, 482}, and it is clearly involved in the pathogenesis of the majority of B-cell lymphomas arising in iatrogenically immunosuppressed patients. Other viruses implicated in the pathogenesis of mature B-cell neoplasms include human herpesvirus-8 (HHV8) / Kaposi sarcoma herpesvirus

(KSHV) in primary effusion lymphoma and the lymphomas associated with multicentric Castleman disease in HIV-infected patients {198}, and hepatitis C virus in lymphoplasmacytic lymphoma associated with type II cryoglobulinemia and with some lymphomas of the liver and salivary glands {13, 1054, 843, 605, 50, 1447, 273}.

Bacteria, or at least immune responses to bacterial antigens, have also been implicated in the pathogenesis of B-cell lymphoma of extranodal marginal zone/ mucosa-associated lymphoid tissue (MALT). Gastric MALT lymphomas in patients infected with *H. pylori* depend on the presence of T cells activated by *H. pylori* antigens for proliferation {553}, and treatment of *H. pylori* infection causes regression of the lymphoma in many patients {1417, 1415, 943}. Similarly, *B. Burgdorferi* has been implicated in the pathogenesis of cutaneous MALT lymphoma {192}, and mixed bacterial infections in intestinal MALT lymphoma associated with immunoproliferative small intestinal disease (IPSID)/alpha heavy chain disease {1083, 1059}.

Pathophysiology

Mature B-cell neoplasms tend to mimic stages of normal B-cell differentiation, and the resemblance to normal cell stages is one basis for their classification and nomenclature. Normal B-cell differentiation begins with precursor B lymphoblasts (blast cells that are the precursors of the entire B-cell line), which undergo immunoglobulin *VDJ* gene rearrangement and differentiate into mature surface immunoglobulin (sIg) positive (IgM+ IgD+) naive B cells that are often CD5+ {658}. Naive B cells are small resting lymphocytes that circulate in the blood and also occupy primary lymphoid follicles and follicle mantle zones (so-called recirculating B cells) {658, 559}. tumours of these cells are usually histologically low grade, clinically indolent and often widespread and leukaemic, consistent with the recirculating behaviour of normal naive B cells. Two neoplasms are thought to correspond to CD5 positive B cells: B-cell chronic lymphocytic leukaemia (50%) and most cases of mantle cell lymphoma {323, 550}.

On encountering antigen, naive B cells undergo blast transformation, proliferate, and ultimately mature into IgG or IgA anti-

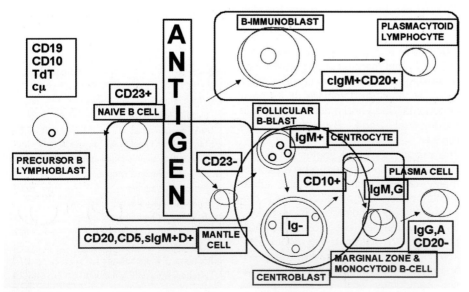

Fig. 6.03 Scheme of B-cell differentiation, showing changes in antigen expressio at various stages.

body-secreting plasma cells and memory B cells. Blast cells formed from naive B cells that have encountered antigen migrate into the centre of a primary follicle and fill the follicular dendritic cell (FDC) meshwork, forming a germinal centre {799, 779}. Germinal centre blast cells are called centroblasts (blast cells of the germinal centre); they are large proliferating cells with vesicular nuclei, one to three prominent, peripheral nucleoli, and a narrow rim of basophilic cytoplasm. Many lack sIg, and also switch off expression of BCL2 protein; thus, they and their progeny are susceptible to death through apoptosis {526, 848, 959}. Centroblasts express BCL6 protein, a nuclear zinc-finger transcription factor that is expressed by both centroblasts and centrocytes, but not by naive or memory B cells, mantle cells or plasma cells {187, 1046}, and also CD10 {497}.

In the germinal centre, somatic mutations occur in the immunogobulin variable (IGV) region gene, which alter the affinity for antigen of the antibody that will be produced by the cell {405, 575}. This results in marked intraclonal diversity in a population of cells derived from only a few precursors. In addition, some cells switch from IgM to IgG or IgA production. Through these mechanisms, the germinal centre reaction gives rise to the better-fitting IgG or IgA antibody of the late primary or secondary immune response {800}. The BCL6 gene also undergoes somatic mutation in the germinal centre, at a lower frequency than is seen in the Ig genes {1003}. Ongoing IGV region gene mutation with intraclonal diversity is a hallmark of germinal centre cells, and both IGV region gene mutation and BCL6 mutation serve as markers of cells that have been through the germinal centre. Most large B-cell lymphomas are composed of cells that at least in part resemble centroblasts and that have mutated IGV-region and often BCL6 genes, consistent with a derivation from cells that have been exposed to the germinal centre. Burkitt lymphoma cells are BCL6+ and have mutated IG genes, and are thus also thought to correspond to a germinal centre blast cell. Both Burkitt and large B-cell lymphoma correspond to proliferating cells, and tend to be clinically aggressive tumours.

Centroblasts mature to centrocytes (cleaved follicle centre cells), which are medium-sized cells with irregular nuclei,

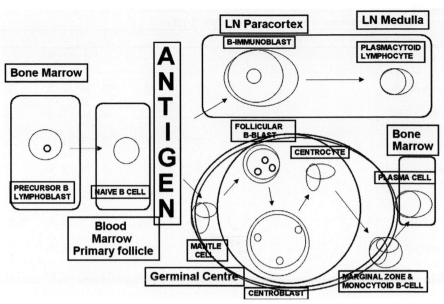

Fig. 6.04 Scheme of B-cell differentiation, showing anatomical sites of various stages.

inconspicuous nucleoli, and scant cytoplasm. Centrocytes express sIg that has an altered antibody combining site compared with its progenitor cell, because of the somatic mutations, and which may have undergone heavy chain class switch. Centrocytes with mutations that result in decreased affinity for antigen rapidly die by apoptosis, while centrocytes with mutations that result in increased affinity are able to bind to antigen trapped on the processes of FDC's. This process "rescues" them from apoptosis and they re-express BCL2 protein {799}. Through

interaction with surface molecules on FDC's and T cells, such as CD23 and CD40 ligand, centrocytes switch off BCL6 protein expression {187, 1046}, and differentiate into either memory B cells or plasma cells {799, 779}. Follicular lymphomas are believed to be tumours of germinal centre B cells (centrocytes and centroblasts), in which centrocytes fail to undergo apoptosis because they have a chromosomal rearrangement, t(14;18), that prevents the normal switching off of BCL2 protein expression. Since they are composed predominantly of centrocytes,

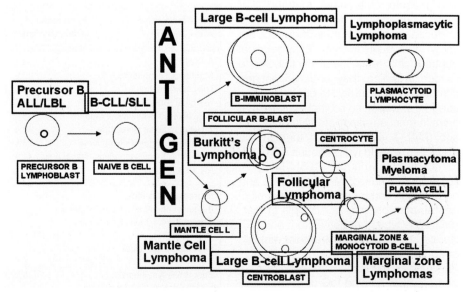

Fig. 6.05 Scheme of B-cell differentiation, showing postulated normal counterpart of B-cell neoplasms.

Table 6.02
Presenting features of common B and T/NK cell neoplasms {1, 70}.

Neoplasm	Frequency	Age	Male	Stage I	II	III	IV	B	EN*	BM	GI	IPI 0/1	2/3	4/5
Large B-cell	31	64	55	25	29	13	33	33	71	16	18	35	46	9
Mediastinal	2	37	34	10	56	3	31	38	56	3	0	52	37	11
Follicular	22	59	42	18	15	16	51	28	64	42	4	45	48	7
SLL/CLL	6	65	53	4	5	8	83	33	80	72	3	23	64	13
MALT	8	60	48	39	28	2	31	19	98	14	50	44	48	8
Mantle cell	6	63	74	13	7	9	71	28	81	51	9	23	54	23
Peripheral T-cell	7	61	55	8	12	15	65	50	82	36	15	17	52	31
ALCL	2	34	69	19	32	10	39	53	59	13	9	61	18	21

which are resting cells, they tend to be indolent.

Memory B cells typically reside in the follicle marginal zones (marginal zone B-cells); they have round to slightly irregular nuclei, moderately condensed chromatin, and a moderate amount of pale cytoplasm. They typically express surface IgM without IgD, pan-B antigens, and lack CD5, and CD10 {1215, 1327, 1326, 1332}. Plasma cells home to the bone marrow; they have condensed chromatin and abundant, basophilic cytoplasm that contains predominantly IgG or IgA; they lack surface immunoglobulin and pan-B antigens, but express CD79a and CD138. Both memory B cells and plasma cells have mutated IGV region genes, but do not continue to undergo mutations; thus they do not show intraclonal diversity. Post-germinal centre B cells retain the ability to home to tissues in which they undergo antigen stimulation, probably through surface integrin expression, so that B cells that arise in mucosa-associated lymphoid tissue (MALT) tend to return there, while those that arise in lymph nodes will home to nodal sites marrow {165}. Marginal zone lymphomas of MALT, splenic, and nodal types correspond to post germinal centre, possibly memory B cells of marginal zone type, that derive from and proliferate specifically in extranodal, splenic or nodal tissues.

Plasma cell myeloma corresponds to a bone-marrow homing IgG or IgA-producing plasma cell.

Genetics

Several mature B-cell neoplasms have characteristic genetic abnormalities that are important in determining their biologic features and that can be useful in differential diagnosis. These include the t(11;14) in mantle cell lymphoma, t(14;18) in follicular lymphoma, t(8;14) in Burkitt lymphoma, and t(11;18) in MALT lymphoma. The first three place a cellular proto-oncogene under the control of the immunoglobulin promotor on chromosome 14q, resulting in constitutive activation of the gene, while the t(11;18) results in a fusion protein. In follicular lymphoma and MALT lymphoma, these translocations result in overexpression of an anti-apoptosis gene (BCL2 or API2), while in mantle cell and Burkitt lymphoma, they result in overexpression of genes associated with proliferation (CYCLIN D1 or MYC).

Principles of classification

The classification of mature B-cell neoplasms is based on utilization of all available information to define disease entities {496}. Morphology and immunophenotype are sufficient for the diagnosis in most of these diseases. Immunophenotyping is used to distinguish the lymphomas of small cell types (chronic lymphocytic leukaemia/small lymphocytic lymphoma, follicular lymphoma, MALT lymphoma, plasma cell neoplasms) from reactive processes, the proliferating types (large B-cell lymphoma and Burkitt lymphoma) from nonlymphoid tumours, and to subclassify morphologically overlapping neoplasms {8}. In general, no one antigen is specific for any of these neoplasms, and a combination of morphologic features and a panel of antigens is necessary for the correct diagnosis. In some diseases, knowledge of clinical features is essential, such as marginal zone lymphoma of MALT type vs nodal or splenic marginal zone lymphoma, and mediastinal large B-cell lymphoma. Molecular genetic analysis, cytogenetic analysis, and fluorescence *in situ*

Table 6.03
Reproducibility of lymphoma diagnosis {1}.

Reproducibility >85% (86-96%)	Contribution of immunophenotype
B-CLL/SLL	3%
Mantle cell lymphoma	10%
Follicular lymphoma	0%
Marginal zone/MALT	2%
Diffuse large B-cell lymphoma	15%
T-Lymphoblastic lymphoma	40%
Anaplastic large-cell lymphoma	39%
Peripheral T-cell lymphoma, unspecified	41%
Mycosis fungoides	
Reproducibility 80%	
Angioimmunoblastic T-cell lymphoma	
Extranodal NK/T-cell lymphoma	
Reproducibility <50%	
Burkitt-like lymphoma	6%
Lymphoplasmacytic lymphoma	

hybridization (FISH) can be helpful in difficult cases, both for determination of clonality in small B-cell neoplams in the distinction from reactive processes, and in detection of specific rearrangements such as the t(11;14), t(14;18) and t(8;14) for subclassification.

In the WHO classification, the mature B-cell neoplasms are listed according to their major clinical presentations: predominantly disseminated, often leukemic types, primary extranodal lymphomas, and predominantly nodal lymphomas (which may involve extranodal sites as well).

Predominantly disseminated lymphoma/leukemia

These tumours usually present with involvement of bone marrow, with or without peripheral blood and solid tissues such as lymph nodes and spleen. B-cell neoplasms include chronic lymphocytic leukaemia (CLL), lymphoplasmacytic lymphoma/Waldenstrom's macroglobulinemia, hairy cell leukaemia, splenic marginal zone lymphoma, and plasma cell myeloma. In general, the disseminated B-cell neoplasms are relatively indolent.

Primary extranodal lymphomas

These are lymphomas that virtually always present in extranodal sites, and appear to correspond to normal lymphoid cells specific for extranodal immunologic reactions. In the B-cell neoplasms, this category is represented by extranodal marginal zone B-cell lymphoma of mucosa-associated lymphoid tissue (MALT lymphoma). Because its clinical presentation and treatment options differ dramatically from the more common nodal or leukemic lymphoid neoplasms, it is considered in a distinct clinical category. MALT lymphomas are less likely to disseminate, and when they do, it is more often to other extranodal sites than to lymph nodes and bone marrow. Exposure to antigen may play a part in pathogenesis of MALT lymphomas.

Predominantly nodal lymphomas

Two B cell neoplasms comprise the majority of nodal small B-cell lymphomas: follicle centre lymphoma (follicular lymphoma) and mantle cell lymphoma. A third type, nodal marginal zone B-cell lymphoma, is rare, but appears to behave similarly to other indolent nodal lymphomas. These neoplasms typically present with disseminated disease involving predominantly lymph nodes, but with frequent involvement of bone marrow, spleen, and liver; they may involve other extranodal sites as part of disseminated disease, but rarely present with localised extranodal disease. Follicular lymphoma comprises the vast majority (80% or more) of lymphomas reported in most American and European clinical trials of Working Formulation low-grade lymphoma. Thus, our understanding of the clinical features and response to treatment of "low-grade lymphoma" is essentially that of follicular lymphoma. Mantle cell lymphoma has been recognized relatively recently; it can be classified as indolent since its survival is measured in years, but its median survival is significantly shorter than that of follicular lymphoma. Removal of this distinctive entity from studies of follicular lymphoma is essential if treatment modalities are to be studied and defined for each type of tumour.

Two aggressive B-cell lymphomas may present with either nodal or extranodal disease, which may be either localised or disseminated. Diffuse large B-cell lymphoma is the most common lymphoma worldwide, accounting for about 30% of the cases. It may involve lymph nodes or extranodal sites; patients typically present with rapidly growing masses at a localised nodal or extranodal site. An important clinical subtype of large B-cell lymphoma is primary mediastinal (thymic) large B-cell lymphoma, an aggressive tumour of young adults with a slight female predominance. Other distinctive clinical entities include primary effusion lymphoma and intravascular lymphoma. Morphologic variants of large B-cell lymphoma exist (centroblastic, immunoblastic, T-cell-rich, anaplastic); the clinical relevance of

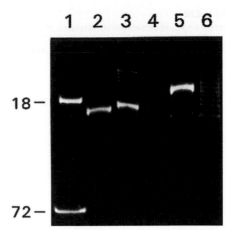

Fig. 6.06 Immunoglobulin gene VJ-PCR analysis in B-cell lymphomas. Lanes 2, 3 and 5 each show a clonal band. Lane 6 (control) shows a polyclonal ladder pattern from a reactive lymph node. Molecular weight markers are shown in lane 1.

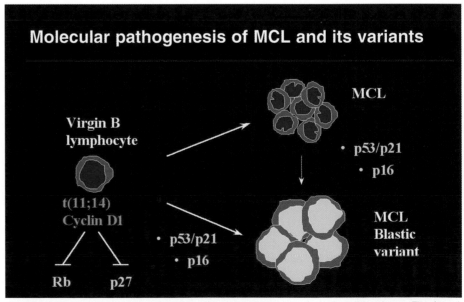

Fig. 6.07 Schematic diagram illustrates the molecular pathogenesis of mantle cell lymphoma. The t(11;14) results in inappropriate expression of the G1 cyclin, CYCLIN D1. The interactions of CYCLIN D1 with the G1/S chedpoint protein Rb and the CDK inhibitor p27 are thought to contribute to the pathogenesis of the lymphoma. Reproduced from Campo et al. {174}.

Table 6.04
Immunophenotype and genetic features of common B-cell neoplasms.

Neoplasm	SIg; CIg	CD5	CD10	CD23	CD43	CD103	BCL6	Cyclin D1	Genetic abnormality	Immunoglobul in genes
B-CLL/SLL	+;–/+	+	–	+	+	–	–	–	trisomy 12; 13q	R, U/M
Lymphoplasmacytic lymphoma	+; +	–	–	–	–/+	–	–	–	t(9;14)	R,M
Splenic marginal zone B-cell lymphoma	+; –/+	–	–	–	–	–	–	–	none known	R,M
Hairy cell leukaemia	+; –	–	–	–	–	++	–	+/–	none known	R,M
Plasma cell myeloma	–; +	–	–/+	–	–/+	–	–	–/+		

debate. Burkitt lymphoma is a highly aggressive tumour of medium-sized, rapidly proliferating B cells, typically with translocations resulting in deregulation of the c-myc oncogene. Major clinical subtypes include endemic, sporadic, and immunodeficiency-associated. Some tumours that have morphologic features intermediate between typical Burkitt lymphoma and large B-cell lymphoma have been called "Burkitt-like". In the WHO classification, this category is considered a subtype of Burkitt lymphoma: so-called atypical Burkitt/Burkitt-like lymphoma.

Clinical features and survival

The clinical presentations, natural histories, and responses to treatment of the mature B-cell neoplasms are extremely heterogeneous, and knowledge of the correct diagnosis is essential to predict outcome and direct therapy. In addition, recognition of new disease entities can pave the way for the development of new therapeutic options. Patients with indolent lymphomas such as chronic lymphocytic leukaemia/small lymphocytic lymphoma, follicular lymphoma, or smoldering plasma cell myeloma are considered incurable and may be observed without treatment until they become symptomatic, with median survival expectations of 5 or more years. Another indolent lymphoma, MALT lymphoma, may be cured with localised radiation therapy. One of the major advances in the past decade was the recognition that MALT lymphoma differed from other small B-cell lymphomas in both its morphology, immunophenotype, and natural history. This opened the door for the discovery that it is related to *H. pylori* infection and could be potentially cured with antibiotics to eradicate *H. pylori* {1417, 553}. Another recently-defined lymphoma of small B cells, mantle cell lymphoma, combines the worst features of indolent and aggressive lymphomas, in being incurable by currently available chemotherapy but clinically aggressive, with a median survival of 3 years. Its recognition by pathologists was essential for the development of new, potentially curative therapies.

Diffuse large B-cell lymphomas are likely heterogeneous, and clinical risk factors are used to stratify patients for treatment; currently approximately 40% overall appear to be cured with aggressive chemotherapy containing adriamycin. New approaches using DNA microarray analysis to assess gene expression suggest that a patterns of gene expression may identify subtypes with differing prognosis, which may lead to advances in therapy {19}. Burkitt lymphoma tends to be highly aggressive and is often treated with more aggressive chemotherapy regimens {306}. Monoclonal antibodies against B-cell surface antigens such as CD20 are being increasingly used as an adjuvant to therapy for mature B-cell neoplasms. Further refinements of disease categories, particularly large B-cell lymphoma, and investigation of potential genetic targets will likely lead to improvements in therapy. Close collaboration between pathologists and oncologists is essential for future progress in the cure of these common neoplasms.

Chronic lymphocytic leukaemia / small lymphocytic lymphoma

H.K. Müller-Hermelink   E. Montserrat
D. Catovsky   N.L. Harris

Definition
Chronic lymphocytic leukaemia / small lymphocytic lymphoma (SLL/CLL) is a neoplasm of monomorphic small, round B-lymphocytes in the peripheral blood, bone marrow and lymph nodes, admixed with prolymphocytes and paraimmunoblasts (pseudofollicles), usually expressing CD5 and CD23. The term SLL, consistent with CLL, is restricted to cases with the tissue morphology and immunophenotype of CLL, but which are non-leukaemic.

ICD-O codes
CLL   9823/3
B-SLL   9670/3

Synonyms
Rappaport: well-differentiated lymphocytic, diffuse
Kiel: CLL; immunocytoma, lymphoplasmacytoid type
Lukes-Collins: small lymphocyte B, CLL
Working Formulation: small lymphocytic, consistent with CLL
REAL: B-cell chronic lymphocytic leukaemia
FAB: B-cell chronic lymphocytic leukaemia

Epidemiology
CLL comprises 90% of chronic lymphoid leukaemias in the United States and Europe. In a recent international study, 6.7% of non-Hodgkin lymphomas were classified as SLL/CLL {8}. The majority of patients are >50 years old (median age 65), with a male: female ratio of 2:1.

Sites of involvement
All the patients with a diagnosis of CLL have, by definition, involvement of bone marrow and peripheral blood at the time of the diagnosis and a lymphocyte count >10x10⁹/l. A diagnosis is possible with lymphocytes <10x10⁹/l, provided the morphology and immunophenotype are typical of CLL. Lymph nodes, liver, and spleen are typically infiltrated, and extranodal sites such as skin, breast, and ocular adnexae may occasionally be involved. A diagnosis of SLL (but not CLL) can be made histologically in the absence of bone marrow or blood involvement.

Clinical features
Most patients are asymptomatic, but some patients present with fatigue, autoimmune hemolytic anaemia, infections, splenomegaly, hepatomegaly, lymphadenopathy or extranodal infiltrates {1074, 109, 112}. Rare patients with CLL present with aleukaemic nodal involvement, but usually develop marrow and blood infiltration. A small M-component may be found in some patients.

Morphology
Lymph nodes and spleen
Enlarged lymph nodes in patients with CLL show effacement of the architecture, with a pseudofollicular pattern of regularly-distributed pale areas containing larger cells in a dark background of small cells {89, 747}. Occasionally, involvement is interfollicular. The predominant cell is a small lymphocyte, which may be slightly larger than a normal lymphocyte, with clumped chromatin, usually a round nucleus, and occasionally a small nucleolus. Mitotic activity is usually very low. Pseudofollicles (also known as proliferation centres, or growth centres) contain a continuum of small, medium and large cells. Prolymphocytes are medium-sized cells with dispersed chromatin and small nucleoli; para-immunoblasts are medium to large cells with round to oval nuclei, dispersed chromatin, central eosino-

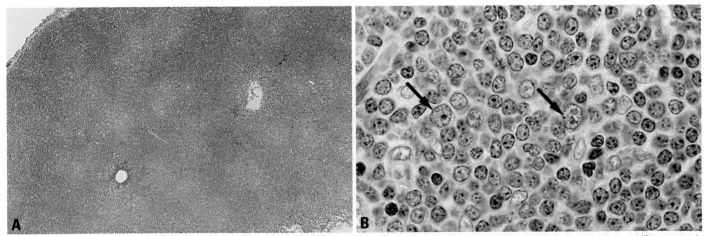

Fig. 6.08 A Lymph node involved by chronic lymphocytic leukaemia, showing a pseudofollicular pattern, with regularly-spaced areas in a dark background (Giemsa stain). **B** High magnification illustrating a mixture of small lymphocytes with scant cytoplasm and clumped chromatin, some sligtly larger prolymphocytes with more dispersed chromatin and small nucleoli, and single paraimmunoblasts (arrows), which are larger cells with round to oval nuclei dispersed chromatin and a central nucleolus.

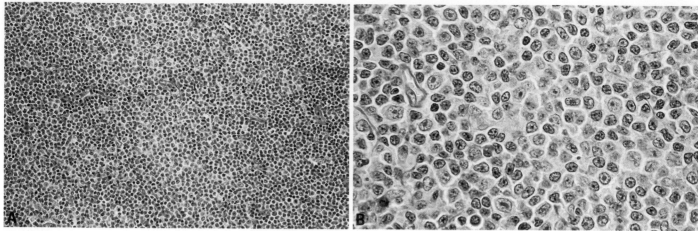

Fig 6.09 Chronic lymphocytic leukaemia, lymph node. **A** A pseudofollicle (proliferation center) corresponding to the pale areas in Fig. 6.08 embedded in a darker background of small lymphocytes (PAS stain). **B** High magnification showing a clustering of larger lymphoid cells (prolymphocytes and paraimmunoblasts) in the pseudofollicle.

philic nucleoli, and slightly basophilic cytoplasm. The size of pseudofollicles and number of para-immunoblasts vary from case to case, but there is no well-documented correlation between lymph node histology and clinical course {89}. In the spleen, white pulp involvement is usually prominent, but the red pulp is also involved; pseudofollicles may be seen but are less conspicuous than in lymph nodes.

In some cases, the small lymphoid cells show moderate nuclear irregularity, which can lead to a differential diagnosis of mantle cell lymphoma; if pseudofollicles and/or prolymphocytes and para-immunoblasts are present, a diagnosis of CLL should be made {1027 115}. Some cases show plasmacytoid differentiation; these are synonymous with the lympho-plasmacytoid immunocytoma of the Kiel classification {752}.

Bone marrow and blood
On bone marrow and peripheral blood smears, CLL cells are small lymphocytes with clumped chromatin and scant cytoplasm, which is clear to lightly basophilic with a regular outline {94}. Nucleoli are usually indistinct or absent. Smudge or basket cells are typically seen in blood smears. The proportion of prolymphocytes (larger cells with prominent nucleoli) in blood films is usually less than 2%. Increasing numbers correlate with a more aggressive disease course, p53 abnormalities and trisomy of chromosome 12 {839}. The variant, CLL with increased prolymphocytes (CLL/PL), is defined by more than 10% prolymphocytes but less than 55% {94}.

Bone marrow involvement may be nodular, interstitial, diffuse, or a combination of the three; pseudofollicles are less common in the marrow than in lymph nodes, but may be found; paratrabecular aggregates are not typical. Bone marrow trephine patterns correlate with prognosis; the nodular and interstitial patterns are seen mainly in early CLL. Advanced disease and bone marrow failure are associated with a diffuse pattern of infil-

tration {1121, 894}.

Some cases of CLL show atypical morphology. There may be a variable proportion of atypical lymphocytes (e.g. prolymphocytes; large lymphocytes; rarely cleaved cells) in blood but with the characteristic CLL immunophenotype. An increased proportion (>10%) of prolymphocytes identifies a clinically aggressive variant designated CLL/PL {94, 839}.

Transformation to diffuse large B-cell lymphoma (DLBCL) (Richter syndrome) {1100} is characterised by confluent sheets of large cells that may resemble paraimmunoblasts, but are more often centroblast- or immunoblast-like. CLL may be associated with Hodgkin lymphoma (HL) {1122, 136, 890}; this may be manifested as scattered Reed-Sternberg cells and variants in a background of CLL, or may occur as discrete areas of classical HL {890}.

Immunophenotype

The tumour cells express weak or dim surface IgM or IgM and IgD, CD5, CD19,

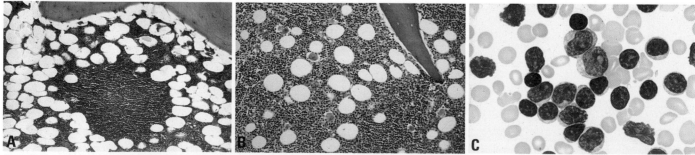

Fig. 6.10 Bone marrow trephine section illustrating (**A**) a nodular pattern of infiltration (**B**) an interstitial pattern of lymphocytic infiltration. **C** In the peripheral blood, lymphocytes are small, round with distinct clumped nuclear chromatin. Nucleoli are visible only in the larger prolymphocytes and smudge or basket cells are common.

CD20 (weak), CD22 (weak), CD79a, CD23, CD43, CD11c (weak), and are CD10- and cyclin D1-; FMC7 and CD79b are as a rule negative or weakly expressed in typical CLL. The immunophenotype of blood lymphocytes has been integrated into a scoring system that helps in the differential diagnosis between CLL and other B-cell leukaemias {840, 895}. Cases with unmutated Ig variable region genes have been reported to be CD38+ {263}. The antigen specificity of the sIg in many cases has been shown to be against self antigens, and these antibodies often have broad specificity – so-called cross-reactive idiotypes {659}. Cytoplasmic Ig is detectable in about 5% of the cases. CD23 and cyclin D1 are useful in distinguishing CLL/SLL from mantle cell lymphoma {1449}; however, some cases of CLL are CD23- or only partially positive, and rare cases of mantle cell lymphoma may partially express CD23; thus, cyclin D1 should be assessed in lymphomas that are CD5+ CD23- {1431}. Some cases with typical CLL morphology may have a departure from the typical immunophenotype (e.g. CD5- or CD23-, FMC7+ or CD11c+, or strong sIg, or CD79b+) {839, 254}.

Genetics

Antigen receptor genes

Ig heavy and light chain genes are rearranged. Recent data suggest that there are two distinct types of CLL defined by the mutational status of the Immunoglobulin *VH* genes: 40-50% percent show no somatic mutations of their variable region genes, consistent with naïve B cells, while 50-60% have somatic mutations, consistent with a derivation from post-germinal center B cells {263 983, 481}. Variable region usage is non-random, and those associated with autoantibodies are often found in CLL cases {983}.

Cytogenetic abnormalities and oncogenes

About 80% of the cases have abnormal karyotypes when examined by FISH analysis {311}. Trisomy 12 is reported in 20% of cases {839, 312}, and deletions at 13q14 in up to 50% {311, 312}. Cases with trisomy 12 have predominantly unmutated immunoglobulin variable region genes, while those with 13q14 abnormalities more often have mutations {983}. Deletions at 11q22-23 are found in

20% of the cases {313}, and somatic mutations have been found in the other allele in these cases {1153}. Deletions at 6q21 or 17p13 (p53 locus) are seen in 5% and 10% of cases respectively {311, 310}. p53 is also expressed in 10% of cases {247}. t(11;14) and *BCL1* gene rearrangement have been reported but most of these cases may be examples of leukaemic mantle cell lymphoma {834}.

Postulated cell of origin

Many cases of CLL are thought to correspond to the recirculating CD5+ CD23+ IgM+ IgD+ naive B cells, which are found in the peripheral blood, primary follicle, and follicle mantle zone {800, 559}. It has been suggested that they are an anergic, self-reactive CD5+ B-cell subset {169, 170}. Cases that show V region mutations may correspond to a subset of peripheral blood CD5+ IgM+ B cells that appear to be memory B cells {666}.

Prognosis and predictive factors

The clinical course is indolent, but CLL is not usually considered to be curable with available therapy. Purine nucleoside analogues, such as fludarabine, may result in sustained remissions {645}. The 5 year overall actuarial survival of SLL in a recent study {8} was 51%, with a failure-free survival (FFS) of 25%. The overall median survival of CLL is 7 years. Clinical staging systems – Rai (0-IV) and Binet (A-C) – are the best predictors of survival {1074, 109}. Cases of CLL/PL, and those with diffuse bone marrow involvement, may have a worse prognosis {894, 861}.

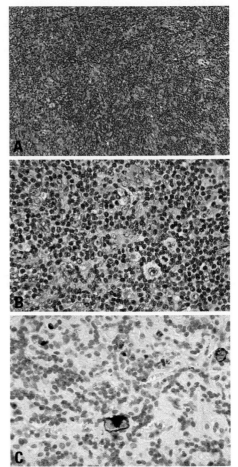

Fig 6.11 Hodgkin lymphoma in CLL. **A** Classical HL in a patient with CLL. The dark area represents the infiltrate of CLL, while the pale are represents HL. **B** At higher magnification, there are classical RS cells in a background of lymphocytes and histiocytes. **C** Immunoperoxidase stain for CD15, showing typical membrane and Golgi region staining of the large cells.

Table 6.05
Immunophenotype in the diagnosis of CLL {311, 1153}.

Marker	CLL	score	other B-cell leukaemias	score
SIg	Weak	1	Strong	0
CD5	Positive	1	Negative*	0
CD23	Positive	1	Negative	0
CD79b/CD22	Weak	1	Strong	0
FMC7	Negative	1	Positive	0
	CLL score 4-5		Usual score	0-2

*Except mantle cell lymphoma

A rapid lymphocyte doubling time (<12 months) is a prediction of poor prognosis in stage A CLL.

Chromosomal abnormalities and immunophenotype seem also to contribute prognostic information. Trisomy 12 correlates with atypical morphology and an aggressive clinical course {839, 311, 609}. Abnormalities of 13q14 are reported associated with long survival. Patients whose tumours have mutations in the Ig genes variable regions have a better prognosis than those with germline VH regions (median survival 7 vs 3 years) {263, 481}. In addition, patients with tumour cells that express CD38 appear to have a worse prognosis {263, 481}.

Cases with 11q22-23 deletions have extensive lymphadenopathy and poor survival {313}, and cases with *TP53* abnormalities have also been reported to have a poor prognosis {310, 247}.

Transformation to high grade lymphoma (Richter Syndrome) occurs in approximately 3.5% of the cases; these are usually diffuse large B-cell lymphomas (3%), but cases resembling Hodgkin disease also occur (0.5%), particularly in patients treated with purine nucleotide analogues. Molecular genetic analysis suggests that in about 50% of the cases, the aggressive lymphoma represents transformation of the original neoplastic clone, while in the remainder, the aggressive lymphoma maybe be a second, unrelated neoplasm {436, 965}.

Variant: Mu heavy chain disease

Mu heavy chain disease is usually associated with a neoplasm resembling CLL, in which a defective mu heavy chain lacking a variable region is produced (see also plasma cell neoplasms). The bone marrow has characteristic vacuolated plasma cells, admixed with small, round lymphocytes. Patients are adults with hepato-splenomegaly, absence of peripheral lymphadenopathy, and a slowly progressive course {376, 400}.

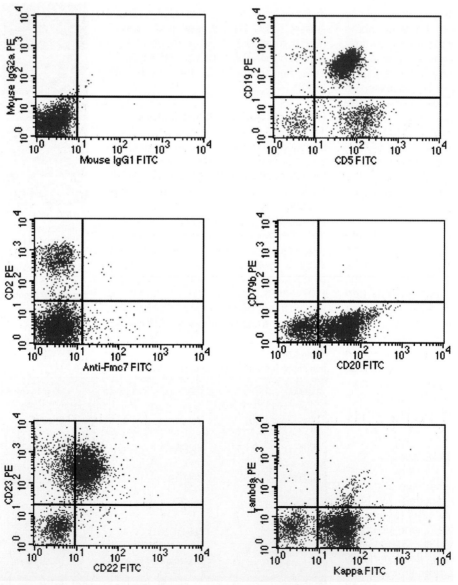

Fig. 6.12 Chronic lymphocytic leukaemia, flow cytometry of a typical case (score 5). From top left to right: Negative control; CD5 and CD19 positive; FMC7 and CD2 negative (20% T-cells +); CD79b negative and CD20 weakly positive; CD23 positive and CD22 weakly positive; SIg weakly positive (kappa).

B-cell prolymphocytic leukaemia

D. Catovsky   H.K. Müller-Hermelink
E. Montserrat   N.L Harris

Definition
B-cell prolymphocytic leukaemia (B-PLL) is a malignancy of B-prolymphocytes (medium-sized, round lymphoid cells with prominent nucleoli) affecting the blood, bone marrow, and spleen. Prolymphocytes must exceed 55% of lymphoid cells in the blood. Cases of transformed chronic lymphocytic leukaemia (CLL) and CLL with increased prolymphocytes are excluded.

ICD-O code   9833/3

Synonyms
Kiel: B-cell prolymphocytic leukaemia
WF: Not classified
FAB: B-cell prolymphocytic leukaemia
REAL: B-cell prolymphocytic leukaemia

Epidemiology
B-PLL is an extremely rare disease, comprising approximately 1% of lymphocytic leukaemias. Most patients are over 60 years old, with a median age of 70 and a male predominance (male:female ratio 1.6:1) {860}.

Sites of involvement
The leukaemic cells are found in the peripheral blood, bone marrow and spleen.

Clinical features
Most patients have marked splenomegaly without peripheral lymphadenopathy, and a rapidly rising lymphocyte count, usually over 100×10^9/l {410}. Anaemia and thrombocytopenia are seen in 50%. A serum M-component is found in some patients.

Morphology
Peripheral blood and bone marrow
The majority (>55% and usually >90%) of the circulating cells are prolymphocytes – medium-sized cells (twice the size of a lymphocyte) with a round nucleus, moderately condensed nuclear chromatin, a prominent central nucleolus, and a relatively small amount of faintly basophilic cytoplasm {860, 418, 94}.

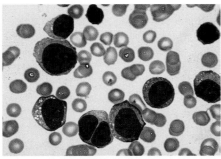

Fig. 6.13 B-cell prolymphocytic leukaemia peripheral blood smear. The cells are medium to large, twice the size of small lymphocytes with moderately condensed nuclear chromatin and prominent vesicular nucleoli. The nuclear outline is usually regular and the cytoplasm weakly basophilic.

Although the nucleus is typically round, there may be some indentation in some cases. The bone marrow shows diffuse intertrabecular infiltration by similar cells.

Tissues other than bone marrow
The morphology of B-PLL in tissues other than bone marrow has not been well studied. The spleen is reported to show extensive white and red pulp involvement, with prolymphocytes present in the red pulp as well as in expanded white pulp nodules. The nodules in the white pulp may show a bizonal appearance with more packed cells in the centre and larger ones on the periphery {728}. The morphology of prolymphocytes is best visualised in the red pulp. Lymph nodes show diffuse or vaguely nodular infiltrates of similar cells. Pseudofollicles are not seen.

Distinction from blastoid variants of mantle cell lymphoma, splenic marginal zone lymphoma, and CLL with increased number of prolymphocytes may be difficult, and some cases reported in the literature as B-PLL may thus be heterogeneous.

Immunophenotype
The cells of B-PLL strongly express surface IgM +/- IgD as well as B-cell antigens (CD19, CD20, CD22, CD79a and b, FMC7); CD5 is present in 1/3 of cases and CD23 is typically absent {840}.

Genetics
Antigen receptor genes
Immunoglobulin genes are clonally rearranged. Information about the muta-

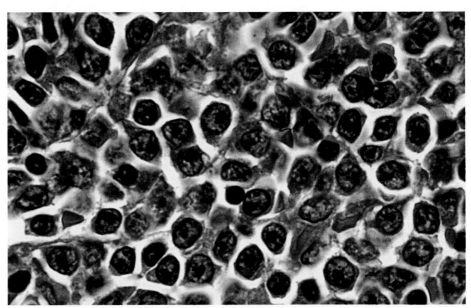

Fig. 6.14 B-cell prolymphocytic leukaemia. Spleen, showing an infiltrate of prolymphocytes.

tional status of the variable region genes is not available.

Cytogenetic abnormalities and oncogenes

Many cases have been reported with breakpoints involving 14q32, particularly with t(11;14)(q13;q32), which is found in up to 20% of typical cases {141, 139}. However, there is still some confusion in the literature about distinguishing B-PLL from cases of the leukaemic blastoid variant of mantle cell lymphoma (MCL). Given the difficulty in distinguishing them

morphologically or immunophenotypically, it is possible that some of the cases reported as B-PLL with t(11;14) may be examples of leukaemic MCL rather than B-PLL. Abnormalities of the *TP53* gene (loss of heterozygosity, p53 protein expression and mutations) have been reported in 53% of cases {753}, the highest incidence observed in lymphoid malignancies. This probably underlies the progressive course and relative treatment resistance of B-PLL. Deletions at 11q23 and 13q14 have also been demonstrated by FISH analysis {754}

Postulated cell of origin
Unknown peripheral B cell stage.

Prognosis and predictive factors
B-PLL responds poorly to therapies for CLL, and survival is short {861}. Responses have been recorded with the combination CHOP (cytoxan, adriamycin, vincristine, and prednisone), the nucleoside analogs fludarabine and cladribine and splenic irradiation. Splenectomy may improve the patient's general condition but does not delay disease progression.

Lymphoplasmacytic lymphoma / Waldenström macroglobulinemia

F. Berger
P.G. Isaacson
M.A. Piris
N.L. Harris

H.K. Müller-Hermelink
B.N. Nathwani
S.H. Swerdlow

Definition
Lymphoplasmacytic lymphoma / Waldenström macroglobulinemia (LDL) is a neoplasm of small B lymphocytes, plasmacytoid lymphocytes, and plasma cells, usually involving bone marrow, lymph nodes and spleen, usually lacking CD5, which has a serum monoclonal protein with hyperviscosity or cryoglobulinemia in most cases. Plasmacytoid/cytic variants of other lymphomas are excluded.

ICD-O code   9671/3

Synonyms
Rappaport: well-differentiated lymphocytic, plasmacytoid
Kiel: immunocytoma, lymphoplasmacytic type
Lukes-Collins: plasmacytic-lymphocytic
Working Formulation: small lymphocytic, plasmacytoid
Waldenström macroglobulinemia

Epidemiology
Lymphoplasmacytic lymphoma (LPL) is a rare disease (1.5% of nodal lymphomas in a recent study) {8} that occurs in older adults, with a median age of 63 and a slight male predominance (53%) {8, 305}.

Sites of involvement
Tumour infiltrates commonly involve the bone marrow, lymph nodes and spleen; peripheral blood may also be involved. Although extranodal infiltrates may occur, including lung, gastrointestinal tract, and skin, most cases previously diagnosed as LPL or immunocytoma in extranodal sites are examples of marginal zone B-cell lymphoma of mucosa-associated lymphoid tissue (MALT) type.

Clinical features
The majority of patients have a monoclonal IgM serum paraprotein (>3gm/dl, Waldenström macroglobulinemia) with

consequent hyperviscosity symptoms. In the cases without a serum M-component the tumour cells usually produce but do not secrete immunoglobulin. The paraprotein may have autoantibody or cryoglobulin activity, resulting in autoimmune phenomena or cryoglobulinemia. Hyperviscosity occurs in 10-30% of patients and results in erythrocyte sludging or rouleaux formation, reduced visual acuity and increased risk of cerebrovascular accidents {305}. Neuropathies occur in about 10% and may result from reactivity of the IgM paraprotein with myelin sheath antigens (myelin-associated glycoprotien or gangliosides), cryoglobulinemia, or paraprotein deposition {305}. Deposits of IgM may occur in the skin or the gastrointestinal tract, where they may cause diarrhoea. Coagulopathies may be caused by IgM binding to clotting factors, platelets, and fibrin. IgM paraproteins may be present in patients with diseases other than LPL, including splenic marginal zone lymphoma, B-cell chronic lymphocytic leukaemia, and even, rarely in patients with extranodal marginal zone B-cell lymphoma of MALT type {934, 98}. Thus, Waldenström macroglobulinemia is not synonymous with LPL.

Aetiology

Recently, several studies from Italy suggest that most cases of type II mixed cryoglobulinemia are associated with hepatitis C virus (HCV) infection, even in patients who have demonstrable lymphoplasmacytic lymphoma in the bone marrow {13, 1054}. Treatment of patients with HCV and cryoglobulinemia with interferon to reduce viral load has been associated with regression of the lymphoma {843}. Hepatitis C virus infection has also been documented in patients with B-cell lymphoma without cryoglobulinemia, most commonly in MAL -lymphomas and in lymphomas of the salivary gland and liver (two sites of chronic viral infection) {605, 50, 1447, 273}. Hepatitis C virus is an RNA virus that cannot integrate into the host genome, but it does infect lymphocytes, and viral proteins have been detected in lymphoid cells in these patients {1144}. It is not clear at this point whether HCV has transforming potential, or whether these neoplasms are antigen-driven, similar to MALT lymphomas.

Genetic susceptibility has been suggested by the occasional occurrence in families. Occupational exposures have also been postulated {305}.

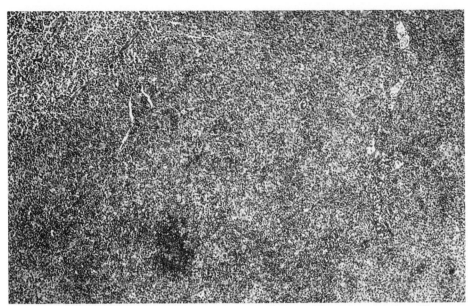

Fig. 6.15 Low-power view of lymph node involved by lymphoplasmacytic lymphoma, showing a diffuse pattern with scattered epithelioid histiocytes.

Morphology

Many B-cell lymphomas can show maturation to plasmacytoid or plasma cells containing cytoplasmic immunoglobulin (CIg), particularly B-cell chronic lymphocytic leukaemia (B-CLL), marginal zone B-cell, and follicular lymphomas. The term LPL is restricted to tumours that lack features of other lymphomas (e.g. pseudofollicles, neoplastic follicles, marginal zone or monocytoid B cells). Defined in this restrictive manner, LPL is an exceedingly rare neoplasm {8}

Lymph nodes

In lymph nodes, the growth pattern of LPL is diffuse, without pseudofollicles, and it may be interfollicular with sparing of the sinuses.

The neoplastic cells are small lymphocytes, plasmacytoid lymphocytes (cells with abundant basophilic cytoplasm, but lymphocyte-like nuclei), and plasma cells, with or without PAS+ intranuclear inclusions (Dutcher bodies). Rare immunoblasts are often present, and there may be reactive epithelioid histiocytes and/or mast cells. Occasional cases show an increase in the number of immunoblasts and mitoses; there is some evidence that these may have a worse prognosis than typical cases {97}, but validated criteria for grading have not been established. Progression to diffuse

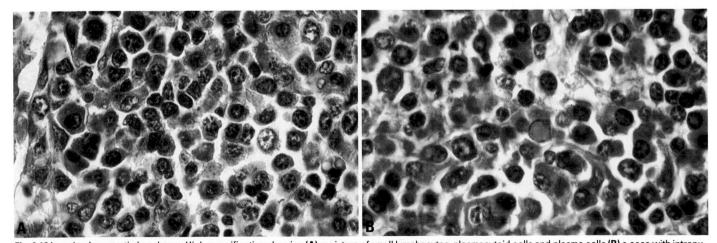

Fig. 6.16 Lymphoplasmacytic lymphoma. High magnification showing **(A)** a mixture of small lymphocytes, plasmacytoid cells and plasma cells **(B)** a case with intranuclear inclusions (Dutcher bodies).

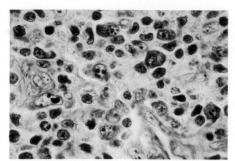

Fig. 6.17 Lymphoplasmacytic lymphoma with increased immunoblasts (Giemsa).

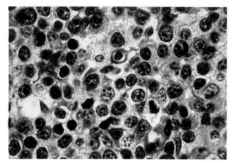

Fig. 6.18 Lymphoplasmacytic lymphoma with progression to immunoblastic lymphoma.

large cell (immunoblastic) lymphoma may occur.

Bone marrow and peripheral blood
Nodular lymphoid aggregates and/or a diffuse interstitial lymphoid infiltrate may be present in the bone marrow. Neoplastic cells may be present in the peripheral blood, but the white blood count is typically lower than in CLL. On smears, a mixture of small lymphocytes, plasma cells, and plasmacytoid lymphocytes are seen.

Immunophenotype
The cells have surface and cytoplasmic (some cells) Ig, usually of IgM type (sometimes G, rarely A), are typically IgD-, express B-cell-associated antigens (CD19, CD20, CD22, CD79a) and are CD5-, CD10-, CD23-, CD43+/-, and CD38+. Lack of CD5 and the presence of strong cytoplasmic Ig are useful in distinction from CLL.

Genetics
Antigen receptor genes
Immunoglobulin heavy and light chain genes are rearranged, and variable (V)-region genes show somatic mutations, suggesting that these cells arise from a population of B cells that have undergone antigen-driven selection {1353}.

Cytogenetic abnormalities and oncogenes
Translocation t(9;14)(p13;q32) and re-arrangement of the *PAX-5* gene is reported in up to 50% of the cases {555, 554}, as well as in other lymphomas with plasmacytoid differentiation {898}. *PAX-5* encodes a protein, B-cell-specific activator protein (BSAP), which is important in early B-cell development. Expression of BSAP is restricted to B cells and appears to be independent of the translocation {692}.

Postulated cell of origin
Peripheral B lymphocyte stimulated to differentiate to a plasma cell, possibly corresponding to the primary immune response to antigen, or to a post germinal centre B cell that has undergone somatic mutation but usually not heavy chain class switch.

Prognosis and predictive factors
The clinical course is typically indolent, with median survival averaging 5 years {305}. Asymptomatic patients are typically not treated. Advanced age, peripheral blood cytopenias, neuropathies, and weight loss are associated with a poorer prognosis. Symptomatic patients are typically treated with alkylating agents and prednisone, or with purine nucleotide analogues. IgM-related complications are treated with plasmapheresis. The disease is not generally considered to be curable with available treatment. Transformation to diffuse large B-cell lymphoma, as in CLL, occurs in a small proportion of the cases and is associated with poor survival.

Variant: Gamma heavy chain disease
Gamma heavy chain disease results from secretion of a truncated gamma chain, which lacks light-chain binding sites (See plasma cell neoplasms). It is usually associated with a tumour resembling lymphoplasmacytic lymphoma, involving lymph nodes, marrow, liver, spleen and peripheral blood.

Most patients are adults with systemic symptoms, including autoimmune manifestations such as haemolytic anaemia and autoimmune thrombocytopenia, arthritis, with lymphadenopathy, splenomegaly, hepatomegaly, involvement of Waldeyer's ring, and peripheral eosinophilia {377}. There is typically a polymorphous proliferation of lymphocytes, plasmacytoid lymphocytes, plasma cells, immunoblasts and eosinophils. Some cases resemble plasma cell myeloma. The clinical course is variable, but probably more aggressive than that of typical IgM-producing LPL {377, 16, 356, 552}.

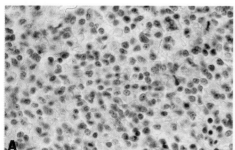
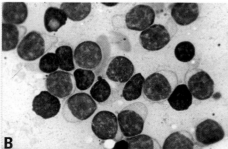
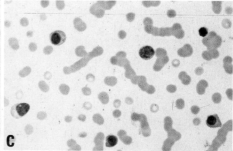

Fig. 6.19 A Bone marrow involvement by lymphoplasmacytic lymphoma: There is an increase in interstitial small lymphocytes and plasma cells (Giemsa). **B** The bone marrow aspirate shows an increase in lymphocytes, many of which are plasmacytoid, with eccentric nuclei and abundant, basophilic cytoplasm. **C** Lymphoplasmacytic lymphoma with Waldenström macroglobulinemia: Peripheral blood showing circulating lymphocytes, plasma cells, and plasmacytoid lymphocytes, with rouleaux formation by red blood cells as a consequence of the IgM paraprotein.

Splenic marginal zone lymphoma

P.G. Isaacson
M.A. Piris
D. Catovsky
S. Swerdlow
E. Montserrat

F. Berger
H.K. Müller-
Hermelink
B. Nathwani
N.L. Harris

Definition
Splenic marginal zone lymphoma (SMZL) is a B-cell neoplasm comprising small lymphocytes which surround and replace the splenic white pulp germinal centres, efface the follicle mantle and merge with a peripheral (marginal) zone of larger cells including scattered transformed blasts; both small and larger cells infiltrate the red pulp. Splenic hilar lymph nodes and bone marrow are often involved; lymphoma cells may be found in the peripheral blood as villous lymphocytes.

ICD-O code   9689/3

Synonyms
Rappaport: well-differentiated lymphocytic lymphoma
Kiel: not listed
Lukes-Collins: small lymphocytic lymphoma
Working Formulation: small lymphocytic lymphoma
FAB: splenic lymphoma with circulating villous lymphocytes (SLVL)

Epidemiology
SMZL is a rare disorder, comprising less than 1% of lymphoid neoplasms {46}, but it may account for most cases of other-wise unclassifiable chronic lymphoid leukaemias that are CD5-. Most patients are over 50 and there is an equal sex incidence {98}.

Sites of involvement
The tumour involves the spleen and splenic hilar lymph nodes, bone marrow, and often the peripheral blood. The liver may be involved. Peripheral lymph nodes are not typically involved {98, 886}.

Clinical features
Patients present with splenomegaly, sometimes accompanied by autoimmune thrombocytopenia or anaemia and variable presence of peripheral blood villous lymphocytes. The bone marrow is usually positive, but peripheral lymphadenopathy is uncommon. Extranodal infiltration is extremely uncommon. About 1/3 of the patients may have a small monoclonal serum protein, but marked hyperviscosity and hypergammaglobulinemia are uncommon {98, 886}.

Morphology
In the splenic white pulp a central zone of small round lymphocytes surrounds, or, more commonly replaces reactive germinal centres with effacement of the normal follicle mantle {565, 886}. This

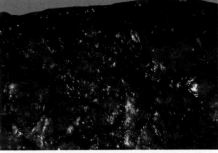

Fig. 6.20 Splenic marginal zone lymphoma, gross photograph of spleen, showing marked expansion of the white pulp, as well as infiltration of the red pulp.

zone merges with a peripheral zone of small to medium-sized cells with more dispersed chromatin and abundant pale cytoplasm, which resemble marginal zone cells and are interspersed with transformed blasts. The red pulp is always infiltrated, with both small nodules of the larger cells and sheets of the small lymphocytes, which often invade sinuses. Epithelioid histiocytes may be present in the lymphoid aggregates. Plasmacytic differentiation may occur. In rare cases, clusters of plasma cells may be present in the centres of the white pulp follicles. In splenic hilar lymph nodes the sinuses are dilated and lym-

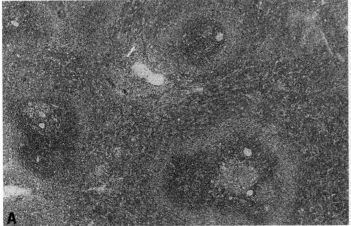
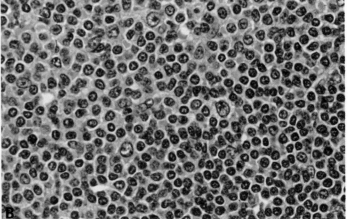

Fig. 6.21 Splenic marginal zone lymphoma showing infiltration of white and red pulp. **A** The white pulp nodules show a central dark zone of small lymphocytes sometimes surrounding a residual germinal centre giving way to a paler marginal zone. **B** High magnification of white pulp nodule showing the central small lymphocytes (lower right) merging with a marginal zone comprising larger cells with pale cytoplasm and occasional transformed blasts.

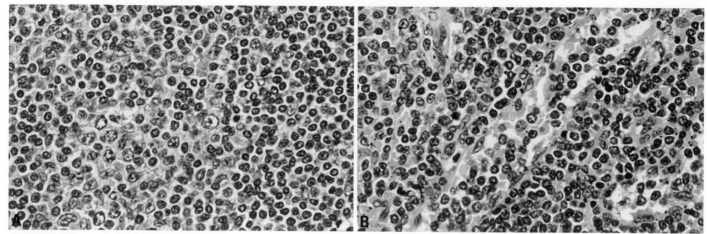

Fig. 6.22 Splenic marginal zone lymphoma. **A** Small lymphocytes invading splenic red pulp with an ill-defined nodule of larger cells. **B** Infiltration of red pulp sinuses.

phoma surrounds and replaces germinal centres, but the two cell types (small lymphocytes and marginal zone cells) are often more intimately mixed without the formation of a distinct "marginal" zone.

In the bone marrow there is a nodular interstitial infiltrate cytologically similar to that in the lymph nodes. Occasionally, neoplastic cells surround reactive follicles, but this is not a consistent finding. Intrasinusoidal lymphoma cells are characteristic {397}.

When lymphoma cells are present in the blood, they are usually, but not always characterised by the presence of short polar villi. Some may appear plasmacytoid {862}.

The differential diagnosis includes other small B-cell lymphoma/leukaemias, inclu-

ding chronic lymphocytic leukaemia, hairy cell leukaemia, mantle cell lymphoma, follicular lymphoma, and lymphoplasmacytic lymphoma. The nodular pattern on marrow biopsy excludes hairy cell leukaemia, but the morphologic features on bone marrow examination may not be sufficient to distinguish between the other subtypes. If villous lymphocyes are present in the blood, this is a helpful feature. Immunophenotyping by flow cytometry on peripheral blood or bone marrow can be helpful. SMZL may be a diagnosis of exclusion in the absence of splenectomy.

Immunophenotype

Tumour cells have surface IgM and IgD, and are CD20+, CD79a+, CD5-, CD10-, CD23-, CD43- {565, 838}. Nuclear cyclin

D1 is absent {1149}. The absence of CD5 and CD43 are useful in excluding CLL and MCL, absence of CD103 in excluding hairy cell leukaemia, and absence of CD10 in excluding follicular lymphoma. On tissue sections, cyclin D1 is also useful in distinguishing between SMZL and MCL {1149}.

Genetics

Antigen receptor genes

Immunoglobulin heavy and light chain genes are rearranged and most cases have somatic mutations. In addition, intraclonal variation has been detected, suggesting ongoing mutations {1438, 324}.

Cytogenetic abnormalities and oncogenes

Allelic loss of chromosome 7q21-32 has been described in up to 40% of SMZL cases {828}. Dysregulation of the *CDK6* gene located at 7q21 has been reported in several cases of SLVL with translocations involving this region {246}. *BCL2* rearrangement and t(14;18) have not been described.

BCL1 rearrangement, t(11;14) and cyclin D1 expression have been reported in a small proportion of the cases; however, the possibility that these cases represent examples of mantle cell lymphoma has not been excluded, since cyclin D1 expression is absent from well-characterised cases of SMZL {1149}.

Trisomy 3 and t(11;18), common in extranodal marginal zone lymphoma of MALT type, are uncommon in SMZL {302, 1098}; trisomy 3 has been described in 17% of cases of SLVL {469}, but no confirmed cases with t(11;18) have been reported.

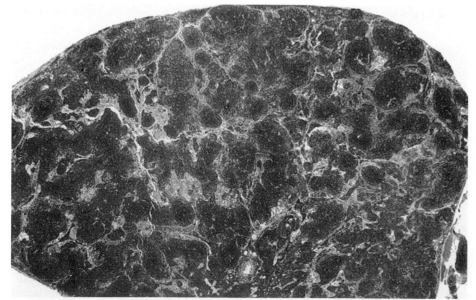

Fig. 6.23 Splenic marginal zone lymphoma. Splenic hilar lymph node showing a nodular infiltrate.

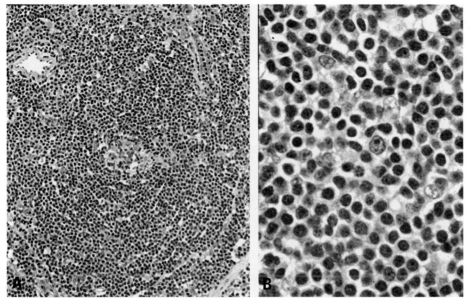

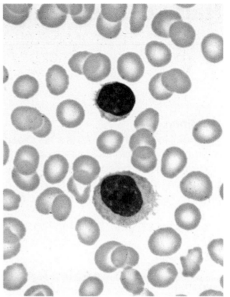

Fig. 6.24 Splenic marginal zone lymphoma. Splenic hilar lymph node nodule showing a small residual germinal centre (**A**) with no evidence of a marginal zone. High magnification shows a mixture of small lymphocytes and larger cells (**B**).

Fig. 6.26 Splenic marginal zone lymphoma. Peripheral blood containing tumour cells with polar villi (villous lymphocytes).

Postulated cell of origin

Post-germinal centre B cell of unknown differentiation stage.

Prognosis and predictive factors

The clinical course is indolent, even with bone marrow involvement {98, 904}. Response to chemotherapy of the type that is typically effective in other chronic lymphoid leukaemias is often poor, but patients typically have haematologic responses to splenectomy, with long-term survival. Transformation to large B-cell lymphoma may occur, as in other indolent B-cell neoplasms {904}.

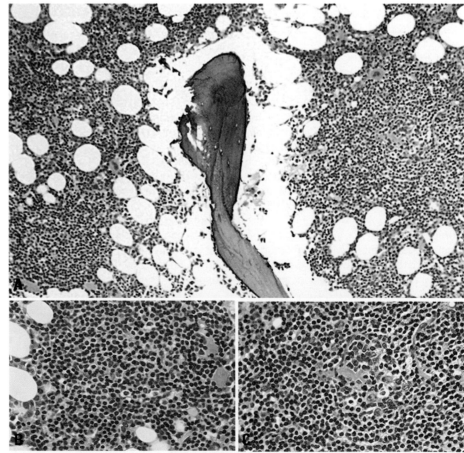

Fig. 6.25 Bone marrow involvement in splenic marginal zone lymphoma. **A** Two large lymphoid aggregates are present in the interstitium. **B** A nodule of small lymphoid cells with rare large cells. **C** A lymphoid aggregate with a small residual germinal centre.

Hairy cell leukaemia

K. Foucar
D. Catovsky

Definition
Hairy cell leukaemia (HCL) is a neoplasm of small B lymphoid cells with oval nuclei and abundant cytoplasm with "hairy" projections in bone marrow and peripheral blood, diffusely infiltrating bone marrow and splenic red pulp, and strongly expressing, CD103, CD22 and CD11c.

ICD-O code
9940/3

Synonym
Leukaemic reticuloendotheliosis.

Epidemiology
Hairy cell leukaemia is a rare disease, comprising 2% of lymphoid leukaemias. Patients are predominantly middle-aged to elderly adults with a median age of 55 years. The male female ratio is 5:1 {130, 129, 403}.

Sites of involvement
Tumour cells are found predominantly in the bone marrow and spleen. Typically a small number of circulating cells are noted. Tumour infiltrates may occur in the liver and lymph nodes, and occasionally also in the skin {130, 129, 403}. Rare patients demonstrate prominent abdominal lymphadenopathy, which is associated with large hairy cells; this may represent a form of transformation {866}.

Clinical features
Most patients present with splenomegaly and pancytopenia and may have few circulating neoplastic cells. Monocytopenia

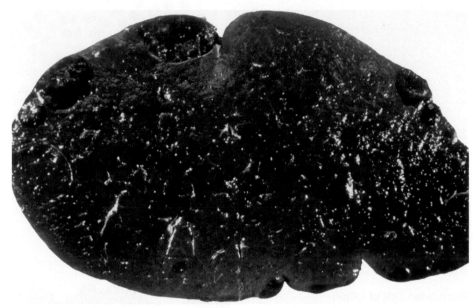

Fig.6.27 Hairy cell leukaemia. The spleen is markedly enlarged (3000g) with diffuse expansion of the red pulp. White pulp is not discernable. Numerous blood cell lakes of varying size are visible.

is characteristic {130, 129, 403}. Other distinctive manifestations include recurrent opportunistic infections, vasculitis or other immune dysfunction.

Morphology
Peripheral blood and bone marrow
Hairy cells are small to medium-sized lymphoid cells with an oval or indented (bean-shaped) nucleus, with homogeneous, spongy, ground-glass chromatin that is slightly less clumped than that of a normal lymphocyte. Nucleoli are typically absent or inconspicuous. The cytoplasm

is abundant and pale blue, with circumferential "hairy" projections on smears {129, 392, 695}. Occasionally the cytoplasm contains discrete vacuoles or rod-shaped inclusions that represent the ribosome lamellar complexes that have been identified by electron microscopy {129}. Hairy cells are characterised by strong, diffuse tartrate resistant acid phosphatase (TRAP) positivity in a variable proportion of the cells {129, 392, 695}. The diagnosis is best made on bone marrow biopsy. The extent of bone marrow effacement in HCL is variable. The

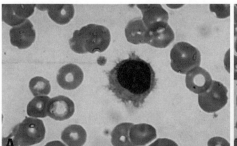
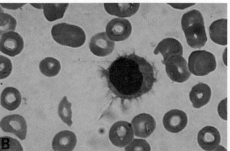
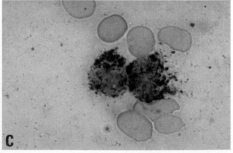

Fig. 6.28 Hairy cell leukaemia, smears. **A** and **B** illustrate the typical morphologic features of two hairy cells. **C** There is strong tartrate resistant acid phosphatase positivity, which is characteristic of hairy cell leukaemia.

primary pattern is interstitial or patchy with some preservation of fat and haematopoietic elements. The infiltrate is characterised by widely spaced, small, round or bean-shaped nuclei, in contrast to the closely packed nuclei of most other low-grade lymphoid neoplasms involving the marrow. The abundant cytoplasm and prominent cell borders may produce a "fried-egg" appearance {130, 129, 695}. Mitotic figures are virtually absent. When infiltration is minimal, the subtle clusters of hairy cells can be overlooked. In patients with advanced disease, a diffuse solid infiltrate may be evident. The obvious discrete aggregates that typify bone marrow infiltrates of many other chronic lymphoproliferative disorders are not a feature of HCL. An increase in reticulin fibers is associated with all hairy cell infiltrates in bone marrow and other sites. This increase in reticulin often results in a "dry tap". In a proportion of patients, the bone marrow is hypocellular with a loss of haematopoietic elements, especially the granulocytic lineage, which can lead to an erroneous diagnosis of aplastic anaemia. In such cases immunostaining for a B-cell antigen such as DBA.44 is essential for the identification of the hairy cells. The production of cytokines by the hairy cells is presumed to be the cause of this haematopoietic suppression {593}.

Spleen and other tissues

In the spleen, HCL infiltrates localise to the splenic red pulp. The white pulp is typically atrophic. The cells fill the red pulp cords and exhibit widely spaced nuclei, inconspicuous nucleoli, and variable nuclear indentations. Red blood cell lakes, collections of pooled erythrocytes surrounded by elongated hairy cells, are the presumed consequence of disruption of normal blood flow in the red pulp {130, 129}. The liver may show infiltrates of hairy cells, predominantly in the sinusoids. Lymph node infiltration may occur, and is predominantly paracortical, with sparing of follicles.

Hairy cell variant

HCL variant is a rare disease, in which bone marrow and spleen histology resemble typical HCL, but the circulating cells have a round or oval nucleus and a prominent nucleolus (resembling prolymphocytes) and moderately basophilic villous cytoplasm {1131}. Patients typically

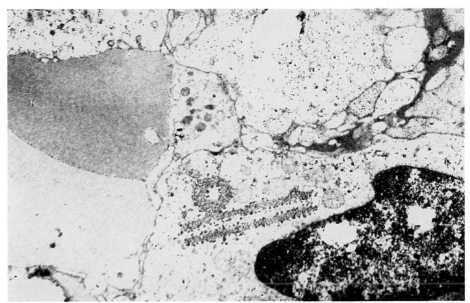

Fig. 6.29 Hairy cell leukaemia. Electron micrograph showing two ribosome lamellar complexes, one in cross section and one in longitudinal section.

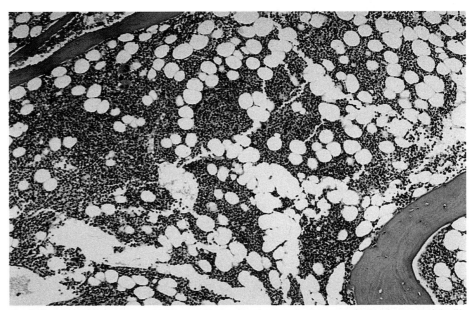

Fig. 6.30 Hairy cell leukaemia, bone marrow biopsy. This low power photomicrograph shows a subtle diffuse, interstitial infiltrate of hairy cells.

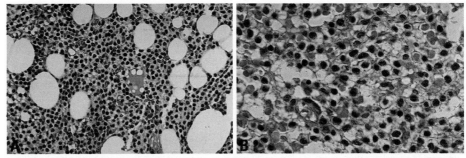

Fig. 6.31 Hairy cell leukaemia, bone marrow biopsy. **A** This medium power photomicrograph shows extensive diffuse infiltration of hairy cell leukaemia. Note widely spaced oval nuclei and paucity of mitotic activity. **B** A "fried egg" appearance of hairy cells is evident on high magnification.

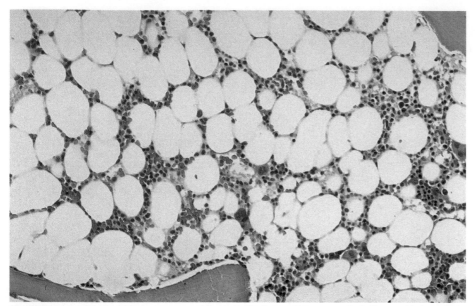

Fig. 6.32 Hairy cell leukaemia, bone marrow biopsy. In this hypocellular case, the infiltrate of hairy cells is subtle; immunohistochemical staining for a B-cell antigen would be useful to identify the hairy cells.

present with a high WBC (50x10⁹/l), and monocytopenia is absent. The cells have a B-cell phenotype and often IgG on the cell membrane but lack the typical hairy cell antigens, such as CD25 and sometimes also CD103, and are often TRAP negative. Differential diagnostic considerations include splenic marginal zone B-cell lymphoma with circulating villous lymphocytes (SLVL) and B-prolymphocytic leukaemia. The response to treatment with agents effective in typical HCL

is usually poor and, as a result, the median survival is significantly shorter in the HCL variant. The relationship of this disorder to typical HCL is not known.

Immunophenotype
The tumour cells are SIg+ (M+/-D, G, or A), and express B-cell-associated antigens (CD19, CD20, CD22, CD79a but not CD79b). They are typically CD5-, CD10-, and CD23-, and express CD11c (strong), CD25 (strong), FMC7, and

CD103 {403, 392, 695}. Tartrate resistant acid phosphatase is present in most cases, but is neither necessary nor specific for the diagnosis. No one marker is specific for distinguishing HCL from other B-cell leukaemias, since CD22, CD11c, CD25, FMC7 and even TRAP can be present in disorders other than HCL. Strong expression of these markers in association with CD103, together with the characteristic morphologic features, are most useful.

In tissue sections, the monoclonal antibody DBA.44 gives strong staining of hairy cells, but other lymphomas may also express this antigen, as well as normal B cells {453}.

Genetics
Antigen receptor genes
Ig heavy and light chain genes are rearranged in HCL. Although studies are limited, Ig variable region genes are mutated, consistent with a post-germinal center cell {1353, 809}.

Cytogenetic abnormalities and oncogenes
No specific cytogenetic abnormality is described. Cyclin D1 is overexpressed in about 50-75% of the cases, but this does not appear to be associated with t(11;14) or BCL1 rearrangement {121}.

Postulated cell of origin
Peripheral B cell of unknown post-germinal centre stage {809}.

Prognosis and predictive factors
HCL does not respond well to conventional lymphoma chemotherapy, but interferon-alpha 2b, deoxycoformycin, or 2-chlorodeoxyadenosine can induce long-term remissions {1262, 275, 1045, 458, 1148, 388}. However, superior response rates are achieved with these two purine nucleoside analogues compared to interferon-alpha 2b. Prolonged remission may also follow splenectomy.

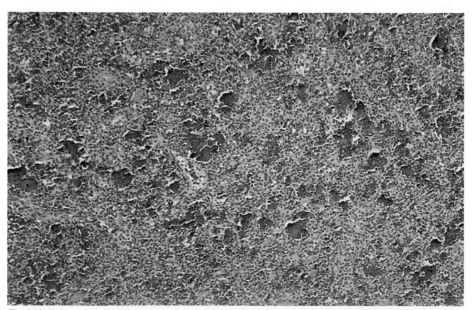

Fig. 6.33 Hairy cell leukaemia. Low power photomicrograph of a spleen extensively infiltrated by hairy cell leukaemia showing obliteration of the white pulp by the infiltrate of hairy cells.

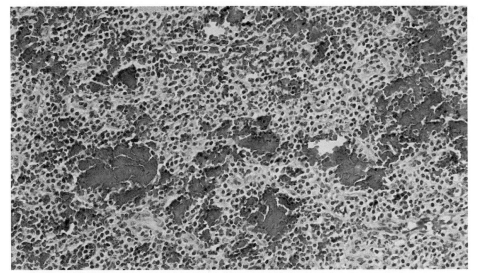

Fig. 6.34 Hairy cell leukaemia, spleen. Red pulp infiltration with numerous red blood cell lakes.

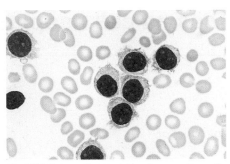

Fig. 6.37 Hairy cell variant, blood smear. The cells have abundant moderately basophilic cytoplasm with villous projections, but in contrast to typical HCL, they have visible nucleoli, resembling prolymphocytes.

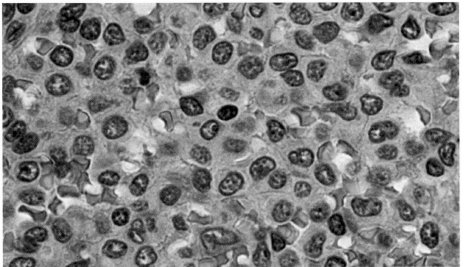

Fig. 6.35 Hairy cell leukaemia, spleen. The hairy cells have oval nuclei that are widely spaced because of their abundant cytoplasm.

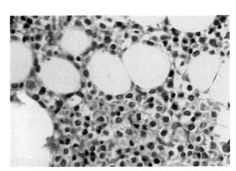

Fig. 6.38 Hairy cell variant. The bone marrow biopsy shows a diffuse, interstitial pattern of infiltration similar to that of typical HCL.

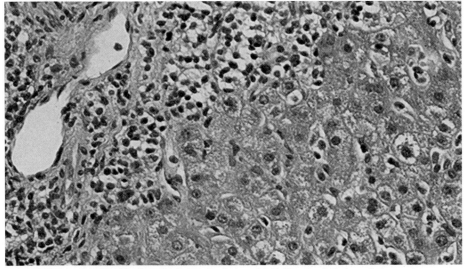

Fig. 6.36 Hairy cell leukaemia, liver. Both portal and sinusoidal infiltration by hairy cells is present.

Plasma cell neoplasms

T.M. Grogan   H.K. Müller-Hermelink
B. Van Camp   N.L. Harris
R.A. Kyle

Introduction

The immunosecretory disorders result from the expansion of a single clone of immunoglobulin secreting, terminally differentiated, end-stage B cells. These monoclonal proliferations of either plasma cells (historically known as plasma cell dyscrasias) or plasmacytoid lymphocytes are characterised by secretion of a single homogeneous immunoglobulin product known as an M-component or monoclonal component. The prominence of the M-component in serum and urine protein electrophoresis (SPE, UPE) has led to various designations for these disorders including monoclonal gammopathies, dysproteinemias and paraproteinemias. The M-components, although monoclonal, may be seen in malignant conditions (plasma cell myeloma and Waldenström macroglobulinemia) and benign or premalignant disorders (monoclonal gammopathy of undetermined significance [MGUS]).

Among these gammapathies are a number of clinicopathological entities, some being primarily plasmacytic, including plasma cell (multiple) myeloma and plasmacytoma; while others contain both lymphocytes and plasma cells, including the heavy chain diseases and Waldenström macroglobulinemia.

Variants of plasma cell myeloma include syndromes defined by the consequence of tissue immunoglobulin deposition, including primary amyloidosis (AL) and light and heavy chain deposition diseases. This chapter will deal specifically with the true plasma cell entities, and will also review the heavy chain diseases. Lymphoplasmacytic lymphoma and other B-cell neoplasms that may have M-components are discussed in other chapters.

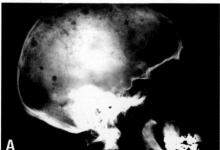

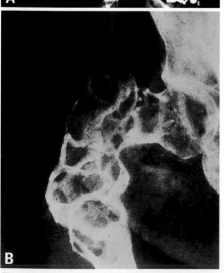

Fig. 6.39 Radiographs of **(A)** skull and **(B)** femoral head demonstrate multiple lytic bone lesions.

Plasma cell myeloma

Definition

Plasma cell myeloma is a bone marrow-based, multifocal plasma cell neoplasm characterised by a serum monoclonal protein and skeletal destruction with osteolytic lesions, pathological fractures, bone pain, hypercalcemia, and anaemia. The disease spans a spectrum from localised, smoldering or indolent to aggressive, disseminated forms with plasma cell infiltration of various organs, plasma cell leukaemia, and disorders due to deposition of abnormal immunoglobulin chains in tissues {465}. The diagnosis is based on a combination of pathological, radiological, and clinical features.

ICD-O code   9732/3

Synonyms
Multiple myeloma
Myelomatosis
Medullary plasmacytoma
Kahler's disease

Epidemiology

In the United States, plasma cell myeloma is the most common lymphoid malignancy in Blacks and the second most common in Whites, representing 15% of all haematological malignancies {290}. The higher incidence in Blacks mirrors their higher physiologic immunoglobulin level relative to Whites, suggesting a larger B-cell population at risk for malignant change. From 1940 to the 1970's the incidence of plasma cell myeloma has shown a net increase of 45% {290}. The median age at diagnosis is 68 years in males and 70 in females, and the male:female ratio is approximately 1.1 {290}.

Sites of involvement

Generalised bone marrow involvement is typically present. Lytic bone lesions and

Table 6.06
Plasma cell neoplasms.

Plasma cell neoplasms
Plasma cell myeloma
Variants:
Non-secretory myeloma
Indolent myeloma
Smoldering myeloma
Plasma cell leukaemia
Plasmacytoma
Solitary plasmacytoma of bone
Extramedullary plasmacytoma
Immunoglobulin deposition diseases:
Primary amyloidosis
Systemic light and heavy chain deposition diseases
Osteosclerotic Myeloma (POEMS syndrome)
Heavy chain diseases (HCD):
Gamma HCD
Mu HCD
Alpha HCD

tumoural masses of plasma cells also occur. The most common sites are in marrow areas of most active haematopoiesis, including in order of frequency, the vertebrae, ribs, skull, pelvis, femur, clavicle, and scapula {465, 1136}.

Clinical features

A constellation of radiological, clinical laboratory and pathological findings are combined to provide diagnostic criteria for plasma cell myeloma.

The extensive skeletal destruction by neoplastic plasma cells results in bone pain, pathological fractures, hypercalcemia and anaemia {1136}. Recurrent bacterial infections and renal insufficiency are common. The recurrent infections are in part a consequence of depressed normal immunoglobulin production due to displacement by the neoplastic clone. Renal failure follows the tubular damage resulting from monoclonal light chain proteinuria. Anaemia is due both to marrow replacement and renal damage with resultant loss of erythropoietin {1136}.

An M-component is found in the serum or urine in 99% of patients {1136}. The serum protein electrophoretic pattern shows a peak or localised band in 80% of patients. In most patients, there is hypogammaglobulinemia (>50% reduction in normal serum Ig); rarely a normal Ig profile is seen. Monoclonal IgG accounts for 50% and IgA for approximately 20% of the cases {1136}. A monoclonal light chain (Bence-Jones protein) is found in the serum of 15% of patients. IgD accounts for 2% while bi-clonal gammopathies are found in 1%. The serum M-protein is usually >3 g/dl of IgG and

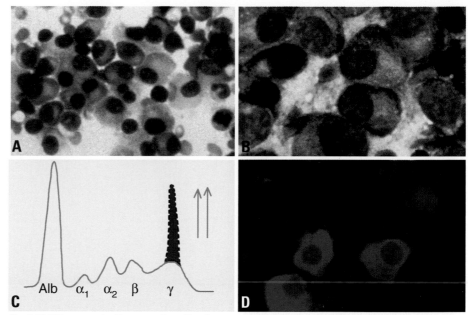

Fig. 6.40 This composite illustrates the salient features of plasma cell myeloma pathology: **A, B** Aggregates of immature plasma cells. **C** A monoclonal gammopathy evidenced by a "spike" in the gamma region of a serum protein electrophoresis densitometry profile. **D** Monotypic cytoplasmic immunoglobulin light chain expression shown by immunofluorescence.

>2g/dl of IgA. A Bence-Jones protein is found in the urine in 75% of patients {1136}.

Clinical variants

Non-secretory myeloma
Rare cases (1%) of plasma cell myeloma have plasma cells that synthesise but do not secrete Ig molecules, leading to the absence of a M-component {123, 128}. Monoclonal cytoplasmic Ig is typically present in the neoplastic plasma cells when evaluated with immunofluorescence or immunoperoxidase studies, indicating a failure to secrete Ig. In rare

cases, no cytoplasmic Ig synthesis is detected. The clinical features are generally identical to plasma cell myeloma except for a lower incidence of renal insufficiency. However, the nonsecretory variant may have a lower level of plasmacytosis and less depression of normal Ig. Due to the lack of serum or urine monoclonal Ig, the diagnosis can be missed, unless bone marrow biopsy with analysis of cytoplasmic Ig staining or other markers of plasma cells is performed {123, 128}.

Two clinical variants, smoldering and indolent myeloma, represent variants of

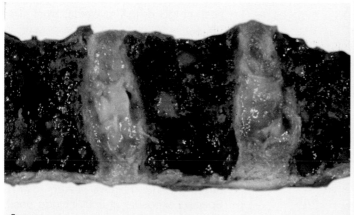

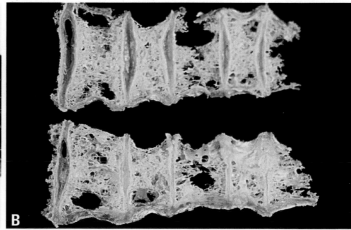

Fig. 6.41 A Plasma cell myeloma, gross photograph of vertebral column, showing multiple lytic lesions, filled with grey, fleshy tumour. **B** Vertebral column, after maceration showing multiple lytic lesions.

plasma cell myeloma in which the diagnostic criteria for myeloma are met, but the patients are asymptomatic and the disease may be stable for long periods.

Smoldering myeloma
These patients have higher levels of M-component and marrow plasmacytosis than patients with MGUS, and fulfil the

minimal criteria for the diagnosis of plasma cell myeloma, but are asymptomatic and have no lytic bone lesions or other clinical features of myeloma, including anaemia, renal insufficiency, or hypercalcemia {17}. A small M-protein may be found in the urine and the concentration of normal serum immunoglobulins is often reduced. In some patients, symptomatic plasma cell myeloma does not develop for years. These patients are typically not treated unless progression occurs {718}.

Indolent Myeloma
This variant is similar to smoldering myeloma in that the diagnostic criteria for plasma cell myeloma are met, but differs from it in that (1) the patients have up to three lytic bone lesions, without bone pain; (2) the M-component is at intermediate levels; (3) like smoldering myeloma patients the patients have a normal haemoglobin, serum calcium and creatinine; and (4) there is no evidence of infection. As with smoldering myeloma, these patients are typically not treated, but are followed until symptoms develop {17}.

Plasma cell leukaemia (PCL)
Peripheral blood involvement (plasma cell leukaemia) occurs rarely in plasma cell myeloma (2%), and is defined as circulating peripheral blood plasma cells exceeding 2×10^9/liter or 20% of peripheral blood white cells. It may occur at the time of diagnosis (primary PCL) or evolve as a terminal complication during the course of plasma cell myeloma (secondary PCL) {421}. Plasma cell leukaemia is more frequent in light-chain only, IgE and IgD myeloma and is less frequently seen in IgG or IgA myeloma. Most clinical signs of myeloma are also seen in PCL, although osteolytic lesions and bone pain are less frequent and lymphadenopathy and organomegaly are more frequent. Renal failure is common. This is an aggressive disease with short survival {421}.

Aetiology
An increased risk (3-4 times) of myeloma has been described in cosmetologists, farmers, and laxative takers {771}. Specific exposure agents include pesticides, petroleum products, asbestos, rubber, plastic and wood products {771}. In addition, high dose radiation (100

Table 6.07
Diagnostic criteria for plasma cell myeloma.

A. The diagnosis of myeloma requires a minimum of one major and one minor criteria or three minor criteria which must include (1) and (2). These criteria must be manifest in a symptomatic patient with progressive disease.

B. Major criteria:
 – Marrow plasmacytosis (>30%)
 – Plasmacytoma on biopsy
 – M-component:
  Serum: IgG >3.5g/dl, IgA >2g/dl
  Urine >1g/24hr of Bence-Jones [BJ] protein

C. Minor criteria:
 – Marrow plasmacytosis (10-30%)
 – M-component: present but less than above
 – Lytic bone lesions
 – Reduced normal immunoglobulins (<50% normal):
  IgG <600 mg/dl, IgA <100 mg/dl, IgM <50mg/dl

Modified from references {83, 333, 1136}.

Table 6.08
Diagnostic criteria for Monoclonal Gammopathy of Undetermined Significance (MGUS), indolent and smoldering myeloma.

A. MGUS:
 – M-component present, but less than myeloma levels
 – Marrow plasmacytosis <10%
 – No lytic bone lesions
 – No myeloma-related symptoms

B. Smoldering Myeloma: same as MGUS except:
 – Serum M-component at myeloma levels
 – Marrow plasmacytosis 10-30%

C. Indolent Myeloma: same as myeloma except:
 – M-component: IgG <7g/dl, IgA <5g/dl
 – Rare bone lesions (≤3 lytic lesions), without compression fractures
 – Normal haemoglobin, serum calcium and creatinine
 – No infections

Modified from references {17, 718, 713, 714}.

Table 6.09
Comparison of MGUS, indolent and smoldering myeloma.

	MGUS	SMM	IMM
Plasma cells (BM)	<10%	10-30%	>30%
M-component	IgG<3.5, IgA<2	IgG>3.5, IgA>2	IgG 3,5-7, IgA 2-5
Lytic bone lesions	None	None	≤3
Symptoms/infection	None	None	None

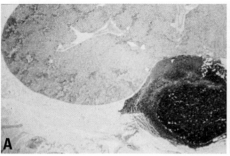
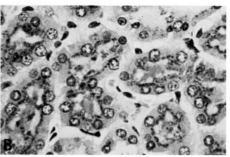

Fig 6.42 **A** Perirenal involvement (extramedullary plasmacytoma) in a patient with plasma cell myeloma. Immunohistochemical assay reveals lambda light chain-bearing perirenal plasmacytoma. **B** Section of kidney showing renal tubular lambda deposition with casts reflecting renal tubular Bence-Jones protein reabsorption. (Immunoperoxidase, anti-lambda light chain).

Polyclonal vs. monoclonal Ig production

Fig 6.43 Diagrammatic demonstration of polyclonal (yellow) versus monoclonal (blue) immunoglobulin production in serum protein electrophoresis profile.

cGy) in survivors of the atomic bomb at Hiroshima and Nagasaki resulted in a myeloma rate 4.7 times greater than controls. Low level radiation exposure is implicated finding increased incidence of myeloma among radiologists and nuclear plant workers {762}. Long-standing, chronic infection such as osteomyelitis or chronic antigenic stimulation such as rheumatoid arthritis has been considered a possible predisposing factor {771}. A possible role for virus has been postulated with the finding of the Kaposi sarcoma-associated Human Herpesvirus 8 (HHV8) in myeloma marrow samples {1128}, but this finding has not been reproducible {245}. The occurrence of plasma cell myeloma in HIV-infected patients also suggests a possible aetiologic association. In some instances the HIV-mediated immunosuppression may result in emergence of Epstein-Barr virus (EBV)-infected B-cell clones. In one reported case an HIV+ patient with myeloma produced an M-component directed against the HIV-1 p24 antigen {685}.

Development of plasma cell myeloma is postulated to follow the "two-hit hypothesis": initial antigenic stimulus giving rise to multiple benign clones with a second hit representing an "accident" or mutagenic event causing malignant transformation {1137, 480}. While the initial antigenic stimulus may be well established in occasional instances (e.g., mineral oil, petroleum, asbestos, etc.) {1053, 771}, in most cases of myeloma the initial antigenic stimulus is unknown. Most myeloma proteins are autoantibodies {1445}. It has been postulated that they may be directed against immunoregulatory autoantibodies {1445}. Thus, myeloma may arise from B cells within the idiotypic network

postulated by Jerne {597}. Although most myeloma proteins lack specificity for foreign antigen, there are rare documented instances of such specificity, including the remarkable case of an M-component in a canary breeder directed against canary droppings {592} and an M-component to horse alpha-macroglobulin 30 years post passive serotherapy with horse serum for tetanus {1174}.

Precursor lesion: Monoclonal gammopathy of undetermined significance (MGUS)

ICD-O code 9765/1

MGUS denotes the presence of a monoclonal (M-) protein in persons without evidence of plasma cell myeloma, Waldenström macroglobulinemia, primary amyloidosis (AL), or other related disorders {713, 714}. This disorder was considered to be benign and often called benign monoclonal gammopathy. However, a pro-portion of patients will evolve to

symptomatic plasma cell myeloma or amyloidosis, so the term MGUS is considered more appropriate {713, 714}. Patients with MGUS are asymptomatic, and the M-component is discovered unexpectedly during serum protein electrophoresis of the blood {713, 714}.

The prevalence of MGUS is 1% in patients older than 50 years of age and 3% in those older than 70 years. About 75% of MGUS paraproteins are IgG with IgM in 15% and IgA in 10% {713, 714}.

Approximately 25% of patients with MGUS develop plasma cell myeloma, primary amyloidosis, macroglobulinemia, or other lymphoproliferative disease after follow-up for more than 20 years {713, 714}. The actuarial risk of malignant transformation is unrelated to the type of M-protein. The median interval from the recognition of the M-protein to diagnosis of myeloma, macroglobulinemia, or amyloidosis is approximately 10 years. Thus, patients with MGUS must be followed indefinitely for evidence of progressive disease {713, 714}.

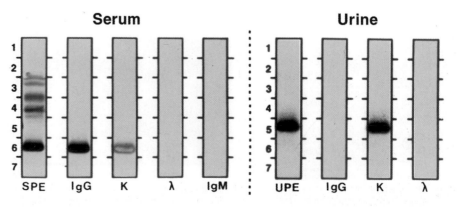

Fig. 6.44 Demonstration of serum and urine "M-component" using the immunofixation technique. As shown, the patient has an IgG kappa serum M-component and a kappa Bence-Jones proteinuria.

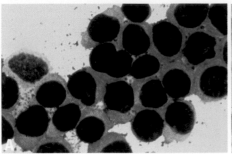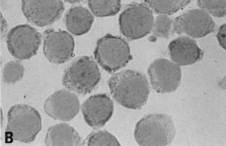

Fig. 6.45 Plasma cell leukaemia, cytospin preparation showing (A) neoplastic plasma cells with (B) expression of CD38 plasma cell antigen.

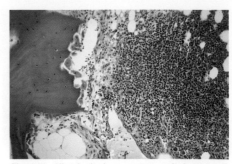

Fig. 6.46 Histological appearance of plasma cell myeloma in a bone marrow biopsy. A discrete plasma cell mass displaces normal marrow fat cells and haematopoietic elements. Near the myeloma mass note prominent osteoclastic activity in the trabecular bone.

MGUS plasma cells resemble normal-appearing mature plasma cells, without nucleoli. They constitute <10% of the nucleated cells in the bone marrow. The plasma cells in MGUS express monotypic cIg of the same isotype as the M-component in the serum and urine, but often a small clone is present in a background of reactive plasma cells, and monotypic Ig is not detectable by routine immuno-histochemistry {1029, 1402}. The immunophenotype is otherwise identical to that of normal plasma cells {772, 490}.

Macroscopy

In plasma cell myeloma, the bone defects on gross examination are filled with a soft gelatinous, fish-flesh, haemorrhagic tissue.

Morphology

The diagnosis of plasma cell myeloma requires integration of morphologic features, laboratory data, and radiological findings. The specific diagnostic criteria for plasma cell myeloma are shown in Table 6.07.

Bone marrow biopsy

Plasma cell myeloma is characterised by an excess of marrow plasma cells {76}. In contrast to normal or reactive plasma cells, which usually occur in small clusters of five or six cells around marrow arterioles, myeloma-associated plasma cells frequently occur in larger foci, nodules or sheets. This "mass" effect of plasma cells strongly favours neoplasia {465, 76}.

A diagnosis of myeloma is favoured when a tumoural mass of plasma cells is seen, which displaces normal marrow elements. Counting plasma cells is not practical on biopsy specimens, but the volume of marrow occupied by plasma cells can be estimated. In general, when 30% of the marrow volume is comprised of plasma cells, a diagnosis of plasma cell myeloma is likely although rare cases of reactive plasmacytosis with >50% plasma cells are described {465, 76}. In histological sections of marrow, the myeloma mass may occasionally be associated with prominent osteoclastic activity resulting in the lytic lesions seen on X-rays.

Bone marrow aspiration

Myeloma plasma cells vary from mature forms indistinguishable from normal plasma cells to immature, pleomorphic, or anaplastic plasma cells {76, 456}. The mature plasma cells are usually oval, with a round eccentric nucleus with "spoke wheel" or "clock-face" chromatin without nucleoli, with abundant baso-philic cytoplasm and a marked perinuclear hof. In contrast, immature forms have dispersed nuclear chromatin, a high nuclear/cytoplasmic ratio, and prominent nucleoli (plasmablasts). Almost 10% of patients with plasma cell myeloma exhibit plasmablastic morphology which is associated with a poorer prognosis {76, 456}. Multinucleated, polylobated, pleomorphic plasma cells also occur {76, 465}. Because nuclear immaturity and pleomorphism rarely occur in reactive plasma cells, they are reliable indicators of neoplastic plasmacytosis.

The cytoplasm of myeloma cells contains abundant endoplasmic reticulum (ER), which may contain retained, condensed or crystallised cytoplasmic Ig producing a variety of morphologically distinctive findings, including: multiple pale bluish-white, grape-like accumulation (Mott cells, Morula cells), cherry-red refractive round bodies (Russell bodies), vermilion staining glycogen-rich IgA (flame cells), overstuffed fibrils (Gaucher-like cells, thesaurocytes) and crystalline rods {465}. These changes are not pathognomonic of myeloma since they may be found in reactive plasma cells.

Peripheral blood

Circulating plasma cells in plasma cell leukaemia span a broad morphologic

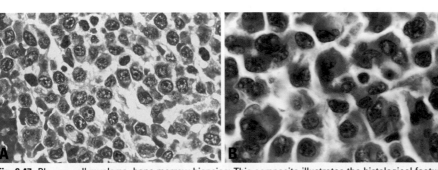

Fig. 6.47 Plasma cell myeloma, bone marrow biopsies: This composite illustrates the histological features of both a mature (A) and an immature (B) myeloma. The mature type has the archetypal "clock-face" chromatin within eccentric nuclei, with low N/C ratio, and abundant cytoplasm with a prominent Hof (Golgi). In contrast, the immature myeloma is profoundly pleomorphic with frequent multinucleate cells consistent with the term "anaplastic plasma cell myeloma".

spectrum from mature to immature blastic forms not distinguishable from myeloblasts. In some instances plasma cells have lymphoid-like morphology {421}.

Kidney
Bence-Jones protein accumulates as aggregates of eosinophilic material in the lumina of the renal tubules. Renal tubular reabsorption of Bence-Jones protein is largely responsible for renal damage in plasma cell myeloma.

Immunophenotype
Plasma cell myeloma typically expresses monotypic cytoplasmic immunoglobulin (Ig) and lacks surface immunoglobulin {696}. The Ig is most commonly IgG, occasionally IgA, and rarely IgD, IgE, or IgM. In 85% both heavy and light chains are produced; in 15% light chain only is expressed representing the circumstance of Bence-Jones myeloma. Most but not all cases lack the pan-B cell antigens CD19 and CD20, while CD38 and the Ig-associated antigen CD79a are expressed in the majority of cases {772}. In contrast with normal plasma cells which express CD19 and lack expression of CD56/58, malignant plasma cells lack CD19 and usually express CD56/58 {1325}. The collagen-1 binding proteoglycan, syndecan-1 (CD138) is found on most cases of myeloma, and may be important for plasma cell anchoring in the bone marrow {1102}. The antigen detected by the monoclonal antibody VS38c is typically expressed. Circulating monoclonal idiotype-identical B lymphocytes have been reported in myeloma patients {697, 463}. Occasional cases of myeloma and plasmacytoma may express CD10 {463}. The phenotype of plasma cell leukaemia is comparable to that of myeloma (monoclonal CIg+, CD38+), except for loss of some adhesion molecules (CD56) {421, 1325}; in primary plasma cell leukaemia the cells often express light chains only, IgE or IgD {421}. Occasionally myeloma may present with aberrant coexpression of myelomonocytic antigens {464}.

Genetics
Antigen receptor genes
Molecular studies of immunoglobulin (Ig) genes commonly reveal clonal rearrangements. While a single, monoclonal rearranged Ig band is the rule in myeloma, multiple rearranged Ig bands are found in

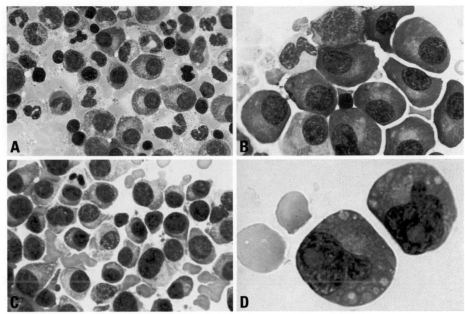

Fig. 6.48 Plasma cell myeloma: cytologic features in marrow aspirations showing variation from mature (**A, B**) to immature (**C, D**) plasma cells. The more mature cells have clumped nuclear chromatin, abundant cytoplasm, low nuclear-cytoplasmic ratio and only rare nucleoli compared to the less mature cells, which have more prominent nucleoli, loose reticular chromatin and a higher nuclear-cytoplasmic ratio. **D** illustrates plasmablasts from a plasmablastic myeloma with prominent nucleoli, reticular chromatin and high nuclear-cytoplasmic ratio.

5% of myeloma patients {74}. There is a high frequency of Ig *VH* gene somatic mutation consistent with derivation from a post-germinal centre, antigen-driven B-cell {67}. Immunoglobulin gene deletion is sometimes found; in patients with light chain only disease or Bence Jones proteinuria, *JH* segments and/or parts or all of chromosome 14 may be lost {74}.

Genetic abnormalities and oncogenes
Cytogenetic analysis in plasma cell myeloma is hampered by the low proliferation fraction in most cases {293, 330}. Recent studies using cytokine-stimulated bone marrow cultures and in situ hybridisation have increased the proportion of

informative cases {1150, 720, 684}. Structural and numerical chromosomal abnormalities are described in 20-60% of newly diagnosed patients, with a mean of 30-40% {330} and in 60-70% of patients with progressive disease, indicating an ascending scale of chromosomal aberration in pathogenesis {74, 720}. Complex karyotypes with multiple chromosomal gains and losses are the most frequent changes, but translocations, deletions and mutations are all reported {293}. Gains in chromosomes 3, 5, 7, 9, 11, 15, and 19, and losses in chromosomes 8, 13, 14, and X are most common. Among losses, monosomy or partial deletion of 13 (13q14) is the most common finding,

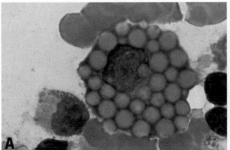
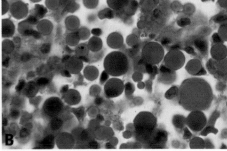

Fig 6.49 Plasma cell myeloma, morphologic variants based on cytoplasmic features. **A** illustrates a so-called Mott cell with abundant "grape-like" cytoplasmic inclusions of immunoglobulin and **B** the presence of numerous Russell bodies.

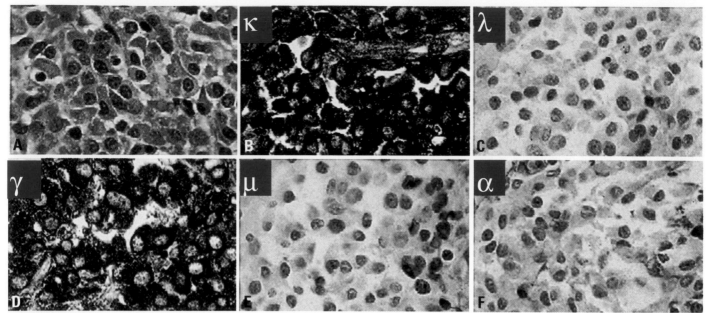

Fig. 6.50 Plasmacytoma composite figure illustrates monotypic immunoglobulin expression. **A** Typical plasma cell morphology. **B** Cytoplasmic kappa light chain positivity. **C** Absence of Lambda light chain expression. **D** Expression of cytoplasmic gamma heavy chain. **E, F** Absence of mu and alpha heavy chains.

occurring in 15-40% of newly diagnosed cases {1150, 720, 684}. The most common structural abnormalities are described in chromosomes 1 (15%), 11 (10%), and 14 (10%). A t(11;14)(q13;q32) translocation, involving rearrangement of the BCL1 locus, is the most common {293, 1150, 720}. This translocation transposes the *CYCLIN D1* gene into an IgH gamma switch region resulting in overexpression of *CYCLIN D1* {219, 1335, 1450}. Altered expression of the *PAX-5* gene on chromosome 9 is thought to result in the loss of CD19, heralding the transition from normal CD19+ plasma cells to CD19- myeloma cells {805}. Deletion at 17p13 associated with allelic loss of P53 is reported in 25% of the cases and may predict a poor outcome {684, 319}. Deletion of the long arm of chromosome 7 has also been related to alteration of the multidrug resistance

gene conferring an increased clinical drug resistant phenotype relevant to myeloma survival {262}.

Postulated cell of origin
Bone marrow-homing plasma cell.

Prognosis and predictive factors
Plasma cell myeloma is usually incurable, with a median survival of 3 years, and 10% survival at 10 years {1136, 74}. Using the myeloma staging scheme shown in Table 6.10, increased tumour burden and poor function are associated with shorter survival time {329, 332}. Patients in stage I have a median survival of >60 months, stage II of 41 months, and stage III of 23 months {329, 332, 1078}. Myeloma patients with normal renal function experienced a 37-month median survival versus 8 months for those with renal insufficiency {329, 332,

1078}. Other prognostic factors include haemoglobin, serum calcium, lytic bone lesions, and amount of the M-component beta-2-microglobulin (B2M) {1078}.
Estimation of the degree of marrow replacement by plasma cells In marrow core biopsies also has prognostic value {76}. Three stages have been defined (Stage I <20%, Stage II 20-50%, and Stage III >50% plasma cells), which predict progressively poorer prognosis {76}. Plasmablastic morphology is also associated with a poorer prognosis {1137}. The proliferation antigen Ki-67 also identifies patients with a poor prognosis {465, 74}. Genetic abnormalities associated with a poorer prognosis include deletions of 13q14 and 17p13 {684}.

Plasmacytoma

Definition
Plasmacytomas are clonal proliferations of plasma cells that are cytologically and immunophenotypically identical to those of plasma cell myeloma, but manifest a localised osseous or extraosseous growth pattern.

Solitary plasmacytoma of bone

Definition
Solitary plasmacytoma of bone (osseous plasmacytoma) is a localised bone

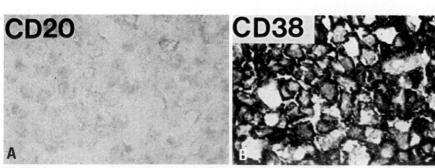

Fig. 6.51 Plasmacytoma showing **A** absence of CD20 and **B** expression of CD38.

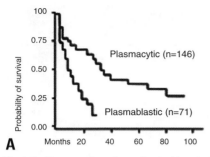 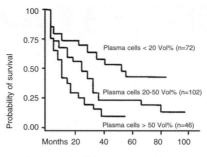 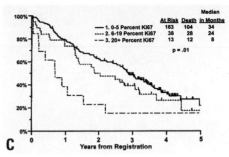

Fig. 6.52 Plasma cell myeloma: Survival in relation to **(A)** cytological maturity, **(B)** the volume of bone marrow biopsy occupied by plasma cells (Reproduced from Bartl R. et al. {76}) and **(C)** growth fraction as measured by Ki-67. Reproduced from Rimsza L.M. et al. {1105}.

tumour consisting of plasma cells identical to those seen in plasma cell myeloma, which appears as a solitary lytic lesion on radiological examination {715}. Complete skeletal radiographs must show no other lesions, and the bone marrow away from the solitary lesion contains no evidence of plasmacytosis.

ICD-O code   9731/3

Epidemiology
This is a rare lesion, comprising 5% of plasma cell neoplasms {715}.

Sites of involvement
The most common sites are in marrow areas of most active haematopoiesis, including in order of frequency, the vertebrae, ribs, skull, pelvis, femur, clavicle, and scapula {465, 715}.

Clinical features
The patients present with bone pain or a pathological fracture from a single bone lesion consisting of monoclonal plasma cells. While the serum and urine typically show no M-protein, some patients may have low level gammopathies. If an M-protein is found in the serum or urine, it usually disappears following local treatment. Immunofixation of serum and urine are essential in following the course of a patient with solitary plasmacytoma. MRI is useful to exclude additional lesions {767}.

Morphology, immunophenotype and genetics
The gross and microscopic features, immunophenotype and genetic features are identical to those of plasma cell myeloma.

Prognosis and predictive factors
Treatment for solitary osseous plasmacytoma is typically radiation therapy.

At 10 years, about 35% of the patients appear to be cured, while 55% develop plasma cell myeloma, and 10% have either local recurrence of the plasmacytoma or another solitary plasmacytoma {715}.

Extraosseous plasmacytoma

ICD-O code   9734/3

Definition
Extraosseous plasmacytoma is a neoplasm of plasma cells forming a tumour at an extraosseous and extramedullary site.

Epidemiology
Extraosseous (extramedullary) plasmacytomas constitute 3-5% of all plasma cell neoplasms {18}. Patients are typically adults (median age 55) with a 2:1 male:female ratio.

Sites of involvement
Approximately 80% occur in the upper respiratory tract including the oropharynx, nasopharynx, sinuses and larynx {1136, 18}, but they may occur in a variety of sites, including the gastrointestinal tract, urinary bladder, central nervous system, breast, thyroid, testis, parotid gland, lymph nodes, and skin.

Table 6.10
Myeloma staging system.

Stage I:
– Low M-component levels: IgG <5g/dl, IgA <3g/dl; Urine BJ <4g/24hr
– Absent or solitary bone lesions.
– Normal haemoglobin, serum calcium, Ig levels (non-M component).
Stage III: Any one or more of the following:
– High M-component: IgG >7g/dl, IgA>5g/dl; Urine BJ 12g/24hr
– Advanced, multiple lytic bone lesions.
– Haemoglobin <8.5g/dl, serum calcium >12mg/dl.
Stage II: Overall values between I and III
Subclassification: Based on renal function
A = serum creatinine <2mg/dl
B = serum creatinine >2mg/dl
Examples:
Stage IA = low myeloma mass (<0.6x1012/m2) with normal renal function
Stage IIIB = high myeloma mass (<1.2x1012/m2) with abnormal renal function
Modified from references {1136, 329, 332}.

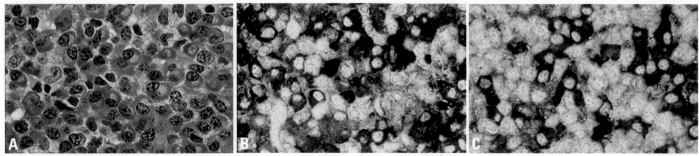

Fig. 6.53 Plasma cell granuloma. **A** The "mass effect" of plasma cells simulates a neoplasm. Immunoperoxidase stains show polytypic cytoplasmic immunoglobulin with some plasma cells expressing **(B)** kappa light chains and some expressing **(C)** lambda light chains.

Clinical features

By definition, there is no evidence of plasma cell myeloma on bone marrow examination or by radiography, 15-20% of patients may have a monoclonal gammopathy. There is no evidence of anaemia, hypercalcemia, or renal insufficiency.

Morphology

The morphologic features are similar to those of osseous plasmacytoma. Some of these cases, particularly in the gastrointestinal tract, may represent extranodal marginal zone B-cell lymphoma of mucosa-associated lymphoid tissue (MALT) type with extreme plasmacytic differentiation.

The differential diagnosis includes reactive plasma cell infiltrates. Immunohistochemistry is sometimes critical in correct diagnosis as shown in. Fig. 6.53 shows an example of a benign, reactive plasma cell granuloma, in which there is a notable "mass effect" suggesting a plasma cell neoplasm (plasmacytoma).

However, polyclonal kappa and lambda light chain expression indicates a polyclonal reactive process, in contrast with the monoclonal pattern shown in. In cases in which immunohistochemistry is unsuccessful, the diagnosis is sometimes greatly aided by analysis of immunoglobulin mRNA.

Immunophenotype and genetic features

The immunophenotype and genetic features are not extensively studied but appear to be identical to those of plasma cell myeloma.

Prognosis and predictive factors

Treatment typically consists of radiation therapy. Regional recurrences develop in approximately 25% of patients, but the development of typical plasma cell myeloma is uncommon, occurring in approximately 15% {18}.

Monoclonal immunoglobulin deposition diseases

Introduction

The monoclonal immunoglobulin deposition diseases (MIDD) are closely-related disorders that are characterised by visceral and soft tissue Ig deposition, resulting in compromised organ function {717, 331, 1178, 716, 1085, 1056, 53, 618, 417, 517, 166, 1403}. Although these are plasma cell neoplasms and thus part of the spectrum of plasma cell myeloma, they produce an immunoglobulin molecule that accumulates in tissue prior to the development of a large tumour burden. Thus, these patients typically do not have overt myeloma at the time of the diagnosis. The MIDD appear to be chemically different manifestations of similar pathological processes, resulting in clinically similar but not identical conditions. There are two major categories of MIDD: primary amyloidosis and light chain deposition disease. Primary amyloidosis is characterised by deposition of a fibrillary protein with a β-pleated sheet structure, which binds Congo red with apple-green birefringence, and contains amyloid-P component {717, 331, 716, 1178}. Light chain deposition disease (LCDD) and its variants, light and heavy chain deposition disease (LHCDD) and heavy chain deposition disease (HCDD), are characterised by deposition of a nonfibrillary, amorphous material that does not have a β-pleated sheet configuration and does

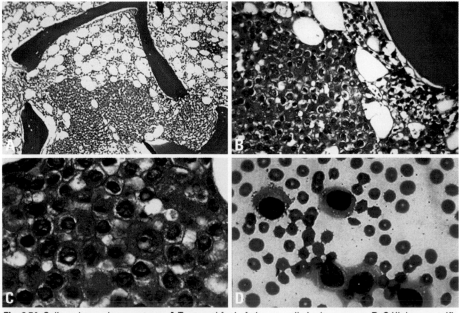

Fig. 6.54 Solitary bone plasmacytoma. **A** Tumoural foci of plasma cells in the marrow. **B, C** Higher magnification showing typical cytology. **D** Touch preparation.

not bind Congo red nor contain amyloid P-component {1085, 1056, 53, 618, 417, 517, 166, 1403}. The Ig isotype differs between the MIDD variants: primary amyloidosis deposits consist most frequently of lambda light chain with over-representation of the $V_{\lambda VI}$ variable region, while LCDD consists most frequently of kappa light chains (80%) with over-representation of the $V_{\kappa IV}$ variable region {1178}.

Primary Amyloidosis

Definition
Primary amyloidosis is a plasma cell neoplasm that secretes an abnormal immunoglobulin, which deposits in various tissues and forms a β–pleated sheet structure that binds Congo red dye with characteristic birefringence {717, 331, 716, 1178}.

ICD-O code   9769/1c

Epidemiology
Primary amyloidosis is a rare disease of adults. In the majority (80%) of patients a monoclonal immunoglobulin is found, with 20% having overt plasma cell myeloma. Among myeloma patients, approximately 15% have or will develop primary amyloidosis {717, 331, 716, 1178}.

Sites of involvement
Plasma cell-related amyloid (AL) accumulates: in the heart, resulting in congestive heart failure; in the liver, resulting in hepatomegaly; in the kidneys, resulting in nephrotic syndrome and or renal failure; in the gut, resulting in malabsorption; in the tongue, resulting in macroglossia; in the nerves, resulting in sensorimotor peripheral neuropathy and loss of sphincter control. Amyloid deposits may also occur in bone.
The diagnostic biopsy site generally is the abdominal subcutaneous fat-pad, bone marrow, or the rectum {717, 331, 716, 1178}.

Clinical features
Clinical findings are related to deposition of amyloid in organs, resulting in organomegaly. Bleeding may occur due to increased fragility of blood vessels from amyloid deposits, binding of coagulation factor X and/or vascular structures to amyloid proteins.

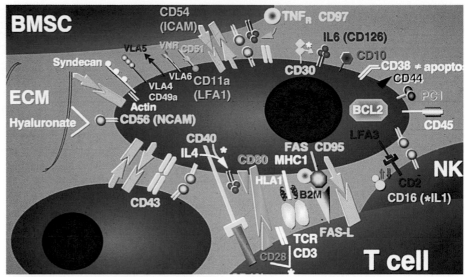

Fig. 6.55 Plasma cell myeloma: diagram of cell surface molecules and their ligands (BMSC = bone marrow stromal cell; ECM = extracellular matrix; NK = NK cell).

Pathophysiology
Amyloid is a fibrillary protein that is deposited in organs leading to organ failure {717, 331, 716, 1178}. Several types of protein can form amyloid, and amyloidosis is classified into 4 major types based on the type of fibrillary protein: 1. primary or immunoglobulin-light chain (AL) amyloidosis (myeloma-associated), 2. secondary (AA) amyloidosis (inflammation associated), 3. familial (AF) amyloidosis, and 4. β-2 microglobulin (β2M) amyloidosis (hemo-dialysis-associated) {1178}.

AL amyloid is composed of intact immunoglobulin light chains that are secreted by monoclonal plasma cells and then ingested, processed and discharged by macrophages into the extracellular matrix. The accumulated AL amyloid includes both intact light chain and fragments of the variable (V) NH_2-terminus region {331}. All light chain V region fragments are amyloidogenic,

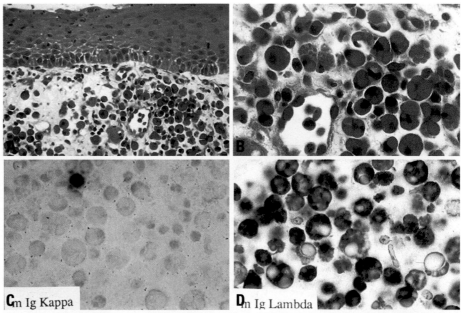

Fig. 6.56 Extramedullary plasmacytoma of the skin with abundant Russell body formation (**A, B**) which can produce nonspecific staining by immunohistochemistry. Monoclonality is demonstrated by non-radioactive in situ hybridisation showing absence of kappa (**C**) and presence of lambda mRNA transcripts (**D**).

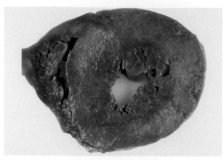

Fig. 6.57 Primary amyloidosis in a patient with plasma cell myeloma. Gross photograph of a section of heart shows the diffuse enlargement characteristic of amyloid deposition, especially notable in the left ventricle. It is pale and has a waxy consistency.

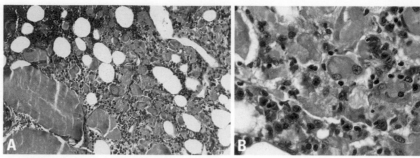

Fig. 6.58 Primary amyloidosis: bone marrow biopsy showing **(A)** characteristic pale, waxy amorphous deposits and **(B)** associated histiocytes, often multinucleated, and neoplastic plasma cells.

with $V_{\lambda VI}$ fragments most frequently found.

Macroscopy

On gross inspection amyloid has a dense "porcelain-like" or waxy appearance.

Morphology

Amyloid stains pink with H & E and is most commonly seen as an amorphous, eosinophilic, waxy-appearing substance, with a characteristic cracking artifact, focally in thickened blood vessel walls, on basement membranes, and in the interstitium of tissues such as adipose tissue or bone marrow {1403}. Macrophages may be present around deposits, as well as foreign-body type giant cells. Organ parenchyma may be massively replaced by amyloid deposits (amyloidoma). Plasma cells may be increased in the adjacent tissues, and in the marrow in particular.

When stained with Congo red, the amyloid appears a pinkish red by standard light microscopy and by polarisation microscopy shows an "apple-green" birefringence. The birefringence results from the stacked β-pleated sheets caused by juxtaposed immunoglobulin molecules.

Immunophenotype

Antibodies to kappa and lambda can be useful in positive identification of primary as opposed to secondary amyloidosis; however, in paraffin-embedded sections, antibodies to light chains may give excess background staining, so that they are often uninterpretable.

The associated plasma cells show monoclonality with either anti-kappa or lambda Ig antibodies {1403}. Antibodies to amyloid P component are also positive.

Prognosis

Patients with plasma cell myeloma and amyloidosis have a shorter survival period than those with myeloma alone {716}.

Monoclonal light and heavy chain deposition diseases

Definition

Monoclonal light and heavy chain deposition diseases are plasma cell neoplasms that secrete an abnormal light or less often heavy chain or both, which do not form amyloid β-pleated sheets, bind Congo red or contain amyloid P-component {1085, 1056, 53, 618, 417, 517, 166}, but deposit in tissues causing organ dysfunction.

These disorders include light chain deposition disease (LCDD) {1085, 1056, 417, 166}, heavy chain deposition disease (HCDD) {53, 618, 517}, and light and heavy chain deposition disease (LHCDD) {166}.

Synonyms

Randall disease {1085}.

Epidemiology

These are rare diseases (<70 cases described) of adults (age range 33-79

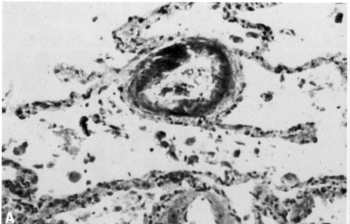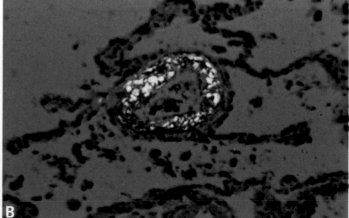

Fig. 6.59 Primary amyloidosis. Pulmonary blood vessel with amyloid deposition, showing **(A)** Congo Red staining and **(B)** apple-green birefringence in polarized light.

years, 56 year median) which usually occur in association with either MGUS or overt myeloma {1056, 618, 166}. There is no evidence of an ethnicity effect and the male/female incidence is nearly equal (9/7) {1056, 618, 166}.

Sites of involvement
Deposition in LCDD and HCDD may involve many organs, most commonly the kidneys, the liver, the heart, the nerves, blood vessels and occasionally the joints {1085, 1056, 53, 618, 417, 517, 166, 1403}. There is prominent deposition of the aberrant Ig on basement membranes, elastic and collagen fibers. Vascular occlusion and microaneurysm formation may occur {1085, 1056, 53, 618, 417, 517, 166, 1403}.

Clinical features
Patients present with symptoms of organ dysfunction as a result of diffuse, systemic immunoglobulin deposits, including nephotic syndrome, renal failure, arthritis, congestive heart failure, and coagulopathy (factor X deficiency) due to liver involvement {166}. HCDD of IgG3 or IgG1 isotypes result in hypocomplementemia since the G3 and G1 subclasses most readily fix complement {517}. There is a monoclonal gammopathy in 85% of cases. The 15% without an m-component reflects strong tissue binding of the aberrant Ig.

Pathophysiology
Non amyloid MIDD are plasma cell neoplasms whose monoclonal Ig product has undergone structural change due to deletional and mutational events {1056, 618, 166}.
In HCDD the critical event is deletion of the CH1 constant domain {53, 618, 517}. When a mutant heavy chain lacks CH1 domain, it fails to associate with heavy

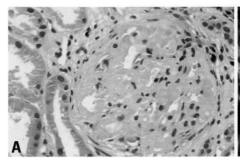
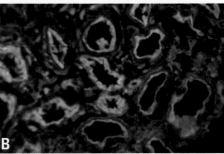

Fig. 6.60 Light chain deposition disease in kidney showing (**A**) pale amorphous patches within glomeruli (nodular glomerulosclerosis) and (**B**) immunofluorescence stain showing renal tubular and extratubular deposition of kappa light chain in a smooth linear pattern.

chain binding protein (BiP), resulting in premature secretion into the circulation {1056, 53, 618}. In HCDD the variable regions also contain amino acid substitutions, that cause an increased propensity for tissue deposition and for binding blood elements. {53, 618}. In LCDD the primary defect involves multiple mutations of the Ig light chain variable region with kappa light chain of $V_{\kappa IV}$ type notably overrepresented {1056, 166}.
These disruptive substitutions in the amino acid sequence result in an Ig with altered physiochemical properties (e.g. more cationic with altered hydro-phobia) or aberrant glycosylation, which favour tissue binding and deposition {417, 166}. There is some suggestion that the mutagenic events in LCDD can be induced by alkylating agent chemo-therapy {1056}.

Morphology
There are prominent tissue monoclonal Ig deposits of a non-amyloid, nonfibrillary, amorphous eosinophilic material, which do not stain with Congo red. They are often seen as refractile eosinophilic material in the glomerular and tubular basement membranes, but may also be seen in bone marrow and other tissues. These deposits by electron microscopy

are typically discrete, dense punctate, granular, nonfibrillary deposits, with an absence of the β-pleated sheet structure by x-ray diffraction. Although in some cases plasma cells are found in the vicinity of deposits, it is more common to find Ig deposition in visceral organs with few if any plasma cells. Thus in general the physiochemically altered Ig is produced in the bone marrow and travels to distant sites via the circulation. Bone marrow plasmacytosis is found in 50-60% of the cases.

Immunophenotype
In contrast with primary amyloidosis, which has a predominance of lambda light chain with over-representation of the $V_{\lambda VI}$ variable region, LCDD has a prevalence of kappa light chains (80%) with overrepresentation of the $V_{\lambda IV}$ variable region {166}. Typically, the kappa chains are demonstrated by immunoflourescence in the renal glomerular and tubular basement membrane. In particular, the hallmark of the disease are the prominent, smooth, ribbon-like linear peritubular deposits of monotypic immuno-globulin along the outer edge of the tubular basement membrane. Even in cases without overt bone marrow plasmacytosis

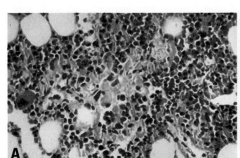
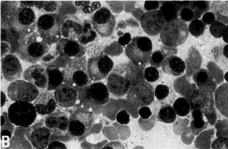
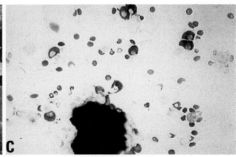

Fig. 6.61 Light chain deposition disease. **A** Bone marrow biopsy showing patches of pale amorphous material. **B** Bone marrow aspirate showing numerous plasma cells. **C** Joint fluid aspirate showing clumps of amorphous material and plasma cells, both staining for kappa light chain by immunoperoxidase.

immunohistochemistry reveals an aberrant kappa/lambda ratio {1403}.

Prognosis

The prognosis is usually very poor with a fatal outcome within 1-2 years even in the absence of aggressive plasma cell proliferation.

Osteosclerotic myeloma (POEMS syndrome)

Definition

Osteosclerotic myeloma is a plasma cell proliferative disorder, which is often a component of a rare syndrome that includes polyneuropathy (sensorimotor demyelination), organomegaly (hepatosplenomegaly), endocrinopathy (diabetes, gynecomastia, testicular atrophy, impotence), monoclonal gammopathy, and skin changes (hyperpigmentation, hypertrichosis) otherwise known as POEMS syndrome {879}. It is characterised by a plasma cell infiltrate in the marrow accompanied by thickened bone trabeculae, and often lymph node changes resembling the plasma cell variant of Castleman disease (angiofollicular hyperplasia). The relationship of this disease to typical plasma cell myeloma is not known.

Synonyms

Crow-Fukase syndrome
Multicentric Castleman disease

Epidemiology

This is a rare disease, occurring predominantly in adults, and estimated to comprise between 1 and 2% of plasma cell dyscrasias {879}. Many cases have been reported from Asia. Males are affected slightly more often than women (M:F=1.4) and the median age is 50 years, younger than that for typical plasma cell myeloma.

Aetiology

Some reported cases have been associated with Kaposi sarcoma herpesvirus/ human herpesvirus 8 (KSHV/HHV-8) {879, 83}.

Clinical features

Patients present with polyneuropathy and a variety of symptoms related to endocrine dysfunction and skeletal lesions, as well as lymphadenopathy. In one report of patients with osteosclerotic myeloma and neuropathy, only 13% had the features of POEMS syndrome. Anaemia is rare, and erythrocytosis may occur. Thrombocytosis is common. Hypercalcemia, renal insufficiency, and pathological fractures are rare. A paraprotein is typically present, and is of either IgG or IgA lambda type. The level of the M-component in serum and urine is usually low. Radiographic studies reveal single or multiple sclerotic bone lesions.

Morphology

The characteristic lesion is an osteosclerotic plasmacytoma, which may occur singly or multiply in the marrow. The lesion is comprised of focally thickened trabecular bone with closely associated peritrabecular fibrosis with entrapped plasma cells.

The bone marrow away from the osteosclerotic lesion usually contains fewer than 5% plasma cells, which are typically mature. Lymph node biopsies show a follicular proliferation with regressed (hyaline vascular) and reactive follicles and interfollicular plasma cell accumulation, consistent with the plasma cell variant of Castleman disease {879}.

Immunophenotype

The plasma cells contain monoclonal cytoplasmic Ig which may be of IgG or IgA heavy chain type. The light chain is lambda in >90% of patients.

Prognosis

The survival appears to be better than that for typical plasma cell myeloma (60% at 5 years) {879}.

Heavy chain diseases

These are rare B cell neoplasms that exclusively produce monoclonal heavy chains and no light chains {402, 399, 1355, 1173, 16, 356, 377, 552, 68, 1354, 376, 400, 1172, 1083, 1059, 564, 87}. They are morphologically and clinically heterogenous and do not appear to be true plasma cell neoplasms. They are discussed here because of the unifying feature of the presence of an abnormal serum immunoglobulin component.

The pathological monoclonal immunoglobulin component is composed of either IgG (Gamma heavy chain disease), IgA (Alpha heavy chain disease) or IgM (Mu heavy chain disease). The heavy chain immunoglobulin is usually an incomplete truncated heavy chain incapable of full assembly, producing variably sized immunoglobulin molecules. It may consequently present without a characteristic serum protein electrophoresis "spike" and requires immunoelectrophoresis or immunofixation to establish heavy chain specificity.

Each of these diseases appears to represent an unusual variant of a type of lymphoma, and are also discussed in the respective section. Gamma HCD is a variant of lymphoplasmacytic lymphoma, mu HCD appears to be a variant of CLL, and alpha HCD is a variant of extranodal marginal zone lymphoma of mucosa-associated lymphoid tissue (MALT).

ICD-O code   9762/3

Gamma heavy chain disease

Definition

Gamma heavy chain disease (GHCD) is a lymphoplasmacytic neoplasm that produces a truncated gamma chain, which lacks light-chain binding sites and does not bind to light chains to form a complete immunoglobulin molecule {402, 399, 1355, 1173, 16, 356, 377, 552}.

Synonym

Franklin disease

Epidemiology

This is a rare disease of adults with a median age of 60 {377}.

Sites of involvement

The tumour may involve the lymph nodes, Waldeyer's ring, bone marrow, liver, spleen and peripheral blood.

Clinical features

Most patients have systemic symptoms (anorexia, weakness, fever, weight loss and recurrent bacterial infections) and autoimmune manifestations such as hemolytic anaemia, autoimmune thrombocytopenia, with lymphadenopathy, splenomegaly, hepatomegaly, involvement of Waldeyer's ring, and peripheral eosinophilia {377}. Circulating plasma cells or lymphocytes may give a plasma cell leukaemia or chronic lymphocytic leukaemia-like (CLL-like) appearance. The patients generally have no lytic bone

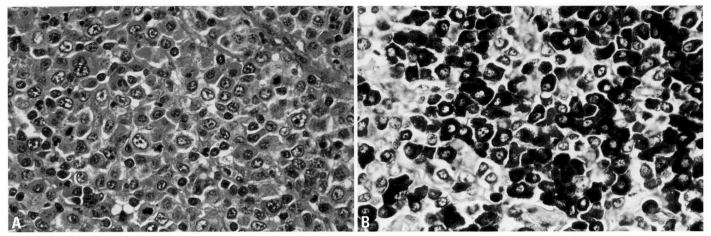

Fig. 6.62 Gamma heavy chain disease. **A** This polymorphous lymphoplasmacytic proliferation is comprised of admixed plasma cells, plasmacytoid lymphocytes and lymphoid cells. **B** Immunohistological assay shows monotypic staining for gamma heavy chain. There was no light chain staining.

lesions. Clinical and laboratory distinction from an infection/inflammatory process is difficult given this constellation of symptoms and the sometimes broad band or near-normal serum protein electrophoresis. The diagnosis is made by immunofixation demonstration of IgG without light chains. Urine protein is usually less than 1g/24 hours.

Morphology
Lymph nodes typically show a polymorphous proliferation with admixed lymphocytes, plasmacytoid lymphocytes, plasma cells, immunoblasts and eosinophils. In some cases plasma cells predominate, and may resemble plasma cell myeloma. There may be a chronic lymphocytic leukaemia (CLL)-like picture, with involvement of the peripheral blood, and rarely, nodal large cell lymphoma.

Immunophenotype
Monoclonal cytoplasmic gamma chain without light chain, Pan B-cell antigen +, CD5-, CD10-.

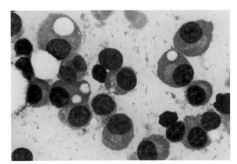

Fig. 6.63 Mu heavy chain disease. Bone marrow aspirate shows predominantly plasma cells with prominent cytoplasmic vacuolation.

Postulated cell of origin
Lymphocyte or plasma cell with defective gamma heavy chain gene.

Prognosis and predictive factors
The clinical outcome is variable, ranging from indolent to rapidly progressive, with a median survival of 12 months {376}.

Mu heavy chain disease

Definition
Mu heavy chain disease is a B-cell neoplasm resembling chronic lymphocytic leukaemia (CLL), in which a defective mu heavy chain lacking a variable region is produced {68, 1354, 376, 400}. The bone marrow has characteristic vacuolated plasma cells, admixed with small, round lymphocytes.

Epidemiology
This is an extremely rare disease of adults.

Sites of involvement
Spleen, liver, bone marrow and peripheral blood are involved; peripheral lymphadenopathy is usually not present.

Clinical features
Most patients present with a slowly progressive chronic lymphocytic leukaemia. Mu chain disease differs from most cases of CLL in the high frequency of hepatosplenomegaly and the absence of peripheral lymphadenopathy. Routine serum protein electrophoresis is frequently normal.
Immunoelectrophoresis reveals reactivity to anti-mu in polymers of diverse sizes.

Although mu chain is not found in the urine, Bence Jones light chains are commonly (50%) found in the urine, particularly kappa chains. The latter, while still produced in mu-HCD, are not assimilable because of heavy chain gene aberrancies leading to truncated forms {68, 1354}.

Morphology
The bone marrow has characteristic vacuolated plasma cells which are typically admixed with small, round lymphocytes similar to chronic lymphocytic leukaemia cells.

Imunophenotype
Monoclonal cytoplasmic mu heavy chain without light chain, Pan B-cell antigen+, CD5-, CD10-.

Prognosis
The clinical course is slowly progressive {68, 1354, 376, 400}.

Alpha heavy chain disease

Definition
Alpha heavy chain disease (αCHD)is a variant of extranodal marginal zone B-cell lymphoma of mucosa-associated lymphoid tissue (MALT), in which defective alpha heavy chains are secreted, which occurs in young adults and involves the gastrointestinal tract resulting in malabsorption and diarrhoea {1172, 1083, 1059, 87}. It begins as a process sometimes reversible by antibiotics but may eventuate as high grade lymphoma.

Table 6.11
Immunosecretory disorders and corresponding neoplasms

Clinical syndrome	Neoplasm
Multiple myeloma	Plasma cell myeloma
Immunoglobulin deposition diseases	
Primary AL amyloidosis	Plasma cell myeloma
Light chain deposition disease	Plasma cell myeloma
P.O.E.M.S. syndrome	Osteosclerotic myeloma; multicentric Castleman disease
Waldenström macroglobulinemia	Lymphoplasmacytic lymphoma
Heavy chain diseases	
Gamma heavy chain disease	Lymphoplasmacytic lymphoma
Mu heavy chain disease	Chronic lymphocytic leukaemia
Alpha heavy chain disease	Extranodal marginal zone (MALT) lymphoma

POEMS = polyneuropathy, organomegaly, endocrine abnormalities, M-component, skin changes;
MALT = mucosa-associated lymphoid tissue

Synonyms
Mediterranean abdominal lymphoma
Immunoproliferative small intestinal disease (IPSID)

Epidemiology
Unlike the other HCD, αCHD involves a young age group with a peak incidence in the second and third decades. It is most common in areas bordering the Mediterranean including Israel, Egypt, Saudi Arabia, and North Africa. It is associated with low socioeconomic standards including poor hygiene, malnutrition and frequent intestinal infections {1172, 1083, 1059}.

Sites of involvement
This disorder involves the gastrointestinal tract, mainly the small intestine, and mesenteric lymph nodes. The bone marrow and other organs are usually not involved, although rare respiratory tract involvement is described {1172}.

Clinical features at presentation
Patients typically present with malabsorption, diarrhoea, hypocalcemia, abdominal pain, wasting, fever and steatorrhoea. Because of defective heavy chain assembly and consequent diversity of IgA molecular forms, the serum protein electrophoresis (SPE) in αCHD is usually normal or shows hypogammaglobulinemia. Typically, specific anti-IgA antibody is required to detect aberrant IgA by immunofixation {1172}.

Morphology
The lamina propria of the bowel is heavily infiltrated with plasma cells and admixed small lymphocytes; marginal zone B cells may be present with formation of lymphoepithelial lesions.
The lymphoplasmacytic infiltrate separates the crypts, and villous atrophy may be present {1083, 564}.

Immunophenotype
The plasma cells and marginal zone cells express monoclonal cytoplasmic alpha chain without light chain, Pan B-cell antigens and are CD5-, CD10- {564}.

Prognosis and predictive factors
In the early phase, αCHD may completely remit with antibiotic therapy. Many patients, however, experience transformation to large B-cell lymphoma, and a fatal outcome is frequent {1172, 87}.

Extranodal marginal zone B-cell lymphoma of mucosa-associated lymphoid tissue (MALT lymphoma)

P.G. Isaacson
H.K. Müller-Hermelink
M.A. Piris
F. Berger
B.N. Nathwani
S.H. Swerdlow
N.L. Harris

Definition

Extranodal marginal zone B-cell lymphoma of mucosa-associated lymphoid tissue (MALT lymphoma) is an extranodal lymphoma comprising morphologically heterogeneous small B-cells including marginal zone (centrocyte-like) cells, cells resembling monocytoid cells, small lymphocytes, and scattered immunoblast and centroblast-like cells. There is plasma cell differentiation in a proportion of the cases. The infiltrate is in the marginal zone of reactive B-cell follicles and extends into the interfollicular region. In epithelial tissues, the neoplastic cells typically infiltrate the epithelium, forming lymphoepithelial lesions.

ICD-O code   9699/3

Synonyms

Rappaport: well-differentiated lymphocytic, plasmacytoid lymphocytic, poorly-differentiated lymphocytic
Kiel: immunocytoma
Lukes-Collins: lymphocytic, plasmacytic-lymphocytic, small cleaved cell
Working Formulation: small lymphocytic, lymphoplasmacytoid, diffuse small cleaved cell

Epidemiology

MALT lymphoma comprises 7-8% of all B-cell lymphomas {8}, and up to 50% of primary gastric lymphoma {1073, 309}. Most cases occur in adults with a median age of 61 and a slight female preponderance (male:female ratio 1:1.2) {8}. There appears to be a higher incidence of gastric MALT lymphomas in north-east Italy {309} and a special sub-type previously known as α chain disease and now called immunoproliferative small intestinal disease (IPSID) occurs in the Middle East {1038} and the Cape region of South Africa {1059}.

Precursor lesions/conditions

In many cases of MALT lymphoma, there is a history of chronic inflammatory, often autoimmune disorders that result in accumulation of extranodal lymphoid tissue. Examples include Helicobacter pylori associated chronic gastritis, Sjögren syndrome or Hashimoto thyroiditis. In the first study in which the association of gastric MALT lymphoma with *H. pylori* infection was examined the organism was present in over 90% of cases {1417}. Subsequent studies have shown

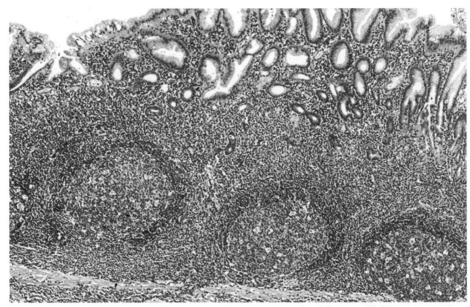

Fig. 6.64 Gastric MALT lymphoma. The tumour cells surround reactive follicles and infiltrate the mucosa. The follicles have a typical starry-sky appearance.

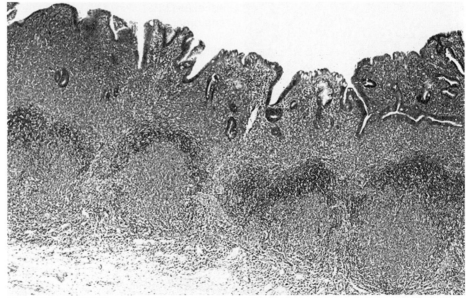

Fig 6.65 Gastric MALT lymphoma. The marginal zone cells infiltrate the lamina propria in a diffuse pattern and have colonised the germinal centres of reactive B-cell follicles. In contrast to the case illustrated above, the colonised follicles do not show a starry-sky pattern.

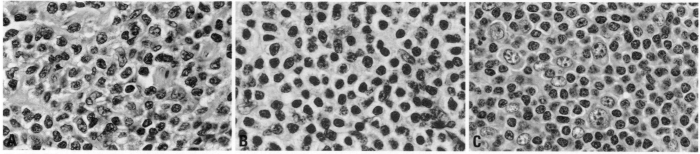

Fig. 6.66 This composite illustrates the morphologic spectrum of MALT lymphoma cells. **A** Neoplastic marginal zone B-cells with nuclei resembling those of centrocytes, but wih more abundant cytoplasm. **B** The cells of this MALT lymphoma have abundant pale staining cytoplasm leading to a monocytoid appearance. **C** MALT lymphoma comprised of cells resembling small lymphocytes. There are scattered transformed blasts.

a lower incidence {930} but also that the density and detectability of *H. pylori* decreases as lymphoma evolves from chronic gastritis {922}. The organism may be undetectable using histopathological techniques in patients who are seropositive {335}.

Patients with certain autoimmune diseases – Sjögren syndrome and Hashimoto thyroiditis – are at increased risk of developing MALT lymphoma. Patients with Sjögren syndrome (SS) or lymphoepithelial sialadenitis (LESA) have a 44-fold increased risk of developing overt lymphoma, comprising about 4-7% of patients {1260, 637}. Approximately 85% of lymphomas in patients with SS/LESA

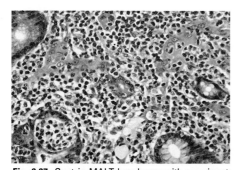

Fig. 6.67 Gastric MALT lymphoma with prominent lymphoepithelial lesions.

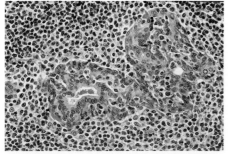

Fig. 6.68 MALT lymphoma of salivary gland showing lymphoepithelial lesions.

are MALT lymphomas. Patients with Hashimoto thyroiditis have a 3-fold excess risk of developing lymphoma and a 70-fold increased risk of thyroid lymphoma, for an overall lymphoma risk of 0.5-1.5% of the patients {638, 531, 37}. 94% of thyroid lymphomas have evidence of thyroiditis in the adjacent gland {289}. Chronic intestinal infections are postulated to be an underlying cause of IPSID {1083, 1059}.

Sites of involvement

The gastrointestinal (GI) tract is the most common site of MALT lymphoma, comprising 50% of all cases, and within the GI tract, the stomach is the most common location (85%) {1073}. The small intestine and colon are typically involved in patients with IPSID. Other common sites include lung (14% of a recent series), head and neck (14%), ocular adnexae (12%), skin (11%), thyroid (4%), and breast (4%) {1283}.

Clinical features

The majority of patients present with stage I or II disease. Approximately 20% of the patients have bone marrow involvement {46, 1284}, but the frequency seems to vary among primary sites, being lower for gastric cases and higher for primary ocular adnexal or pulmonary cases {1284, 1283}. Multiple extranodal sites may be involved in up to 10% of the cases at the time of presentation. Multifocal nodal involvement is rare (7.5% of the cases in a recent series) {1283}. Application of staging systems for nodal lymphomas can be misleading in MALT type lymphomas, since involvement of multiple extranodal sites, particularly within the same organ (e.g. salivary gland, skin), may not reflect truly disseminated disease.

Despite plasmacytic differentiation in many of the cases, a serum paraprotein (M-component) is rare in MALT lymphomas. The major exception is IPSID, in which an aberrant alpha heavy chain can usually be found in the peripheral blood {1059}.

Aetiology

Hussell and colleagues have shown that continued proliferation of gastric MALT lymphoma cells from patients infected with *H. pylori* depends on the presence of T cells specifically activated by *H. pylori* antigens {553}. The importance of this stimulation *in vivo* has been clearly demonstrated by the induction of remissions in gastric MALT lymphomas with antibiotic therapy to eradicate *H. pylori* {1415}. A role for antigenic stimulation by *Borrelia burgdorferi* has been proposed for some cases of cutaneous MALT lymphoma {192}. Isaacson has suggested that "acquired MALT" secondary to autoimmune disease or infection in these sites may form the substrate for lymphoma development {563}.

Morphology

The lymphoma cells infiltrate around reactive B-cell follicles, external to a preserved follicle mantle, in a marginal zone distribution and spread out to form larger confluent areas which eventually overrun some or most of the follicles {569, 570}. The characteristic marginal zone B cells have small to medium-sized, slightly irregular nuclei with moderately dispersed chromatin and inconspicuous nucleoli, resembling those of centrocytes; they have relatively abundant, pale cytoplasm. The accumulation of more pale-staining cytoplasm may lead to a monocytoid appearance. Alternatively, the marginal zone cells may more closely

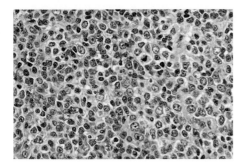

Fig. 6.69 MALT lymphoma with an increased number of large cells.

resemble small lymphocytes). Plasmacytic differentiation is present in approximately one third of gastric MALT-type lymphomas and is a constant and often striking feature in thyroid MALT-type lymphomas and in IPSID {1059, 87}. Large cells resembling centroblasts or immunoblasts are usually present, but are in the minority. In glandular tissues epithelium is often invaded and destroyed by discrete aggregates of lymphoma cells resulting in the so-called lymphoepithelial lesions. Lymphoepithelial lesions are aggregates of three or more marginal zone cells with distortion or destruction of the epithelium, often together with eosinophilic degeneration of epithelial cells. The lymphoma cells sometimes specifically colonise the germinal centres of the reactive follicles and in extreme examples, this can lead to a close resemblance to follicular lymphoma. MALT lymphoma is defined as a lymphoma composed predominantly of mall cells. Transformed centroblast- or immunoblast-like cells may be present in variable numbers in MALT lymphoma but

when solid or sheet-like proliferations of transformed cells are present the tumour should be diagnosed as diffuse large B-cell lymphoma and the presence of accompanying MALT lymphoma noted. The term "high-grade MALT lymphoma" should not be used, and the term "MALT lymphoma" should not be applied to a large B-cell lymphoma even if it has arisen in a MALT site.

The histological features of IPSID are similar to those of other cases of MALT lymphoma, but typically show striking plasmacytic differentiation {87, 564}.

In lymph nodes, MALT lymphoma invades the marginal zone with subsequent interfollicular expansion. Discrete aggregates of monocytoid B cells may be present in a parafollicular and perisinusoidal distribution. Cytological heterogeneity is still present and both plasma cell differentiation and follicular colonisation may be seen.

Differential diagnosis

The differential diagnosis of MALT lymphoma includes reactive processes (Helicobacter pylori gastritis, lymphoepithelial sialadenitis, Hashimoto thyroiditis) and other small B-cell lymphomas (follicular lymphoma, mantle cell lymphoma, small lymphocytic lymphoma). Distinction from reactive processes is based mainly on the presence of destructive infiltrates of extrafollicular B cells, typically with the morphology of marginal zone cells {1415}. In borderline cases, immunophenotyping or molecular genetic analysis to assess B-cell clonality are necessary to establish or exclude

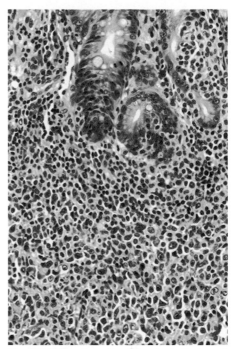

Fig. 6.70 Diffuse large B-cell lymphoma (bottom of field) with residual MALT lymphoma in the superficial mucosa.

a diagnosis of MALT lymphoma. Distinction from other small B-cell lymphomas is based on a combination of the characteristic morphologic and immunophenotypic features.

Immunophenotype

Tumour cells typically express IgM, and less often IgA or IgG, and show light chain restriction. In IPSID, both the plasma cells and marginal zone cells express α heavy chain without any light chain

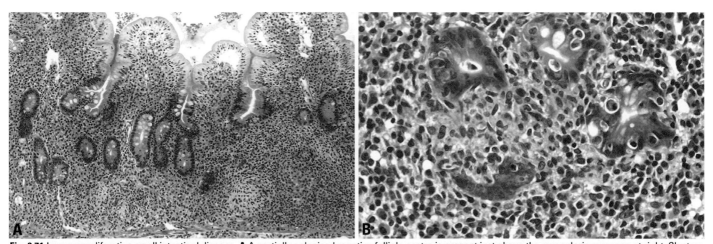

Fig. 6.71 Immunoproliferative small intestinal disease. **A** A partially colonised reactive follicle centre is present just above the muscularis mucosae at right. Clusters of pale staining marginal zone cells are present adjacent to the follicle and elsewhere in the biopsy. The lamina propria and small intestinal villi are expanded by plasma cells. **B** A lymphoepithelial lesion in a case of IPSID showing destruction of intestinal crypts by marginal zone cells with surrounding plasma cells.

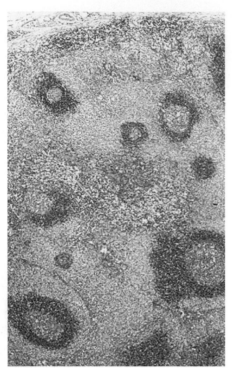

Fig. 6.72 Gastric lymph node involved by MALT lymphoma. The tumour cells infiltrate the marginal zones and spread into the interfollicular areas.

{564}. The tumour cells of MALT lymphoma are CD20+, CD79a+, CD5-, CD10, CD23-, CD43+/-, CD11c+/- (weak).

The lymphoma cells express the marginal zone cell-associated antigens CD21 and CD35. Staining for CD21 and CD35 typically reveals expanded meshworks of follicular dendritic cells corresponding to colonised follicles. There is no specific marker for MALT lymphoma at present. The demonstration of immunoglobulin light chain restriction is important in the differential diagnosis with benign lymphoid infiltrates. In the differential diagnosis with other small B-cell lymphomas, absence of the characteristic markers for those neoplasms is important: lack of CD5 is ueful in distinction sfrom mantle cell and small lymphocytic lymphomas, cyclin D1 in distinction from mantle cell lymphoma, and CD10 in the differential diagnosis with follicular lymphoma.

Genetics

Antigen receptor genes
Immunoglobulin heavy and light chain genes are rearranged and show somatic mutation of variable regions, consistent with derivation from a post-germinal centre, memory B cell {322, 1066}.

Cytogenetic abnormalities and oncogenes
Trisomy 3 is found in 60% and t(11;18) (q21;q21) has been observed in 25-50% of the cases {1416, 156, 989}. In con-trast, the t(11;18) is not found in primary large B cell gastric lymphoma. Recently, analysis of the t(11;18) breakpoint has shown fusion of the apoptosis-inhibitor gene *API2* to a novel gene at 18q21, named MLT {301}. Neither t(14;18) nor t(11;14) is present.

Postulated cell of origin
Post germinal centre, marginal zone B-cell.

Prognosis and predictive factors
MALT lymphomas run an indolent natural course and are slow to disseminate; recurrences may involve other extranodal sites. The tumours are sensitive to radiation therapy, and local treatment may be followed by prolonged disease-free intervals. Involvement of multiple extranodal sites and even bone marrow involvement do not appear to confer a worse prognosis {1284}. Protracted remissions may be induced in *H. pylori*-associated gastric MALT lymphoma by antibiotic therapy for H. pylori {1415, 943}. Cases with the t(11;18)(q21;q21) appear to be resistant to *H. pylori* eradication therapy {778}. In IPSID, remissions have followed therapy with broad spectrum antibiotics {87}. Transformation to diffuse large B-cell lymphoma may occur.

Table 6.12
Criteria for histologic differential diagnosis of gastric MALT lymphoma {119}.

Score	Diagnosis	Histological features
0	Normal	Scattered plasma cells in lamina propria. No lymphoid follicles
1	Chronic active gastritis	Small clusters of lymphocytes in lamina propria. No lymphoid follicles. No lymphoepithelial lesions
2	Chronic active gastritis with florid lymphoid follicle formation	Prominent lymphoid follicles with surrounding mantle zone and plasma cells. No lymphoepithelial lesions
3*	Suspicious lymphoid infiltrate, probably reactive	Lymphoid follicles surrounded by small lymphocytes that infiltrate diffusely in lamina propria and occasionally into epithelium
4*	Suspicious lymphoid infiltrate, probably lymphoma	Lymphoid follicles surrounded by marginal zone cells that infiltrate diffusely in lamina propria and into epithelium in small groups
5	MALT lymphoma	Presence of dense diffuse infiltrate of marginal zone cells in lamina propria with prominent lymphoepithelial lesions

* For categories 3 and 4, immunophenotyping or molecular genetic analysis to assess B-cell clonality are required to confirm or exclude MALT lymphoma.

Nodal marginal zone B-cell lymphoma

P.G. Isaacson
B.N. Nathwani
M.A. Piris
F. Berger

N.L. Harris
H.K. Müller-Hermelink
S. Swerdlow

Definition
Nodal marginal zone B-cell lymphoma (NMZL) is a primary nodal B-cell neoplasm that morphologically resembles lymph nodes involved by marginal zone lymphomas of extranodal or splenic types, but without evidence of extranodal or splenic disease. Monocytoid B-cells may be prominent.

ICD-O code   9699/3

Synonyms
Rappaport: well-differentiated lymphocytic, poorly-differentiated lymphocytic, mixed lymphocytic-histiocytic
Kiel: monocytoid B-cell
Lukes-Collins: parafollicular B-cell
Working Formulation: small lymphocytic, plasmacytoid; follicular or diffuse small cleaved cell; follicular or diffuse mixed small and large cell

Epidemiology
Nodal marginal zone lymphoma is a rare disease, comprising only 1.8% of lymphoid neoplasms in a recent study {8, 46}. Clinical investigation revealed evidence of an extranodal lymphoma in approximately 1/3 of the cases in one recent series {173}.

Sites of involvement
Peripheral lymph nodes, occasionally bone marrow and peripheral blood.

Clinical features
Most patients present with localised or generalised peripheral lymphadenopathy, with good performance status {98}.

Morphology
The marginal zone and interfollicular areas of the lymph node are infiltrated by marginal zone (centrocyte-like) B-cells, monocytoid B-cells, or small B-lymphocytes, with scattered centroblast and immunoblast-like cells present {954, 1182}. Two types have been described, one that closely resembles nodal involvement by MALT lymphoma, and one that resembles splenic marginal zone lymphoma {173}. Plasma cell differentiation is a feature of some cases. Follicular colonisation may be present. Transformation to large B-cell lymphoma may occur.

In patients with extranodal (MALT) lymphoma, Hashimoto thyroiditis or Sjogren syndrome, nodal involvement by marginal zone lymphoma should be considered secondary involvement by MALT lymphoma.

Immunophenotype
Most cases are similar to extranodal marginal zone (MALT) lymphoma; some are reported to be IgD+ CD43-, similar to splenic MZL {173}.

Genetics
These have not been well studied. However, the t(11;18)(q21;q21) and trisomy 3 associated with extranodal marginal zone lymphoma are not frequent {302, 1098}.

Postulated cell of origin
Marginal zone B-cell of nodal type.

Prognosis and predictive factors
The clinical course has not been well studied. In two recent series, the majority of the patients responded to chemotherapy, but with a high early relapse rate; nonetheless, the median survival was approximately 5 years, consistent with an indolent lymphoma {98, 934}.

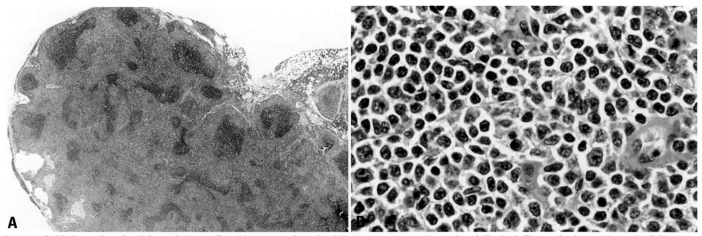

Fig. 6.73 A Whole section of nodal marginal zone B-cell lymphoma. Reactive follicles are separated by an interfollicular infiltrate of paler staining cells. **B** The neoplastic cells in nodal marginal zone B-cell lymphoma have irregularly shaped nuclei and moderately abundant pale cytoplasm. Occasional plasma cells and transformed blasts are present.

Follicular lymphoma

B.N. Nathwani
N.L. Harris
D. Weisenburger
P.G. Isaacson

M.A. Piris
F. Berger
H.K. Müller-Hermelink
S.H. Swerdlow

Definition

Follicular lymphoma (FL) is a neoplasm of follicle centre B cells (centrocytes/cleaved follicle centre cells (FCC) and centroblasts/noncleaved FCC), which has at least a partially follicular pattern.

ICD-O codes:

Follicular lymphoma	9690/3
Grade 1	9691/3
Grade 2	9695/3
Grade 3	9698/3

Synonyms

Rappaport: nodular poorly differentiated lymphocytic, mixed lymphocytic-histiocytic, histiocytic, or undifferentiated
Kiel: centroblastic/centrocytic (CB/CC) follicular, follicular and diffuse; centroblastic, follicular
Lukes-Collins: small cleaved, large cleaved, small noncleaved or large noncleaved follicular centre cell (follicular)
Working Formulation: follicular small cleaved, mixed, large, or small noncleaved cell
REAL classification: Follicle centre lymphoma, follicular

Epidemiology

Follicular lymphoma comprises about 35% of adult non-Hodgkin lymphomas in the U.S. and 22% worldwide {8}; the incidence is lower elsewhere in Europe, in Asia, and in underdeveloped countries {27}. Follicular lymphoma comprises up to 70% of "low grade" lymphomas

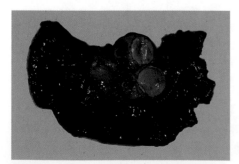

Fig. 6.74 Follicular lymphoma, gross photograph. There is involvement of mesenteric lymph node, but adjacent bowel wall is not affected.

enrolled in U.S. clinical trials {440}. It affects predominantly adults, with a median age of 59 years and a male:female ratio of 1:1.7 {8}. Follicular lymphoma rarely occurs in individuals under age 20 years; paediatric patients are predominantly males with early-stage disease, often localised to the head and neck, including tonsils, and approximately 50% of the tumours are of large cell (grade 3) type {384, 1042}.

Sites of involvement

Follicular lymphoma predominantly involves lymph nodes, but also spleen, bone marrow, peripheral blood, and Waldeyer's ring. Involvement of non-haematopoietic extranodal sites, such as the gastrointestinal tract, soft tissue, skin, and other sites may occur, but this is usually in a setting of widespread nodal disease. Primary follicular lymphoma of the skin ("cutaneous follicle centre lymphoma") represents one of the most common types of cutaneous B-cell lymphoma {1387}.

Clinical features

Most patients have widespread disease at diagnosis, including peripheral and central (abdominal and thoracic) lymph nodes and spleen; the bone marrow is involved in 40%. Only 1/3 of patients are in Stage I or II at the time of the diagnosis {8}. Despite widespread disease, patients are usually asymptomatic except for lymph node enlargement.

Morphology

Most cases of follicular lymphoma have a predominantly follicular pattern. Neoplastic follicles are often poorly defined and often lack mantle zones; they are closely packed, efface the nodal architecture, and have neither polarisation nor a prominent starry-sky pattern. Diffuse areas may be present, often with sclerosis. The pattern is reported as follicular (>75% follicular), follicular and diffuse (25-75% follicular), or minimally follicular (<25% follicular). Interfollicular involvement by neoplastic cells is com-

mon; this does not constitute a diffuse pattern. The neoplastic centrocytes in the interfollicular regions are often smaller than those in the follicles, with less nuclear irregularity.

Most cases of follicular lymphoma are composed of two types of cells normally found in follicle centres (germinal centres). Small to medium sized cells with angulated, elongated, twisted or cleaved nuclei, inconspicuous nucleoli and scant pale cytoplasm are known as centrocytes or cleaved FCC. Large transformed cells with usually round or oval, but occasionally indented nuclei, vesicular chromatin, one to three peripheral nucleoli and a narrow rim of cytoplasm, which is basophilic on Giemsa stain are known as centroblasts or noncleaved FCC. In some cases, neoplastic centroblasts may have hyperchromatic, irregular or lobulated nuclei. Centrocytes typically predominate; centroblasts are always present, but are usually in the minority, so that most cases have a monomorphic appearance, in contrast to the mixed appearance of reactive follicles. Some cases show increased centroblasts, giving a "mixed" appearance, and a smaller number have a predominance of centroblasts. Rare cases consist entirely of large or small centroblasts (large noncleaved or small noncleaved cells).

In about 10% of the cases, FL may show discrete foci of marginal zone or monocytoid-appearing B cells, typically at the periphery of the neoplastic follicles {933}. Plasmacytoid differentiation or signet ring cells may rarely occur.

Follicular lymphoma is graded by the proportion of centroblasts. Histological grading can predict clinical outcome, but the optimal method and clinical significance are still debated. We recommend a 3-grade system (Grades 1-3), based on counting the absolute number of centroblasts in ten neoplastic follicles, expressed per 40x high-power microscopic field (hpf) {811, 870, 935}. Grade 1 cases have 0-5 centroblasts/hpf; Grade 2 cases have 6-15 centroblasts /hpf; Grade 3 cases have >15 centroblasts/hpf. Ten high power fields within different follicles are counted; these are representative follicles, not selected for those with the most numerous large cells. If discrete areas of grade 3 FL are present in an otherwise Grade 1 or Grade 2 case, a separate diagnosis should be made, and the approximate amount of each grade reported. Grade 3 FL can be further subdivided for investigational purposes according to the number of centroblasts. In Grade 3a there are >15 centroblasts/hpf, but centrocytes are still present, while Grade 3b has solid sheets of centroblasts.

The above counts are based on a high-power field of 0.159 mm² (1 ocular with an 18 mm field of view at 1x magnification, and a 40x objective). Oculars with wider fields of view produce a larger 40x hpf. For example, an ocular with a 20 mm in diameter field of view at 1x gives a 0.196 mm² hpf, 1.2 times as large as the standard 0.159 mm² field, and an ocular

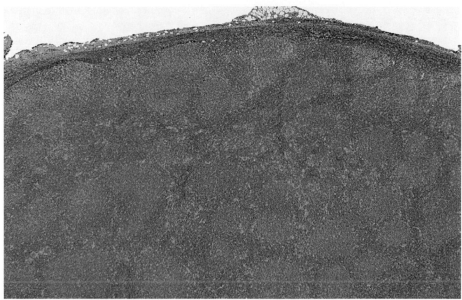

Fig. 6.75 Follicular lymphoma: The neoplastic follicles are closely packed, focally show an almost back-to-back pattern, and lack mantle zones.

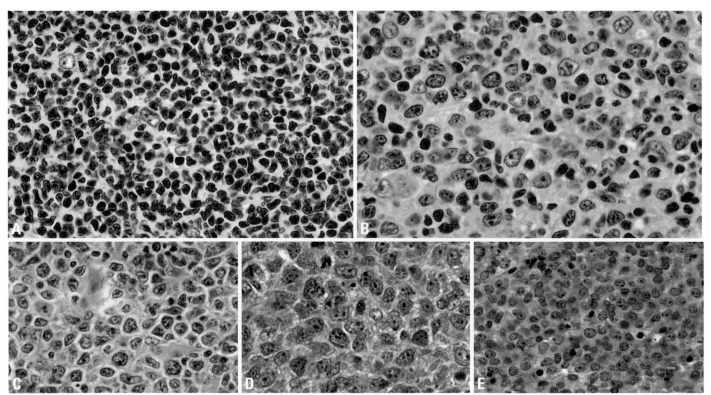

Fig. 6.76 A Follicular Lymphoma, Grade 1. Note the monotonous population of small lymphoid cells with irregular, angulated nuclei, dispersed chromatin, inconspicuous nucleoli, and scant cytoplasm. No centroblasts are shown in this picture, but they were scattered in many follicles. The three large cells are follicular dendritic cells (also shown in figure 8). **B** Follicular Lymphoma, Grade 2. Note the mixture of small, medium and large lymphoid cells. The small cells are consistent with centrocytes (small cleaved cells). Small centroblasts (small noncleaved cells) and large centroblasts (large noncleaved cells) have round nuclei with vesicular chromatin and one to three prominent basophilic nucleoli, usually located adjacent to the nuclear membranes. **C** Follicular Lymphoma, Grade 3A. Although there are many centroblasts (>15 per hpf), there are admixed centrocytes. **D** Follicular Lymphoma, Grade 3B. Note the monotonous population of centroblasts (noncleaved cells) without admixed centrocytes (cleaved cells). **E** Follicular lymphoma, grade 3B with small centroblasts. Note the medium sized cells whose nuclei have a variable number of nucleoli, resembling Burkitt lymphoma cells.

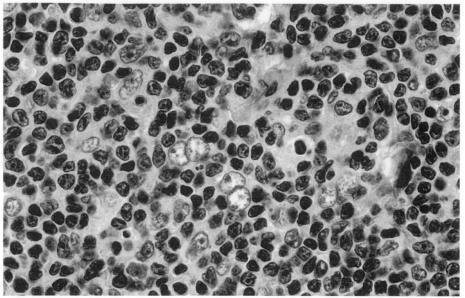

Fig. 6.77 Follicular lymphoma, illustrating follicular dendritic cells (FDC). Four FDC, arranged in the form of two pairs, are present in the centre of the field. The nuclei are round, but with flattening of adjacent nuclear membranes, and have bland, dispersed chromatin with one small, centrally located nucleolus. The cytoplasm is not seen in H&E or Giemsa-stained sections. Centroblasts, in contrast to FDC, have vesicular chromatin, and multiple distinct nucleoli that are usually located adjacent to the nuclear membranes.

Table 6.13
Follicular lymphoma: grading and variants.

Grading	Definition
Grade 1	0-5 centroblasts per hpf*
Grade 2	6-15 centroblasts per hpf*
Grade 3	>15 centroblasts per hpf*
3a	Centrocytes present
3b	Solid sheets of centroblasts
Reporting of pattern	**Proportion follicular**
Follicular	>75%
Follicular and diffuse	25-75% **
Focally follicular	<25% **
Follicular lymphoma: variants	
Diffuse follicle centre lymphoma	
Grade 1	0-5 centroblasts/hpf*
Grade 2	6-15 centroblasts/hpf*
Cutaneous follicle centre lymphoma	(see text for definition)

*hpf = high-power field of 0.159 mm2 (40X objective, 18 mm field of view ocular; count 10 hpf and divide by 10).
If using a 10 mm field of view ocular, count 8 hpf and divide by 10 or count 10 hpf and divide by 12 to get the number of centroblasts/0.159 mm2 hpf.
If using a 22 mm field of view ocular, count 7 hpf and divide by 10 or count 10 hpf and divide by 15 to get the number of centroblasts/0.159 mm2 hpf.

**give approximate % in report

with a 22 mm in diameter field of view gives a 0.237 mm2 hpf, which is 1.5 times as large as the 0.159 mm² hpf). This may result in a proportion of the cases being given a higher grade if oculars with a wider field of view are used. These differences can be eliminated by using a factor to compensate for different oculars. Thus, if using an ocular with a 20 mm field of view, the final count should be divided by 1.2 (or count 10 hpf and divide by 12 instead of 10); if using a 22 mm field of view ocular, the final count is divided by 1.5 to get a count equivalent to that in 10 hpf using an 18 mm field of view ocular. Note that the ocular magnification (e.g. 10x, 15x) does not affect the calculation.

In grading follicular lymphoma, care must be taken to distinguish between centroblasts and large centrocytes (large cleaved cells), counting only centroblasts. In addition, follicular dendritic cells (FDC) have nuclei that are similar in size to those of centroblasts; they have pale, greyish chromatin, small, central eosinophilic nucleoli, often double nuclei, with flattening of the adjacent nuclear membranes. Their cytoplasm is indistinct and not basophilic, in contrast to that of centroblasts, and forms long processes best seen on stains for CD21 or CD23.

Since both pattern and cytology vary among follicles, lymph nodes must be adequately sampled (all submitted for microscopy in most cases) and all sections carefully reviewed. Variation between grades in different areas should be noted (e.g. follicular lymphoma, predominantly grade 1 with focal areas of grade 3). Any area of diffuse large B-cell lymphoma in a follicular lymphoma indicates transformation to an aggressive phase and should be reported as a separate diagnosis, with an estimate of the proportion of each.

Examples:
1. The lymphoma is >75% follicular, and there are 45 centroblasts in 10 high-power fields.
Diagnosis: Follicular lymphoma, grade 1/3, predominantly follicular

2. The lymphoma is 50% follicular, and there are 100 centroblasts in 10 high-power fields; however, in one section, about 20 follicles show 20-30 centroblasts per hpf.

Diagnosis: Follicular lymphoma, grade 2/3, follicular and diffuse, with focal progression to follicular lymphoma, grade 3/3

3. The lymph node is over 75% follicular, and the follicles contain 120 centroblasts in 10 high-power fields, but there is a diffuse area in which there is a predominance of centroblasts, comprising about 25% of the examined area.
Diagnosis: Diffuse large B-cell lymphoma (25%) and follicular lymphoma, grade 2/3 (75%)

Immunophenotype

The tumour cells are usually SIg+ (IgM +/- IgD, IgG or rarely IgA) Bcl2+ CD10+ CD5- and CD43- and express B-cell associated antigens (CD19, CD20, CD22, CD79a). Occasional cases of grade 3 follicular lymphoma are CD43+ {723}. The tumour cells express the nuclear protein BCL6 {187, 1046}. Tight meshworks of CD21+ CD23+ FDC are present in follicular areas {1449}. CD10 expression is often stronger in the follicles than in interfollicular neoplastic cells {497, 307}. BCL2 protein is expressed in the majority of the cases, ranging from nearly 100% in grade 1 to 75% in grade 3 follicular lymphoma {721}. BCL2 protein is useful in distinguishing neoplastic from reactive follicles, but is not useful in distinguishing follicular from other types of low-grade B-cell lymphoma, most of which also express BCL2 protein. Cutaneous follicular lymphoma is frequently BCL2 negative.

Genetics

Antigen receptor genes
Immunoglobulin heavy and light chains are rearranged; variable region genes show extensive somatic mutations with intraclonal heterogeneity, consistent with a derivation from follicle centre cells {230, 990}.

Cytogenetic abnormalities and oncogenes
Virtually all cases of follicular lymphoma have cytogenetic abnormalities {1297}. The most common, t(14;18)(q32;q21), involving rearrangement of the *BCL2* gene, is present in 70-95% of the cases {1119, 542}. The t(14;18) is not associated with either a better or worse prognosis. Rare cases have a t(2;18)(p12;q21), which places the *BCL2* gene with the

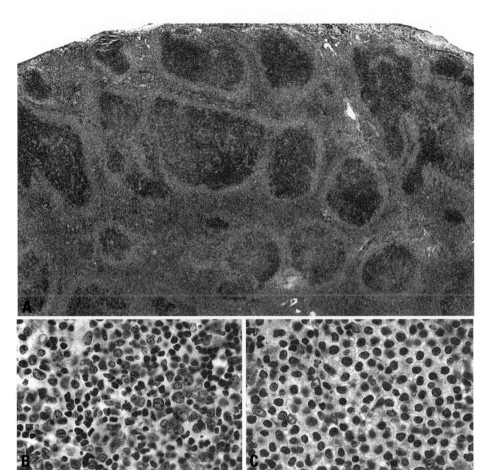

Fig. 6.78 Follicular lymphoma with marginal zone differentiation. **A** At the periphery of the follicles, there is a pale rim corresponding to marginal zone differentiation. **B** The centres of the follicles contain the typical mixture of centrocytes and centroblasts. **C** The cells at the periphery of the follicles are medium sized cells with slightly irregular nuclei and abundant lightly eosinophilic to pale staining cytoplasm, consistent with marginal zone or monocytoid B cells.

light chain gene on chromosome 2. The *BCL2* translocation appears to occur at an early stage of B-cell development, during immunoglobulin gene rearrangement. The BCL2 protein is expressed by resting and B and T cells, but not by normal germinal centre cells, cortical thymocytes {526}, or monocytoid B cells {721}. Transgenic mice expressing the *BCL2* gene develop massive follicular lymphoid hyperplasia, with persistence of a mature B cell population {848}. Overexpression of BCL2 protein confers a survival advantage on B cells in vitro, by preventing apoptosis under conditions of growth factor deprivation {959}. When a resting B cell that carries the *BCL2* translocation undergoes blast transformation in response to antigen, failure to switch off the *BCL2* gene may contribute to development of lymphoma.
In cases with t(14;18), it is the sole abnormality in only 10%; the remainder have

Table 6.14
Follicular lymphoma: genetic abnormalities.

	% positive (approximate)
Cytogenetic Abnormalities	100
t(14;18)(q32;q21)	80
+7	20
+18	20
3q27-28	15
6q23-26*	15
17p*	15
Oncogene abnormalities	
BCL2 rearranged	80
BCL6 rearranged	15
BCL6 5' mutations	40

*Associated with a worse prognosis {1297}

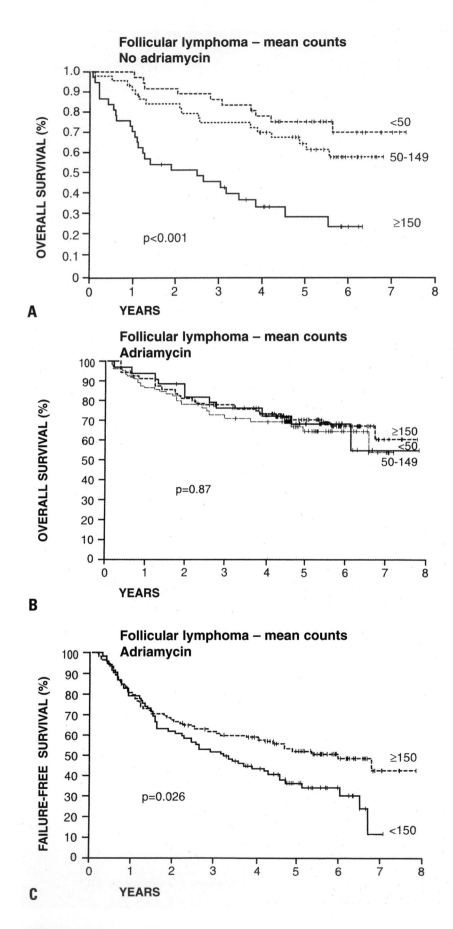

Fig 6.79 Survival curves for patients with follicular lymphoma, graded according to the proposed WHO scheme (Data from {1366}) **A** Overall survival of patients treated with regimens not containing adriamycin (palliative therapy): there is no difference in survival for patients with grade 1 vs grade 2 follicular lymphoma (0-50 and 51-150 centroblasts/10 hpf), while those with grade 3 (>150 centroblasts/10 hpf) had a significantly worse overall survival. **B** Overall survival of patients treated with adriamycin-containing regimens (curative intent): the 3 survival curves are identical, indicating that there is no survival benefit for patients with grade 1 and grade 2 FL treated with adriamycin, but that the adverse prognosis of grade 3 FL is eliminated by aggressive therapy. **C** Failure-free survival of patients treated with adriamycin: there is a suggestion of a plateau in the curve for grade 3 FL (>150 CB/10 hpf), suggesting the possibility of cure for some of these patients; in contrast, patients with grade 1 and grade 2 FL continue to experience relapses.

additional breaks (median of 6 in one recent study), most commonly involving chromosomes 1, 2, 4, 5, 13, and 17, or additions of X, 7, 12, or 18 {1297}. The 17p abnormalities may reflect alterations in the *TP53* gene at 17p13, which have been shown to be associated with transformation in follicular lymphoma {1141}. Abnormalities at 6q23-36 are found in 10-40% of B-cell lymphomas of all types, and are the most common second abnormality in cases with the t(14;18). Three distinct deletions have been described, at 6q21, 6q23, and 6q25-27, suggesting the presence of 3 distinct tumour suppressor genes {964}. Deletions and other alterations of chromosome 9p, involving the p15 and p16 gene loci have been reported in cases of follicular lymphoma that transform to DLBCL {1043, 339}. Abnormalities of 3q27 and/or *BCL6* rearrangement are found in about 15% of follicular lymphomas, while 5' mutations of the *BCL6* gene are found in approximately 40% {1020}.

Postulated cell of origin
Germinal centre B cells.

Prognosis and predictive factors
One difficulty in interpreting clinical studies of follicular lymphoma is the fact that many did not include immunologic analysis and preceded recognition of mantle cell lymphoma and marginal zone B-cell lymphomas. Some cases of these lymphomas are likely to have been included in some earlier studies of follicular lym-

phoma, and may have influenced the survival data.

Histological grade correlates with prognosis in follicular lymphoma, with grades 1 and 2 being indolent and not usually curable, and grade 3 being more aggressive and having a potential for cure with aggressive therapy, similar to diffuse large B-cell lymphoma. The curability of grade 2 follicular lymphoma remains a subject of debate, with most studies showing decreased survival for grade 2 cases, and some showing a potential for cure in grade 2 but not grade 1 cases {30, 786, 602, 441}. The vast majority of published studies show a significantly more aggressive clinical course for grade 3 cases {30, 818, 852, 78}. These cases are typically treated with combination chemotherapy as for diffuse large B-cell lymphoma; their prognosis appears to be slightly better than that for DLBCL, but with an increased likelihood of relapse {78, 28, 1378, 630, 442}. In the recent study of the REAL classification, grade 3 follicular lymphoma had a significantly worse overall survival when treated with non-adriamycin-containing regimens; the survival in the group treated with adriamycin was identical to that of grade 1 and grade 2 cases {1366}.

Many studies have indicated {1090, 747, 3, 1360} that the presence of even very large diffuse areas in a follicular lymphoma of grade 1 or 2 (small cleaved or mixed small and large cell) does not significantly alter the prognosis; therefore, if any definite follicular areas are seen in a lymphoma of follicle centre type, the tumour is classified as follicular lymphoma. However, some studies have suggested that the degree of nodularity does have an impact on survival {352, 547}. For this reason, we suggest that the proportion of follicular and diffuse components be estimated in the pathology report. In grade 3 follicular lymphoma (follicular large cell), the presence of diffuse areas is more common, and most {78, 1360} but not all {28, 1351} studies show that this finding is associated with a worse outcome. In a recent study, cases with monocytoid B-cell differentiation had a worse prognosis than other cases, but this result requires confirmation {933}.

The presence of more than 6 chromosomal breaks was associated with a poor outcome in one study; in addition, breaks at 6q23-26 or 17p conferred a worse prognosis and a shorter time to transformation {1297, 759}.

The prognosis of paediatric patients appears to be good, with the majority of reported cases disease free at the time of last follow-up {384, 1042}. Clinical factors included in the International Prognostic Index, such as LDH and performance status, are as important as grade in predicting outcome in follicular lymphoma {8, 7}.

In 25-35% of patients with follicular lymphoma, transformation or "progression" to a large B-cell lymphoma, usually diffuse, occurs {416, 534}. This occurrence is usually associated with a rapidly progressive clinical course and death from tumour that is refractory to treatment {416, 49}.

Variants

Cutaneous follicle centre lymphoma
Many cases of primary cutaneous B-cell lymphoma have a partially follicular pattern and/or are composed of cells that resemble centrocytes (often large) and centroblasts {1387}. These tumours are often *BCL2* negative, and their relationship to nodal FL is not known. They occur on the head and trunk, and tend to remain localised to the skin, where they are amenable to local therapy, unlike primary nodal FL {1104}.

Diffuse follicle centre lymphoma
Rare lymphomas appear to be composed of centrocytes and centroblasts, similar to follicular lymphoma, but do not form follicles and therefore cannot be called follicular lymphoma. The term diffuse follicle centre lymphoma (FCL) is used for these cases. Diffuse FCL is defined as a lymphoma composed of cells resembling centrocytes, with a minor component of centroblasts, and an entirely diffuse pattern; both the small and large cells must have the immunophenotype of follicle centre cells (pan-B antigen expression, typically SIg+ CD10+ BCL2+ BCL6+).

Synonym
Kiel: Diffuse centroblastic/centrocytic lymphoma (CB/CC).

These cases comprise about 40% of diffuse "mixed" lymphomas in the Rappaport classification and the Working Formulation {393, 854}, and only 4% of CB/CC lymphomas in the Kiel classification {747}. In some cases it is likely that focal follicular areas are present, and that a sampling problem results in a purely diffuse pattern. Diffuse follicle centre lymphoma should be graded as for follicular lymphoma, grades 1 and 2. If centroblasts predominate, or if the small cells are T cells, the tumour is classified as diffuse large B-cell lymphoma. Thus, a diagnosis of diffuse follicle centre lymphoma can rarely be made without immunophenotyping.

Studies using the Kiel classification {142} suggest that purely diffuse cases of centroblastic/centrocytic lymphoma have a significantly worse prognosis than cases with a follicular or follicular and diffuse pattern.

Mantle cell lymphoma

S.H. Swerdlow
F. Berger
P.I. Isaacson
H.K. Müller-Hermelink

B.N. Nathwani
M.A. Piris
N.L. Harris

Definition
Mantle cell lymphoma (MCL) is a B-cell neoplasm composed of monomorphous small to medium-sized lymphoid cells with irregular nuclei, which morphologically most closely resemble centrocytes/ cleaved follicular centre cells (FCC) but which often have at least slightly less irregular nuclear contours {751, 1300, 1252, 731, 70, 174}. Neoplastic transformed cells (centro-blasts / noncleaved FCC), paraimmunoblasts and pseudofollicles / proliferation centres are absent.

ICD-O code   9673/3

Synonyms
Rappaport: intermediately or poorly differentiated lymphocytic lymphoma, diffuse or nodular
Kiel: centrocytic (mantle cell) lymphoma
Working formulation: malignant lymphoma, diffuse, small cleaved cell type (rarely follicular, small cleaved or diffuse, mixed small and large cell or large cell type).

Epidemiology
MCL comprises approximately 3-10% of non-Hodgkin lymphomas {8}. It occurs in middle aged to older individuals with a median age of about 60 and a variably marked male predominance (at least about 2:1) {1252, 731, 8, 42, 46, 1338, 122}.

Sites of involvement
Lymph nodes are the most commonly

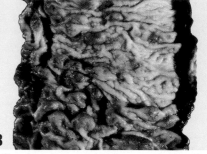
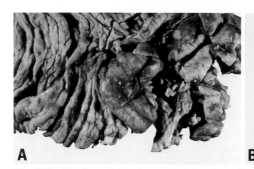

Fig. 6.80 Mantle cell lymphoma involving the colon (lymphomatous polyposis), gross photograph. **A** Overview showing one large and multiple small polypoid mucosal lesions. **B** Closeup showing tiny polypoid mucosal lesions.

involved site; the spleen and bone marrow (with or without blood involvement) are other important sites of disease {1252, 42, 122, 956}. The most commonly involved other extranodal sites are the gastrointestinal tract (reported in up to almost 30% of patients) and Waldeyer's ring. Most cases of multiple lymphomatous polyposis (multiple gastrointestinal tract lesions demonstrating lymphoma) represent mantle cell lymphoma {1125, 702, 960}.

Macroscopy
Multiple lymphomatous polyposis associated with mantle cell lymphoma demonstrates multiple variably sized polyps in any part of the gastrointestinal tract {1125, 702, 960}.

Clinical features
Most patients present with stage III or IV disease with lymphadenopathy, hepato-

splenomegaly, frequently with massive splenomegaly and marrow involvement (>50%) {174, 8, 46, 1338, 122, 956}. Peripheral blood involvement is found in at least about 25% of cases. Some patients have marked lymphocytosis mimicking prolymphocytic leukaemia {42, 122, 956}. A minority of patients present with extranodal disease, often of the gastrointestinal tract or involving Waldeyer's ring.

Morphology
MCL demonstrates architectural destruction by a monomorphic lymphoid proliferation with a vaguely nodular, diffuse, or mantle zone growth pattern {751, 1300, 1252, 731, 70}. Rarely a true follicular growth pattern is seen. Most cases are composed of small to medium sized lymphoid cells with slightly to markedly irregular nuclear contours, most closely resembling centrocytes. The nuclei have

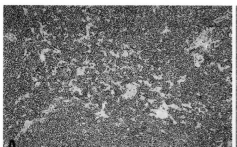
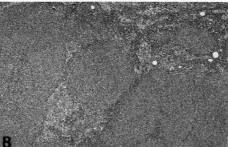
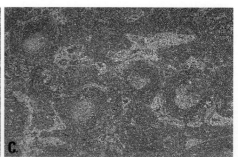

Fig. 6.81 Mantle cell lymphoma, lymph nodes. **A** There is diffuse architectural effacement and typical pale hyalinised vessels. **B** In addition to diffuse areas, note the prominent vague neoplastic nodules. **C** A mantle zone growth pattern is seen in this lymph node with an intact architecture.

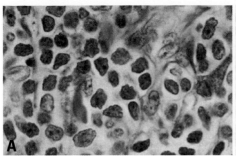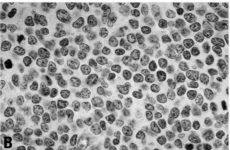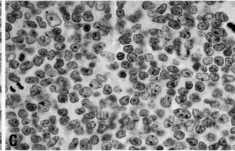

Fig. 6.82 Mantle cell lymphoma. **A** In this case, the cells closely resemble centrocytes / cleaved follicle centre cells even though the neoplastic cells are not of follicle centre origin. There is also a typical hyalinized vessel present (PAS stain). **B** Blastoid mantle cell lymphoma: In this classic case, the tumour cells resemble lymphoblasts. **C** This blastoid mantle cell lymphoma is pleomorphic and has prominent nucleoli.

moderately dispersed chromatin but inconspicuous nucleoli. Neoplastic transformed cells resembling centroblasts, immunoblasts or paraimmunoblasts and pseudofollicles are absent. Hyalinized small vessels are commonly seen. Many cases have scattered single epithelioid histiocytes which in occasional cases can give a "starry sky" appearance. Plasma cells may be present but are non-neoplastic. Histological transformation to typical large cell lymphoma does not occur; however, loss of a mantle zone growth pattern, an increase in nuclear size, pleomorphism and chromatin dispersal, and an increase in mitotic activity may be seen in some cases at relapse {1252, 731, 42, 956}. Some of the latter cases will fulfil the criteria for a blastoid mantle cell lymphoma.

Several types of morphologic variants are recognised (Table 6.15); however, only the two blastoid variants are considered to be of potential clinical significance (see grading of mantle cell lymphoma below) {731, 1446, 1254, 988, 987, 1444}.

Grading
Although mantle cell lymphoma is not formally graded for clinical purposes at present, if blastoid features are present, they should be noted in the diagnosis.

Immunophenotype
The neoplastic cells are monoclonal B-cells with relatively intense surface IgM ± IgD {1252, 1300, 174, 1446}. They are typically CD5 positive, usually CD10 negative, bcl-6 negative, CD23 negative to weakly positive, FMC-7 positive and usually CD43 positive {1252, 1446, 226, 1444, 1449, 497, 315, 700, 1317}. CD5 negative cases do exist and may be more indolent {635}. Immunohistological

stains for CD21 or CD35 demonstrate loose meshworks of follicular dendritic cells. All cases are bcl-2 protein positive and virtually all express cyclin D1, including the rare cases that are CD5 negative {1431, 1450, 1253, 268}. Cases with gastrointestinal tract involvement express the α4β7 homing receptor {424}.

Genetics
Antigen receptor genes
Immunoglobulin heavy and light chain genes are rearranged. Variable region genes are unmutated in the majority of the cases, consistent with a pre-germinal centre B cell, but a small proportion of the cases show somatic mutation suggesting a follicular/post-follicular genotype {323, 550, 1047}.

Cytogenetic abnormalities and oncogenes
Southern blot analysis or conventional cytogenetics demonstrate 70-75% of

cases with the t(11;14)(q13;q32) translocation between the immunoglobulin heavy chain and the *CYCLIN D1 (CCND1, PRAD1, BCL-1)* genes {1111, 1390, 1389, 1334}. Virtually all cases show this rearrangement using fluorescence in situ hybridisation {763, 1318}. Almost all cases also show overexpression of CYCLIN D1 mRNA {269}. Many cases also have point mutations and/or deletion of the *ATM* (ataxia telangiectasia mutated) gene {1238, 1152}. A minority of cases especially of blastoid type and other more aggressive cases show additional mutations, deletion or other abnormalities in negative cell cycle regulatory proteins such as TP53, p16, and p18 {174, 987, 1444, 80, 454, 791, 1392, 1391}. There are also other relatively frequent cytogenetic abnormalities, some of which are also seen in chronic lymphocytic leukaemia. These include 13q14 deletion, total or partial trisomy +12,17p deletion, and many others {80, 257}. Some are

Table 6.15
Morphologic variants of mantle cell lymphoma.

Blastoid variants
– Usual: Cells resemble lymphoblasts with dispersed chromatin and a high mitotic rate (>10/10 hpf and usually at least 20-30/10hpf).
– Pleomorphic: Heterogeneous cells with large cleaved to oval nuclei and pale cytoplasm on Giemsa (or MGP) stain. Nucleoli may be prominent.
Other variants
– Small round lymphocytes with more clumped chromatin, either admixed or predominant, mimicking small lymphocytic lymphoma.
– Prominent foci of cells with abundant pale cytoplasm resembling marginal zone or monocytoid B-cells and mimicking a marginal zone B-cell lymphoma; sometimes these paler foci may also resemble proliferation centres of a small lymphocytic lymphoma.

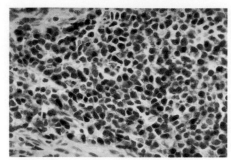

Fig. 6.83 The cyclin D1 immunostain shows nuclear positivity.

more often associated with blastoid mantle cell lymphoma {98}. The pleomorphic blastoid variant has a high incidence of tetraploidy {988, 987}. *BCL2* and *C-MYC* rearrangements are absent.

Postulated cell of origin
Peripheral B-cell of inner mantle zone (precise cell type uncertain).

Prognosis and predictive factors
Mantle cell lymphoma has a median survival of 3-5 years, but the vast majority of patients cannot be cured {1446, 42, 1338, 122, 956, 386}. More successful therapeutic regimens have been reported {652, 651}. The most consistently reported adverse histopathological prognostic parameter is a high mitotic rate although the definition varies (>10-37.5/15 hpf) {1252, 42, 122}. Some report the blastoid variant to have a more aggressive course and whether a mantle

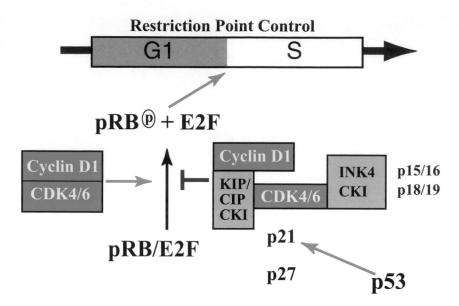

Fig. 6.84 Cell cycle regulatory proteins involved in restriction point control between G1 and S phase. The cyclin D1/cyclin dependent kinase (CDK) 4/6 complex promotes phosphorylation of the retinoblastoma protein (pRB). This leads to release of the E2F transcription factors which then leads to progression of the cell cycle into the S phase. There are two families of negative cell cycle regulatory proteins that inhibit the cyclin D1/cdk4/6 activity – the INK4 family that includes p15/p16 and p18/p19 and the KIP/CIP family that includes p21 and p27. P53 protein leads to increased expression of p21. Although not illustrated, it has been suggested that p27 in mantle cell lymphomas is bound by the increased amounts of cyclin D1 so that there is loss of its inhibitory effect on cyclin E and then further phosphorylation of pRB.

zone pattern is a good prognostic indicator is controversial {731, 122, 956, 807}. Peripheral blood, but not marrow involvement, is another agreed upon adverse prognostic indicator {1252, 122, 1048}. Other adverse prognostic indicators that have been reported include tri-

somy 12, karyotypic complexity, some other cytogenetic abnormalities, p53 mutation/overexpression and a variety of clinical parameters {174, 1338, 122, 80, 454, 791, 257}.

Diffuse large B-cell lymphoma

K.C. Gatter
R.A. Warnke

Definition
Diffuse large B-cell lymphoma (DLBCL) is a diffuse proliferation of large neoplastic B lymphoid cells with nuclear size equal to or exceeding normal macrophage nuclei or more than twice the size of a normal lymphocyte. The cytologic features differ among the variants described below.

ICD-O code
9680/3

Synonyms
Rappaport: diffuse histiocytic, diffuse mixed lymphocytic and histiocytic
Kiel: centroblastic, B-immunoblastic, B-large cell anaplastic
Lukes-Collins: large cleaved follicular centre cell (FCC), large noncleaved FCC, B-immunoblastic
Working Formulation: diffuse large cell, large cell immunoblastic, diffuse mixed small and large cell
REAL: diffuse large B-cell lymphoma

Epidemiology
Diffuse large B-cell lymphomas (DLBCL) constitute 30-40% of adult non-Hodgkin lymphomas in western countries. In developing countries they constitute an even higher proportion of lymphomas. The median age is in the 7th decade, but the range is broad, and these tumours may be seen in children {8, 46}. They are slightly more common in males than females. Over the past few decades the incidence has been increasing, independent of HIV as a risk factor.

Sites of involvement
Patients may present with nodal or extranodal disease. Up to 40% are at least initially confined to extranodal sites {496}. The most common extranodal site is the gastrointestinal tract (stomach or ileocoecal region) but virtually any extranodal location may be a primary site including the skin, central nervous system (CNS), bone, testis, soft tissue, salivary gland, female genital tract, lung, kidney, liver, Waldeyer's ring, and spleen. Primary presentation with bone marrow

and/or peripheral blood involvement is rare. Certain morphologic variants are more prevalent at particular extranodal sites. For example, DLBCL primary in bone often exhibit multilobated nuclei {1324, 1033}.

Clinical features
Patients typically present with a rapidly enlarging, often symptomatic mass at a single nodal or extranodal site. However, with staging evaluation, many patients have disseminated disease {8, 46}.

Aetiology
The cause or causes of diffuse large B-cell lymphoma remain unknown. They usually arise *de novo* (referred to as primary) but can represent progression / transformation (referred to as secondary) of a less aggressive lymphoma, e.g. chronic lymphocytic leukaemia / small lymphocytic lymphoma (CLL/SLL), follicular lymphoma, marginal zone B-cell lymphoma or nodular lymphocyte predominant Hodgkin lymphoma (NLPHL). Underlying immunodeficiency is a significant risk factor (see chapter 9). DLBCL in the setting of immunodeficiency are more often Epstein-Barr virus (EBV)-positive than sporadic DLBCL.

Macroscopy
In lymph nodes DLBCL usually present with homogeneous fish-flesh replacement of most if not all of the structure. Occasionally the involvement is only partial. In all cases the appearance of the lesion can be modified by haemorrhage or necrosis. In extranodal sites, DLBCL usually form a tumour mass with or without fibrosis.

Morphology
Diffuse large B-cell lymphoma typically replaces the normal architecture of the underlying lymph node or extranodal tissue in a diffuse pattern. Lymph node involvement may be complete, partial, interfollicular, or, less commonly, sinusoidal. The perinodal soft tissue is often infiltrated; broad or fine bands of sclero-

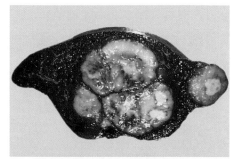
Fig. 6.85 Spleen involved by diffuse large B-cell lymphoma contains large tumor nodules.

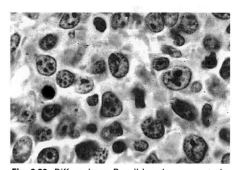
Fig. 6.86 Diffuse large B-cell lymphoma, centroblastic variant.

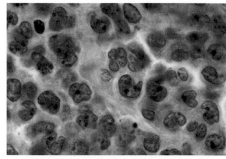
Fig. 6.87 Diffuse large B-cell lymphoma, centroblastic variant. In this example, the tumor cells have a polymorphic and polylobated appearance.

sis may be observed. DLBCL are composed of large transformed lymphoid cells. Cytologically, they are diverse and can be divided into morphologic variants. However, distinction among these variants has generally met with poor intraobserver and interobserver reproducibility {496}. Immunophenotypic and genotypic parameters have not helped to delineate distinctive morphologic subtypes, with rare exceptions. Thus, pathologists have the choice to use only the term diffuse large B-cell lymphoma or to use one of the specific morphologic variants listed below.

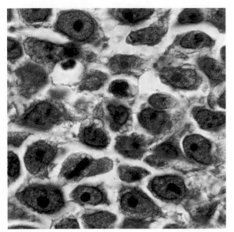

Most cases will conform to one of the morphologic variants, with centroblastic being the most common. Unusual variants have been described with myxoid stroma, a fibrillary matrix, pseudorosettes, spindly cells, signet ring cells, cytoplasmic granules, microvillous projections, and intercellular junctions. Cases of lymphomatoid granulomatosis with sheeting out of malignant cells represent progression to a variant of DLBCL (see below). Prominence of medium-sized cells may require special studies to exclude extra-medullary leukaemias and Burkitt lymphoma variants.

Morphologic variants
Centroblastic
This variant is composed of medium-sized to large lymphoid cells with oval to round, vesicular nuclei with fine chromatin and 2-4 membrane bound nucleoli. The cytoplasm is generally scanty and amphophilic to basophilic. This variant may have a monomorphic or polymorphic appearance. It includes both the monomorphic and polymorphic variants of centroblastic lymphoma, as defined in the Kiel classification {346, 749}. In some cases the cells may be multilobated. In still other cases, centroblast-like cells may be admixed with multilobated cells and up to 90% immunoblasts, producing a markedly polymorphous cellular infiltrate.

Immunoblastic
The majority of the cells (>90%) in this variant are immunoblasts with a single centrally located nucleolus and an appreciable amount of basophilic cytoplasm. Immunoblasts with plasmacytoid differentiation may also be present. Centroblasts must represent <10% of the population. Clinical and/or immunophenotypic findings may be essential in differentiating this variant from extramedullary involvement by a plasmablastic variant of plasma cell myeloma.

T-cell/histiocyte rich
In this variant the majority of cells are non-neoplastic T-cells with or without histiocytes and fewer than 10% large neoplastic B-cells are present. The histiocytes may or may not be epithelioid in appearance. The large cells may resemble L&H cells, centroblasts, immunoblasts, or Reed-Sternberg cells {223, 278}. Small B-cells are rare to infrequent. Areas with increased numbers of small B-cells may raise the possibility of asso-

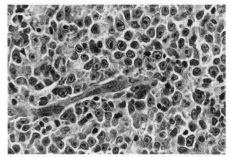

ciated NLPHL, especially if a vaguely nodular growth pattern is present. The growth pattern is predominantly diffuse and a fine reticular fibrosis is often present. Immunophenotypic studies may be essential in the differential diagnosis with classical Hodgkin lymphoma. Many cases formerly designated as diffuse mixed lymphoma in the working formuation represent the T-cell/histiocyte-rich variant of DLBCL {1084}.

Anaplastic
This variant of DLBCL is characterised by very large round, oval, or polygonal cells with bizarre pleomorphic nuclei which may resemble Reed-Sternberg cells. The cells may grow in a cohesive pattern mimicking carcinoma and may show a sinusoidal pattern of growth {491}. These cases are biologically and clinically unrelated to anaplastic large cell lymphoma of cytotoxic T-cell derivation (see chapter 7).

Immunophenotype
Diffuse large B-cell lymphomas express various pan-B markers such as CD19, CD20, CD22, and CD79a, but may lack one or more of these. Surface and/or cytoplasmic immunoglobulin (IgM> IgG

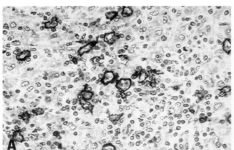
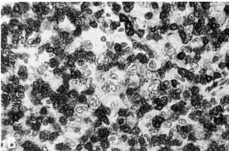
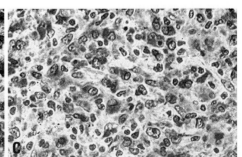

>IgA) can be demonstrated in 50-75%. Cytoplasmic immunoglobulin is often seen in cases exhibiting plasmacytic differentiation {1232, 308}. While the vast majority of anaplastic large B-cell lymphomas express CD30, non-anaplastic cases may occasionally stain for CD30 {1044}. Some cases express CD5 (10%) or CD10 (25-50%). CD5+ DLBCL are negative for cyclin D1 expression distinguishing them from blastoid variants of mantle cell lymphoma. CD5+ DLBCL may arise *de novo* rather than as a manifestation of progression of SLL/CLL {830}. BCL2 is positive in approximately 30-50% of cases. Nuclear expression of BCL6 is found in a very high proportion of cases. P53 protein expression, usually associated with *TP53* mutations, is found in a minority of cases. Expression of plasma cell-associated markers such as syndecan (CD138) is seen in a minority of cases. The proliferative fraction as detected by Ki-67 staining is usually high (>40%) and may be greater than 90% in some cases {878}.

Genetics

Most cases have rearranged immunoglobulin heavy and light chain genes and show somatic mutations in the variable regions. Translocation of the *BCL2* gene, i.e. t(14;18), a hallmark of follicular lymphoma, occurs in 20-30% of cases {1370, 773}. Up to 30% of cases show abnormalities of the 3q27 region involving the candidate protooncogene *BCL6*. *MYC* rearrangement is uncommon {1437}. Many cases exhibit complex cytogenetic abnormalities. Infection of the neoplastic cells by EBV may be seen and is more common in cases associated with underlying immunodeficiency. A recent study employing DNA microarrays identified two major molecular categories with gene expression patterns suggestive of different stages of B-cell develop-

Table 6.16
Prognostic factors and risk score comprising the International Prognostic Index.

Prognostic factors	Risk score	
Age (> 60 yrs)	Low	0, 1
LDH (> nl)	Low, Int	2
Performance status (2-4)	High, Int	3
Stage (III, IV)	High	4, 5
Extranodal (> 1 site)		

ment. One type had an expression profile characteristic of germinal centre B-cells, whereas the other type had a profile similar to that of *in vitro* activated peripheral blood B-cells {19}.

Postulated cell of origin

Peripheral B-cells of either germinal centre or post germinal centre origin.

Prognosis and predictive factors

DLBCL are aggressive but potentially curable with multiagent chemotherapy. The International Prognostic Index based on clinical parameters is strongly predictive of outcome {46}. A high proliferative rate has been associated with worse survival in some series {878} while BCL2 expression has been associated with an adverse disease free survival {513, 522, 422, 1398}. P53 overexpression in a majority of the malignant cells is another adverse prognostic indicator {1398}. Although several studies have reported a slightly worse prognosis for immunoblastic over centroblastic variants {142, 346}, other studies have failed to confirm this {858, 1133}. In some studies *BCL6* translocation has been reported to be associated with a better prognosis {963}. Patients with germinal centre B-like DLBCL had a significantly better overall survival than those whose lymphomas were activated B-like {19}.

Other rare variants / subtypes with distinctive immunophenotypic features

Plasmablastic

This rare variant of DLBCL typically presents in the oral cavity in the setting of HIV infection. The cells in approximately 60%

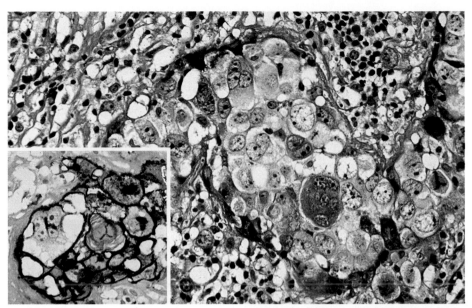

Fig. 6.91 Diffuse large B-cell lymphoma, anaplastic variant. Large lymphoma cells with pleomorphic nuclei infiltrate the sinus. The inset shows strong membranous and paranuclear labeling of the lymphoma cells for CD20.

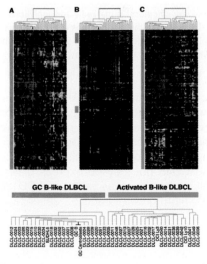

Fig. 6.92 Two major patterns of gene expression can be identified in diffuse large B-cell lymphomas by gene array technology. One group displays a germinal centre B-cell signature, whereas a second group displays an activated B-cell signature. The analysis is based on the expression of approximately 12,000 genes. Reproduced from Alizadeh et al. {19}.

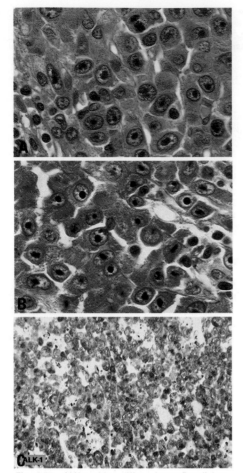

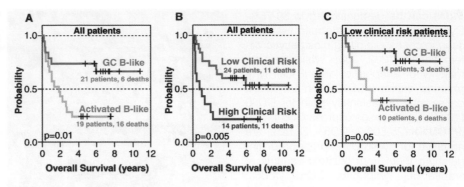

Fig. 6.93 Clinically distinct subgroups of DLBCL were defined by gene expression profiling. Kaplan-Meier plots are grouped according to the International Prognostic Index (IPI Score). Low risk and high risk patients are plotted separately. Reproduced from Alizadeh et al. {1155}.

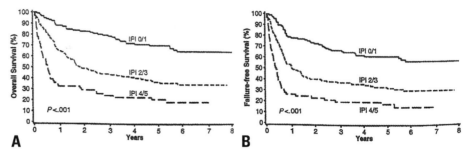

Fig. 6.94 Diffuse large B-cell lymphoma. Overall survival and failure-free survival according to the International Prognostic Index (IPI Score) in the study conducted by the Non-Hodgkin's Lymphoma Classification Project {1}.

Fig. 6.95 ALK-positive diffuse large B-cell lymphoma. This rare variant of diffuse large B-cell lymphoma has a plasmablastic appearance and expresses full length ALK-protein. **A** In an H&E stain, the cytoplasm is markedly eosinophilic. **B** In a Giemsa stain, the cytoplasm is more basophilic. Cells have prominent central nucleoli. **C** Strong cytoplasmic staining for ALK may be seen.

of cases contain EBV. Although these lymphomas are indistinguishable from some examples of immunoblastic lymphoma on morphologic grounds, few if any of the lymphoma cells stain for CD20 and CD45 but they do express plasma cell markers such as vs38c and CD138. The high growth fraction, absence of mature monoclonal plasma cells, and the characteristic clinical features help to distinguish this variant from plasma cell myeloma {149, 325, 1052, 279}.

Diffuse large B-cell lymphoma with expression of full-length ALK

This lymphoma is composed of monomorphic large immunoblast-like cells, with round pale nuclei containing large central nucleoli and an abundant amphophilic cytoplasm (basophilic with the Giemsa stain) with sometimes plasmablastic differentiation {283}. Some Reed-Sternberg-like cells are often seen. Lymph nodes are massively infiltrated with invasion of the sinuses. Tumour cells lack CD30 but express CD45 (weakly), EMA (strongly), as well as VS38 (endoplasmic reticulum-associated marker). They contain intracytoplasmic IgA with light chain restriction. They lack other B or T associated antigens with the exception of CD4 and CD57. Antibodies detecting the ALK protein show a granular cytoplasmic and dot-like positivity in the Golgi area. The t(2;5) and the resultant *NPM-ALK* fusion gene cannot be demonstrated. The mechanism of upregulation of the ALK kinase is unknown. This type of lymphoma seems to occur more frequently in adults and in males. The disease follows an aggressive course.

Mediastinal (thymic) large B-cell lymphoma

P.M. Banks
R.A. Warnke

Definition

Mediastinal (thymic) large B-cell lymphoma (Med-DLBCL) is a subtype of DLBCL arising in the mediastinum of putative thymic B-cell origin with distinctive clinical, immunophenotypic and genotypic features {888, 1026, 660, 567, 934, 266}.

ICD-O code   9679/3

Synonyms

Large-cell lymphoma of the mediastinum
Primary mediastinal clear-cell lymphoma of B-cell type
Mediastinal diffuse large-cell lymphoma with sclerosis
REAL: Primary mediastinal (thymic) large B-cell lymphoma

Epidemiology

Most patients are in their third to fifth decade with a female predominance {1026, 739, 189}

Clinical features

Patients present with localised disease and signs and symptoms relating to large anterior mediastinal masses, sometimes with impending superior vena cava syndrome. When disseminated, other extranodal sites are often involved, such as kidney, adrenal, liver, skin and brain {660, 739, 189, 111}.

Aetiology

No epidemiologic clustering or evidence of risk factors for the development of this type of lymphoma has been identified. EBV is not present {189}.

Morphology

There is a massive diffuse proliferation associated with variably dense compartmentalising fibrosis. The identification of thymic remnants may be facilitated by immunohistochemical staining. These remnant clusters may be organised in lobules sometimes mimicking a carcinoma. The neoplastic cells vary in size and nuclear shape, both within and among cases. However, in most cases, the cells

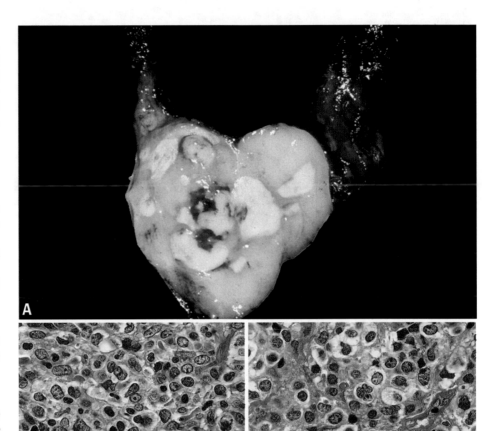

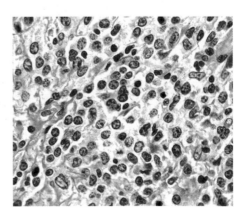

Fig. 6.96 Mediastinal large B-cell lymphoma. **A** Cut surface showing fleshy tumor with necrosis. **B** Sheets of large cells with abundant pale cytoplasm, separated by collageneous fibrosis. **C** Nuclei are round (centroblast-like) or sometimes multilobated.

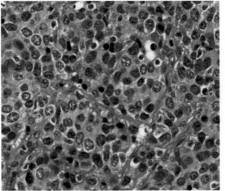

Fig. 6.97 Mediastinal (thymic) large B-cell lymphoma. This example has centroblastic cells with abundant cytoplasm. The lymphoma cells are compartmentalised into groups by fine bands of sclerosis.

Fig. 6.98 Mediastinal large B-cell lymphoma. Typical histology of DLBCL thymic.

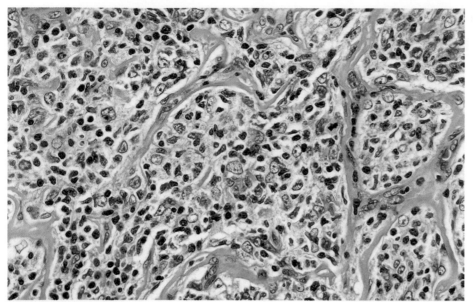

Fig. 6.99 Mediastinal large B-cell lymphoma. Classic clear-cell appearance with associated delicate interstitial fibrosis.

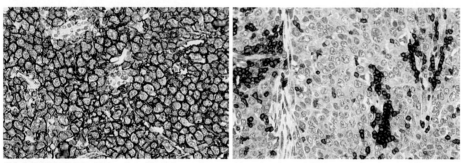

Fig. 6.100 Mediastinal large B-cell lymphoma. Immunohistochemistry. **A** All large cells express CD20 on the membrane. **B** Nests of CD3 positive lymphocytes are present with a perivascular distribution.

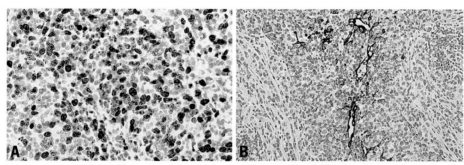

Fig. 6.101 Mediastinal large B-cell lymphoma. Immunohistochemistry. **A** More than 60% of the large cells express nuclear KI-67. **B** Thymic remnants infiltrated by tumour cells, the epithelial component is positive for cytokeratin.

have abundant pale cytoplasm. Small numbers of interspersed benign lymphocytes and eosinophils may raise suspicion of Hodgkin lymphoma (HL) {1026, 1012} and an association with nodular sclerosis HL (so-called "composite lymphoma") has been seen in rare cases {591, 1123a}. Because of its mediastinal location, biopsy samples of this tumour are often small and obscured by profuse sclerosis with associated cellular crush artifact.

Immunophenotype

Mediastinal (thymic) large-cell lymphomas are of B-cell phenotype, expressing markers such as CD19 and CD20; however, both immunoglobulin (Ig) and HLA class I and II molecules are frequently incompletely expressed or absent {624, 887}. CD10 and CD5 are also absent. Expression of CD30 is often present but is weak. The CD30-staining may be focal or extensive {521}. Tumour cells express leukocyte common antigen CD45, in contrast to the cells of classical Hodgkin lymphoma which are typically negative.

Genetics

Immunoglobulin gene rearrangements are demonstrable in these tumours, even when immunoglobulin is not phenotypically expressed {624, 887, 889}. The hyperdiploid karyotypes, often with gains in chromosome 9p and amplification of the *REL* gene, support the concept that this subtype of DLBCL is distinct from those arising in other sites {604}. Recently, overexpression of the *MAL* gene has been identified in a high proportion of cases {242}. The cells lack *BCL2*, *BCL6* and *MYC* rearrangements {1312}.

Postulated cell of origin

Thymic B-cell {567, 604, 266}.

Prognosis and predictive factors

Response to intensive chemotherapy, with or without radiotherapy, is usually good; however, chances for long-term remission correlate strongly with the initial stage of disease. Those patients with disease extending into adjacent thoracic viscera have a poorer prognosis than those patients with disease confined to the mediastinum. Spread to infradiaphragmatic organs predicts an unfavourable outcome {1026, 660, 189}. Variations in microscopic appearance do not predict differences in survival {1012}.

Intravascular large B-cell lymphoma

K.C. Gatter
R.A. Warnke

Definition
Intravascular large B-cell lymphoma is a rare subtype of extranodal DLBCL characterised by the presence of lymphoma cells only in the lumina of small vessels, particularly capillaries.

ICD-O code   9680/3

Synonyms
Angioendotheliomatosis proliferans systemisata; malignant angioendotheliomatosis; intravascular lymphomatosis.
Kiel: angio-endotheliotropic (intravascular) lymphoma
Lukes-Collins: angiotropic large cell lymphoma
REAL: diffuse large B-cell lymphoma.

Epidemiology
Intravascular large B-cell lymphomas occur in adults. Based on the small number of cases reported in the literature, no distinctive epidemiological features have been identified.

Sites of involvement
This lymphoma is usually widely disseminated in extranodal sites at presentation (CNS, skin, lung, kidneys, adrenals). Intravascular involvement may also be seen in the marrow.

Clinical features
Symptoms are highly variable since most result from occlusion of small vessels by tumour cells in a variety of organs. Intravascular large B-cell lymphoma most commonly presents with skin lesions (skin plaques and nodules) or neurological symptoms (dementia, focal symptoms). About 9% of patients present with "B symptoms". Multiple organs may be involved and a variety of clinical presentations have been described. These include nephrotic syndrome, pyrexia and hypertension, breathlessness and haematologic abnormalities (autoimmune haemolytic anaemia, leukopenia, pancytopenia and disseminated intravascular coagulation).

Pathophysiology
The intravascular growth pattern has been hypothesised to be secondary to a defect in homing receptors on the neoplastic cells {379}. Some evidence in favour of this comes from a recent study showing a lack of CD29 (beta1 integrin) and CD54 (ICAM-1) adhesion molecules in 6 of 6 cases of intravascular large B-cell lymphoma {1050}.

Macroscopy
The gross features often only appreciated at post mortem are mostly those of haemorrhage, thrombosis and necrosis in a wide range of tissues. Actual

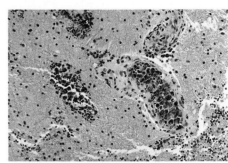

Fig. 6.102 Intravascular large B-cell lymphoma. The large lymphoma cells fill the vessels in this brain biopsy.

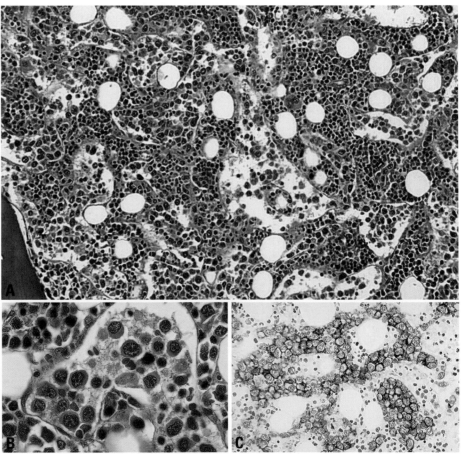

Fig. 6.103 Intravascular large B cell lymphoma. Bone marrow biopsy. **A** Active haematopoiesis between distended sinuses containing large lymphomatous cells. **B** The tumour cells are large with abundant cytoplasm surrounding a more or less irregular nucleus. **C** The tumour cells are highlighted by staining for CD20.

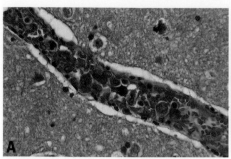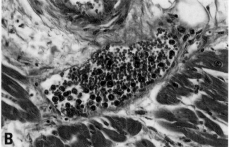

Fig. 6.104 Intravascular large B cell lymphoma. The large tumour cells are present in the lumen of small vessels (**A**) in the central nervous system and (**B**) in the myocardium.

deposits of tumour may not be visible to the naked eye.

Morphology
The neoplastic lymphoid cells are mainly lodged in the lumina of small vessels in many organs. Fibrin thrombi may be seen in some cases. The tumour cells are large with vesicular nuclei, prominent nucleoli and frequent mitotic figures. Rare cases have cells with anaplastic features.

In organs such as the lung and bone marrow, the involvement may be very subtle. Recognition of single neoplastic cells in small capillaries may be enhanced by immunostains for CD45 and CD20. Malignant cells are rarely seen in cerebrospinal fluid and blood.

Immunophenotype
Tumour cells are usually positive for B-cell associated antigens (e.g. CD19, CD20, CD22, CD79a). CD5 coexpression is seen in some cases. Rare cases of intravascular lymphoma of T-cell phenotype have been reported {1281, 1177}. Factor VIII, an endothelial cell-related antigen, may be detected, but is considered to represent absorption of factor VIII, rather than expression by the neoplastic cells {1422, 821}.

Genetics
The majority of cases studied have had immunoglobulin gene rearrangements. Rare reported cases of intravascular lymphoma have had T-cell receptor gene rearrangements {216, 1025, 1177, 314}. Karyotypic abnormalities have been described but too few cases have been studied for any consistent patterns to emerge {885}.

Postulated cell of origin
Transformed peripheral B-cell.

Prognosis and predictive factors
In general this is an extremely aggressive lymphoma which responds poorly to chemotherapy {304}. Death occurs in most cases within a short time of presentation. The poor prognosis in these patients reflects in part frequent delays in diagnosis due to their protean presentation. There is some evidence for a variant confined to skin which may have a relatively better prognosis but numbers of patients studied are small {216}.

Primary effusion lymphoma

P.M. Banks
R.A. Warnke

Definition

Primary effusion lymphoma (PEL) is a neoplasm of large B-cells usually presenting as serous effusions without detectable tumour masses. It is universally associated with human herpes virus 8 (HHV-8)/Kaposi sarcoma herpes virus (KSHV), most often occurring in the setting of immunodeficiency.

ICD-O code 9678/3

Synonym

Body cavity-based lymphoma.

Epidemiology

The majority of cases arise in the setting of human immunodeficiency virus (HIV) infection {198, 914, 1129}. Most patients are young to middle aged homosexual males {914, 1129}.

This neoplasm is rare even in the setting of HIV infection (see chapter 9) {668}. At least one case has been reported in an HIV negative allograft recipient. The disease also occurs in the absence of immunodeficiency especially in elderly males most often from areas with high prevalence for HHV-8/KSHV infection such as the Mediter-ranean {1278, 233}

Sites of involvement

The most common sites of involvement are the pleural, pericardial and peritoneal cavities. Typically only one body cavity is involved. Other sites of involvement

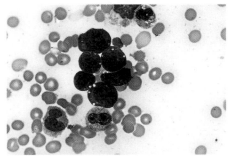

Fig. 6.106 Primary effusion lymphoma. The cells exhibit pleomorphism, basophilic cytoplasm with clear vacuoles and prominent nucleoli. Wright stain.

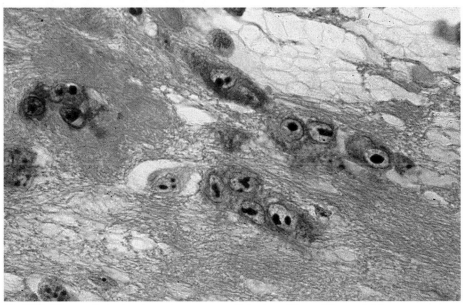

Fig. 6.105 Primary effusion lymphoma. Large tumor cells in pleural biopsy (Giemsa stain).

include the gastrointestinal tract, soft tissue and other extranodal sites {986, 81, 287}.

Clinical features

Patients typically present with effusions in the absence of lymphadenopathy or organomegaly. Some patients have pre-existent Kaposi sarcoma {34}. Rare cases may be associated with multicentric Castleman disease {1278}.

Aetiology

The neoplastic cells are positive for HHV-8/KSHV in all cases. Most cases are coinfected with EBV {34, 48, 533, 1129}. High levels of cytokines, in particular IL-6 and IL-10 may be found in the effusions {36}.

Morphology

With Wright or May Grunwald Giemsa staining performed on cytocentrifuge preparations, the cells exhibit a range of appearances, from large immunoblastic or plasmablastic cells to cells with more anaplastic morphology. Nuclei are large, round to more irregular in shape, with prominent nucleoli. The cytoplasm can

be very abundant and is deeply basophilic with the presence of vacuoles in occasional cells. A perinuclear hof consistent with plasmacytoid differentiation may be seen. Some cells can resemble Reed-Sternberg cells.

The cells often appear more uniform in histological sections than in cytospin preparations. However, the cells are generally large, with some pleomorphism, ranging from large cells with round or ovoid nuclei to very large cells having irregular nuclei and abundant cytoplasm {34, 914, 287}. Pleural biopsies show tumour cells adherent to the pleural surface often embedded in fibrin and occasionally invading the pleura. This disease should be distinguished from pyothorax associated DLBCL which usually presents with a pleural mass lesion. The cells of that tumour are EBV positive and HHV8/KSHV negative {243}.

Immunophenotype

Lymphoma cells usually express leukocyte common antigen (CD45) but are usually negative for pan-B-cell markers such as CD19, CD20 and CD79a {672, 914}. Surface and cytoplasmic expression of immunoglobulin is likewise often absent. Activation and plasma cell-related markers such as CD30, CD38, and CD138 are usually demonstrable. Aberrant cytoplasmic CD3 expression has been reported {81}. Because of the markedly aberrant phenotype, it is often difficult to assign a lineage with immunophenotyping. The nuclei of the neoplastic cells are positive by immunohistochemistry for the HHV8/KSHV-associated latent protein {326}. This is very useful in establishing a diagnosis. Despite the usual presence of EBV, staining for LMP1 is negative.

Genetics

Immunoglobulin genes are rearranged and are mutated {831}. Some cases also have aberrant rearrangement of T-cell receptor genes {529}. No characteristic chromosomal abnormalities have been identified. Comparative genomic analysis has revealed gain in sequence of chromosomes 12 and X, in common with other HIV-associated lymphomas {903}.

HHV-8/KSHV viral genomes are present in all cases. EBV is found in most cases and is most reliably detected by EBER in-situ hybridisation {34, 533}. EBV tends to be absent in elderly HIV-negative patients {1278, 233}.

Postulated cell of origin

Post-germinal centre B-cell.

Prognosis

The clinical outlook is extremely unfavourable, with or without therapy; median survival is less than six months.

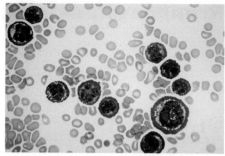

Fig. 6.107 Primary effusion lymphoma. The lymphoma cells vary in size with some having round nuclei and prominent nucleoli and others having irregular nuclear outlines and less conspicuous nucleoli. Cytoplasmic vacuoles are evident in the basophilic cytoplasm.

Burkitt lymphoma

J. Diebold
E.S. Jaffe
M. Raphael
R.A. Warnke

Definition

Burkitt lymphoma (BL) is a highly aggressive lymphoma often presenting at extranodal sites {162, 163} or as an acute leukaemia {1212}, composed of monomorphic medium-sized B-cells with basophilic cytoplasm and numerous mitotic figures {1, 496, 549, 748, 1419}. Translocation involving *MYC* is a constant genetic feature {495, 1019, 1419, 1421}. Epstein-Barr Virus (EBV) is found in a variable proportion of cases.

ICD-O code   9687/3 (lymphoma)
                  9826/3 (leukaemia)

Synonyms

Rappaport: undifferentiated lymphoma, Burkitt type
Lukes-Collins: small non-cleaved follicular centre cell
WF: small non-cleaved cell, Burkitt type
Kiel: Burkitt and Burkitt lymphoma with intracytoplasmic immunoglobulin
REAL: Burkitt lymphoma
FAB: L3 ALL

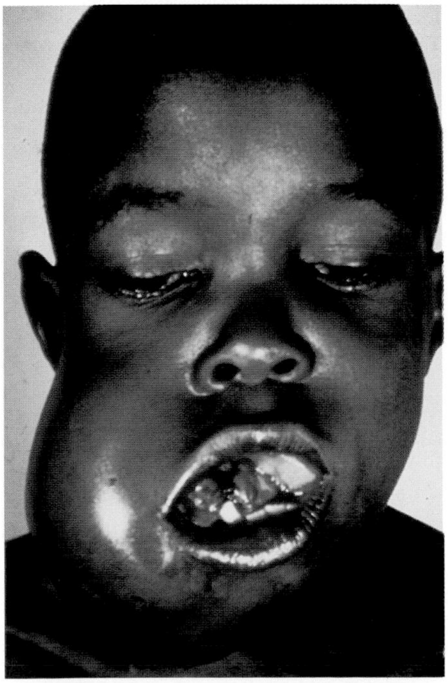

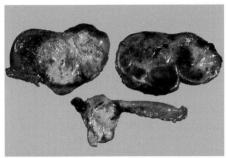
Fig. 6.109 Sporadic Burkitt lymphoma with bilateral ovarian tumours.

Epidemiology

Three clinical variants of Burkitt lymphoma are recognised, each manifesting differences in clinical presentation, morphology and biology.

1. Endemic BL

This variant occurs in equatorial Africa, representing the most common malignancy of childhood in this area with an incidence peak at 4 to 7 years and a male to female ratio of 2 to 1 {163, 1361, 1419}. BL is also endemic in Papua, New Guinea. In endemic regions there is a correlation between the geographical occurrence and some climatic factors (rainfall, altitude, etc.) which correspond to the geographical distribution of endemic malaria {163, 354, 1419}.

2. Sporadic BL

This variant is seen throughout the world, mainly in children and young adults {163, 306, 761, 804, 812, 1361, 1418}. The incidence is low, 1-2% of all lymphomas in Western Europe and in USA. BL accounts for approximately 30 to 50% of all childhood lymphoma. The median age of the adult patients is about 30 years {306, 3}. The male to female ratio is about 2 or 3 to 1. In some parts of the world, e.g. in South America and North Africa, the incidence is intermediate between true sporadic and endemic variants. Low socio-economic status and early EBV infection are associated with a higher prevalence of EBV positive BL {35, 1361}.

3. Immunodeficiency associated BL

This variant is seen primarily in association with the human immunodeficiency virus (HIV) infection, occurring often as the initial manifestation of the acquired immunodeficiency syndrome (AIDS) {1087}. EBV is identified in 25-40% of the cases {482, 1087}. BL is less often seen in other immunodeficiency states.

Sites of involvement

Extranodal sites are most often involved with some variation according to the clinical variants. However, in all three clinical variants, patients are at risk for central nervous system involvement {1440}.

In endemic BL, the jaws and other facial bones (orbit) are the site of presentation in about 50% of the cases {162, 163, 1419} Distal ileum, coecum and/or omentum, ovaries, kidneys, and breast may also be involved {163, 1361, 1419}.

In sporadic BL, jaw tumours are less common. The majority of the cases presents with abdominal masses {306, 804, 1361, 1418}. The ileo-coecal region represents the most frequent site of involvement {761}. Similar to endemic BL, ovaries, kidneys and breasts are also frequently involved. Breast involvement, often bilateral and massive, has been associated with onset during puberty, pregnancy or lactation. Retro-peritoneal masses may result in spinal cord compression with paraplegia. Lymph node

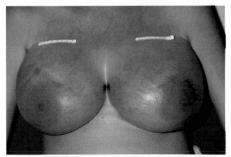
Fig. 6.110 Bilateral breast involvement may be the presenting manifestation during pregancy, and puberty. BL cells have prolactin receptors.

Fig. 6.108 Endemic Burkitt lymphoma. This African patient presented with a large jaw tumour.

presentation can be seen, more commonly in adults than in children. Waldeyer's ring and mediastinal involvement are rare. A leukaemic phase can be observed in patients with bulky disease, but only rare cases present purely as acute leukaemia (Burkitt leukaemia, L3/ALL) with bone marrow involvement and circulating B-blasts resembling Burkitt cells {803, 804, 1057, 1212}.

In immunodeficiency-associated BL, nodal localisation is frequent as well as bone marrow involvement {482, 1087, 1439}.

Clinical features

Patients present with bulky disease, often with a high tumour burden due to the short doubling time of the tumour. The clinical presentation varies according to the epidemiologic subtype and the site of involvement. Some patients, mainly males, present as acute leukaemia, with peripheral blood and bone marrow involvement. Bone marrow involvement is a poor prognostic sign and is often found in patients with a high tumour burden. In patients with bulky tumours or acute leukaemia, high uric acid and high LDH level are usually seen. BL is staged according to the system of Murphy et al (see table 6.17) {911}. Localised stages (I and II) are found in approximately 30% of the patients, while advanced stages (III and IV), are seen in 70% of patients at presentation.

The tumour lysis syndrome is due to rapid tumour cell death upon institution of therapy. It is most characteristic of BL, but also may be seen in other lymphomas with a high growth fraction. Tumour cell death is associated with release of intracellular components composed of purines, xanthine, hypoxanthine, uric acid, phosphates and potassium into the blood stream. It results in severe hyperkalemia, with possible cardiac arrest, hyperphosphataemia with secondary hypocalcemia, precipitation of uric acid, xanthine and/or phosphate in the renal tubules, causing severe renal failure {235, 1374}. In patients at risk of tumour lysis syndrome, very careful monitoring should be done during the initial period of treatment {1374}.

Aetiology

Epstein-Barr virus (EBV) plays an important role in endemic BL {35, 354, 475, 1269, 1419}. EBV was first discovered

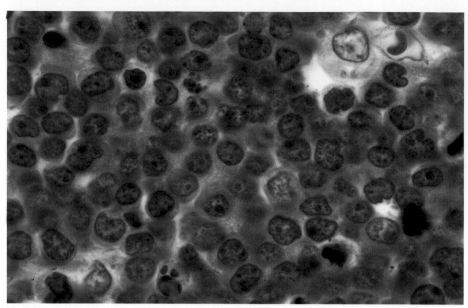

Fig. 6.111 Classical Burkitt lymphoma. The cells are uniform in size and shape with multiple small basophilic nucleoli. The nuclear diameter of the tumour cells is similar to that of the starry sky histiocytes (upper right).

from a BL cell line {347}. In endemic BL, the EBV genome is present in the majority of the neoplastic cells in all patients {1058, 1269, 1419}. The lymphoma is preceded by a long period of polyclonal B-cell activation due to multiple bacterial, viral (EBV, HIV) and parasitic infections (particularly malaria) which may favour the development of the lymphoma, due to defective T-cell regulation of EBV-infected B-cells {354, 1419}.

In sporadic BL, the frequency of EBV association is low, less than 30% of the cases. Low socio-economic status and early EBV infection are associated with a higher prevalence of EBV positive BL {35, 475}. In immunodeficiency-associated cases, EBV is identified only in 25 to 40% of the cases {482, 1087} (see chapter 9).

As in endemic BL, antigenic stimulation and abnormal B-cell expansion also play a role in the development of BL in this setting {1019}. That EBV is not associated with many cases of BL leads to the hypothesis that the virus is not essential for the pathogenesis of BL, but rather may represent only a co-factor. In the absence of EBV or in concert with EBV, other environmental factors (immunosuppression, antigenic stimulation, etc.) probably play a role.

Genetic abnormalities involving the *MYC* gene at chromosome 8q24 play an essential role in BL pathogenesis {181, 475, 942, 1019, 1189, 1432}.

Macroscopy

Involved organs are replaced by masses of fish flesh-appearing tissue, often associated with haemorrhage and necrosis. Adjacent organs or tissues are compressed and/or infiltrated. Nodal involvement is rare in endemic and sporadic BL, and in fact uninvolved lymph nodes may be surrounded by tumour.

Morphology
Classical BL

This morphologic type of BL is observed in endemic BL and in a high percentage of sporadic BL cases, particularly in children {1, 496, 495, 549, 748, 3, 1361, 1419}. The medium-sized cells show a diffuse monotonous pattern of infiltration. Sometimes after fixation the cells exhibit squared off borders of retracted cyto-

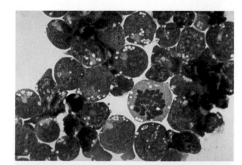

Fig. 6.112 Classical Burkitt lymphoma, touch imprint. The deeply basophilic cytoplasm can be appreciated, as well as abundant lipid vacuoles in the cytoplasm.

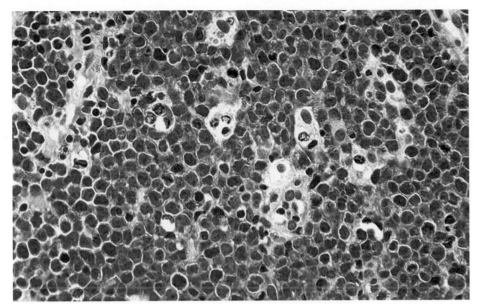

Fig. 6.113 Atypical Burkitt lymphoma. A prominent starry sky pattern in apparent.

plasm and may appear cohesive, particularly in mercury-based fixatives. The nuclei are round with clumped chromatin and relatively clear parachromatin, and contain multiple basophilic medium sized, centrally situated nucleoli. The cytoplasm is deeply basophilic and usually contains lipid vacuoles. Such cellular details are better perceived in imprints. The tumour has an extremely high proliferation rate (many mitotic figures) as well as a high rate of spontaneous cell death. A «starry sky» pattern is usually present, imparted by numerous benign macrophages that have ingested apoptotic tumour cells. The nuclei of the tumour cells approximate in size those of

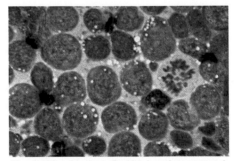

Fig. 6.114 Atypical Burkitt lymphoma, the nuclei are slightly irregular, and nucleoli are more prominent than in classical BL.

the admixed starry-sky histiocytes.

Variant:
BL with plasmacytoid differentiation
In this variant {496, 495, 549, 748}, some tumour cells exhibit eccentric basophilic cytoplasm with often a single central nucleolus; monotypic intracytoplasmic immunoglobulin can be demonstrated. As in the atypical/Burkitt-like variant, a certain degree of pleomorphism in nuclear size and shape can be recognised {549, 748}. This variant can be observed in children {748} but is more common in immunodeficiency states {1087} (see chapter 9).

Variant: atypical Burkitt/Burkitt-like
This variant is predominantly composed of medium-sized Burkitt cells and shows other features of BL (high degree of apoptosis, high mitotic index) {496, 495, 1218}.
The diagnosis requires a growth fraction of nearly 100% {1218}. However, in contrast to classical BL, this variant shows greater pleomorphism in nuclear size and shape. Nucleoli are more prominent and fewer in number {370, 496, 495}. Finally the term «atypical Burkitt/Burkitt-like» is reserved for cases with proven or with a strong presumptive evidence of MYC translocation.

Immunophenotype
Tumour cells express membrane IgM with light chain restriction and B-cell-associated antigens (e.g. CD19, CD20, CD22), CD10 and BCL6 {496, 495, 549, 665, 748, 812, 1218, 1361, 1419}. The cells are negative for CD5, CD23 and TdT. BCL2 is not expressed. The expression of CD10 and BCL6 point towards a germinal centre origin for the tumour cells. CD21, the receptor for C3d, can be expressed in the endemic form, but sporadic cases are usually negative {803}. Monotypic intracytoplasmic immunoglobulins may be demonstrated in the plasmacytoid variant {549, 748}. A very high growth fraction is observed: nearly 100% of the cells are positive for Ki-67 {496, 495, 549, 748, 1218}. Infiltrating T cells are less common than in diffuse large B-cell lymphomas.
Blasts of BL presenting with leukaemia have a mature B-cell phenotype, in contrast to the blasts of precursor B-ALL, including brighter CD45 expression. They are CD34 negative and usually TdT negative. They express membrane light chain restricted Ig and usually are positive for CD19, CD20, CD22 and CD79a.

Genetics
The tumour cells show clonal rearrangements of the immunoglobulin (Ig) heavy and light chain genes. Somatic mutations of the Ig genes are found, consistent with a germinal centre stage of differentiation {665, 1263}.
All cases have a translocation of MYC at band q24 from chromosome 8 to the Ig heavy chain region on chromosome 14 [t(8;14)] at band q32 or less commonly to light chain loci on 2p12 [t(2;8)] or 22q11[t(8;22)]. In endemic cases, the breakpoint on chromosome 14 involves the heavy chain joining region (early B-cell) whereas in sporadic cases, the translocation involves the Ig switch

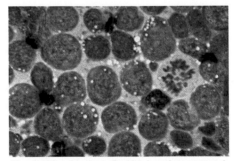

Fig. 6.115 Atypical Burkitt lymphoma, touch imprint. As in classical BL the cells have deeply basophilic cytoplasm and cytoplasmic lipid vacuoles.

region (later stage of B-cell) {181, 475, 942, 1019, 1189, 1212, 1432}. The *MYC* gene is constitutively expressed secondary to the influence of the promoters of the Ig genes on chromosomes 14, 2 or 22, encoding for immunoglobulin heavy chain, or the light chains kappa or lambda, respectively. The deregulation of *MYC* plays a decisive role in lymphomagenesis by driving the cells through the cell cycle {411, 475}. *MYC* also activates target genes specifically involved in apoptosis. Mutations in *MYC* may further enhance its tumourigenicity {1432}. Other genetic lesions in BL include inactivation of *TP53*, secondary to mutations in up to 30% of sporadic and endemic BL {107, 411, 1057}.

It should ne noted that *MYC* translocations are not entirely specific for BL. For example, the *MYC* translocation has been reported in secondary precursor B-lymphoblastic leukaemia / lymphoma following follicular lymphoma {271}.

EBV genomes can be demonstrated in the tumour cells in nearly all endemic cases {1058} and in 25-40% of immunodeficiency-associated cases {482, 1087}, but are less frequent in sporadic cases (<30%). As noted above, the exact role of EBV in the pathogenesis of BL is not understood.

Postulated cell of origin

Germinal centre B-cell.

Prognosis and predictive factors

In endemic and sporadic BL, the tumour is highly aggressive but potentially curable. The treatment should begin as early as possible, due to the short doubling time of the tumour.

Staging is performed according to the scheme proposed by Murphy and Hustu {911} and modified by Magrath {803}. Staging is largely related to tumour burden, and identifies patients with limited stage disease and patients with extensive intraabdominal or intrathoracic tumour {1374}. Reduction of tumour mass by surgical resection has been shown to be of value in some cases. Bone marrow and central nervous system involvement, unresected tumour greater than 10 cm, a high LDH serum level are recognised as poor prognostic factors, particularly in sporadic BL. Endemic BL is highly sensitive to polychemotherapy. Intensive combination chemotherapy regimens result in cure rates of up to 90% in patients with low stage disease and 60-80% in patients with advanced disease {803, 1212}. The results are better in children than in adults {1008, 1009}. However, even patients with advanced stage, including bone marrow and central nervous system involvement, may be cured with a high dose treatment program {306}.

Relapse, if it occurs, usually is seen within the first year after diagnosis. Patients without relapse for 2 years can be regarded as cured {803, 1374}. However, rare instances of a recurrence due to the development of a second neoplastic clone (a second BL) have been seen.

In Burkitt leukaemia, the treatment consists of very intensive chemotherapy of relatively short duration which differs substantially from current treatment of acute lymphoblastic leukaemia. With such treatment, most patients have a very good prognosis with 80-90% survival {1212, 1374}.

Table 6.17
Staging system for Burkitt lymphoma {803, 911, 1374}.

Stage	Definition
I	A single tumour (extranodal) or single anatomic area (nodal) with the exclusion of mediastinum or abdomen.
II	A single tumour (extranodal) with regional node involvement. Two or more nodal areas on the same side of the diaphragm. Two single (extranodal) tumours with or without regional node involvement on the same side of the diaphragm. Primary gastrointestinal tract tumour, usually in the ileocoecal area, with or without involvement of associated mesenteric nodes only.
II R	Completely resected abdominal disease.
III	Two single tumours (extranodal) on opposite sites of the diaphragm. Two or more nodal areas above and below the diaphragm. All primary intrathoracic tumours (mediastinal, pleural, thymic). All paraspinal or epidural tumours, regardless of other tumour site(s). All extensive primary intraabdominal disease.
III A	Localized but non resectable abdominal disease.
III B	Widespread multiorgan abdominal disease.
IV	Any of the above with initial CNS and/or bone marrow involvement (< 25%).

Lymphomatoid granulomatosis

E.S. Jaffe
W.H. Wilson

Definition

Lymphomatoid granulomatosis (LYG) is an angiocentric and angiodestructive lymphoproliferative disease involving extranodal sites, comprised of Epstein Barr virus (EBV)-positive B cells admixed with reactive T cells, which usually numerically predominate. The lesion has a spectrum of histological grade and clinical aggressiveness, which is related to the proportion of large B cells. LYG may progress to an EBV+ diffuse large B-cell lymphoma (DLBCL).

ICD-O code   9766/1

Synonyms and historical annotation

Angiocentric immunoproliferative lesion
Lymphomatoid granulomatosis must be distinguished from extranodal NK/T-cell lymphoma, nasal-type, which often has an angiodestructive growth pattern, and is also associated with EBV {584} (see chapter 7).

Epidemiology

Lymphomatoid granulomatosis is a rare condition. It usually presents in adult life, but may be seen in children with immunodeficiency disorders. It affects males more often than females (at least 2:1) {640}.

Sites of involvement

The most common site of involvement is lung, and most patients have pulmonary disease at some point during the clinical course. Other common sites of involvement include brain (26%), kidney (32%), liver (29%), and skin (25-50%). Upper respiratory tract and the gastrointestinal tract may be affected {255}. Lymph nodes and spleen are very rarely involved {640, 590, 686, 853}.

Clinical features

Patients frequently present with signs and symptoms related to the respiratory tract, such as cough (58%), dyspnoea (29%), and chest pain (13%). Other constitutional symptoms are common,

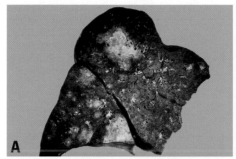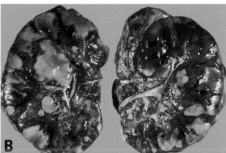

Fig. 6.116 Lymphomatoid granulomatosis. **A** Lung involved by lymphomatoid granulomatosis. Large nodules show central cavitation. **B** Large necrotic nodules also are found in the kidney.

including fever, malaise, weight loss, neurological symptoms, arthralgias, myalgias, and gastrointestinal symptoms. Very few patients present with asymptomatic disease (<5%) {590}.

Aetiology

Lymphomatoid granulomatosis is an EBV-driven lymphoproliferative disorder. Patients with underlying immunodeficiency are at increased risk for lymphomatoid granulomatosis {470, 489}. Predisposing conditions include allogeneic organ transplantation, Wiskott-Aldrich syndrome, human immunodeficiency virus (HIV) infection, and X-linked lymphoproliferative syndrome. However, patients presenting without evidence of underlying immunodeficiency usually manifest reduced immune function upon careful clinical or laboratory analysis {1397, 1208}.

Genetic susceptibility

As noted above, patients with genetically acquired immunodeficiency resulting in ineffective immunosurveillance for EBV are at increased risk.

Macroscopy

Lymphomatoid granulomatosis most commonly presents as pulmonary nodules that vary in size. The lesions are most often bilateral in distribution, involving mid and lower lung fields. Larger nodules frequently exhibit central necrosis, and may cavitate. Nodular lesions

are found in the kidney and brain, usually associated with central necrosis. Skin lesions are extremely diverse in appearance. Nodular lesions are found in the subcutaneous tissue. Dermal involvement may also be seen, sometimes with necrosis and ulceration. Cutaneous plaques or a maculopapular rash are less common cutaneous manifestations {640, 590, 853}.

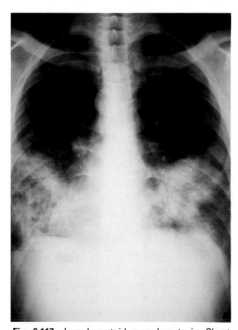

Fig. 6.117 Lymphomatoid granulomatosis. Chest radiograph identifies multiple nodules, mainly affecting the lower lung fields.

Morphology

Lymphomatoid granulomatosis is characterised by an angiocentric and angio-destructive polymorphous lymphoid infiltrate {640, 686}. Lymphocytes predominate, and are admixed with plasma cells, immunoblasts, and histiocytes. Neutrophils and eosinophils are usually inconspicuous. Well-formed granulomas are usually absent {775}. The background small lymphocytes may show some atypia or irregularity, but do not appear overtly neoplastic. Lymphomatoid granulomatosis is comprised of a usually small number of EBV-positive B cells admixed with a prominent inflammatory background {470, 641}. The EBV-positive cells usually show some atypia. They may resemble immunoblasts, or less commonly have a more pleomorphic appearance reminiscent of Hodgkin cells. Multinucleated forms may be seen. However, classical Reed-Sternberg cells are not present, and if seen, should raise the diagnosis of Hodgkin lymphoma.

Vascular changes are prominent in lymphomatoid granulomatosis. Lymphocytic vasculitis, with infiltration of the vascular wall is seen in most cases. The vascular infiltration may compromise the vascular integrity, leading to infarct-like tissue necrosis. More direct vascular damage in the form of fibrinoid necrosis is also common, and is mediated by chemokines induced by EBV {1274}.

Grading

Early studies showed the value of histological grading in the management of lymphomatoid granulomatosis {640}. Large numbers of atypical lymphoid cells were associated with a worse prognosis. Lipford et al. proposed a grading scheme using three histological grades {775}. It is now apparent that the grading of lymphomatoid granulomatosis relates to the proportion of EBV-positive B-cells relative to the reactive lymphocyte background {471}.

Grade I lesions contain a polymorphous lymphoid infiltrate without cytologic atypia. Large transformed lymphoid cells are absent or rare, and necrosis is usually not prominent. By in-situ hybridisation with EBER1/2 probe only infrequent EBV-positive cells are identified (<5 per high power field) {1397}. In some cases, EBV-positive cells may be absent. Grade II lesions contain occasional large lymphoid cells or immunoblasts in a poly-

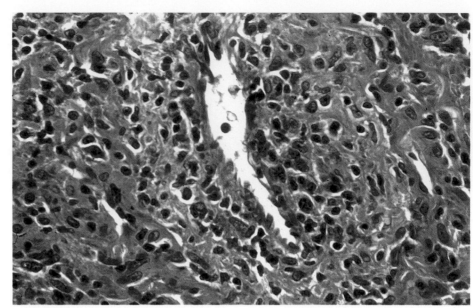
Fig. 6.118 Lymphomatoid granulomatosis. Grade I lesion of the lung shows a polymorphous infiltrate in the vascular wall.

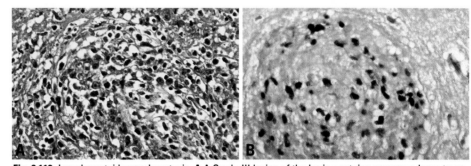
Fig. 6.119 Lymphomatoid granulomatosis. **A** A Grade III lesion of the brain contains numerous large transformed lymphoid cells. **B** These cells are positive for Epstein Barr virus by *in situ* hybridisation with the EBER probe .

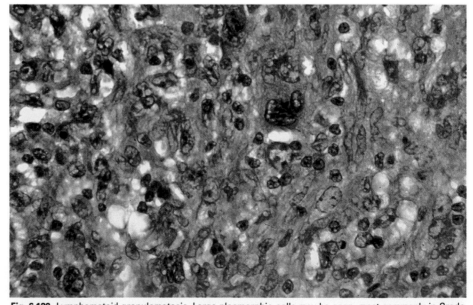
Fig. 6.120 Lymphomatoid granulomatosis. Large pleomorphic cells may be seen, most commonly in Grade III lesions, rarely in Grade II.

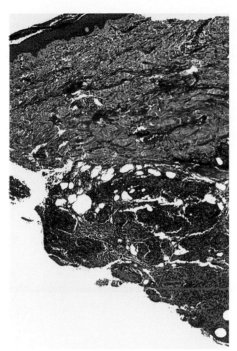

Fig. 6.121 Lymphomatoid granulomatosis. Cutaneous manifestations are diverse, but most often show subcutaneous infiltration, sometimes with fat necrosis and a granulomatous response.

morphous background. Necrosis is more commonly seen. *In situ* hybridisation for EBV readily identifies EBV-positive cells, which usually number 5-20/high power field. Grade III lesions are readily identified as malignant lymphomas on histo-logical grounds. Large lymphoid cells are numerous, although an inflammatory background is still present. Markedly pleomorphic and Hodgkin-like cells are often present, and necrosis is usually extensive. By *in situ* hybridisation, EBV-positive cells are extremely numerous, and focally may form small confluent sheets. Grade III lymphomatoid granulomatosis is considered a subtype of diffuse large B-cell lymphoma, and should be approached as such clinically {775, 1397}. However, some cases may still show spontaneous regression with immunotherapy or alteration in the immune state.

Immunophenotype

The EBV-positive B-cells usually express CD20; however, CD79a is more variably positive {471, 1397, 1267}. The cells are variably positive for CD30, but negative for CD15. LMP1 is usually positive in the larger atypical and more pleomorphic cells. Stains for cytoplasmic immunoglobulin are frequently non-informative, although in rare cases monoclonal cytoplasmic immunoglobulin expression may be seen {1397}. The background lymphocytes are CD3-positive T cells, with CD4+ cells more frequent than CD8+ cells.

Genetics

In most cases of Grade II or Grade III disease, clonality of the immunoglobulin genes can be demonstrated by molecular genetic techniques, such as VJ-PCR {853, 470}. In some cases different clonal populations may be identified in different anatomic sites {1397, 883}. Southern blot analysis also may show clonality of EBV {855}. Demonstration of clonality in Grade I cases is more inconsistent, an observation which may be related to the relative rarity of the EBV-positive cells in these cases. Alternatively, some cases of lymphomatoid granulomatosis may be polyclonal. Alterations of oncogenes have not been identified. T-cell receptor gene analysis shows no evidence of monoclonality {853, 855}.

Postulated cell of origin

Mature B lymphocyte, transformed by EBV.

Prognosis and predictive factors

The natural history of lymphomatoid granulomatosis is variable {365}. In some patients it may follow a waxing and waning clinical course, with spontaneous remissions without therapy. However, in most patients the disease is more aggressive, with a median survival of under two years {640}. More recent series have shown responses to aggressive chemotherapy for Grade III lesions {775}. Grade I and II lesions may respond to interferon-alpha 2b {1397}. The most common cause of death is progressive pulmonary involvement.

CHAPTER 7

Mature T-Cell and NK-Cell Neoplasms

Mature T-cell and NK-cell neoplasms are relatively uncommon, but show significant differences in incidence in different parts of the world. In general, they are more common in Asians than in other races. Epstein-Barr virus is associated most often with extranodal NK/T-cell lymphomas and NK-cell leukaemias. The human T-cell leukaemia virus (HTLV-1) is aetiologically linked to adult T-cell leukaemia/lymphoma, and the incidence of this disease closely correlates with the distribution of the virus. However, for most T-cell and NK-cell neoplasms, the cause is unknown.

Clinically, they are among the most aggressive of all haematopoietic and lymphoid neoplasms, although some diseases have a more protracted clinical course. A variety of factors contribute to the aggressive clinical behaviour including advanced clinical stage and chemotherapeutic resistance for many of these neoplasms. However, exceptions occur, and one disease, anaplastic large cell lymphoma, is generally responsive to chemotherapy.

The definition of T-cell and NK-cell neoplasms based on morphological, immunophenotypic and genetic features is generally imprecise. Therefore, currently clinical features play an important part in the definition of these diseases.

WHO histological classification of mature T-cell and NK-cell neoplasms

Leukaemic / disseminated

T-cell prolymphocytic leukaemia	9834/3
T-cell large granular lymphocytic leukaemia	9831/3
Aggressive NK cell leukemia	9948/3
Adult T-cell leukaemia/lymphoma	9827/3

Cutaneous

Mycosis fungoides	9700/3
Sézary syndrome	9701/3
Primary cutaneous anaplastic large cell lymphoma	9718/3
Lymphomatoid papulosis[1]	9718/1

Other extranodal

Extranodal NK/T cell lymphoma, nasal type	9719/3
Enteropathy-type T-cell lymphoma	9717/3
Hepatosplenic T-cell lymphoma	9716/3
Subcutaneous panniculitis-like T-cell lymphoma	9708/3

Nodal

Angioimmunoblastic T-cell lymphoma	9705/3
Peripheral T-cell lymphoma, unspecified	9702/3
Anaplastic large cell lymphoma	9714/3

Neoplasm of uncertain lineage and stage of differentiation

Blastic NK cell lymphoma	9727/3

---

[1] Clinically not considered a neoplastic disorder.

Mature T-cell and NK-cell neoplasms: Introduction

E.S. Jaffe
E. Ralfkiaer

Definition

Mature T-cell neoplasms are derived from mature or post-thymic T cells. Because NK-cells are closely related, and share some immunophenotypic and functional properties with T-cells, these two classes of neoplasms are considered together {1221}.

Incidence

Mature T-cell and NK-cell neoplasms are relatively uncommon. In a large international study that evaluated lymphoma cases from the United States, Europe, Asia, and South Africa, T-cell and NK-cell neoplasms accounted for only 12% of all non-Hodgkin lymphomas {8}. The most common subtypes of mature T-cell lymphomas are peripheral T-cell lymphoma, unspecified (3.7%) and anaplastic large cell lymphoma (2.4%).

Epidemiology

T-cell and NK-cell lymphomas show significant variations in incidence in differ-

ent geographical regions and racial populations. In general, T-cell lymphomas are more common in Asia {616}. These differences result from both a true increased incidence, as well as a relative decrease in the frequency of many B-cell lymphomas, such as follicular lymphoma, seen commonly in North America and Europe. One of the main risk factors for T-cell lymphoma in Japan is the virus, HTLV-1. In endemic regions of southwestern Japan, the seroprevalence of HTLV-1 is 8-10%. The cumulative life-time risk for the development of adult T-cell leukaemia/lymphoma (ATLL) is 6.9% for a seropositive male and 2.9% for a seropositive female {683}. Other regions with a relatively high seroprevalence for HTLV-1 include the Caribbean basin, where Blacks are primarily affected over other racial groups {760}. Differences in viral strain also may affect the incidence of the disease {523, 1345}. Another major factor affecting the incidence of T-cell and NK-cell lymphomas is racial predisposition. Nasal and nasal-type NK/T-cell lymphomas, and aggressive NK/T-cell leukaemia are much more

common in Asians than they are in other races {27}. In Hong Kong, nasal NK/T-cell lymphoma is one of the more common subtypes, accounting for 8% of cases. By contrast, in Europe and North America, it accounts for less than 1% of all lymphomas. Other peoples at increased risk for this disease are individuals of Native American descent in Central and South America, and Mexico {40, 341}. These populations are genetically linked to Asians, and are believed to have emigrated to the American continent from Asia, either over the Aleutician land bridge or a water route {892}. Overall, the incidence of T-cell and NK-cell malignancies does not appear to be changing, although long term epidemiological data are not available, as it is only recently with modern immunophenotypic and molecular tools that these neoplasms have been reliably distinguished from B-cell lymphomas.

Pathophysiology

Mature T-cell lymphomas manifest the immunophenotypic features of post-thymic T lymphocytes. There are two

Table 7.01
Incidence of peripheral T-cell lymphomas.

Diagnosis	% of total cases
Diffuse large B-cell	30.6%
Follicular lymphoma	22.1%
Marginal zone B-cell lymphoma, MALT	7.6%
Peripheral T-cell lymphomas (PTL)	7.6%
PTL, NOS	3.7%
Nasal NK/T	1.4%
Angioimmunoblastic T-cell	1.2%
Enteropathy-type	<1
Hepatosplenic	<1
Adult T-cell leukaemia/lymphoma*	<1
CLL/SLL	6.7%
Mantle cell lymphoma	6.0%
Mediastinal large B-cell lymphoma	2.4%
Anaplastic large cell lymphoma/T-null	2.4%
Burkitt lymphoma/Burkitt-like	2.5%
Nodal marginal zone lymphoma	1.8%
Precursor T-cell lymphoblastic	1.7%
Lymphoplasmacytic lymphoma	1.2%
Other types	7.4%

* Data taken from the International Non-Hodgkin's Lymphoma Classification study {8}. Case series did not include regions endemic for HTLV-1.

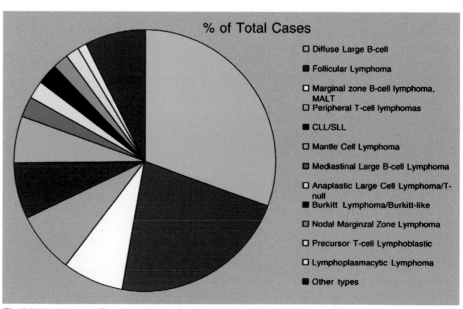

Fig. 7.01 Incidence of T-cell lymphomas, in relationship to other lymphoma subtypes.

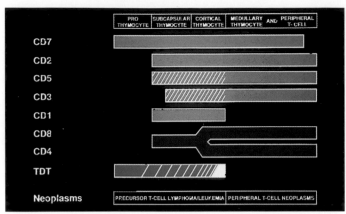

Fig. 7.02 T-cell differentiation scheme. Antigen expression changes during T-cell differentiation. Cortical thymocytes coexpress CD4 and CD8, but at the medullary stage of differentiation, only CD 4 or CD 8 is expressed.

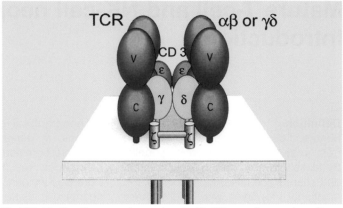

Fig. 7.03 The T-cell receptor is complexed with CD3 as a dimer at the cell surface. It is composed of either αβ or γδ chains, each having an external V and C domain. The CD3 complex contains γ, δ and ε chains.

major classes of T cells: αβ T cells and γδ T cells {284}. This distinction is based on the structure of the T-cell receptor. The αβ and γδ chains are each composed of an external variable (V) and constant (C) portion. They both are associated with CD3, which is identical in both T-cell subsets. CD3 contains γ, δ, and ε chains. NK cells do not have a complete T-cell receptor complex, but usually express the ε chain of CD3 in the cytoplasm, which can be recognised by polyclonal antibodies to CD3.

Table 7.02
Mature T-cell and NK-cell neoplasms.

Leukaemic or disseminated
T-cell prolymphocytic leukaemia
T-cell granular lymphocytic leukaemia
Aggressive NK-cell leukaemia
Adult T-cell lymphoma/leukaemia

Extranodal
Extranodal NK/T-cell lymphoma, nasal type
Enteropathy-type T-cell lymphoma
Hepatosplenic T-cell lymphoma
Subcutaneous panniculitis-like T-cell lymphoma

  Cutaneous
  Blastic NK-cell lymphoma*
  Mycosis fungoides/Sezary syndrome
  Primary cutaneous anaplastic large cell lymphoma

Nodal
Peripheral T-cell lymphoma, unspecified
Angioimmunoblastic T-cell lymphoma
Anaplastic large cell lymphoma

_____
* Neoplasm of uncertain lineage and stage of differentiation

Gamma-delta T cells are negative for both CD4 and CD8, and also usually negative for CD5. A subpopulation expresses CD8. Gamma-delta T cells represent a more primitive type of immune response. They comprise less than 5% of all normal T cells, and show a restricted distribution, being found mainly in the splenic red pulp, intestinal epithelium, and other epithelial sites. It is notable that these sites are more commonly affected by γδ T-cell lymphomas, which are relatively rare {241, 47, 1303}. Gamma-delta T cells have a restricted range of antigen recognition. They are not MHC restricted in their function, and represent a first line of defense against bacterial peptides, such as heat shock proteins {284}. They are often involved in responses to mycobacterial infections, and in mucosal immunity.

Alpha-beta T cells are divided into two major subtypes, CD4-positive and CD8-positive. In normal lymphoid tissues, CD4-positive cells exceed CD8-positive cells, and a similar ratio is seen among malignant diseases. CD4-positive T cells or "Helper T cells" are mainly cytokine secreting cells, whereas CD8-positive T cells are mainly involved in cytotoxic immune reactions. CD4-positive cells are divided into two major types, based on their cytokine secretion profile. Th1 cells secrete interleukin (IL)-2 and interferon γ, but not IL-4, 5, or 6. By contrast, Th2 cells secrete IL-4, 5, 6, and 10 {284}. Th1 cells provide help mainly to other T cells and macrophages, whereas Th2 cells provide help mainly to B-cells, in their production of antibodies {285}.

These various immune profiles have not yet been related to the subtypes of T-cell lymphomas and leukaemias, and there have been relatively few studies correlating the subclassification of T cell lymphomas with specific profiles of cytokine or chemokine expression {601}. Nevertheless, many of the clinical manifestations of T cell lymphomas can be related to cytokine expression by the neoplastic cells. For example, the hypercalcemia associated with ATLL has been linked to secretion of factors with osteoclast-activating activity {664, 1358}. The haemophagocytic syndrome seen in many T cell and NK-cell malignancies has been associated with secretion of both cytokines and chemokines {737, 1276}.

NK cells share some functions and markers with cytotoxic T cells. They can express CD2, CD7, CD8, CD56, and CD57, all of which can be seen in some T-cell subsets. As noted above, they also are often positive for the epsilon chain of

Table 7.03
Frequent features of mature extranodal T/NK-cell lymphomas.

– Broad cytologic spectrum
– Disease definition is heavily dependent upon clinical features, not morphology
– Infrequent lymph node involvement, even with recurrences
– Frequent spread to other extranodal sites
– Cytotoxic T-cell or NK-cell phenotype
– Frequent apoptosis and/or necrosis, with or without angioinvasion
– Increased incidence of a haemophagocytic syndrome
– Presence of EBV correlates with both anatomic site, and geographic factors

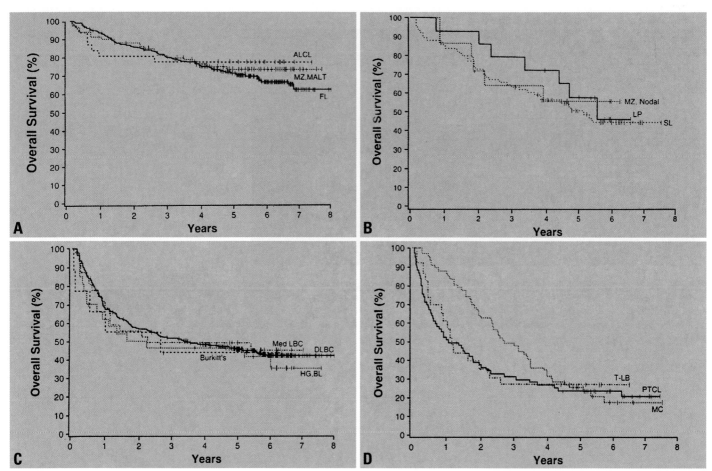

Fig. 7.04 Survival of Non-Hodgkin lymphoma subtypes according to the REAL classification. Most peripheral T-cell lymphomas (PTCL) fall into Group D, with less than 30% 5 year overall survival. The one exception is anaplastic large cell lymphoma, T/null, which is in Group A, with a 5 year median survival of greater than 70%. Abbreviations: ALCL, anaplastic large cell lymphoma; MZ, MALT, extranodal marginal zone lymphoma of MALT type; FL, follicular lymphoma; MZ, nodal, nodal marginal zone lymphoma; LP, lymphoplasmacytic lymphoma; SL, B-cell chronic lymphocytic leukaemia/small lymphocytic lymphoma; Med LBC, mediastinal large B-cell lymphoma; DLBC, diffuse large B-cell lymphoma; HG, BL, high grade B-cell lymphoma, Burkitt-like; T-LB, precursor T-cell lymphoblastic lymphoma/leukaemia MC, mantle cell lymphoma. Reproduced from {8}.

Table 7.04
Extranodal T/NK-cell lymphomas of cytotoxic lineage.

Subtype	EBV	CD3	TIA-1	GranB / Per	CD56	Major	Minor
SPTCL	−	+s	+	+	−/+	αβ	γδ
ETTL	−/+	+s	+	+	−/+	αβ	γδ / NK
Nasal	+	+c	+	+	+	NK	γδ / αβ
Hep/spl	−	+s	+	−	+	γδ	αβ

SPTCL, subcutaneous panniculitis-like T-cell lymphoma
ETTL, enteropathy-type T-cell lymphoma
Extranodal NK/T-cell lymphoma, nasal-type
Hep/spl, hepatosplenic T-cell lymphoma
GranB/Per, Granzyme B, perforin
s, surface CD3
c, cytoplasmic CD3

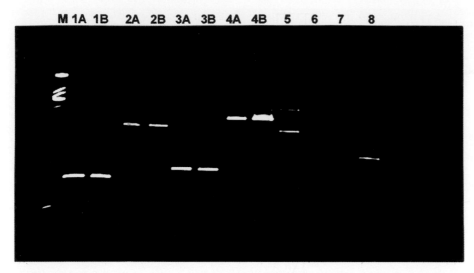

Fig. 7.05 T-cell receptor PCR analysis performed by DGGE gradient gel electrophoresis in clinical samples with a suspected diagnosis of T-cell lymphoma. Clonal rearrangement of the T-cell receptor gamma chain gene is illustrated by discrete bands in lanes 1-6 and 8. Lanes coded A and B represent sequential samples from the same patient and show identical rearrangements Clonal bands were not detected in lanes 6 and 7. Modified from {455}.

CD3. However, they are usually positive for CD16, which is less often positive on T cells. Both NK cells and cytotoxic T cells express cytotoxic proteins, including perforin, granzyme B, and T-cell intracellular antigen (TIA)-1 {588}. These antigens are also seen on cytotoxic T-cell and NK-cell malignancies {580}.

The classification of T-cell and NK-cell neoplasms proposed by the WHO emphasises a multiparameter approach, integrating morphologic, immunophenotypic, genetic, and clinical features. Clinical features play particular importance in the subclassification of these tumours, in part due to the lack of specificity of other parameters. T-cell lymphomas show great morphological diversity, and a spectrum of histological appearances can be seen within individual disease entities. The cellular composition can range from small cells with minimal atypia to large cells with anaplastic features. Such a spectrum is seen in anaplastic large cell lymphoma, adult T-cell lymphoma/leukaemia, and nasal NK/T cell lymphoma, as selected examples. Moreover, there is morphological overlap between disease entities. Many of the extranodal cytotoxic T-cell and NK-cell lymphomas share similar appearances, including prominent apoptosis, necrosis, and angioinvasion {587}. In contrast to B-cell lymphomas, specific immunophenotypic profiles are not associated with most T-cell lymphoma sub-

types. While certain antigens are commonly associated with specific disease entities, these associations are not entirely disease-specific. For example, CD30 is a universal feature of anaplastic large cell lymphoma, but can be expressed, usually to a lesser extent, in other T-cell and B-cell lymphomas. CD30 is of course also positive in Hodgkin lymphoma. Similarly, while CD56 is a characteristic feature of nasal NK/T-cell lymphoma, it can be seen in other T-cell lymphomas, and even in plasma cell neoplasms {208, 701, 1325}. Additionally, within a given disease entity, variation in the immunophenotypic features can be seen. For example, hepatosplenic T-cell lymphomas are usually of γδ T-cell phenotype, but a minority of cases are of αβ derivation.

Finally, in contrast to B-cell lymphomas, there are no convenient immunophenotypic markers of monoclonality, although the presence of an aberrant immunophenotype may point towards a diagnosis of malignancy {1034}. Therefore, molecular genetic studies, most commonly PCR studies for rearrangement of the T-cell receptor genes, are generally required in order to evaluate the clonality of a T-cell proliferative process {455, 689}. Presently, specific genetic abnormalities have not been identified for many of the T-cell and NK-cell neoplasms. One of the few exceptions is anaplastic large cell lymphoma, which is strongly associated

with the t(2;5) and other variant translocations {582, 1229}. However, the molecular pathogenesis of most T-cell and NK-cell neoplasms remains to be defined. For all of the above reasons, clinical features play a major role in the subclassification of T-cell and NK-cell neoplasms {667}. Several broad clinical groups are delineated: 1) leukaemic or disseminated; 2) nodal; 3) extranodal; and 4) cutaneous.

Survival

T-cell and NK-cell lymphomas as a group are clinically aggressive and have a much poorer response to therapy, and shorter survival than either B-cell lymphomas or Hodgkin lymphoma {8}. One of the few T-cell lymphomas with a good response to therapy is anaplastic large cell lymphoma. The poor response to therapy may be due to an intrinsic drug resistance for many of these neoplasms {320}. In addition, many T-cell and NK-cell neoplasms present with advanced stage disease, which also confers a poor prognosis {787}. T-cell lymphomas have been most commonly treated with standard chemotherapeutic protocols largely developed for B-cell lymphomas, and then empirically applied to T-cell diseases. Few clinical trials have been restricted to the T-cell lymphomas, in part due to the relative rarity of these neoplasms.

T-cell prolymphocytic leukaemia

D. Catovsky
E. Ralfkiaer
H.K. Müller-Hermelink

Definition

T-cell prolymphocytic leukaemia (T-PLL) is an aggressive T-cell leukaemia characterised by the proliferation of small to medium sized prolymphocytes with a mature post-thymic T-cell phenotype involving the blood, bone marrow, lymph nodes, liver, spleen and skin.

ICD-O code   9834/3

Synonyms

Lukes: "Knobby" type of T-cell leukaemia
Kiel: T-prolymphocytic leukaemia/T-cell lymphocytic leukaemia
REAL: T-cell-prolymphocytic leukaemia / T-cell chronic lymphocytic leukaemia

Epidemiology

T-PLL is a relatively rare condition, representing approximately 2% of cases of small lymphocytic leukaemia in adults over the age of 30 {833}.

Sites of involvement

Leukaemic T cells are found in the peripheral blood, bone marrow, lymph nodes, spleen, liver and skin.

Clinical features

Most patients present with hepatosplenomegaly and generalised lymphadenopathy. Skin infiltration, but not erythroderma, is seen in 20% of patients, and serous effusions, chiefly pleural, in a minority {833}. Anaemia and thrombocytopenia are common and the lymphocyte count is high, usually over 100 x 10⁹/l {833}. Serum immunoglobulins are normal and there is no M component in the serum. Serology for HTLV-1 is always negative.

Morphology

Peripheral blood and bone marrow

The diagnosis is made on peripheral blood films which show a predominance of small to medium-sized lymphoid cells with non-granular basophilic cytoplasm, round, oval or markedly irregular nuclei and a visible nucleolus. In 25% of cases the cell size is small and the nucleolus

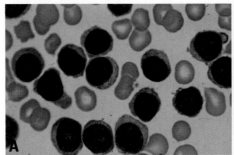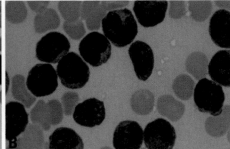

Fig. 7.06 A, B Peripheral blood films from typical cases of T-PLL.

may not be visible by light microscopy (small cell variant) {833, 836}. In a minority of patients the nuclear outline is very irregular and could even be cerebriform (cerebriform or Sézary cell-like variant) {1014}. Irrespective of the nuclear features, a common morphological feature is the presence of cytoplasmic protrusions or blebs. T-prolymphocytes stain strongly with alpha-naphthyl acetate esterase with dot-like staining in the golgi region {835}. The bone marrow is diffusely infiltrated with cells with the same morphology as the peripheral blood, but the diagnosis is difficult to make by bone marrow histology alone.

Other tissues

Cutaneous involvement is seen in 20% of patients and consists of dense dermal infiltrates, often around the skin appendages, but without epidermotropism {833}. The spleen histology shows dense red and white pulp infiltration. In lymph nodes the involvement is diffuse and tends to predominate in the paracortical areas, sometimes with sparing of follicles. Prominent high-endothelial venules may be numerous and are often infiltrated by neoplastic cells.

Variant forms

The small cell variant accounts for 20%

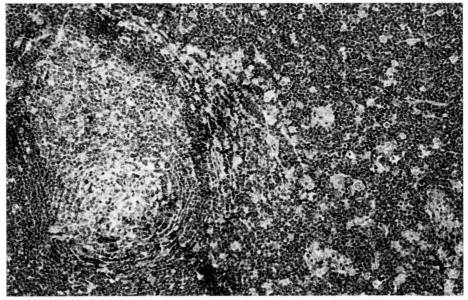

Fig. 7.07 T-PLL. Lymphnode is diffusely infiltrated, but a B-cell follicle is unaffected. Giemsa stain.

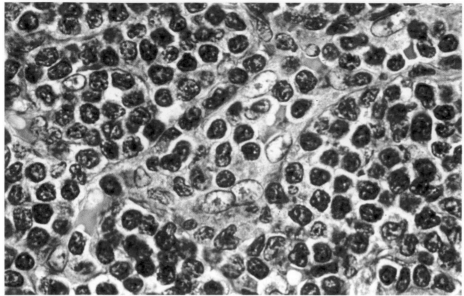

Fig. 7.08 T-PLL. Prominent high endothelial venule showing tumour cells in the lumen (circulating blood), in the wall, and the adjacent paracortex. Giemsa stain.

of T-PLL cases and the cerebriform (or Sézary cell-like) variant for 5% {1014, 140}. Ultrastructural analysis is useful to recognise these T-PLL variants {836}.

Immunophenotype

T-prolymphocytes are peripheral T cells which are TdT and CD1a negative while CD2, CD3 and CD7 are positive; the membrane expression of CD3 may be weak.

In 60% of patients the cells are CD4+,CD8-, and in 25% they coexpress CD4 and CD8, a feature almost unique to T-PLL; 15% are CD4-,CD8+ {833}.

Genetics

Antigen receptor genes

T-cell receptor γ and β chains are clonally rearranged.

Cytogenetic abnormalities and oncogenes.

The most frequent chromosome abnormality in T-PLL involves inversion of chromosome 14 with breakpoints in the long arm at q11 and q32, seen in 80% of patients. In 10% there is a reciprocal tandem translocation t(14;14)(q11;q32) {138, 808}. These translocations juxtapose the TCR α/β locus with the oncogenes *TCL1* and *TCL1b* at 14q32.1 which

are activated through the translocation {1348, 1017}. Abnormalities of chromosome 8, idic (8p11), t(8;8)(p11-12;q12) and trisomy 8q are seen in 70-80% of cases {1210}. Deletions at 12p13 are also a feature of T-PLL when studied by FISH analysis {520}. The translocation t(X;14) (q28;q11) is less common, but it also involves the TCR α/β locus at 14q11 with the *MTCP1* gene, which is homologous to *TCL1*, at Xq28 {1236}. Both *TCL1* and *MTCP1* have oncogenic properties as both can induce a T-cell leukaemia (CD4-/CD8+) in transgenic mice after 15 months incubation {462, 1347}. Molecular and FISH studies also show deletions at 11q23, the locus for the Ataxia Telangiectasia Mutated (*ATM*) gene, and mutational analysis has shown clustering of missence mutations at the *ATM* locus in T-PLL {1237, 1350}.

Postulated cell of origin

Unknown T-cell with a mature (post-thymic) immunophenotype. Immunophenotypic features, e.g. strong CD7, coexpression of CD4 and CD8 and weak membrane CD3 suggest that T-PLL arises from a T-cell at an intermediate stage of differentiation between cortical thymocytes and peripheral blood T-lymphocytes.

Prognostic and predictive features

The course of the disease is progressive and the median survival is less than one year, but presentation with an indolent course has also been documented {420}. Encouraging responses have been reported with the monoclonal antibody CAMPATH-1H {1013} and less frequently with the nucleoside analog pentostatin and the combination chemotherapy regimen CHOP. Autologous and allogeneic stem cell transplants for patients who achieve remission are currently being explored to improve the outlook of this aggressive leukaemia.

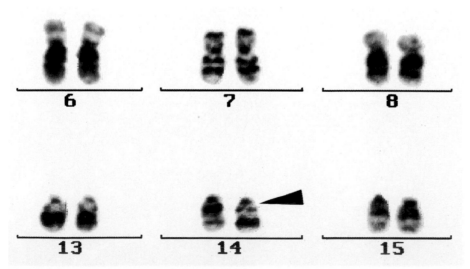

Fig. 7.09 T-PLL. Partial Karyotype showing inv14q (q11;q32).

T-cell large granular lymphocyte leukaemia

W.C. Chan
D. Catovsky
K. Foucar
E. Montserrat

Definition
T-cell large granular lymphocyte leukaemia (T-LGL) is a heterogeneous disorder characterised by a persistent (>6 months) increase in the number of peripheral blood large granular lymphocytes (LGLs), usually between 2-20x10^9/l, without a clearly identified cause.

ICD-O code   9831/3

Synonyms
T-cell chronic lymphocytic leukaemia
Tγ – lymphoproliferative disorder
Proliferation of large granular lymphocytes
LGL leukaemia

Epidemiology
T-LGL leukaemia represents 2-3% of cases of small lymphocytic leukaemia.

Sites of involvement
T-LGL involves the peripheral blood, bone marrow, liver and spleen. Lymphadenopathy is very rare.

Clinical features
Most cases have an indolent clinical course. Severe neutropenia with/without anaemia is a frequent disease feature; 60% of patients are symptomatic at presentation {214, 996, 729}. Lymphocytosis is usually between 2-20x10^9/l. Severe anaemia due to red cell hypoplasia has been reported in association with T-LGL leukaemia {711}.
Moderate spleno-megaly is the main physical finding. Rheumatoid arthritis, the presence of autoantibodies, circulating immune complexes and hypergammaglobulinemia are also common {214, 985, 790, 789, 729}.

Morphology
The predominant cells in blood and bone marrow films are LGLs with abundant cytoplasm and fine or coarse azurophilic granules {146, 851, 1176}. The granules in the lymphocytes often exhibit a characteristic ultrastructural appearance described as parallel tubular arrays {851} and contain a number of proteins that play a role in cytolysis such as perforin and granzyme B. There is no agreement on the level of lymphocytosis required for diagnosis of T-LGL leukaemia {1176}, but reactive lymphocytosis often has a value <5x10^9/l and T-LGL leukaemia >5x10^9/l. However, values of LGLs greater than 2x10^9/l are consistent with this diagnosis. The extent of bone marrow involvement is variable, with often an interstitial and rarely a nodular pattern; lymphocytes frequently comprise less than 50% of the cellular elements.

Variant
Cases morphologically resembling T-LGL leukaemia but with a NK immunophenotype (CD3-, TCRαβ-) are classified with the NK disorders.

Immunophenotype
LGL leukaemia cells have a mature T-cell immunophenotype {214, 996, 985, 1176, 709}. According to the predominant cell markers they can be subdivided in:
a) Common variant (80% of cases):
   CD3+, TCRαβ+, CD4-, CD8+
b) Rare variants:
   i) CD3+, TCR αβ+, CD4+, CD8-
   ii) CD3+, TCRαβ+, CD4+ and CD8+
   iii) CD3+, TCR γδ+ (CD4 and CD8 expression not well defined)

CD11b, CD56 and CD57 are variably expressed; CD57 is often expressed in the common type {729}. TIA-1 is usually positive.

Genetics
Antigen receptor genes
Cases classified as T-LGL leukaemia are, as a rule, clonal as documented by T-cell receptor (TCR) gene rearrangement studies {1082, 790}. Most cases have TCRβ chain gene rearranged and only in a minority the TCRβ is in germline configuration, but have a rearrangement of TCRγ {1346}.

Cytogenetic abnormalities
There is no unique karyotypic abnormality, but chromosomal translocations have been described in a minority of cases {789}. Leukaemic LGLs express constitutively Fas (CD95) and Fas-ligand. Fas ligand is found at high levels in the patients'

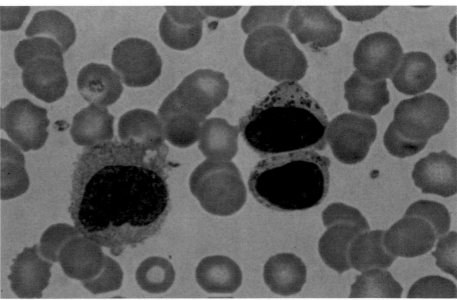

Fig. 7.10 T-cell large granular lymphocyte leukaemia. Two LGLs with prominent granules are seen.

sera. The LGL cells, however, are resistant to Fas-induced apoptosis, due to a defective CD95 apoptotic pathway {729}.

Postulated cell of origin
CD8 positive T-cell subset for the common type and a subset of Tγδ lymphocytes for the rare type expressing the T-cell receptor (TCR) γδ.

Prognosis and predictive factors
Opinion varies with regard to whether all the cases of T-LGL leukaemia represent leukaemic disorders. For cases where the clinical course is indolent and nonprogressive, the possibility of a reactive lymphocytosis, which may be clonal in certain circumstances, has been raised by some investigators. Morbidity is associated with neutropenia, but mortality due to this cause is uncommon. Progression with a more aggressive course is occasionally seen {427} and, in a minority, transformation to a peripheral T-cell lymphoma composed of large cells has been suggested {957}. Patients that require treatment may benefit from cyclosporin A {137, 1207}, methotrexate {214, 729}, cyclophosphamide and corticosteroids; some patients have benefited from pentostatin {865}. Splenectomy has been carried out in patients with a large spleen, but this does not correct the cytopenia.

Aggressive NK-cell leukaemia

J.K.C. Chan
K.F. Wong
E.S. Jaffe
E. Ralfkiaer

Definition
Aggresive NK-cell leukaemia is characterised by a systemic proliferation of NK cells. The disease has an aggressive clinical course {557, 203, 208}.

ICD-O code   9948/3

Synonyms
Kiel, Lukes-Collins, Working Formulation: Not listed
REAL: Large granular lymphocyte leukaemia, NK-cell type
Others: Aggressive NK-cell leukaemia/lymphoma

Epidemiology
This is a rare form of leukaemia/lymphoma which is more prevalent among Asians than Whites. Patients are mostly teenagers and young adults. There is no sex predilection or a slight male predominance {208, 557, 203, 712, 710, 425, 984}.

Sites of involvement
The most commonly involved sites are: peripheral blood, bone marrow, liver and spleen, but any organ can show involvement. Since the number of neoplastic cells in the peripheral blood and bone marrow can be limited, the disease is different from the usual leukaemias and thus has in the past been called "aggressive NK-cell leukaemia/lymphoma". There can be overlap with nasal-type NK/T-cell lymphoma showing multiorgan involvement; in fact NK-cell leukaemia might represent the leukaemic counterpart of extranodal NK/T-cell lymphoma, nasal type {203}.

Clinical features
The patients usually present with fever, constitutional symptoms and a leukaemic blood picture. The number of circulating

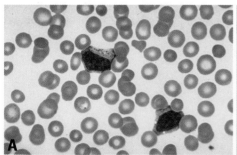 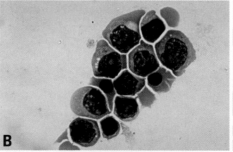 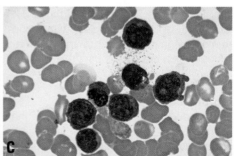

Fig. 7.11 Aggressive NK-cell leukaemia, Giemsa-stained peripheral blood smear or buffy coat smear from three different cases, illustrating the cytologic spectrum of the circulating granular lymphocytes. **A** In this blood smear, the neoplastic cells are very similar to normal large granular lymphocytes. **B** In this example, the neoplastic cells are larger, with more coarse chromatin. **C** In this case, the neoplastic cells have more open chromatin and distinct nucleoli. Azurophilic granules can be observed in the cytoplasm.

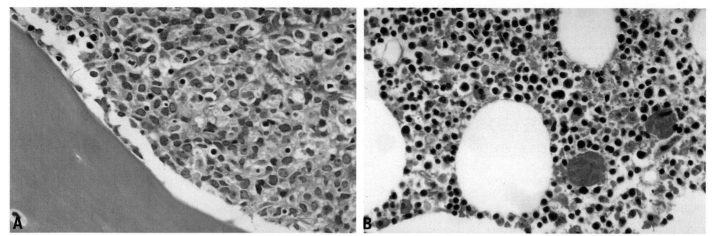

Fig. 7.12 Aggressive NK-cell leukaemia, bone marrow biopsy. **A** This example shows extensive involvement by a monotonous neoplastic cell population. **B** This example shows infiltration by neoplastic cells, which are admixed with erythrophagocytic histiocytes. This patient had features of hemophagocytic syndrome.

leukaemic cells can be low or high (a few percent to >80% of all leukocytes); anaemia, neutropenia and thrombocytopenia are common. Hepatosplenomegaly is common, sometimes accompanied by lymphadenopathy, but skin lesions are uncommon. The disease may be complicated by coagulopathy, haemophagocytic syndrome or multiorgan failure {208, 557, 712, 558, 676, 975, 968}. The serum soluble Fas ligand level is often markedly elevated, and this may contribute to the development of multiorgan failure {639, 1265}. Rare cases may evolve from extranodal NK/T-cell lymphoma or indolent NK-cell lymphoproliferative disorder {985, 967, 1206}.

Aetiology
Little is known about the aetiology of aggressive NK-cell leukaemia, but the strong association with Epstein-Barr virus (EBV) suggests a possible pathogenetic role of the virus. Rare patients may manifest features of hypersensivity to mosquito bites {572, 571}.

Morphology
Circulating leukaemic cells are slightly larger than normal large granular lymphocytes and some may contain irregular, hyperchromatic nuclei. Nucleoli can be inconspicuous or distinct. There is an ample amount of pale or lightly basophilic cytoplasm containing fine or coarse azurophilic granules. The bone marrow shows massive, focal or subtle infiltration by the neoplastic cells and there can be intermingled reactive histiocytes with haemophagocytosis.

In tissue sections, the leukaemic cells show diffuse or patchy destructive infiltrates. They often appear monotonous, with round or irregular nuclei, condensed chromatin and small nucleoli. There are frequently admixed apoptotic bodies. Necrosis is common, and there may or may not be angioinvasion.

Immunophenotype
The neoplastic cells are CD2+, surface CD3-, CD3ε+, CD56+ and positive for cytotoxic molecules. Thus, the immunophenotype is identical to that of extranodal NK/T-cell lymphoma, nasal-type.

CD11b and CD16 may be expressed, while CD57 is usually negative {203, 984}.

Genetics
T-cell receptor (TCR) genes are in germline configuration. Clonality therefore has to be established by other methods, such as cytogenetic studies and pattern of X chromosome inactivation in female patients. The great majority of cases harbour EBV in a clonal episomal form {208, 425, 642, 499, 1185}. A variety of clonal cytogenetic abnormalities have been reported, such as del(6)(q21q25) {1407}.

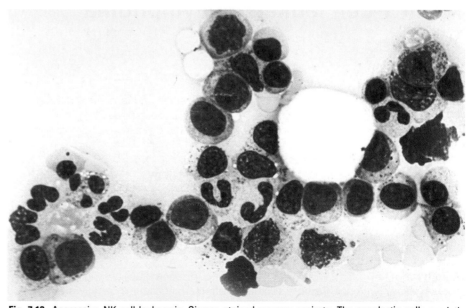

Fig. 7.13 Aggressive NK-cell leukaemia, Giemsa-stained marrow aspirate. The neoplastic cells are intimately intermingled with the haemopoietic cells. It can be difficult to distinguish the neoplastic granular lymphocytes from the myelocytes. In contrast to the latter, the cytoplasm of the former cells often exhibits a bluish rather than reddish tinge.

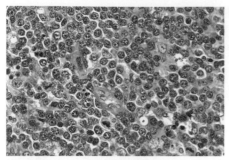

Fig. 7.14 Aggressive NK-cell leukaemia, lymph node. In this example, the neoplastic cells appear monotonous, and possess round nuclei. There are many interspersed apoptotic bodies.

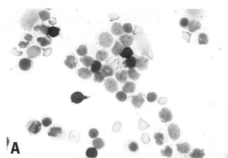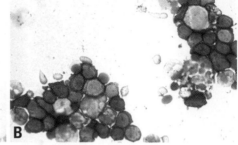

Fig. 7.15 Aggressive NK-cell leukaemia, immunophenotyping on smears. **A** The neoplastic cells are negative for surface CD3 (Leu4), while the normal T lymphocytes are stained. **B** The neoplastic cells show strong immunoreactivity for CD56.

Postulated cell of origin
NK cells.

Prognosis and predictive factors
Most cases pursue an aggressive to fulminant clinical course, resulting in a fatal outcome in one or two years. In fact, many patients die within days to weeks of initial presentation {203}.

Distinction from indolent NK-cell lymphoproliferative disorder
Not all large granular lymphocyte proliferations with an NK-cell phenotype are aggressive. There is a form of indolent NK-cell lymphoproliferative disorder, also known as chronic NK-cell lymphocytosis or NK-cell large granular lymphocyte lymphocytosis, with a nonprogressive course {214, 985, 984, 213, 1072, 1273}. Only exceptional cases transform to an aggressive phase {985, 967}.

Indolent NK-cell lymphoproliferative disorder occurs mostly in adults. Most patients are asymptomatic, although they may rarely have vasculitis or nephrotic syndrome. They show persistent increase in circulating large granular lymphocytes. There is no fever, hepatosplenomegaly or lymphadenopathy. In contrast to T-cell large granular lymphocyte leukaemia, there is no association with red cell aplasia, neutropenia or rheumatoid arthritis. The immunophenotype of the large granular lymphocytes is: CD2+, surface CD3-, CD56+, CD16+, CD57+. EBV is negative. TCR genes do not show rearrangements. It is currently not clear whether this condition is reactive or neoplastic.

Adult T-cell leukaemia/lymphoma

M. Kikuchi
E.S. Jaffe
E. Ralfkiaer

Definition
Adult T-cell leukaemia lymphoma (ATLL) is a peripheral T-cell neoplasm most often composed of highly pleomorphic lymphoid cells. The disease is usually widely disseminated, and is caused by the human retrovirus, human T-cell leukaemia virus type 1 (HTLV-1).

ICD-O code
Adult T-cell leukaemia/lymphoma 9827/3

Synonyms
Lukes-Collins: T-immunoblastic sarcoma.
Kiel: T-cell lymphoma, small cell type, pleomorphic medium and large cell type (HTLV-1+).
Working Formulation: various categories (mixed small and large cell, diffuse large cell, immunoblastic).
REAL: adult T-cell lymphoma/leukaemia (HTLV-1+)

Epidemiology
ATLL is endemic in several regions of the world, in particular Japan, the Caribbean basin and parts of Central Africa. The distribution of the disease is closely linked to the prevalence of HTLV-1 in the population.
The disease has a long latency, and affected individuals usually are exposed to the virus very early in life. The virus may be transmitted in breast milk, and through exposure to blood and blood products. Cumulative incidence of ATLL

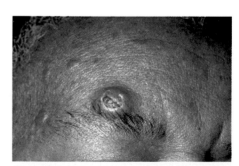

Fig. 7.16 Adult T-cell leukaemia/ lymphoma. Skin lesions can be papular or nodular, or in some patients a diffuse exfoliative rash may be seen.

is estimated to be 2.5% among HTLV-1 carriers in Japan {1258}. Sporadic cases are found in the United States and elsewhere in the world. It occurs in adults with a median age of 55 years. The male to female ratio is 1.5: 1 {1427}.

Sites of involvement
Most patients present with widespread lymph node involvement, and involvement of peripheral blood. The number of circulating neoplastic cells does not correlate with the degree of bone marrow involvement, suggesting that circulating cells are recruited from other organs, such as the skin. The skin is the most common extralymphatic site of involvement (>50%).
The disease is usually systemic in distribution, with involvement of spleen and extranodal sites including skin, lung, liver, gastrointestinal tract, and central nervous system {159}.

Clinical features
Several clinical variants are recognised: acute, lymphomatous, chronic and smoldering {1186}. The most common *acute variant* is characterised by a leukaemic phase, often with a markedly elevated white blood cell count, skin rash and generalised lymphadenopathy. Hypercalcemia, with or without lytic bone lesions, is common.
Patients with acute ATLL have systemic disease, with hepatosplenomegaly, and constitutional symptoms, and elevated LDH. Leukocytosis and eosinophilia are common. Many patients have an associated T-cell immunodeficiency, with frequent opportunistic infections such as *Pneumocystis carinii* pneumonia and Strongyloidiasis.
The *lymphomatous variant* is characterised by prominent lymphadenopathy, without peripheral blood involvement. Most patients have advanced stage disease, similar to the acute form. However, hypercalcemia is less often seen.
The *chronic variant* is associated with skin lesions, most commonly an exfoliative rash. While there may be an absolute lymphocytosis, atypical lymphocytes are not numerous in the blood. Hypercalcemia is absent.
In the *smoldering variant* the white blood cell count is normal with <5% circulating, neoplastic cells. Patients frequently have skin or pulmonary lesions, but hypercalcemia is not present. Progression from chronic and smoldering to acute variants occurs in 25% of the cases, but usually after a long duration {1186}.

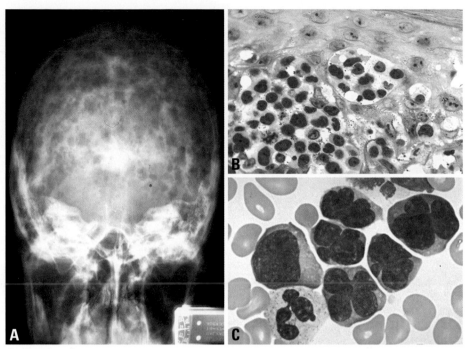

Fig. 7.17 Adult T-cell leukaemia/ lymphoma. **A** Radiograph shows extensive lytic bone lesions. **B** Neoplastic cells infiltrate the epidermis, producing Pautrier-like microabscess. **C** Peripheral blood films with medium-sized to large lymphoid cells with pleomorphic nuclei and basophilic cytoplasm. The nuclear features of ATLL are very variable; cells with many nuclear lobules have been described as "flower cells". (In chronic forms of the disease, the lymphoid cells may be smaller with condensed nuclear chromatin).

Aetiology
HTLV-1 is causally linked to ATLL. The p40 tax viral protein leads to transcriptional activation of many genes in the HTLV-1 infected lymphocytes {395}. HTLV-1 infection alone is not sufficient to result in neoplastic transformation of infected cells. However, additional genetic alternations acquired over time may result in the development of a malignancy.

Morphology
In the acute and lymphomatous subtypes the neoplastic lymphoid cells are medium-sized to large, often with pronounced nuclear pleomorphism. The nuclear chromatin is coarsely clumped,

Table 7.05
Adult T-cell lymphoma/leukaemia: clinical features (U.S. NCI series) {113, 159}.

Clinical feature	At presentation(%)	During course(%)
Leukaemia	62	100
Hypercalcemia	73	83
Lytic bone lesions	36	
Lymphadenopathy	61	85
Hepatosplenomegaly	61	
Skin lesions	61	
Bone marrow +	58	
Stage IV	100	

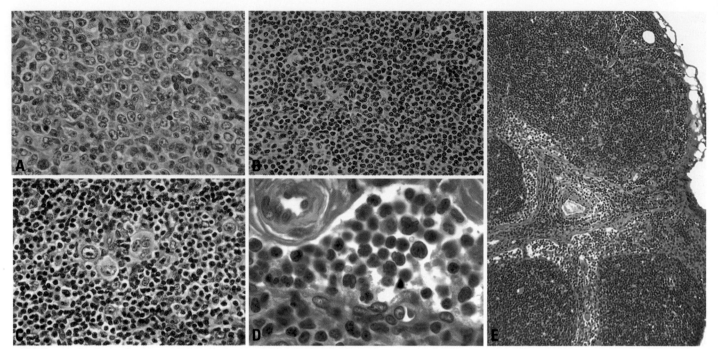

Fig. 7.18 Adult T-cell leukaemia/lymphoma. **A** Proliferation of large atypical cells with irregular and pleomorphic nuclei. Some smaller cells with irregular nuclei are intermingled. **B** This is an example of ATLL of small cell predominance. **C** Hodgkin-like variant. There are interspersed RS-like cells and giant cells with lobulated or convoluted nuclei against the background of small lymphocytes with mild nuclear atypia. **D** Neoplastic cells with polylobated nuclei are within dilated sinus. **E** At low power the lymph node shows open sinuses.

with distinct, sometimes prominent nucleoli. The neoplastic cells are often polylobated and have been termed flower cells in the peripheral blood. These cells may have deeply basophilic cytoplasm, most readily observed with Giemsa stains of the peripheral blood smears. In addition, there is always a small proportion of blast-like cells with transformed nuclei and dispersed chromatin {1186}. Giant cells with convoluted

or cerebriform nuclear contours may be present {972}. Rare cases may be composed of small atypical lymphocytes with nuclear pleomorphism. Cell size does not correlate with the clinical course {583}.

Marrow infiltrates are usually patchy, ranging from sparse to moderate. Osteoclastic activity may be prominent, even in the absence of bone marrow infiltration by neoplastic cells. In the skin epi-

dermal infiltration with Pautrier-like microabscesses are frequently found. In lymph nodes some cases may have a leukaemic pattern of infiltration, with preservation or dilation of lymph node sinuses that may contain malignant cells. The inflammatory background is usually sparse, although eosinophilia may be present in some cases {972}.

In the chronic and smoldering variants the neoplastic cells are usually small with minimal cytologic atypia. The skin shows a sparse dermal infiltrate with hyperkeratosis of the overlying epidermis.

Some patients with early or smoldering adult T-cell lymphoma/leukaemia may reveal a Hodgkin-lymphoma-like histology in the lymph nodes. Involved lymph nodes show expanded paracortical areas with diffuse infiltrates of small to medium-sized lymphocytes with mild nuclear irregularities, indistinct nucleoli and scant cytoplasm. There are interspersed Reed-Sternberg (RS)-like cells and giant cells with lobulated or convoluted nuclei. These cells are EBV-positive B-lymphocytes that express CD30 and CD15. This variant of incipient disease usually progresses to overt ATLL rapidly (within months) {970}. The expansion of EBV+ B-cells is felt to be secondary to

Table 7.06
Clinical features of smoldering and chronic ATLL. Modified from {644, 1428}.

Smoldering ATLL	Chronic ATLL
Normal WBC	Increased WBC
Blood ATLL cells <3%	Blood ATLL cells >10%
No lymphadenopathy	Mild lymphadenopathy
No hepatosplenomegaly	Slight hepatosplenomegaly
Skin rash (erythema, papules)	Skin rash variable
Normal LDH, Ca++	LDH slightly inc, Ca++ nl.
Survival > 2 yrs.	Survival usually > 2 yrs.

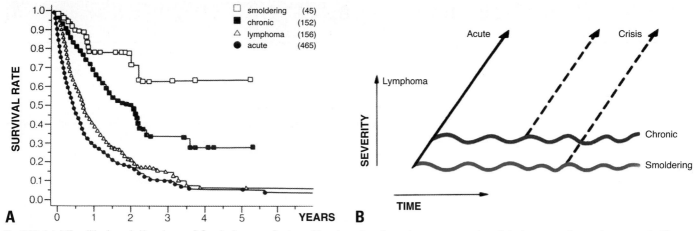

Fig. 7.19 Adult T-cell leukaemia/ lymphoma. **A** Survival curves. Acute and lymphomatous forms have an aggressive clinical course, whereas longer survival in seen in patients with chronic or smoldering disease. **B** Heterogeneity of the clinical course of ATL. Patients with chronic or smoldering disease may develop an acute crisis, with histological and clinical progression.

the underlying immunodeficiency seen in patients with ATLL.

Immunophenotype
Tumour cells express T-cell-associated antigens (CD2, CD3, CD5), but usually lack CD7. Most cases are CD4+, CD8-. Rare cases are CD4-, CD8+ or double positive for CD4 and CD8. CD25 is expressed in nearly all cases. The large transformed cells may be positive for CD30, but are ALK negative {1259}. TIA-1 and granzyme B are negative {972}.

Genetics
Clonally integrated HTLV-1 is found in all cases {1314}. T-cell receptor genes are clonally rearranged {969}.

Postulated cell of origin
Peripheral CD4+ T cells in various stages of activation.

Prognosis and predictive factors
Clinical subtypes, age, performance status, serum calcium and LDH levels are major prognostic factors {1429}. The survival time in acute and in lymphomatous variants ranges from two weeks to more than one year. The causes of death are infectious complications including *Pneumocystis carinii* pneumonia, cryptococcus meningitis, disseminated herpes zoster and hypercalcemia {1186}. Chronic and smoldering forms have a more protracted clinical course and a longer survival, but can transform into an acute phase with an aggressive course {971}.

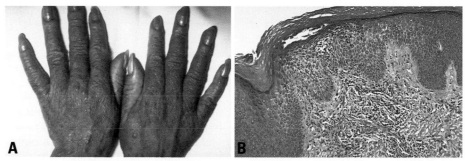

Fig. 7.20 Adult T-cell leukaemia/ lymphoma. Skin findings in smoldering ATLL. **A** Clinical photo shows a diffuse skin rash. **B** A sparse infiltrate is seen in the dermis with minimal cytologic atypia.

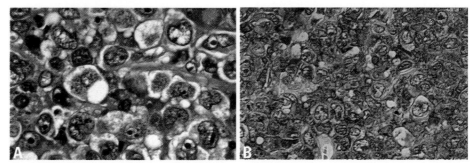

Fig. 7.21 Adult T-cell leukaemia/lymphoma. **A** In this case the infiltrate consists of large cells resembling anaplastic lymphoma. **B** The cells are strongly positive for CD30.

Extranodal NK/T-cell lymphoma, nasal type

J.K.C. Chan
E. S. Jaffe
E. Ralfkiaer

Definition

Extranodal NK/T-cell lymphoma, nasal type, is a predominantly extranodal lymphoma characterised by a broad morphologic spectrum. The infiltrate is often angiocentric, with prominent necrosis and vascular destruction. It is designated NK/T (rather than NK) cell lymphoma because while most cases appear to be NK-cell neoplasms (EBV+ CD56+), rare cases show an EBV+ CD56- cytotoxic T-cell phenotype.

The qualifier "nasal-type" draws attention to the fact that the nasal cavity is the commonest and prototypic site of involvement. However, identical neoplasms may be seen in other extranodal organs. The term "nasal NK/T-cell lymphoma" may be used as a synonym for those cases presenting in the nasal region.

ICD-O code   9719/3

Synonyms and historical annotation

Lukes-Collins: not listed
Kiel: not listed (pleomorphic T-cell lymphoma, small, medium-sized and large cell types)
Working Formulation: not listed (various categories, small lymphocytic, diffuse small cleaved cell, mixed small and large cell, diffuse large cell, immunoblastic)
REAL: angiocentric T-cell lymphoma
Others: malignant midline reticulosis; polymorphic reticulosis; lethal midline granuloma; angiocentric immunoproliferative lesion.

The term "polymorphic reticulosis" was coined in 1966 for nasal lymphoproliferative lesions with a mixed cellular composition, to distinguish them from the more monotonous-appearing conventional malignant lymphomas {337}. This term has been fairly widely used as a pathological diagnosis. Currently there is no doubt that polymorphic reticulosis is a malignant lymphoma, most commonly of NK- or T-cell lineage, and thus this non-specific term should be dropped from usage {203, 1243}.

Lymphomatoid granulomatosis had been considered to belong to the same spectrum as polymorphic reticulosis – angiocentric immunoproliferative lesions. There is now good evidence that lymphomatoid granulomatosis is a different entity, and represents a peculiar form of EBV-positive T-cell rich B-cell lymphoproliferation {581} (see chapter 6).

Epidemiology

NK/T-cell lymphoma is more prevalent in Asia, Mexico, and Central and South America. It occurs most often in adults, and is more common in males than females. These lymphomas have also been described in immunosuppressed patients and post-transplant conditions.

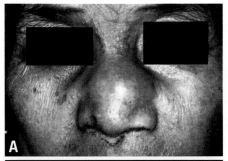
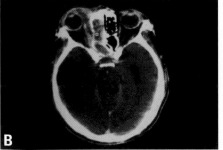

Fig. 7.22 A Patient suffering from nasal NK/T-cell lymphoma shows expansion of the nasal bridge. **B** Computed tomogram from a patient with nasal NK/T-cell lymphoma. The tumour in the nasal cavity extends upward into the orbit, resulting in proptosis.

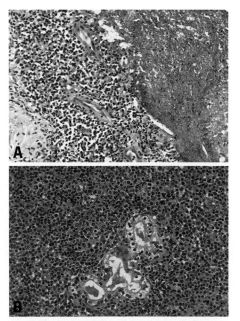

Fig. 7.23 Nasal NK/T-cell lymphoma. **A** There is prominent ulceration and necrosis in the nasal mucosa. **B** The nasal mucosa is diffusely infiltrated and expanded by an abnormal lymphoid infiltrate. The mucosal glands commonly show a peculiar clear cell change.

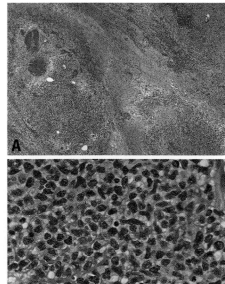

Fig. 7.24 Nasal-type NK/T-cell lymphoma in the testis. **A** There is a diffuse dense lymphoid infiltrate, with prominent coagulative necrosis. **B** In this example, the neoplastic cells appear monotonous and are medium-sized.

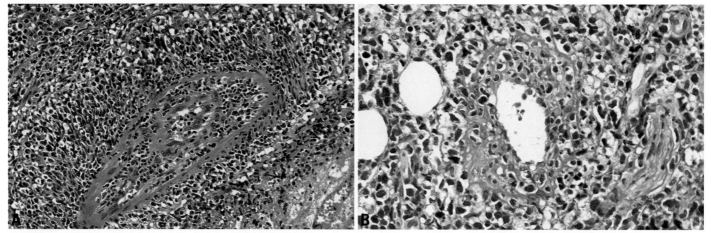

Fig. 7.25 Nasal NK/T-cell lymphoma. **A** The lymphomatous infiltrate shows infiltration and destruction of an artery. **B** In this case involving the skin, the lymphomatous infiltrate has an angiocentric angiodestructive quality.

Sites of involvement

NK/T-cell lymphoma shows an extranodal presentation, the sites of predilection being the nasal cavity, nasopharynx, palate, skin, soft tissue, gastrointestinal tract and testis. Some cases may be accompanied by secondary lymph node involvement {203, 929, 208, 709, 1251, 1301, 648, 1032, 207}.

Clinical features

Patients with nasal involvement present with symptoms of nasal obstruction or epistaxis due to presence of a mass lesion, or with extensive midfacial destructive lesions (so-called lethal midline granuloma). The lymphoma can extend to adjoining tissues such as the nasopharynx, paranasal sinuses, orbit, oral cavity, palate and oropharynx. The disease is often localised to the upper aerodigestive tract at presentation, and marrow involvement is very uncommon. Nonetheless, the disease may disseminate rapidly to various sites, e.g. skin, gastrointestinal tract, testis, or cervical lymph nodes during the clinical course. Some cases may be complicated by a haemophagocytic syndrome {709, 222}. Nasal-type NK/T-cell lymphomas occurring outside the nasal cavity have variable presentations depending upon the major site of involvement. The skin is commonly involved in the form of nodules, often with ulceration. Intestinal lesions often manifest as perforation. The patients commonly have high stage disease at presentation, with involvement of multiple extranodal sites. Systemic symptoms such as fever, malaise and weight loss can be present {208, 648, 929,

1406}. Lymph nodes can be involved as part of disseminated disease. Marrow and blood involvement can occur, and such cases overlap with aggressive NK-cell leukaemia.

Aetiology

Little is known about the aetiology of extranodal NK/T-cell lymphoma. Nasal NK/T-cell lymphoma is almost constantly associated with Epstein-Barr virus (EBV), irrespective of the ethnic origin of the patients, suggesting a probable pathogenic role of the virus {212, 40, 341,

1331, 625, 1069}. Nasal-type NK/T-cell lymphoma presenting in organs other than nose also shows a strong association with EBV in Asian patients, but the strength of association is less clear for White patients {208}.

Morphology

The histological features for extranodal NK/T-cell lymphoma are similar irrespective of the site of involvement. Mucosal sites often show extensive ulceration. The lymphomatous infiltrate is diffuse, but an angiocentric and angiodestructive

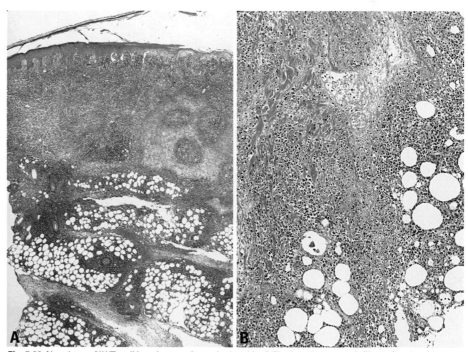

Fig. 7.26 Nasal-type NK/T-cell lymphoma primary in the skin. **A** The lymphomatous infiltrate involves the epidermis, dermis and subcutaneous tissue. **B** Note the presence of coagulative necrosis.

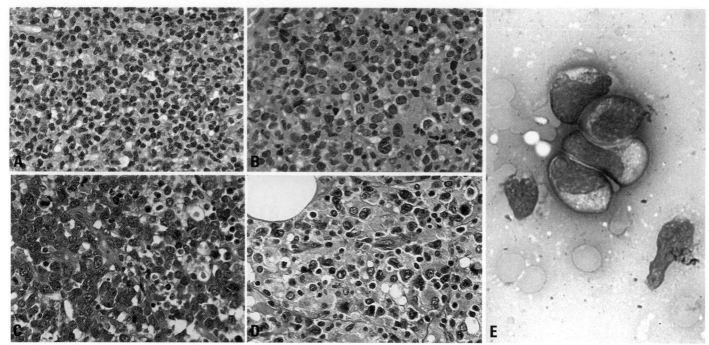

Fig. 7.27 The cytologic spectrum of extranodal NK/T-cell lymphoma. **A** This nasal tumour is composed predominantly of small cells with irregular nuclei. **B** This nasal tumour is composed predominantly of medium-sized cells with pale cytoplasm. **C** This nasal tumour is composed mostly of large cells. There are many apoptotic bodies. **D** Nasal-type NK/T-cell lymphoma of skin, with pleomorphic large cells admixed with smaller cells. **E** Touch preparation of nasal tumour (Giemsa stain). Azurophilic granules are evident in the pale cytoplasm of the lymphoma cells.

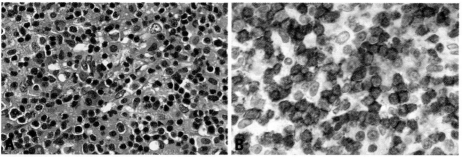

Fig. 7.28 Nasal NK/T-cell lymphoma. **A** This example is difficult to diagnose because the neoplastic cells are practically indistinguishable from normal small lymphocytes. There are many admixed plasma cells. **B** The presence of large numbers of cells staining for CD56 supports a diagnosis of lymphoma.

growth pattern is frequently present. Fibrinoid changes can be seen in the blood vessels. Coagulative necrosis and apoptotic bodies are very common. These have been attributed to vascular occlusion by lymphoma cells, but recent studies have also implicated other factors (such as chemokines, cytokines) {1274}.

The cytological spectrum of extranodal NK/T-cell lymphoma is very broad. Cells may be small, medium-sized, large or anaplastic in appearance. In most cases, the lymphoma is composed of medium-sized cells or a mixture of small and large cells. The cells may have irregular nuclei which can be elongated. The chromatin is granular, except in the very large cells, which may have vesicular nuclei. Nucleoli are generally inconspicuous or small. The cytoplasm is moderate in amount and is often pale to clear. Mitotic figures are easily found, even for small cell-predominant lesions. In touch preparations stained with Giemsa, azurophilic granules are commonly detected. Electron dense granules can be seen by electron microscopy.

NK/T-cell lymphomas, particularly those predominated by small or mixed cell populations, may show a heavy admixture of inflammatory cells, including small

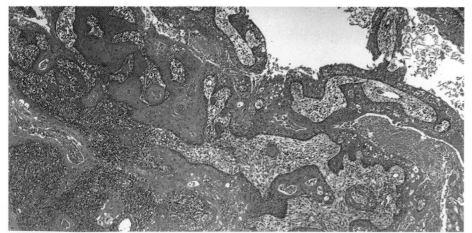

Fig. 7.29 Nasal NK/T-cell lymphoma associated with prominent pseudoepitheliomatous hyperplasia of the mucosal epithelium. This can potentially be misinterpreted as squamous cell carcinoma.

lymphocytes, plasma cells, histiocytes and eosinophils (hence the previously popular term "polymorphic reticulosis"). Such cases may mimic an inflammatory process. The lymphoma can sometimes be accompanied by florid pseudoepitheliomatous hyperplasia of the overlying epithelium, mimicking squamous cell carcinoma.

Immunophenotype

The most typical immunophenotype of extranodal NK/T-cell lymphoma is: CD2+, CD56+, surface CD3-, and cytoplasmic CD3ε+ {203, 584, 1313, 210, 578}. Most cases are also positive for cytotoxic granule associated proteins (such as granzyme B, TIA-1 and perforin). Other T and NK-cell associated antigens are usually negative, including CD4, CD5, CD8, TCRβ, TCRδ, CD16 and CD57. CD43, CD45RO, HLA-DR, interleukin-2 receptor, Fas (CD95) and Fas ligand are commonly expressed {896, 948, 947, 973}. Occasional cases are positive for CD7 or CD30.

Many investigators include lymphomas that demonstrate a CD3ε+, CD56-, cytotoxic molecule+, EBV+ phenotype among the nasal-type NK/T-cell lymphomas, since these cases show a similar clinical disease as cases with CD56 expression. However, the diagnosis should not be made in the absence of cytotoxic molecule expression or EBV positivity. Thus nasal or other extranodal lymphomas that are CD3ε positive, but negative for EBV and cytotoxic molecules should be diagnosed as peripheral T-cell lymphoma, unspecified. It is also emphasised that CD56 (N-CAM), although a highly useful marker for NK/T-cell lymphomas, is not specific and can be expressed in other peripheral T-cell lymphomas, particularly those that express the γδ-T-cell receptor.

Genetics

T-cell receptor and immunoglobulin genes are in germline configuration in a majority of the cases. EBV can be demonstrated in the tumour cells in the great majority of cases. The EBV is usually present in a clonal episomal form {212, 40, 341, 1331, 625, 1069, 525, 855}. A variety of cytogenetic aberrations have been reported, but so far no specific chromosomal translocations have been identified. The commonest cytogenetic abnormality is del(6)(q21q25) or i(6)(p10), but it is currently unclear

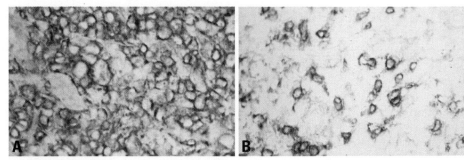

Fig. 7.30 Nasal NK/T-cell lymphoma immunostained for CD2 and surface CD3 on frozen section. **A** Almost all cells are CD2 positive. **B** The neoplastic cells are negative for surface CD3. The positive cells represent the admixed reactive T lymphocytes.

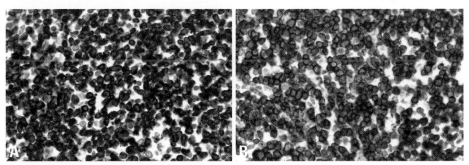

Fig. 7.31 Nasal NK/T-cell lymphoma, immunostaining. **A** The neoplastic cells show strong staining for cytoplasmic CD3ε. **B** They also stain for CD56.

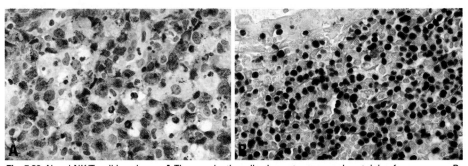

Fig. 7.32 Nasal NK/T-cell lymphoma. **A** The neoplastic cells show strong granular staining for granzyme B. **B** In situ hybridisation for EBV encoded RNA (EBER). In this nasal tumour, practically all the neoplastic cells show nuclear labelling.

whether this is a primary or progression-associated event {1407, 1198}.

Postulated cell of origin

Activated NK cells or (more rarely) cytotoxic T lymphocytes are the most likely normal counterpart.

Prognosis and predictive factors

The prognosis of nasal NK/T-cell lymphoma is variable, with some patients responding well to therapy and others dying of disseminated disease despite aggressive therapy {709, 222, 765}. The prognostic importance of cytological

grade is unclear; some studies suggest that tumours composed predominantly of small cells are less aggressive, but other studies have not shown this feature to be of significance on multivariate analysis {1243, 222, 524}.

Nasal-type NK/T-cell lymphoma occurring outside the nasal cavity is highly aggressive, with short survival times and poor response to therapy {203, 208}. Expression of multi-drug resistance genes may contribute to chemotherapy resistance in a majority of cases {320, 984}.

Enteropathy-type T-cell lymphoma

P. Isaacson
D. Wright
E. Ralfkiaer
E.S. Jaffe

Definition
Enteropathy-type T-cell lymphoma is a tumour of intraepithelial T-lymphocytes, showing varying degrees of transformation but usually presenting as a tumour composed of large lymphoid cells.

ICD-O code   9717/3

Synonyms
Lukes-Collins: not listed (T-immunoblastic)
Kiel: not listed (pleomorphic T-cell lymphoma, medium and large cell)
Working formulation: not listed (diffuse large cell, immunoblastic)
REAL: intestinal T-cell lymphoma (with and without enteropathy)

Epidemiology
The disease is uncommon in most parts of the world, but is seen with increasing frequency in those areas with a high prevalence of coeliac disease.

Sites of involvement
The tumour occurs most commonly in the jejunum or ileum. Presentation in the duodenum, stomach, colon or outside the gastrointestinal tract has been recorded, but is rare.

Clinical features
A small proportion of the patients have a history of childhood onset coeliac disease. Most show adult onset disease or are diagnosed as having coeliac disease in the same clinical episode in which the lymphoma is diagnosed. Patients pres-

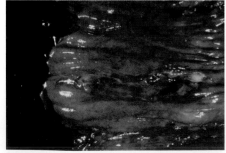

Fig. 7.33 Enteropathy-type T-cell lymphoma: jejunum showing circumferentially-oriented ulcers.

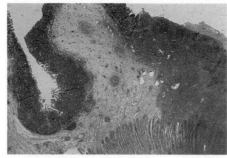

Fig. 7.34 Enteropathy-type T-cell lymphoma showing a deeply infiltrating tumour with adjacent enteropathic mucosa.

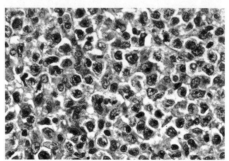

Fig. 7.35 Tumour cells are characterised by moderate amounts of eosinophilic cytoplasm and round or angulated nuclei with prominent nucleoli.

ent with abdominal pain, often associated with intestinal perforation.

Aetiology
There is a clear association with coeliac disease. Some cases, especially in South and Central America have been associated with EBV {1071}. However, extranodal NK/T-cell lymphoma, nasal type, commonly involves the gastrointestinal tract, and must be considered in the differential dignosis {929, 208}.

Precursor lesions
In a proportion of patients there is a prodromal period of refractory coeliac disease that is sometimes accompanied by intestinal ulceration (ulcerative jejunitis).

Macroscopy
The tumour usually presents as multiple ulcerating raised mucosal masses but may present as one or more ulcers or as a large exophytic mass.

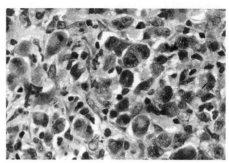

Fig. 7.36 Anaplastic variant of enteropathy-type T-cell lymphoma.

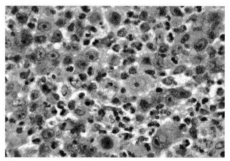

Fig. 7.37 Enteropathy-type T-cell lymphoma. There is a heavy infiltrate of eosinophils between the tumour cells.

Histopathology
The tumour forms an ulcerating mucosal mass that invades the wall of the intestine. There is a wide range of cytomorphological appearances {566, 1420}. Most commonly, the tumour cells are relatively monomorphic medium-sized to large cells with round or angulated vesicular nuclei, prominent nucleoli and moderate to abundant, pale-staining cytoplasm. Less commonly, the tumour exhibits marked pleomorphism with multinucleated cells bearing a resemblance to anaplastic large cell lymphoma.
Most tumours show infiltration by inflammatory cells, including large numbers of histiocytes and eosinophils and in some cases these may be so abundant as to obscure the relatively small number of tumour cells present. Infiltration of the epithelium of individual crypts is present in many cases. In a subset of cases the neoplastic cells are small and monomor-

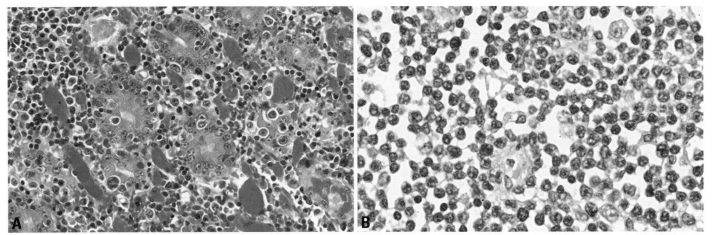

Fig. 7.38 Enteropathy-type T-cell lymphoma. **A** Individual lymphoma cells invading intestinal crypt epithelium. **B** Monomorphic variant composed of small to medium size cells.

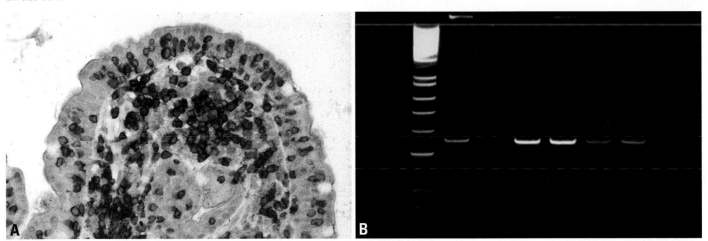

Fig. 7.39 A Small intestinal mucosa from a case of refractory coeliac disease immunostained sequentially for for CD3 (alkaline phosphatase-blue) and CD8 (peroxidase-brown). Most intraepithelial lymphocytes are CD3+, CD8-. **B** Polymerase chain reaction products of DNA extracted from enteropathy-type T-cell lymphoma and adjacent enteropathic mucosa . Lanes from the left are as follows: Lane 1, molecular weight markers; lane 2, positive control; lane 3, negative control; lanes 4 and 5, lymphoma; lanes 6 and 7, adjacent non-lymphomatous mucosa. An identical dominant clone, confirmed by sequencing, is present in the tumour and adjacent mucosa.

phic with darkly staining nuclei and a narrow rim of cytoplasm. The intestinal mucosa adjacent to the tumours, especially those in the jejunum, usually shows enteropathy comprising villous atrophy, crypt hyperplasia, increased lamina propria lymphocytes and plasma cells and intraepithelial lymphocytosis. The degree of enteropathy is highly variable, however, and may consist only of an increase in intraepithelial lymphocytes.

Immunophenotype

Tumour cells are CD3+, CD5-, CD7+, CD8-/+, CD4-, CD103+ and contain cytotoxic granule associated proteins. In almost all cases, a varying proportion of the tumour cells express CD30 {1420, 1214}. In the subset comprised of small to medium-sized cells the tumour cells

are CD8+ and express CD56 {225}. The intraepithelial lymphocytes in the adjacent enteropathic mucosa may show an abnormal immunophenotype, usually CD3+, CD5-, CD8-, CD4-,identical to that of the lymphoma. Likewise the intraepithelial lymphocytes in refractory coeliac disease are usually CD8- {191, 62}.

Genetics

Most patients show the HLA DQA1*0501, DQB1*0201 genotype that characterises coeliac disease {544}. TCR β and γ genes are clonally rearranged {568, 912}. Similar clonal rearrangements may be found in the adjacent enteropathic intestine {544} suggesting that the immunophenotypically aberrant intraepithelial lymphocytes constitute a neoplastic population. In refractory coeliac disease the

intraepithelial lymphocytes also comprise a monoclonal population and share the same clonal TCR gene rearrangement as the subsequent T-cell lymphomas that may develop {191, 51}

Postulated cell of origin

Intraepithelial T-cells of the intestine.

Prognosis

The prognosis is usually poor with death frequently resulting from abdominal complications in patients already weakened by uncontrolled malabsorption. Long-term survivals are recorded. Recurrences are most frequent in the small intestine.

Hepatosplenic T-cell lymphoma

E.S. Jaffe
E. Ralfkiaer

Definition
Hepatosplenic T-cell lymphoma is an extranodal and systemic neoplasm derived from cytotoxic T-cells usually of γδ T-cell receptor type, medium in size, demonstrating marked sinusoidal infiltration of spleen, liver and bone marrow.

ICD-O code   9716/3

Synonyms
Lukes-Collins: not listed
Kiel: not listed (pleomorphic T-cell lymphoma; small cell, medium-sized cell)
Working formulation: not listed
(diffuse small cleaved cell)
REAL: hepatosplenic γδ T-cell lymphoma

Epidemiology
This is a rare form of lymphoma, representing less than 5% of all peripheral T-cell neoplasms. Peak incidence occurs in adolescents and young adults, in males much more commonly than females {241}.

Sites of involvement
Patients present with marked hepatosplenomegaly with no peripheral lymphadenopathy {364}. Bone marrow is nearly always involved, but neoplastic cells may be difficult to detect in routine sections {241}. Lymph node involvement is rarely seen.

Clinical features
Patients usually manifest marked thrombocytopenia, often with anaemia and leukocytosis {241}. Abnormal cells are usually present in the bone marrow, but may be difficult to identify. A bone marrow biopsy with immunohistochemistry to identify neoplastic cells in sinusoids is useful in making the diagnosis. Peripheral blood involvement may occur, especially late in the clinical course.

Aetiology
Gamma delta T-cell lymphomas appear somewhat more common in immunosuppressed patients following solid organ transplantation. Therefore, chronic immune stimulation in the setting of immunosuppression has been postulated as playing a role {47, 1113}.

Macroscopy
The spleen is enlarged with diffuse involvement of the red pulp, without any gross lesions identifiable. Similarly, diffuse hepatic enlargement in the absence of gross lesions is seen.

Morphology
The cells of hepatosplenic T-cell lymphoma are monotonous, medium in size with a rim of pale cytoplasm {241}. The nuclear chromatin is loosely condensed with small inconspicuous nucleoli. Some irregularity of the nuclear contour can usually be seen. The liver and spleen show marked sinusoidal infiltration with sparing of portal triads and white pulp, respectively. Rare cases show greater cytologic atypia {825}.

Immunophenotype
The neoplastic cells are CD3+ and usually TCRδ1+, TCRαβ-, CD56±, CD4-, CD8- and CD5-. The cells express the cytotoxic granule associated protein, TIA-1, but are usually negative for perforin {241, 366}. Therefore, the cells do not appear to be functionally mature or activated cytotoxic T-cells. A minority of cases appear to be of αβ type, which is considered a variant of the more common γδ form of the disease {722}.

Genetics
The cells have rearranged TCR γ genes. TCR β genes may be germline or rearranged in some cases. Isochromosome 7q is present in all cases so-far studied, sometimes in conjunction with other abnormalities, most commonly trisomy 8 {20, 240, 1357}. *In situ* hybridisation for EBV has been negative.

Postulated cell of origin
Immature peripheral γδ (or less commonly αβ) T-cells of cytotoxic type {802}.

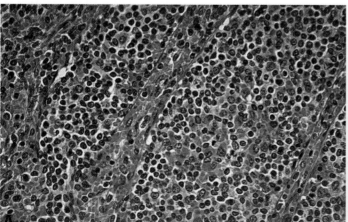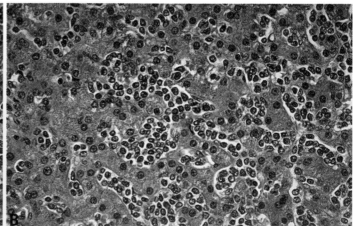

Fig. 7.40 Hepatosplenic T-cell lymphoma. **A** Splenic sinusoids are distended by a monotonous population of neoplastic lymphoid cells with a moderate rim of pale cytoplasm. **B** The neoplastic cells diffusely infiltrate the hepatic sinusoids.

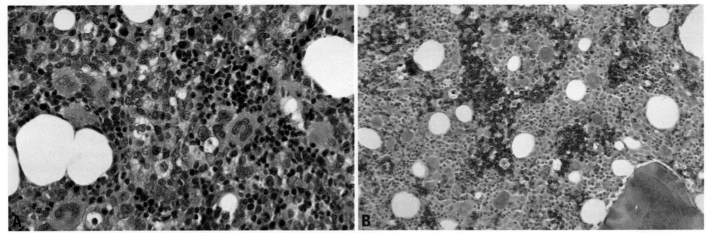

Fig. 7.41 Hepatosplenic T-cell lymphoma. **A** The bone marrow is usually hypercellular with neoplastic cells infiltrating sinusoids. **B** Neoplastic cells are difficult to detect in H&E stained sections, but are highlighted with immunohistochemistry for CD3.

Prognosis and predictive factors

The course is aggressive. Patients may respond initially to chemotherapy, but relapses are seen in the vast majority of cases. The median survival is less than 2 years. Hepatosplenic T-cell lymphomas of αβ type are more common in females, but otherwise have similar clinical features {1441}.

Variants

Other forms of γδ T-cell lymphoma with usually extranodal localisations occur. Frequent sites of involvement include skin and subcutaneous tissue, intestine, or the nasal region {47, 1303}. These do not seem to constitute a single entity, but resemble other forms of extranodal T-cell lymphomas including mycosis fun-goides, pagetoid reticulosis, subcutaneous panniculitis-like T-cell lymphoma, enteropathy-type T-cell lymphoma, and nasal NK/T-cell lymphomas.

Subcutaneous panniculitis-like T-cell lymphoma

E.S. Jaffe
E. Ralfkiaer

Definition
Subcutaneous panniculitis-like T-cell lymphoma (SPTCL) ia a cytotoxic T-cell lymphoma, which preferentially infiltrates subcutaneeous tissue. It is composed of atypical lymphoid cells of varying size, often with marked tumour necrosis and karyorrhexis.

ICD-O code   9708/3

Synonyms
Lukes-Collins: not listed
Kiel: not listed (pleomorphic T-cell lymphoma; small, medium-sized, mixed or large cell, immunoblastic T-cell lymphoma)
Working formulation: various categories (diffuse small cleaved cell, diffuse mixed small and large cell, diffuse large cell, immunoblastic)
REAL: subcutaneous panniculitic T-cell lymphoma

Epidemiology
SPTCL is a rare form of lymphoma, representing less than 1% of all non-Hodgkin lymphomas. It occurs in males and females equally, and has a broad age range. Cases have been reported in children under the age of two years. Most cases occur in young adults {701}.

Sites of involvement
Patients present with multiple subcutaneous nodules, usually in the absence of other sites of disease. The most common sites of localisation are the extremities and trunk. The nodules range in size from 0.5 cm to several centimeters in diameter. Larger nodules may become necrotic.

Clinical features
Clinical symptoms are primarily related to the subcutaneous nodules. Systemic symptoms are variable. Some patients may present with a haemophagocytic syndrome with pancytopenia, fever, and hepatosplenomegaly {447}. Lymphadenopathy is usually absent.

Aetiology
Some subcutaneous panniculitis-like T-cell lymphomas are of gamma delta phenotype, and in these cases immuno-

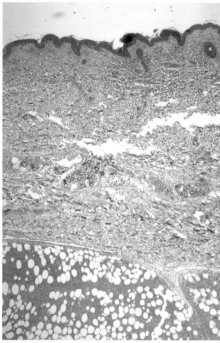

Fig. 7.42 Subcutaneous panniculitis-like T-cell lymphoma. At low power infiltrate is confined to the subcutaneous tissue without involvement of the overlying dermis or epidermis.

Table 7.07
T and NK-cell neoplasms with frequent/preferential cutaneous involvement.

	Clinical features	CD3,CD4,CD8	Cytotoxic granule associated proteins	CD56	EBV	T-cell receptor	Major lineage	Minor lineage
Mycosis fungoides	patches, plaques, tumours	CD3+,CD4+,CD8-	–	–	–	R	T αβ	T γδ
Subcutaneous	Subcutaneous	CD3+,CD4-,CD8+	+	–/+	–	R	T αβ	T γδ
Extranodal T/NK, nasal type	Tumours	sCD3-, cCD3+,CD4-,CD8-	+	+	+	G	NK	T αβ / T γδ
Primary cutaneous ALCL	Tumours (often solitary or localised)	CD3+,CD4+,CD8-	+	–	–	R	T αβ	
Blastic NK-cell lymphoma	Tumours	CD3-,CD4+,CD8-	–	+	–	G	Postulated NK precursor	

* ALCL = anaplastic large cell lymphoma

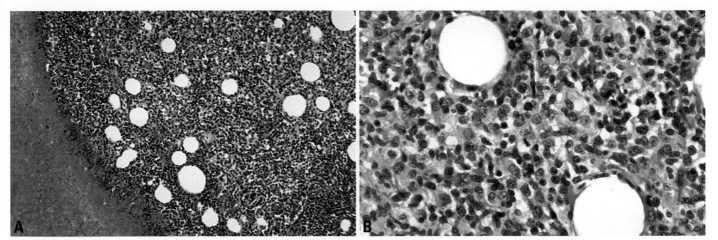

Fig. 7.43 Subcutaneous panniculitis-like T-cell lymphoma. **A** Cells diffusely infiltrate adipose tissue. Necrosis and karyorrhexis are common. **B** Neoplastic cells surround fat cells, often with some admixed histiocytes. However, other inflammatory cells are absent. This case was of T γδ derivation.

suppression appears to be a predisposing factor {47, 633}. In most patients the disease presents sporadically. Epstein Barr virus is absent {701}.

Precursor lesions
There is no evidence that there is a true precursor lesion. However, in initial biopsies the infiltrate may appear deceptively benign.

Histopathology
The infiltrate extends diffusely through the subcutaneous tissue, usually without sparing of septae. The overlying dermis and epidermis are typically uninvolved. The neoplastic cells range in size from small cells with round nuclei and inconspicuous nucleoli to larger transformed cells with hyperchromatic nuclei. The lymphoid cells have a moderate amount of pale-staining cytoplasm. A helpful diagnostic feature is the rimming of the neoplastic cells surrounding individual fat cells. Admixed reactive histiocytes are frequently present, particularly in areas of fat infiltration and destruction.

The histiocytes are frequently vacuolated, due to ingested lipid material. Vascular invasion may be seen in some cases, and necrosis and karyorrhexis are common. However, the infiltrates usually are confined to the subcutaneous tissue, with sparing of the dermis. This feature is helpful in the differential diagnosis from other lymphomas involving skin and subcutaneous tissue. Cases of gamma delta T-cell origin may show both dermal and epidermal involvement {701}.

Immunophenotype
The cells have a mature T-cell phenotype, usually CD8-positive, with expression of cytotoxic molecules including granzyme B, perforin, and T-cell intracellular antigen (TIA-1). Most cases are derived from αβ cells, although 25% of cases may be γδ positive {701, 1134, 366}. Cases of γδ origin are often double-negative for CD4 and CD8, and positive for CD56 {587}.

Possible normal counterpart
Mature cytotoxic T-cell.

Genetic features
The neoplastic cells show rearrangement of T-cell receptor genes, and are negative for Epstein Barr viral sequences. No specific cytogenetic features have been reported.

Prognosis
Dissemination to lymph nodes and other organs is uncommon and usually occurs late in the clinical course. The natural history is aggressive, but patients often respond effectively to combination chemotherapy {447, 1134, 680}. A haemophagocytic syndrome is a frequent complication and usually precipitates a fulminant downhill clinical course. However, if therapy for the underlying lymphoma is instituted and is successful, the haemophagocytic syndrome may remit.

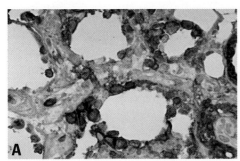
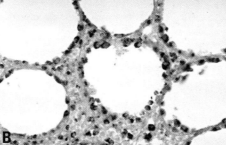
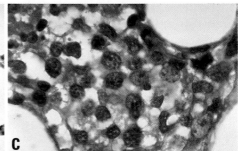

Fig. 7.44 Subcutaneous panniculitis-like T-cell lymphoma. **A, B** Immunohistochemical stains highlight the rimming of individual fat spaces by tumour cells, shown here with staining for CD 8 and TIA-1. **C** Neoplastic cells have round to oval hyperchromatic nuclei with inconspicuous nucleoli and abundant pale cytoplasm.

Blastic NK-cell lymphoma

J.K.C. Chan
E.S. Jaffe
E. Ralfkiaer

Definition

Blastic NK-cell lymphoma is composed of cells with a lymphoblast-like morphology and evidence of commitment to the NK lineage. At least a proportion of cases represent precursor NK-cell lymphoblastic lymphoma/leukaemia {679, 1264}.

The disease overlaps with and may be identical to the entity called primary cutaneous CD4+ CD56+ haematolymphoid neoplasm {1031}. The relationship with cases of acute myeloid leukaemia expressing CD56+ requires clarification {1166, 1250}.

ICD-O code   9727/3

Synonyms

Lukes-Collins, Kiel, Working Formulation, REAL: Not recognised
Others: Lymphoblastoid variant of NK-cell lymphoma, monomorphic NK-cell lymphoma

Epidemiology

This is a rare form of lymphoma. Currently it is unclear whether it shows any racial predilection like extranodal NK/T-cell lymphoma, nasal type. Most patients are middle-aged or elderly, but no age is exempt.

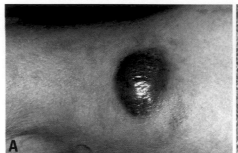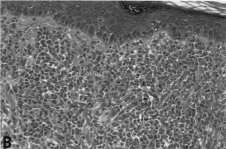

Fig. 7.45 Blastic NK-cell lymphoma. **A** Presenting as a skin tumour. **B** Involving skin. The dermis shows diffuse dense infiltration by lymphoma. Note absence of necrosis or angiocentric growth.

Sites of involvement

The disease tends to involve multiple sites, with a predilection for skin. Lymph node, soft tissue, peripheral blood or bone marrow can be simultaneously involved {929, 208, 203, 145}. Very rarely, the nasal cavity is the primary site of involvement {1069, 924}.

Clinical features

The patients usually present with extranodal tumour, most commonly in the form of skin lesions. There may be accompanying lymphadenopathy, and most patients have disseminated disease at presentation {929, 675, 131, 902}.

Aetiology

There are currently no clues to the aetiology of blastic NK-cell lymphoma. In contrast to extranodal NK/T-cell lymphoma, nasal type, there is no association with Epstein-Barr virus (EBV).

Morphology

Blastic NK-cell lymphoma is characterised by a diffuse monotonous infiltrate of medium-sized cells with fine chromatin, resembling lymphoblastic or myeloblastic leukaemia.

Not uncommonly, a single-file pattern of infiltration can be identified in areas. Coagulative necrosis and an angiocentric infiltrate are uncommon. Exceptionally, tumour cell rosettes resembling Homer-Wright rosettes can be formed {674}.

In Giemsa-stained touch preparations, azurophilic granules may or may not be found {827}.

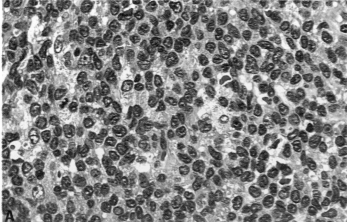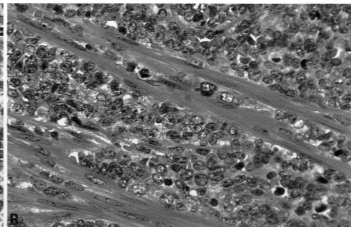

Fig. 7.46 Blastic NK-cell lymphoma. **A** The neoplastic cells are uniform and medium-sized, with fine chromatin and scanty cytoplasm, reminiscent of lymphoblastic lymphoma. **B** The neoplastic cells can be slightly larger, reminiscent of acute myeloid leukaemia.

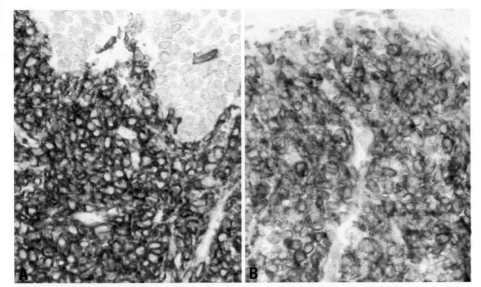

Fig. 7.47 Blastic NK-cell lymphoma. **A** The cells are strongly positive for CD43 and **B** CD56.

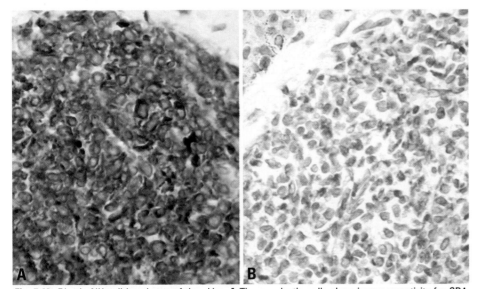

Fig. 7.48 Blastic NK-cell lymphoma of the skin. **A** The neoplastic cells show immunoreactivity for CD4, **B** but not for the cytotoxic marker TIA1.

Immunophenotype

The neoplastic cells are negative for surface CD3 and are positive for CD56. CD4 and CD43 are usually expressed. CD68 is generally negative, or only weakly focally expressed. Expression of CD2, CD7, cytoplasmic CD3ε and cytotoxic molecules is variable, but usually negative. Some cases are TdT and/or CD34-positive {929, 208, 303, 675, 827, 926}. Because of the morphologic similarity to lymphoblastic and myeloblastic neoplasms and the fact that CD56 may be expressed in both myeloblastic and precursor T-lymphoblastic leukaemia / lymphoma, the diagnosis of blastic NK-cell lymphoma should only be made in the absence of commitment to the T-cell or myeloid lineages. Thus the neoplastic cells should be negative for surface CD3, myeloperoxidase and CD33, and the diagnosis is preferably supported by absence of TCR gene rearrangements.

Genetics

T-cell receptor genes are germline, and all cases studied so far have been EBV negative {208, 303, 1069, 924, 827}. Specific chromosomal aberrations have not been observed.

Postulated cell of origin

A precursor NK-cell origin has been proposed. However, the precise lineage of this neoplasm is still unresolved.

Prognosis and predictive factors

The clinical course is aggressive with a poor response to regimens used for non-Hodgkin lymphomas. Partial responses to "acute leukaemia-like" regimens have been seen in rare cases. Cases with localised skin lesions have a better prognosis.

Mycosis fungoides and Sézary syndrome

E. Ralfkiaer
E.S. Jaffe

Mycosis fungoides

Definition
Mycosis fungoides is a mature T-cell lymphoma presenting in the skin with patches/plaques and characterised by epidermal and dermal infiltration of small to medium-sized T-cells with cerebriform nuclei.

ICD-O code   9700/3

Synonyms
Lukes-Collins: cerebriform T
Kiel: small cell, cerebriform
Working Formulation: mycosis fungoides
REAL: mycosis fungoides

Epidemiology
Mycosis fungoides is the most common subtype of the T-cell lymphomas that arise primarily in the skin {1387}. However, with an estimated annual incidence of 0.29 per 100,000 it is overall a rare disease which accounts for no more than 0.5% of all non-Hodgkin lymphomas {655}. Most patients are adults/elderly. The male to female ratio is 2:1 {655}.

Sites of involvement
The disease is as a rule limited to the skin for a protracted period (years). Extracutaneous dissemination may occur in advanced stages, mainly to lymph nodes, liver, spleen, lungs and blood {655}. Involvement of the bone marrow is rare.

Clinical features
The disease has a long natural history. Thus many patients show non-specific scaly eruptions years before a diagnostic histology develops. The initial diagnostic lesions are limited patches and/or plaques, frequently on the trunk. These lesions may persist for years. However, in most patients they progress to more generalised, infiltrated plaques and eventually further on to tumours {1387, 655}. Rare patients may develop a generalised disease with erythroderma, and such cases may overlap with Sézary syndrome. Cases of so-called d'emblee lesions (presenting with skin tumours without a preceding patch/plaque stage) are rare and not entirely well-defined. Indeed it is likely that most such lesions are in reality examples of other subtypes of T-cell lymphoma with preferential cutaneous infiltrates. Extracutaneous dissemination in mycosis fungoides is usually a late event and predominantly occurs in patients with extensive/advanced cutaneous disease {655}.

Aetiology
The pathogenesis of the disease is unknown. HTLV-1 (or a related virus) has been implicated in some studies which have shown that truncated proviral sequences similar to tax and/or pol could be detected by PCR in 30-90% of the patients in a series from the United States {995, 434}. A majority of these patients have antibodies to tax, but unlike adult T-cell leukaemia/lymphoma, not to the

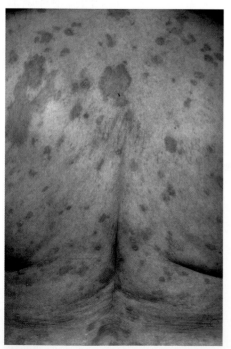

Fig. 7.49 Mycosis fungoides, disseminated plaque stage.

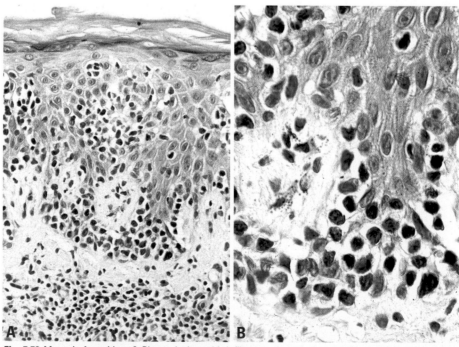

Fig. 7.50 Mycosis fungoides. **A** Plaque lesion with infiltrates of atypical, cerebriform lymphocytes in the upper dermis. **B**. The epidermis is involved, mainly with single cells.

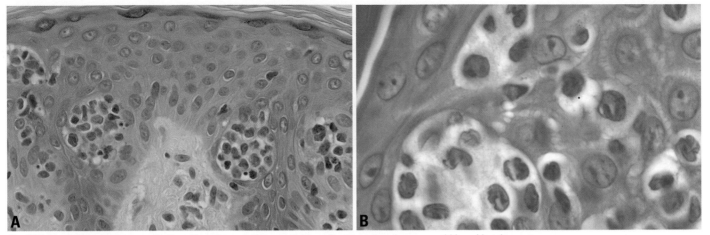

Fig. 7.51 Mycosis fungoides, neoplastic cells with cerebriform nuclei form Pautrier microabscesses within epidermis.

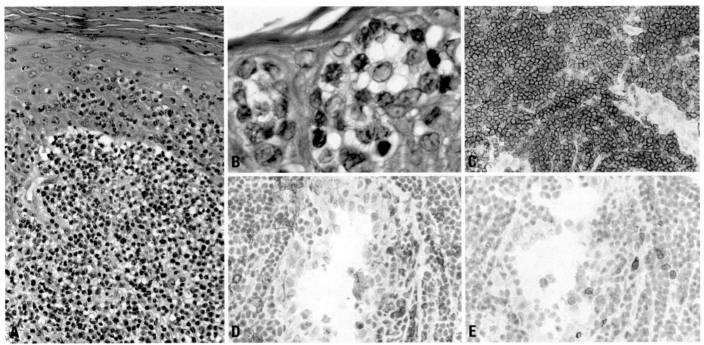

Fig. 7.52 Mycosis fungoides. **A** Tumour lesion with more massive infiltrates involving both the upper and deep dermis. **B** In the epidermis, Pautrier abcesses can be seen. **C** The neoplastic cells show an aberrant phenotype with expression of CD3, but no reaction for either CD4 **(D)** or CD8 **(E)**.

structural proteins of HTLV-1 {995, 994}. Thus, it is possible that HLTV-1 (or a related virus) may be associated with the disease in some patients. Whether this virus is a cause of the disease or is a secondary event is not known {756}. Furthermore, these laboratory findings have shown geographical variation and were not identified in a European series {117}.

Morphology

Skin lesions show epidermotropic infiltrates consisting of small to medium-sized cells with irregular (cerebriform) nuclei {1387}. A minority of larger cells with sim-

ilar nuclei may be present, but are never prominent. So-called Pautrier microabscesses, consisting of aggregates of cerebriform cells in the epidermis, are highly characteristic, but are only seen in a proportion of the cases. Epidermal involvement with single cell exocytosis is more common {1387}. In the dermis, infiltrates may be patchy, band-like or diffuse depending upon the stage of the disease. There is often an associated inflammatory infiltrate consisting of small lymphocytes and eosinophils. These cells are especially numerous in early skin lesions. Enlarged lymph nodes from patients with

mycosis fungoides frequently show dermatopathic lymphadenopathy with paracortical expansion due to the presence of large number of histiocytes and interdigitating cells with abundant, pale cytoplasm. Different histological grades/categories, reflecting the degree of lymph node involvement, have been introduced in some studies, i.e. category I (no involvement); category II (early involvement); and category III (massive involvement) {236, 1155}. In category I, lymph nodes show dermatopathic lymphadenopathy. Scattered cerebriform lymphocytes or small foci of 3-6 atypical

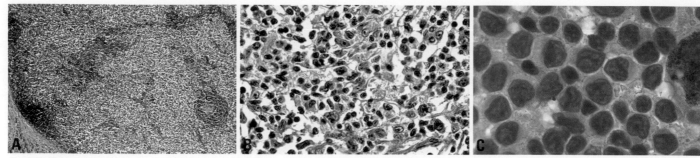

Fig. 7.53 Mycosis fungoides, partial lymph node involvement, corresponding to category II. **A** At low magnification, features of dermatopathic lymphadenopathy are seen with marked expansion of the paracortical area that appears pale due to a large number of histiocytes/interdigitating cells. **B** At higher magnification, sheets of atypical lymphocytes are evident. **C** In touch imprint, atypical cells with cerebriform nuclei are appreciated. Macrophages containing abundant melanin pigment are also present.

Table 7.08
Grading of lymph node involvement in mycosis fungoides (modified from Colby et al., Scheffer et al. {236, 1155}).

Category	Histologic features
I (LN0-2), no involvement by MF	Dermatopathic lymphadenopathy; scattered cerebriform lymphocytes may be present, but clusters are not seen.
II (LN3), early involvement by MF	Focal obliteration of architecture with clusters of atypical, cerebriform lymphocytes, often mainly paracortical in distribution.
III (LN4), massive involvement by MF	Complete replacement of architecture with diffuse infiltrates of atypical, cerebriform lymphocytes.

cells may be present, but larger clusters are not seen. Category II lymph nodes show partial effacement of the architecture with clusters and/or sheets of atypical, cerebriform lymphocytes that are often mainly paracortical in distribution. Lymph nodes in category III show more massive, diffuse infiltrates with complete effacement of the normal architecture {236, 1155}.

Studies of the T-cell receptor genes in lymph nodes classified according to these criteria have shown that clonal T-cells are present in a majority of category II and III lesions, and occasionally in category I lesions {798, 647, 66}. There are indications that the presence of clonal T-cells may be associated with an unfavourable outcome, also in cases that are scored as negative (uninvolved) by conventional examination {798, 647, 66}. It is therefore recommended that T-cell receptor rearrangement analyses are performed in all cases that are not obviously involved by histological examination.

Infiltrates of mycosis fungoides in organs other than the skin and lymph nodes may be massive or interstitial depending upon the degree of infiltration.

Table 7.09
Clinical staging system used for mycosis fungoides {1329}.

Stage I	Disease confined to the skin either with limited patches/plaques (stage Ia); disseminated patches/plaques (stage Ib); or skin tumours (stage Ic)
Stage II	Lymph nodes enlarged, but uninvolved histologically
Stage III	Lymph node involvement documented by histology
Stage IV	Visceral dissemination

Immunophenotype

The typical phenotype is CD2+, CD3+, TCRβ+, CD5+, CD4+, CD8- {1387, 1079}. Rare cases may be positive for CD8 or TCRδ {1079, 905}. A lack of CD7 is frequent in all stages of the disease. However, this feature is of limited value from a diagnostic point of view, since a lack of CD7 may also be seen in benign cutaneous lymphoid lesions {1079}. Aberrant expression of other T-cell antigens may be seen, but mainly occurs in the advanced (tumour) stages {1079}. HECA antigen associated with lymphocyte homing to the skin is expressed in most cases {1387}. Cytotoxic granule associated proteins are not expressed in the early patch/plaque lesions, but may be positive in a fraction of the neoplastic cells in the more advanced lesions {1344}.

Genetics

T-cell receptor genes are clonally rearranged in most cases {99}. Inactivation of *CDKN2A/p16* and *PTEN* has been identified in 2 studies {938, 1151} and may be associated with disease progression. Complex karyotypes are present in many patients, in particular in the advanced stages {1382, 1280}. A vast number of different structural and numerical alterations have been described, but so far no specific abnormality has been identified.

Postulated cell of origin

Peripheral, epidermotropic T-cells.

Prognosis and predictive features

The single most important prognostic factor in mycosis fungoides is the extent of the disease, as reflected in the clinical stage. Patients with limited disease generally have an excellent prognosis with a similar survival as the background population {655, 1387, 1329}. In the more advanced stages, the prognosis is poor, in particular in patients with skin tumours and/or extracutaneous dissemination {655, 1387, 1329}. Age above 60 years and elevated LDH are other adverse prognostic indicators {297}. As a terminal event, transformation to a large T-cell lymphoma may be seen {1343, 296}. Such cases also show an aggressive behaviour.

Sézary syndrome

Definition
Sézary syndrome is a generalised mature T-cell lymphoma characterised by the presence of erythroderma, lymphadenopathy and neoplastic T-lymphocytes in the blood. The neoplastic T-cells have cerebriform nuclei, and the disease is by tradition regarded as a variant of mycosis fungoides. However, the behaviour is usually much more aggressive.

ICD-O code   9701/3

Synonyms
Kiel: small cell, cerebriform
Lukes-Collins: cerebriform T
Working Formulation: mycosis fungoides
REAL: Sézary syndrome

Epidemiology
This is a rare disease. It occurs exclusively in adults {1387}.

Sites of involvement
This is by definition a generalised disease with involvement of skin, lymph nodes and blood. All visceral organs may be involved in the terminal stages. However, there is often a remarkable sparing of the bone marrow {1387, 655}.

Clinical features
Patients present with erythroderma and general enlargement of lymph nodes. Other features are pruritus, alopecia, palmar or plantar hyperkeratoses and onychodystrophy {1387}.

Aetiology
The pathogenesis of the disease is unknown. The association with HTLV-1 is controversial {434}.

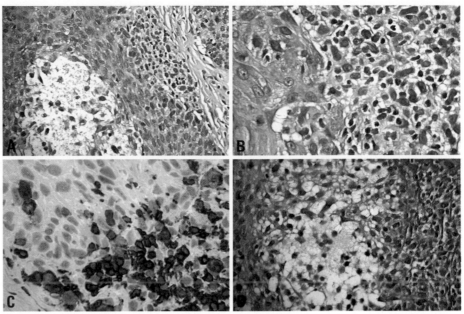
Fig. 7.54 Mycosis fungoides. **A** Mycosis fungoides associated follicular mucinosis with atypical lymphocytes infiltrating a hair follicle. **B** At a higher magnification, cerebriform nuclei are appreciated. **C** The atypical cells are CD3 positive. **D** The involved follicle shows mucinous degeneration with accumulation of Alcian blue-positive material.

Morphology
Skin lesions in Sézary syndrome are similar to those in mycosis fungoides with epidermal and dermal infiltrates of cerebriform T-lymphocytes. Involved lymph nodes show effaced architecture and paracortical or diffuse infiltrates with or without associated features of dermatopathic lymphadenopathy. In the blood neoplastic cells contain markedly convoluted nuclei and may appear either predominantly small (Lutzner cells) or large (classical Sézary cells) {1387}, or there may be a mixture of small and large cells. The proportion of neoplastic cells in the blood varies from few to many. There is no consensus upon the degree of blood lymphocytes required. However, a minimum of 1000 Sézary cells per mm³ blood is required in most studies {1387, 655}. The demonstration of an elevated CD4/CD8 ratio, of increased proportions of CD4+, CD7- T-lymphocytes and of clonal rearrangement of the T-cell receptor genes are other useful diagnostic criteria {1387, 1126}. When the bone marrow is involved, infiltrates are often sparse and mainly interstitial.

Immunophenotype
Tumour cells are CD2+, CD3+, TCRβ+, CD5+ and CD7 ±. Most cases are CD4+. Expression of CD8 is rare {1387}. Aberrant T-cell phenotypes are common.

Genetics
T-cell receptor genes are clonally rearranged {1126}. Consistent cytoge-

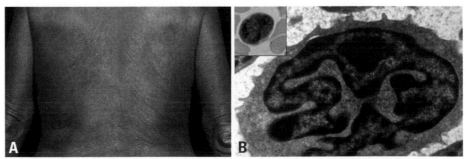
Fig. 7.55 Sézary syndrome. **A** Generalised skin disease with erythroderma. **B** Peripheral blood with typical Sézary cells. The markedly convoluted (cerebriform) nuclei are easily seen by ultrastructural examination. The inset shows the morphology in Giemsa stained blood films.

netic abnormalities have not been identified, but complex karyotypes are frequent, similar to mycosis fungoides {1382, 1280}.

Postulated cell of origin
Peripheral, epidermotropic T-cells.

Prognosis and predictive features
This is an aggressive disease with an overall survival rate at 5 years of between 10 and 20% {1387, 655}. As a terminal event, transformation to a large T-cell lymphoma may be seen {296}.

Variants
Pagetoid reticulosis
Pagetoid reticulosis is a variant of mycosis fungoides in which the infiltrates are strictly epidermal. A distinction is by tradition made between cases with localised (Woringer-Kolopp disease) or multiple (Ketron-Goodman disease) skin lesions. However, it is generally recommended that the designation be restricted to the localised variants which have an excellent prognosis {1387}. The neoplastic T-cells contain cerebriform nuclei, similar to mycosis fungoides. They are often CD30-positive and may be either CD8+, CD4-; CD8-, CD4+; or CD4-, CD8- {479}. Clonal T-cell receptor gene rearrangement has been shown in some cases {479}.

Mycosis fungoides-associated follicular mucinosis
This is a rare disease characterised by follicular (rather than epidermal) infil-

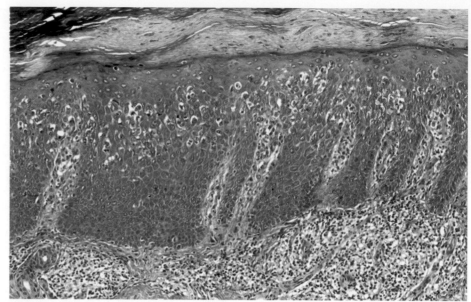

Fig. 7.56 Pagetoid reticulosis with prominent epidermal infiltrates of atypical, cerebriform lymphocytes.

trates of cerebriform T-cells associated with mucinous degeneration of hair follicles {435}. The disease preferentially involves the head and neck area. Clonal T-cell receptor gene rearrangements are found in most cases. The course is indolent, although prognosis seems to be slightly less favourable than in "classical" mycosis fungoides {1387}.

Granulomatous slack skin
Granulomatous slack skin disease is a rare lymphoproliferative disease. It is by tradition regarded as a variant of mycosis fungoides. It may, however, also be seen in association with other types of lymphoma, e.g. Hodgkin lymphoma, and it is possible that it may be a distinct entity. The salient features are slowly developing folds of atrophic skin, preferential involvement of the axillae or groin and a granulomatous infiltrate consisting of atypical T-lymphocytes admixed with macrophages and multi-nucleated giant cells {743}. The latter cells show elastophagocytosis which is highly characteristic. Clonally rearranged TCR genes have been demonstrated in some patients {743}.

Primary cutaneous CD30-positive T-cell lymphoproliferative disorders

E. Ralfkiaer
G. Delsol
R. Willemze
E.S. Jaffe

Three types of primary cutaneous CD30-positive T-cell lymphoproliferative disorders are distinguished. These include:
1. Primary cutaneous anaplastic large cell lymphoma (C-ALCL)
2. Lymphomatoid papulosis
3. Borderline lesions.

These disorders are grouped together because they seem to constitute a spectrum of related conditions originating from transformed or activated CD30-positive T-lymphocytes {1387}. They may coexist in individual patients {844}, they can be clonally related {227} and they often show overlapping clinical and/or histological features {82}. Accordingly, a correct diagnosis always requires assessment of both clinical, histological, and phenotypic features.

Primary cutaneous anaplastic large cell lymphoma (C-ALCL)

Definition

A T-cell lymphoma, presenting in the skin and consisting of anaplastic lymphoid cells, the majority of which are CD30-positive. Distinction from systemic ALCL with cutaneous involvement and secondary high-grade lymphomas with CD30 expression is important clinically. In nearly all patients the disease is limited to the skin at the time of diagnosis as assessed by meticulous staging {1387, 82}. Furthermore, patients should not suffer from other subtypes of lymphoma {1387, 82}.

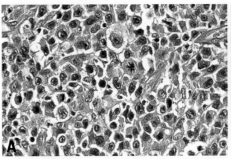
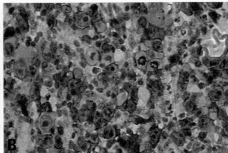

Fig. 7.58 Primary cutaneous anaplastic large cell lymphoma. **A** The infiltrate consists of large lymphoid cells with pronounced nuclear pleomorphism and many mitotic figures. **B** The neoplastic cells are strongly positive for CD30 with both membrane labelling and cytoplasmic dots (CD30).

ICD-O code 9718/3

Synonyms
Lukes-Collins: not listed (T-immuno-blastic)
Kiel: anaplastic large cell
Working Formulation: various categories (diffuse large cell; immunoblastic)
REAL: primary cutaneous anaplastic large cell (CD30+) lymphoma
Related terms: regressing atypical histiocytosis; Ki-1 lymphoma

Epidemiology
The primary cutaneous CD30-positive T-cell lymphoproliferative disorders account for approximately 25% of the T-cell lymphomas which arise primarily in the skin {1387}. They occur predominantly in adults/elderly and are rare in children {1387, 82}. The male to female ratio is 1.5-2.0:1.

Sites of involvement
The disease is nearly always limited to the skin at the time of diagnosis. Extracutaneous dissemination may occur, mainly to regional lymph nodes. Involve-ment of other organs is rare {1387, 82}.

Clinical features
Most patients present with limited disease with solitary or localised skin lesions which may be tumours, nodules or (more rarely) papules {1387, 82}. Multicentric cutaneous disease is seen in approximately 20% of the cases {82}.

Lesions may show partial or complete spontaneous regression, similar to lymphomatoid papulosis. However, cutaneous relapses are frequent {82}. Extracutaneous dissemination occurs in approximately 10% of the patients, mainly to regional lymph nodes and most frequently in patients with multicentric cutaneous disease {844, 82}.

Aetiology
The cause of the disease is unknown.

Morphology
The cytological features are similar to those of systemic ALCL. However, pleomorphic, multinucleated giant cells and Reed-Sternberg-like cells are often more numerous, and resemble the Hodgkin-like cells seen in Type A lesions of lymphomatoid papulosis. The infiltrates are diffuse and usually involve both the upper and deep dermis and the subcutaneous tissue {1387}. Epidermal invasion and ulceration may be seen, but epidermotropism is less common. A modest inflammatory background may be seen, but if the inflammatory background is abundant, the diagnosis of lymphomatoid papulosis should be considered.

Immunophenotype
The neoplastic cells express T-cell antigens and are usually positive for CD4 {1387, 704}. CD30 is expressed by a majority (>75%) of the cells {1387}. Cytotoxic granule associated proteins

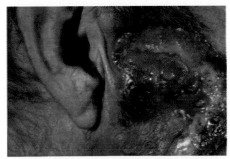

Fig. 7.57 Primary cutaneous anaplastic large cell lymphoma presenting with an ulcerated skin tumour.

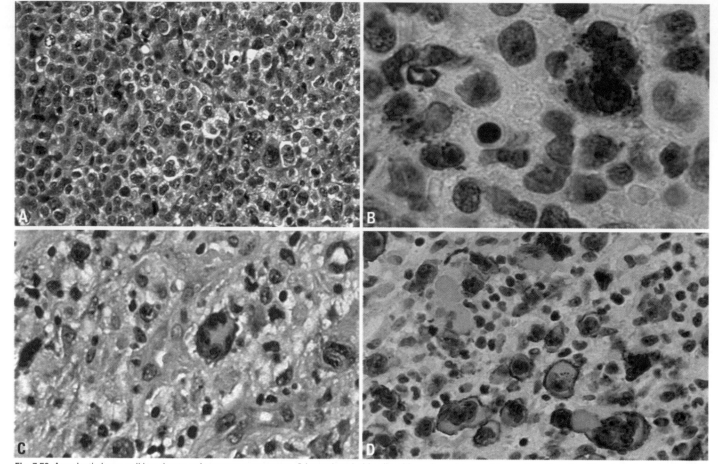

Fig. 7.59 Anaplastic large cell lymphoma, primary cutaneous type. **A** Large lymphoid cells with nuclear pleomorphism and scattered multinucleated giant cells (HE). **B** A fraction of the neoplastic cells are positive for TIA-1. **C** Numerous multinucleated giant cells (HE). **D** The cells are strongly CD30-positive.

(granzyme B, perforin, TIA-1) are positive in 70% of the cases {704, 126}. Aberrant T-cell phenotypes with variable loss of CD2, CD5 and/or CD3 are common, but null cell phenotypes are rare {1387}. Half of the lesions are positive for the cutaneous lymphocyte antigen recognised by HECA-452 {1387}. Unlike systemic neoplasms, most cutaneous cases are negative for epithelial membrane antigen (EMA) {1387}. Staining for the ALK protein is negative {105}.

Genetics
TCR genes are clonally rearranged in most cases {1387}. *NPM-ALK* fusion transcripts have been reported in a few cases by sensitive, nested RT-PCR techniques {105}. However, such cases clearly constitute an extremely small minority, and most likely represent systemic ALCL presenting with cutaneous disease. Thus the t(2;5) translocation is not found in this disease {105, 1409, 1376, 276}.

Postulated cell of origin
Transformed or activated skin-homing T-lymphocyte.

Prognosis and predictive features
The prognosis is favourable with an overall survival rate at 5 years of approximately 90% {82}. The presence of extracutaneous disease is an unfavourable prognostic indicator, whereas spontaneous regression of skin lesions has been associated with a favourable outcome {1342, 1011}. In cases with limited disease, skin-directed therapies are recommended such as radiotherapy or surgical excision. Aggressive, multiagent chemotherapy should be reserved for cases with overt/developing extracutaneous involvement {82}. Multiagent chemotherapy in patients with multifocal skin lesions, but no extracutaneous disease, does not prevent subsequent skin relapses, and should therefore only be given by exception.

Lymphomatoid papulosis

Definition
Lymphomatoid papulosis is a chronic recurrent skin disease characterised by the appearance of spontaneously regressing papules and an atypical T-cell infiltrate which can mimic a T-cell lymphoma histologically.

The disease usually has a benign course and is therefore not a lymphoma strictly speaking, but rather an atypical lymphoproliferation which can be clonal and progress to lymphoma in some instances.

ICD-O code   9718/1

Synonyms
Lukes-Collins: not listed
Kiel: not listed
Working Formulation: not listed
REAL: not listed
Epidemiology

This is a rare disease which predominantly affects adults/elderly. The male to female ratio is 1.5:1 {1387, 82}.

Sites of involvement
This disease is limited to the skin. Extracutaneous dissemination only occurs in cases with progression to lymphoma.

Clinical features
The characteristic skin lesions are recurrent papules and/or nodules which regress spontaneously, typically within 3 to 6 weeks {82}. Larger tumour lesions greater than 2.5 cm showing regression are rarely seen {82}.

Aetiology
The cause of the disease is unknown.

Morphology
Fully developed papular lesions show wedge-shaped, dermal infiltrates consisting of atypical T lymphocytes admixed with varying proportions of inflammatory cells such as neutrophils, eosinophils, macrophages and small lymphocytes. The atypical T-lymphocytes may resemble the cerebriform cells seen in mycosis fungoides or they may assume Reed-Sternberg (RS)-like features. A distinction is made between type A and type B lesions {1387, 82}. In type A lesions many RS-like cells are present together with numerous inflammatory cells. Type B lesions show a predominance of cells with cerebriform nuclei and contain only few inflammatory cells. In individual patients both types of lesions may exist.

Immunophenotype
The atypical T cells are CD4+, CD8-. They often express aberrant phenotypes with variable loss of pan-T-cell antigens, e.g. CD2, CD5 {614, 1081}. CD30 is positive in type A lesions, but often negative in type B lesions {1387}. Cytotoxic granule associated proteins are expressed by the atypical cells in most cases {126}. The ALK protein is consistently absent {105}.

Genetics
Clonally rearranged TCR genes are seen in a majority of type B lesions and occasionally in type A lesions {1371, 1383}. Overall clonal rearrangement of TCR genes can be detected in approximately

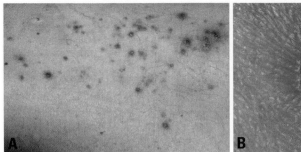
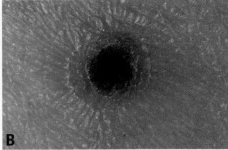

Fig. 7.60 Lymphomatoid papulosis. **A** Numerous skin papules; some are necrotic and ulcerated. **B** A close up of a typical, partially necrotic papule.

half of the patients. Identical patterns of rearrangement have been demonstrated in lymphomatoid papulosis and associated lymphoma lesions in some patients {227}. The t(2;5) translocation does not occur {105, 1409}.

Possibly normal counterpart
Activated skin-homing T-lymphocyte.

Prognosis and predictive features
Most patients follow a benign course, but the disease is often of long duration (years). Low-dose methotrexate (5-20 mg/week) and psoralen/UVA (PUVA) therapy are the best available therapies to reduce the number of skin lesions and recurrences. However, after discontinua-

tion of whatever therapy is selected, the disease continues its natural course. Therefore, treatment should be reserved for patients with large, numerous and/or scarring skin lesions {82}. Association with lymphoma is seen in 10-20% of the patients {1387, 82}. Various lymphomas have been described, including mycosis fungoides, C-ALCL, and Hodgkin lymphoma {1387, 844, 227, 82}. There are as yet no known criteria which can reliably predict which patients will progress to lymphoma {82}. Long term follow-up is therefore recommended.

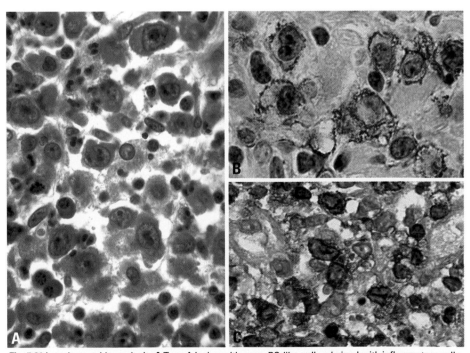

Fig. 7.61 Lymphomatoid papulosis. **A** Type A lesion with many RS-like cells admixed with inflammatory cells. **B** Type A lesion. The RS-like cells shown are strongly positive for CD30. **C** Type B lesion. The infiltrate is composed of cerebriform cells which are strongly positive for CD3.

Borderline lesions

Related term: lymphomatoid papulosis, diffuse large cell type (type C); anaplastic large cell lymphoma, lymphomatoid papulosis-like histology.

Borderline lesions of CD30-positive primary cutaneous T-cell lymphoproliferative disorders are lesions in which there is a discrepancy between the clinical features and the histological appearance {1387}. As a consequence these lesions are difficult to classify as either "classical" lymphomatoid papulosis or frank C-ALCL. Cases that mimic a lymphoma histologically (confluent sheets of CD30-positive atypical/anaplastic lymphoid cells), but resemble lymphomatoid papulosis clinically (regressing papules) have been referred to as lymphomatoid papulosis, type C {1387, 82}. The opposite situation (solitary skin tumours resembling lymphomatoid papulosis histologically) has been termed anaplastic lymphoma, lymphomatoid papulosis-like {82}. Reports of borderline lesions of primary cutaneous CD30-positive T-cell lymphoproliferative disorders are few. The prognosis seems to be favourable {1387, 1011}, but long term follow-up is required.

Angioimmunoblastic T-cell lymphoma

E.S. Jaffe
E. Ralfkiaer

Definition

Angioimmunoblastic T-cell lymphoma (AILT) is a peripheral T-cell lymphoma characterised by systemic disease, a polymorphous infiltrate involving lymph nodes, with a prominent proliferation of high endothelial venules and follicular dendritic cells.

ICD-O code   9705/3

Synonyms

Lukes-Collins: immunoblastic lymphadenopathy
Working Formulation: various categories (diffuse mixed small and large cell, diffuse large cell, immunoblastic, atypical hyperplasia)
Kiel: AILD-type (Lymphogranulomatosis X) T-cell lymphoma
REAL: angioimmunoblastic T-cell lymphoma

Epidemiology

AILT occurs in the middle aged and elderly, with an equal incidence in males and females.
It is one of the more common specific subtypes of peripheral T-cell neoplasms, accounting for approximately 15-20% of cases, or 1-2% of all non-Hodgkin lymphomas {8}.

Sites of involvement

Patients usually present with generalised peripheral lymphadenopathy, hepatosplenomegaly, and frequent skin rash. Bone marrow is commonly involved upon biopsy.

Clinical features

Angioimmunoblastic T-cell lymphoma usually presents with advanced stage disease, systemic symptoms, and polyclonal hypergammaglobulinemia {1194, 576}. Skin rash, often with pruritus, is frequently present. Other common symptoms are oedema, pleural effusion, arthritis, and ascites. An association with drug hypersensitivity reactions was described in early series. Laboratory findings include circulating immune complexes, cold agglutinins with haemolytic anaemia, positive rheumatoid factor, and anti-smooth muscle antibodies.

Aetiology

Patients exhibit immunodeficiency, but the immune abnormalities appear secondary to the neoplastic process, rather than preceding it. Cells positive for Epstein-Barr virus (EBV) are found in the majority of cases (> 75%). However, the EBV-positive cells are for the most part B-cells {1368}. Another study found evidence for EBV localisation in the T-cells as well {24}.

Precursor lesions

AILT was initially felt to be an atypical reactive process, angioimmunoblastic lymphadenopathy, with an increased risk of progression to lymphoma. Currently, most individuals believe that AILT arises de novo as a peripheral T-cell lymphoma. However, some argue that atypical and oligoclonal proliferations may precede the development of lymphoma, and consider that angioimmunoblastic lymphadenopathy may be in some cases a preneoplastic process {408, 1201}.

Histopathology

The lymph node architecture is partially effaced, and regressed follicles are often evident. The paracortex is diffusely infiltrated by a polymorphous population of small to medium-sized lymphocytes, usually with clear to pale cytoplasm and distinct cell membranes {408, 928}. The lymphocytes show minimal cytologic atypia, and this form of lymphoma may be difficult to distinguish from atypical T-zone hyperplasia. The abnormal lymphoid cells are admixed with small, reactive lymphocytes, eosinophils, plasma cells, histiocytes and increased numbers of fol-

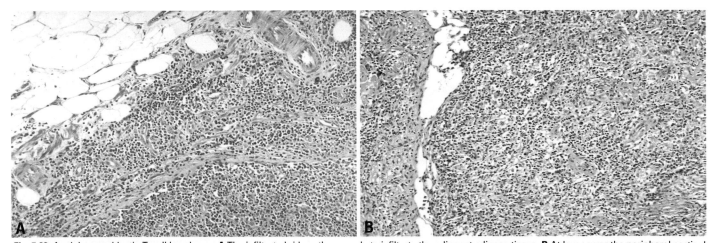

Fig. 7.62 Angioimmunoblastic T-cell lymphoma. **A** The infiltrate bridges the capsule to infiltrate the adjacent adipose tissue. **B** At low power the peripheral cortical sinus is often patent and distended.

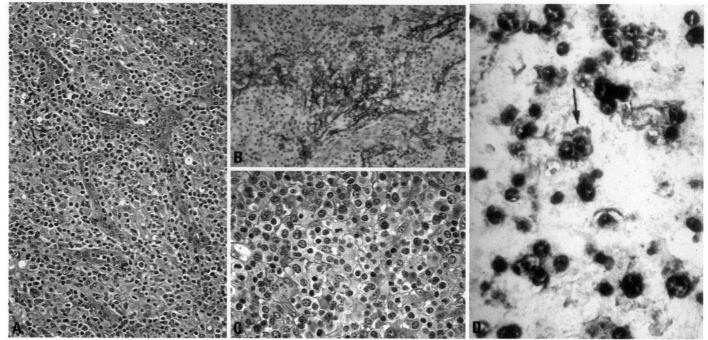

Fig. 7.63 Angioimmunoblastic T-cell lymphoma. **A** Low power shows architectural effacement by a polymorphous lymphoid infiltrate. Prominent arborizing blood vessels are evident. **B** Staining for CD21 highlights the processes of follicular dendritic cells which abut and extend from the post-capillary venules. Remnants of follicular dendritic cells also may be found in residual regressed follicles. **C** The infiltrate is composed of medium to large lymphoid cells with abundant clear cytoplasm. These cells, which are CD3-positive, are associated with a polymorphous inflammatory background. **D** Numerous cells positive for Epstein Barr virus are characteristically present. By double staining, most of the EBER-positive cells are CD20-positive (arrow).

licular dendritic cells (best appreciated by immunohistological examination). Large basophilic blasts of B-cell phenotype may be present. Reed-Sternberg-like cells may be seen {1068}. The infiltrate typically bridges the lymph node capsule, but the peripheral cortical sinus may be patent. High endothelial venules are abundant and show arborisation. In rare cases hyperplastic germinal centres may be seen; such cases may show progression to typical AILT {1093}.

Grading

Grading of AILT is generally not performed. However, individual cases often show variation in the proportion of T-cell immunoblasts. An increase in T-cell immunoblasts may be observed over time.

Immunophenotype

The infiltrates are composed of mature T-cells, usually with an admixture of CD4 and CD8 cells. CD4+ cells usually outnumber CD8+ cells. Plasma cells are polyclonal. Follicular dendritic cells (CD21+) are conspicuous, usually surrounding the high endothelial venules. This latter feature is helpful in differential diagnosis.

It has been proposed that the CD21-positive cells may not be true follicular dendritic cells, but rather fibroblastic reticu-

lum cells showing overexpression of CD21 {600}.

Possible normal counterpart

Mature T-cell of CD4+ phenotype.

Genetics

T-cell receptor genes are rearranged in 75% of cases {1369, 961, 368}. Immunoglobulin gene rearrangement may be found in 10% of cases, and most likely correlates with expanded EBV+ B-cell clones {774}. The most frequent cytogenetic abnormalities are trisomy 3, trisomy 5, and an additional X chromosome {626, 1158}. EBV sequences are frequently present in scattered cells, mainly in B-cells, but perhaps also in T-cells {1368, 24}. EBV-positive B-cells may be numerous.

Prognosis and predictive factors

The clinical course is aggressive with a median survival of less than three years. Patients often succumb to infectious complications, which makes delivery of aggressive chemotherapy difficult {1194, 787}.

Secondary Epstein-Barr virus-positive B-cell lymphomas have been described in some patients {12}.

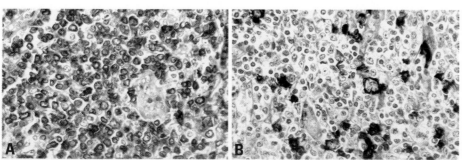

Fig. 7.64 Angioimmunoblastic T-cell lymphoma. **A** CD3 stain identifies neoplastic cells around high endothelial venule. **B** CD20 stains scattered B-cells, some of which are large. These B-cells are often EBV-positive.

Peripheral T-cell lymphoma, unspecified

E. Ralfkiaer
H.K. Müller-Hermelink
E.S. Jaffe

Definition

A number of distinctive entities have been defined which correspond to recognisable subtypes of T-cell neoplasia. Once these have been separated out, there remains a large group of predominantly nodal (and occasionally extranodal) T-cell lymphomas, which constitute a significant proportion of the peripheral T-cell neoplasms seen in Western countries. We collectively refer to these as peripheral T-cell lymphomas with the optional addition of "unspecified" to emphasise that these cases do not belong to any of the better defined entities. We realise that multiple morphological subtypes are distinguished in other classifications (see below). However, evidence that these correspond to distinctive clinicopathological diseases is lacking {496, 49, 438, 787}. This is in addition to the fact that attempts to distinguish between them on a morphological basis have met with poor inter- and intra-observer reproducibility {503, 928}.

ICD-O code   9702/10

Synonyms

Lukes-Collins: T-immunoblastic lymphoma
Kiel: various categories (T-zone lymphoma, lymphoepithelioid cell (Lennert) lymphoma, pleomorphic T-cell lymphoma small, medium-sized, and large cell types, T-immunoblastic lymphoma)
Working Formulation: various categories (diffuse small cleaved cell, diffuse mixed small and large cell, diffuse large cell, immunoblastic)
REAL: peripheral T-cell lymphoma, unspecified (provisional cytological categories: large cell, medium-sized cell, mixed large/medium-sized cell)

Epidemiology

These tumours account for approximately half of the peripheral T-cell lymphomas seen in Western countries {438, 787, 8}. Most patients are adults, but children may also be affected. The male to female ratio is 1:1.

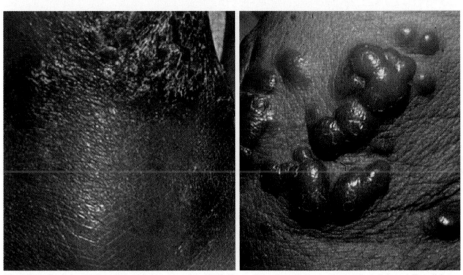

Fig. 7.65 Peripheral T-cell lymphoma, unspecified. Two diverse manifestations of peripheral T-cell lymphoma in the skin. On the left the lesion resembles a scaly plaque, whereas large tumors are present on the right. Both cases were derived from gamma/delta T-cells {1303}. Reproduced from Toro et al. {1303}.

Sites of involvement

Most patients present with nodal involvement, but any site may be affected, and patients often have generalised disease with infiltrates in the bone marrow, liver, spleen and extranodal tissues, including frequently the skin {49, 438, 787}. Peripheral blood is often involved and leukaemic presentation may be seen.

Table 7.10
Differential diagnosis of nodal peripheral T-cell lymphoma, unspecified.

Disease	Immunophenotypic features
PTL, unspec	CD4>CD8, antigen loss frequent (CD7, CD5), CD30-/+
AILT	Mixed CD4/8, Proliferation of FDC, EBV+ blasts
ATLL	CD4+, CD25+, CD7-, CD30-/+, CD15-/+
ALCL	CD30+, ALK+/-, EMA+, CD25+, cytotox. Ag+, CD4+/-, CD3-/+
TCRBCL	Large CD20+ blasts in background of CD3+ reactive T-cells
T-zone hyperplasia	Mixed CD4/CD8, intact architecture, variable CD25, CD30; scattered CD20+

AILT, angioimmunoblastic T-cell lymphoma; PTL, unspec, peripheral T-cell lymphoma, unspecified;
ATLL, adult T-cell leukaemia/ lymphoma; ALCL, anaplastic large cell lymphoma;
TCRBCL, T-cell rich large B-cell lymphoma; +, nearly always positive; +/-, majority positive; -/+, minority positive;
FDC, follicular dendritic cells; cytotox. Ag, cytotoxic granule associated proteins (TIA-1, perforin, granzyme B).

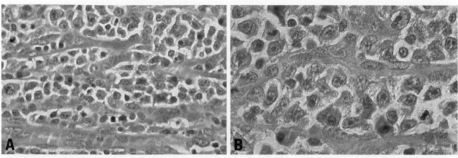

Fig. 7.66 Peripheral T-cell lymphoma, unspecified. **A** Diffuse infiltrates of large lymphoid cells with pleomorphic, irregular nuclei with prominent nucleoli. **B** In between the neoplastic cells, there are scattered eosinophils and numerous arborising vessels.

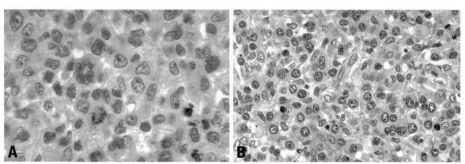

Fig. 7.67 Peripheral T-cell lymphoma, unspecified. **A** Nuclei are markedly pleomorphic with polylobated nuclear features. **B** In some cases nuclei are round and monomorphic in appearance. In such cases the diagnostic of peripheral T-cell lymphoma may not be suspected on histological grounds.

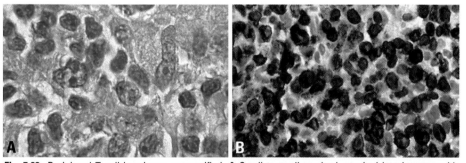

Fig. 7.68 Peripheral T-cell lymphoma, unspecified. **A** Small to medium-sized, atypical lymphocytes with irregular, nuclear outlines. **B** The cells are strongly positive for CD3.

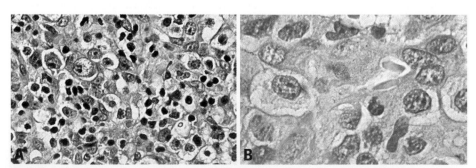

Fig. 7.69 A, B Peripheral T-cell lymphoma, unspecified, with prominent clear cell features.

Clinical features

Patients most often present with lymph node enlargement, but a majority have advanced disease with constitutional symptoms (B-symptoms) and a poor performance status {49, 438, 787}. Paraneoplastic features such as eosinophilia, pruritus or haemophagocytic syndrome may be seen {49}.

Aetiology

The cause(s) is/are unknown. As this category is heterogenous, multiple aetiologies may ultimately be identified.

Morphology

These lymphomas show diffuse infiltrates with effacement of the normal lymph node architecture. The cytological spectrum is extremely broad, but most cases show a predominance of medium-sized or large cells with irregular, pleomorphic nuclei which may be hyperchromatic or vesicular with prominent nucleoli and many mitotic figures {496, 1244}. Clear cells and RS-like cells are often present. Rare cases contain a predominance of small lymphoid cells with atypical nuclei with irregular outlines. High endothelial venules are usually increased, and arborising vessels may be seen {496, 1244}.

An inflammatory, polymorphous background with small lymphocytes, eosinophils, plasma cells and clusters of epithelioid histiocytes, is often present. Rare morphological patterns corresponding to the T-zone and lymphoepithelioid cell (Lennert) lymphomas of the Kiel classification can be recognised, but there is presently no evidence that these show any specific clinical features {298, 1007}.

T-zone variant

The T-zone variant typically shows an interfollicular growth pattern with preserved or even hyperplastic follicles. A diffuse subtype has been described, but is difficult to distinguish with confidence from other variants of T-cell lymphoma. Tumour cells are predominantly small or medium-sized and do not show pronounced nuclear pleomorphism. Clusters of clear cells and scattered RS-like cells are often present. High endothelial venules are prominent and reactive cells are numerous, including eosinophils, plasma cells and epithelioid histiocytes {1244}. Distinction from atypi-

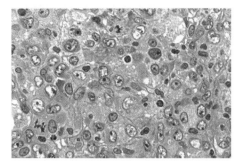

Fig. 7.70 Peripheral T-cell lymphoma, unspecified, consisting of large lymphoid cells with vesicular, immunoblast-like nuclei (HE).

cal T-zone hyperplasia is usually impossible on morphological grounds and requires molecular genetic studies for confirmation.

Lymphoepithelioid cell variant (Lennert lymphoma)

The lymphoepithelioid cell variant (Lennert lymphoma) shows diffuse or (more rarely) interfollicular infiltrates consisting predominantly of small cells with only slight nuclear irregularities. Numerous small clusters of epithelioid histiocytes are present {1244}. Clear cells may be seen, but are less frequent than in peripheral T-cell lymphomas of angioimmunoblastic or T-zone type. High endothelial venules are not prominent. RS-like cells, eosinophils and plasma cells are commonly present.

Immunophenotype

T-cell-associated antigens are positive, but aberrant T-cell phenotypes are common {504, 1039}. Most nodal cases are CD4+, CD8-. CD30 can be expressed by a majority of the tumour cells in large cell variants {496}. Such cases should not be confused with the anaplastic large cell lymphomas.

Expression of cytotoxic granule associated proteins is rare in nodal cases, in contrast to anaplastic large cell lymphoma {125, 202, 694, 390, 366, 587}. Epstein-Barr virus (EBV) is usually absent in the tumour cells, but may be present in reactive, bystander cells of mainly B-cell or more rarely T-cell type {260}.

The EBV-positive cells may assume Reed-Sternberg (RS)-like features mimicking Hodgkin lymphoma {1068}. Some cases may express CD56, a phenomenon more commonly observed in extranodal cases, which often also have a cytotoxic T-cell phenotype {648}.

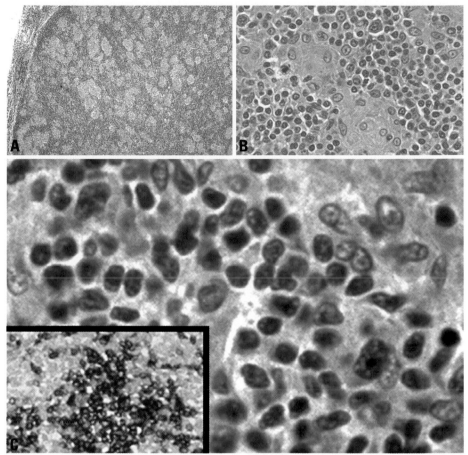

Fig. 7.71 Peripheral T-cell lymphoma, unspecified, of the lymphoepithelioid (Lennert) variant. **A** Clusters of epithelioid histiocytes are present throughout the lymph node. **B** Atypical lymphoid cells are intermixed with histiocytes. **C** The neoplastic lymphocytes are small with irregular nuclei and condensed chromatin. The neoplastic cells are strongly positive for CD3 (inset in **C**).

Genetics

TCR genes are clonally rearranged in most cases {455}. Complex karyotypes, consistent with clonal evolution, are frequent {1156, 755}. A vast number of different numerical and structural alterations have been described. No single consistent abnormality has been identified. Trisomy 3 is frequent in the lymphoepithelioid cell (Lennert) variant {1156}.

Postulated cell of origin

Peripheral T-cells in various stages of transformation.

Prognosis and predictive features

These are among the most aggressive of the non-Hodgkin lymphomas. Patients often respond poorly to therapy, relapses are frequent and the overall and failure-free survival rates at 5 years are low (20-30%) {49, 438, 787, 8}. So far the only factors consistently associated with

the prognosis are stage and the international prognostic index {49, 438, 787, 8}. No significant differences have been detected between the different categories of the updated Kiel classification {49, 438}. It has been suggested that the presence of EBV may be an indication of a poor outcome {260}. However, further studies are needed to substantiate this notion.

Anaplastic large cell lymphoma

G. Delsol
E. Ralfkiaer
H. Stein
D. Wright
E.S. Jaffe

Definition

Anaplastic large cell lymphoma (ALCL) is a T-cell lymphoma consisting of lymphoid cells that are usually large with abundant cytoplasm and pleomorphic, often horseshoe-shaped nuclei. The cells are CD30-positive and most cases express cytotoxic granule-associated proteins. The majority are positive for the anaplastic large cell lymphoma kinase (ALK) protein, but cases without ALK expression are also included in this category. Primary systemic anaplastic large cell lymphoma must be distinguished from primary cutaneous ALCL (see above) and from other subtypes of T- or B-cell lymphoma with anaplastic features and/or CD30 expression.

ICD-O code   9714/3

Synonyms

Lukes-Collins: not listed (T-immunoblastic sarcoma)
Kiel: large cell anaplastic
Working Formulation: various categories (diffuse large cell, immunoblastic)
REAL: anaplastic large cell lymphoma (T/null-cell type) {496}

Related terms: malignant histiocytosis, sinusoidal large cell lymphoma, Ki-1 lymphoma, regressing atypical histiocytosis

Epidemiology

ALCL accounts for approximately 3% of adult non-Hodgkin lymphomas and 10-30% of childhood lymphomas {1234}. ALK-positive ALCL is most frequent in the first three decades of life and shows a male predominance, which is particularly striking in the second and third decades (male/female ratio = 6.5). ALK-negative ALCL are prevalent in older individuals and are associated with a lower male/female ratio (= 0.9).

Aetiology

No causative agent or predisposing factors have so far been demonstrated.

Sites of involvement

Primary systemic ALCL positive for the ALK protein frequently involves both lymph nodes and extranodal sites. Extranodal sites commonly involved include skin (21%), bone (17%), soft tissues (17%), lung (11%) and liver (8%)

{151, 1234}. Involvement of the gut and central nervous system (CNS) is rare. Mediastinal disease is less frequent than in Hodgkin lymphoma. The incidence of bone marrow involvement is approximately 10% when analysed with H&E, but is increased significantly (30%) when immunohistochemical stains for CD30, EMA and/or ALK are used {394}. This is owing to the fact that bone marrow involvement is often subtle with only scattered malignant cells that are difficult to detect by routine examination.
ALK-negative ALCLs show similar features but extranodal involvement is less frequent {1234}.

Clinical features

The majority of patients (70%) present with advanced stage III to IV disease with peripheral and/or abdominal lymphadenopathy, often associated with extranodal infiltrates and involvement of the bone marrow {151, 1234}. Patients often show B symptoms (75%), especially high fever {151, 1234}.

Morphology

Cases of ALCL positive for the ALK protein show a broad morphologic spectrum. {496, 281, 204, 657, 1036, 90, 579}. However, all cases contain a variable proportion of cells with eccentric, horseshoe- or kidney-shaped nuclei often with an eosinophilic region near the nucleus. These cells have been referred to as hallmark cells because they are present in all morphologic variants {90}. Although the hallmark cells are typically large, smaller cells with similar cytological features may be seen and can greatly aid in accurate diagnosis {90}. Depending upon the plane of section, some cells may appear to contain cytoplasmic inclusions, but these are not true inclusions but invaginations of the nuclear membrane. Cells with these features have been referred to as doughnut cells {579}. The tumour cells in the common type of ALCL have more abundant cytoplasm than most other lymphomas. The cytoplasm may appear clear, basophilic or

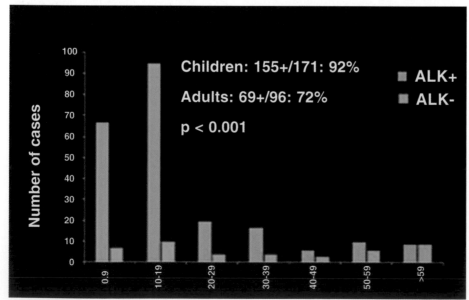

Fig. 7.72 Distribution of ALK-positive and negative ALCL by age.

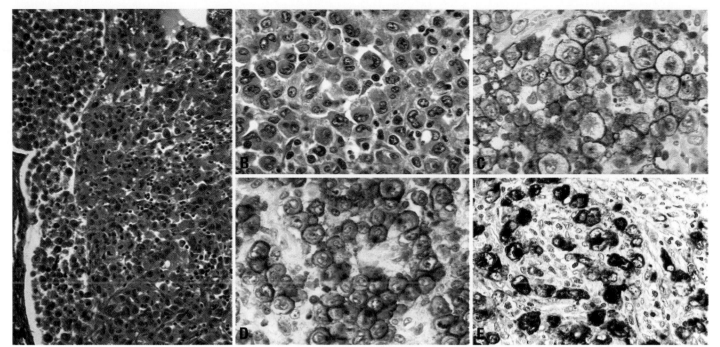

Fig. 7.73 General feature of ALCL common type. **A** The lymph node architecture is obliterated by malignant cells and intrasinusoidal cells are observed. **B** Predominant population of large cells with irregular nuclei. Note large hallmark cells showing eccentric kidney shape nuclei. **C** All malignant cells are strongly positive for CD30 and **D** for the epithelial membrane antigen. **E** All malignant cells are strongly positive for granzyme B.

eosinophilic. Multiple nuclei may occur in a wreath-like pattern and may give rise to cells resembling Reed-Sternberg cells. The nuclear chromatin is usually finely clumped or dispersed with multiple small, basophilic nucleoli. In cases composed of larger cells, the nucleoli are more prominent, but eosinophilic, inclusion-like nucleoli are rarely seen.

When the lymph node architecture is only partially effaced, the tumour characteristically grows within the sinuses and, thus, may resemble a metastatic tumour. Tumour cells may also colonise the paracortex and often grow in a cohesive manner.

Several cytomorphologic variants have been recognised. These include the common, the lymphohistiocytic and the small cell variants. In approximately 10% of the cases more than one variant can be seen in an individual patient {90}. Furthermore, relapses may reveal morphologic features different from those seen initially {90, 527}.

ALCL, common variant (70%) {90} is predominantly composed of pleomorphic large cells with hallmark features as described above. Tumour cells with more monomorphic, rounded nuclei also occur, either as the predominant population or mixed with the more pleomorphic

cells. Rarely, erythrophagocytosis by malignant cells may be seen.

ALCL, lymphohistiocytic variant (10%) is characterised by tumour cells admixed with a large number of histiocytes {1036, 90}. The histiocytes may mask the malignant cells which are often smaller than in the common type. The neoplastic cells often cluster around blood vessels and can be highlighted by immunostaining using antibodies to CD30, ALK and/or cytotoxic molecules. Occasionally, the histiocytes show signs of erythrophagocytosis.

ALCL, small cell variant (5-10%) shows a predominant population of small to medium-sized neoplastic cells with irregular nuclei {657, 579, 90}. Hallmark cells are always present and are often concentrated around blood vessels {90}. This morphologic variant of ALCL is often misdiagnosed as peripheral T-cell lymphoma unspecified by conventional examination. When the blood is involved, atypical cells reminiscent of flower-like cells can be noted in smear preparations.

Other histological patterns can be seen although they are not recognised as distinctive variants. These include a giant cell rich subtype, a sarcomatoid subtype, and a "signet ring"-like subtype {90}. Many cases of ALCL may be asso-

ciated with an oedematous background, often with a myxomatous stroma and prominent fibroblasts {221}. Capsular thickening and vaguely nodular fibrosis are uncommon features, seen in only 1-2% of cases. Other rare cases of ALCL are characterised by an abundant admixture of neutrophils.

ALK-negative ALCL is less well characterised and it is controversial whether tumours with morphologic and phenotypic features of ALCL, but which are negative for ALK, should be considered a phenotypic variant of ALCL or a different entity. There are no clear phenotypic or molecular markers to definitively answer this question, but the older median age and more aggressive clinical course of ALK-negative ALCLs compared to ALK-positive ones supports the idea that they may represent different entities {582}. ALK-negative ALCL is generally composed of larger and more pleomorphic cells with more prominent nucleoli {927}. Large CD30-positive cells resembling the cells of ALK-negative ALCL may be seen as a secondary phenomenon in other T-cell lymphomas, suggesting that the morphology and immunophenotype of ALK-negative ALCL may be a final common pathway in diverse T-cell malignancies. At the very

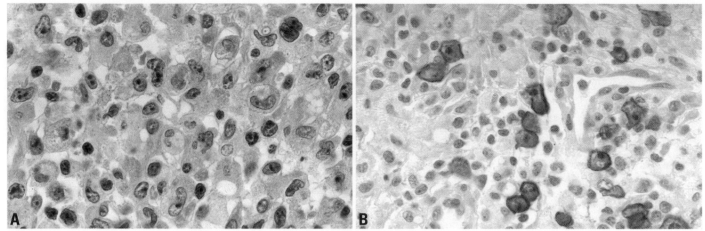

Fig. 7.74 ALCL lymphohistiocytic variant. **A** Large-sized cells (hallmark cells) are admixed with a predominant population of non-neoplastic cells, including histiocytes and plasma cells. **B** Malignant cells are highlighted by CD30 staining.

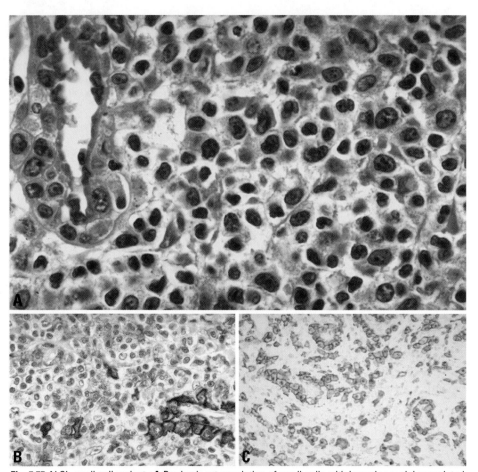

Fig. 7.75 ALCL small cell variant : **A** Predominant population of small cells with irregular nuclei associated with scattered hallmark cells. Note that large-sized cells predominate around the vessel. **B** CD30 staining highlights the perivascular pattern. Note that large cells are strongly positive for CD30 whereas small and medium-sized malignant cells are weakly stained. **C** Characteristic perivascular pattern highlighted by staining for CD30.

least, ALK positivity is an important prognostic factor in ALCL and should be investigated and reported in every case if possible.

Differential diagnosis

In some cases, there may be morphologic overlap between ALCL and Hodgkin lymphoma. Occasional cases of ALCL

with partial nodal involvement may have a vaguely nodular pattern and be associated with some sclerosis. More commonly, cases of Hodgkin lymphoma, particularly nodular sclerosis type, may contain confluent sheets of RS cell variants, and resemble ALCL. However, since Hodgkin lymphoma is in the vast majority of cases a B-cell neoplasm, and since ALCL is a T-cell neoplasm, this does not represent a true biological borderline. In such cases, immunophenotyping for CD15, pan-B and pan-T antigens, EMA, and ALK protein and, if necessary, molecular genetic analysis for antigen-receptor gene rearrangement will usually suffice to place the case in one category or the other. Thus, the category of Hodgkin-like or Hodgkin-related ALCL is not considered to be a "real" entity in this classification {582}.

Immunophenotype

The tumour cells are positive for CD30 on the cell membrane and in the Golgi region (diffuse, cytoplasmic CD30-positivity is of dubious significance). The strongest immunostaining is seen in the large cells. Smaller tumour cells may be only weakly positive or even negative for CD30 {90}. In the lymphohistiocytic and small cell variants, the strongest CD30 expression is also present in the larger tumour cells, which often cluster around blood vessels {90}.

ALK expression is detectable in 60-85% of the cases. The ALK staining may be cytoplasmic and nuclear or it may be restricted either to the nucleus or to the cytoplasm (see below). In the majority of the cases, which have the t(2;5)/*NPM-*

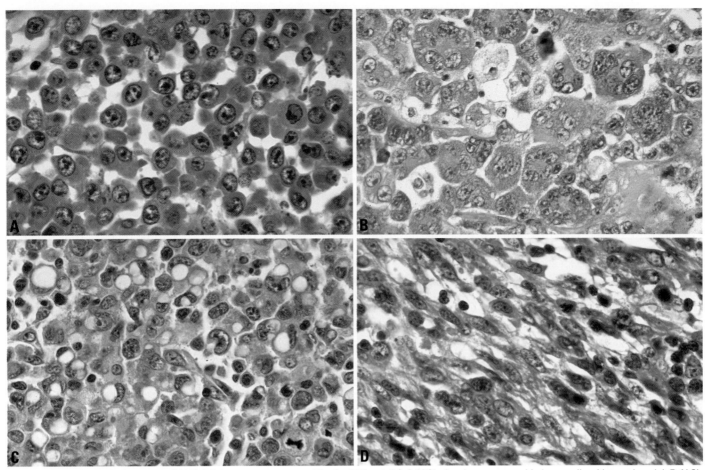

Fig. 7.76 Other histological patterns of ALCL (all these cases were positive for ALK protein): **A** ALCL showing monomorphic large cells with round nuclei; **B** ALCL consisting of pleomorphic giant cells. **C** ALCL rich in signet ring cells. **D** ALCL showing sarcomatous features

ALK translocation, ALK staining is both cytoplasmic and nuclear. This pattern results from the fusion of a portion of the ALK protein, which is normally a transmembrane protein, with nucleophosmin (NPM), a nuclear transport protein. In cases with variant translocations (see Genetics), the ALK staining may be membranous or cytoplasmic. ALK expression is virtually specific for ALCL since it is absent from all postnatal normal human tissues except rare cells in the brain {1062}. It is also absent from human neoplasms other than ALCL with the exceptions of rare diffuse large B-cell lymphomas expressing cytoplasmic IgA and showing an immunoblastic/plasmablastic morphology {283} (see chapter 6). ALK expression may also be seen in rare cases of rhabdomyosarcoma {357, 496} and inflammatory myofibroblastic tumours {459}.

The majority of ALCLs are positive for EMA {281, 90}. The staining pattern for EMA is usually similar to that seen with CD30 although, in some cases, only a proportion of malignant cells is positive.

The great majority of ALCLs express one or more T-cell antigens {90}. However, due to loss of several pan T-cell antigens, some cases may have an apparent "null cell" phenotype, but show evidence for a T-cell lineage at the genetic level {390}. Since no other distinctions can be found in cases with a T-cell versus a null-cell phenotype, T/null ALCL is considered a single entity {90, 496, 586}. CD3, the most widely used pan T-cell marker, is negative in more than 75% of cases {90, 204}. CD5 and CD7 are often negative as well. CD2 and CD4 are more useful and are positive in a significant proportion of cases. Furthermore, most cases exhibit positivity for the cytotoxic associated antigens TIA-1, granzyme B, and/or perforin {390, 694}. CD8 is usually negative, but rare CD8-positive cases exist. CD43 is expressed in two thirds of the cases, but this antigen lacks lineage specificity. Tumour cells are variably positive for CD45 and CD45RO and strongly positive for CD25 on frozen sections {281}. Blood group antigen H and Y (detected with monoclonal BNH.9) have been reported in 50% of the cases {282}. CD15 expression is rarely observed and when present only a small proportion of the neoplastic cells is stained {90}. ALCLs are consistently negative for EBV (i.e. EBER and LMP1) {147}. A recent study employing array technology to detect new genes expressed in ALCL identified clusterin as being aberrantly expressed in all cases of systemic ALCL, but not in primary cutaneous ALCL {1311}.

Enzyme cytochemistry
Early reports of tumours with the features of ALCL found evidence of lysosomal enzyme activity by enzyme histochemistry. The cells were positive for acid phosphatase and non-specific esterase {507, 1377}. However, in contrast to the diffuse cytoplasmic reactivity typical of histiocytes, strong perinuclear reactivity

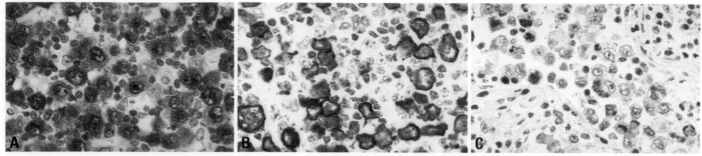

Fig. 7.77 Different ALK staining patterns: **A** Nuclear, nucleolar and cytoplasmic staining associated with the t(2;5) translocation (expression of the NPM-ALK hybrid protein). **B** Strong membranous and cytoplasmic staining sparing the nucleus in a case associated with the t(1;2) translocation (expression of the TPM3-ALK hybrid protein). **C** Finely granular cytoplasmic staining associated with the t(2 :22) translocation (expression of CLTCL-ALK hybrid protein).

was seen {577}. This pattern of staining is characteristic of activated lymphoid cells. Granular staining for some antibodies reactive with CD68, such as KP-1, may be seen, but other antibodies directed against CD68, such as PG-M1, are negative.

Genetics

Approximately 90% of ALCLs show clonal rearrangement of the T-cell receptor (TCR) genes irrespective of whether they express T-cell antigens or not. The remainder show no rearrangement of TCR or Ig genes {390}. EBV sequences are absent, and this feature is helpful in the distinction from CD30-positive, EBV-expressing B-cell lymphomas that have been misinterpreted as "anaplastic large cell lymphomas" in some older series.
Expression of ALK in ALCL is due to

genetic alteration of the *ALK* locus on chromosome 2. Several different abnormalities may be seen. The most frequent alteration is a translocation, t(2;5)(p23;35), between the *ALK* gene on chromosome 2 and the nucleophosmin *(NPM)* gene on chromosome 5 {823, 726}. Variant translocations involving *ALK* and other partner genes on chromosomes 1, 2, 3, and 17 also occur {362, 515, 725, 1112, 1229, 1305, 1396}. The t(2;5) can be detected by RT-PCR, but cases with variant translocations will be negative by standard RT-PCR using primers that are specific for the *ALK* and *NPM* genes {357, 1049}. All result in upregulation of *ALK*, but the distribution of the staining varies depending on the translocation. The classic t(2;5) leads to positive staining for *ALK* in both the nucleolus, nucleus and the cytoplasm. In the variant translocations, often only cytoplas-

mic staining will be observed. Therefore, immunohistochemistry has largely supplanted molecular tests for the diagnosis of ALCL.
The *ALK* gene encodes a tyrosine kinase receptor belonging to the insulin receptor superfamily, which is normally silent in lymphoid cells {897}. In the t(2;5)(p23;35), the nucleophosmin gene, a housekeeping gene *(NPM),* fuses the *ALK* gene to produce a chimeric protein in which the N terminal portion of *NPM* is linked to the intracytoplasmic portion of *ALK* {897}. The particular cytoplasmic, nuclear and nucleolar staining seen in cases associated with the t(2;5) can be explained by the formation of dimers between wild-type nucleophosmin and the fusion NPM-ALK protein. The wild-type nucleophosmin provides nuclear localisation signals whereby the NPM-ALK protein, despite the absence of nuclear localisation signal, can enter the nucleus {824}. On the other hand, the formation of NPM-ALK homodimers using dimerisation sites at the N-terminus of *NPM* mimics ligand binding and is responsible for the activation of the *ALK* catalytic domain, i.e. autophosphorylation of the tyrosine kinase domain of *ALK* which is responsible for the oncogenic properties of the ALK protein.
Some ALK-positive ALCLs are associated with the presence of a t(1;2)(q25;p23) {725, 1112} translocation involving the *TPM3* gene on chromosome 1 (which encodes a non-muscular tropomyosin protein) {725}, In cases associated with the t(1;2) translocation that express the TPM3-ALK protein (104 kD), ALK staining is restricted to the cytoplasm of malignant cells and in virtually all cases one sees a stronger staining on the cell membrane {725, 824}. This staining pattern is found in 10-20% of ALK-positive

	Nucleophosmin	Anaplastic Lymphoma Kinase	Staining	Frequency
t(2;5)	NPM	ALK	cytoplasmic / nuclear / nucleolar	70-80%
	Tropomyosin 3			
t(1;2)	TPM3	ALK	cytoplasmic	10-20%
	Trk Fusion Gene			
t(2;3)	TFG	ALK	cytoplasmic	2-5%
	ATIC (Pur H gene)			
Inv2	ATIC	ALK	cytoplasmic	2-5%
	Clathrin heavy chain			
t(2;17)	CLTC	ALK	cytoplasmic granular	2-5%
t(2;19) /others	?	ALK	?	1-2%

Fig. 7.78 Translocations and fusion proteins involving ALK. Note that Clathrin heavy polypeptide maps to 17q11-ter and not to 22q11.2 as originally reported {1305}

ALCL. Tropomyosins have no nuclear localisation signal but they are known to form dimeric alpha coiled-coil structures that could induce dimerisation of the chimeric TPM3-ALK protein and activation of the *ALK* catalytic domain, i.e. the autophosphorylation of ALK protein {110}.

The genes fused with *ALK* in two other variant translocations, t(2;3)(p23;q35), {1112, 515} and the inv(2)(p23 q35) {1400, 1311} have been recently identified. Two different fusion proteins of 85 and 97 kD (TFG-ALKshort and TFG-ALKlong) are associated with the t(2;3)(p23;q35) which involves the *TFG* (*TRK*-fused gene) {515}. The inv(2)(p23 q35) involves *ATIC* gene (formerly known as pur-H) which encodes the 5-aminoimidazole-4-carboxamide-ribonucleotide transformylase-IMP cyclohydrolase (ATIC) which plays a key role in the de novo purine biosynthesis pathways {1311}. In *TFG-ALK* and *ATIC-ALK* positive ALCLs, ALK staining is restricted to the cytoplasm in a diffuse pattern {515, 1311}. Rare cases of ALCL show a unique granular ALK cytoplasmic staining pattern {1305}. In these cases the ALK gene is fused to *CLTC* gene which encodes the clathrin heavy polypeptide which is the main structural protein of coated vesicles. The sequence of the fusion gene suggests that these tumours might have reciprocal translocations involving breakpoints at 17q11-qter and 2q23 (the site of the *ALK* gene). In CLTC-ALK positive ALCL, the implication of the clathrin heavy polypeptide in the hybrid protein accounts for the granular cytoplasmic staining pattern since the, CLTC-ALK hybrid protein is involved in the formation of the clathrin coat on the surface of vesicles. Moreover, the process of clathrin coat formation mimicks ligand binding and this would allow the autophosphorylation of the carboxy-terminal domain of ALK protein, probably responsible for its oncogenic property {1305}.

Genetic studies of ALK-negative ALCL have not been performed, and may be useful in the future in determining whether ALK-positive and ALK-negative ALCL are part of the same disease entity.

Postulated cell of origin
Activated mature cytotoxic T cell.

Prognosis and predictive factors
The international prognostic index (IPI) appears to be of some value in predicting outcome, although less so than in other variants of lymphoma {361, 423}. The most important prognostic indicator is ALK positivity, which has been associated with a favourable prognosis in series from the United States, Europe, and Japan {361, 423, 1188}. No differences have been found between NPM-ALK positive tumours and tumours showing variant translocations involving *ALK* and fusion partners other than *NPM* {361, 423, 1188}. The overall 5-year survival rate in ALK-positive ALCL is close to 80%, in contrast to only 40% in ALK-negative cases of disease. Relapses are not uncommon (30% of cases), but often remain sensitive to chemotherapy.

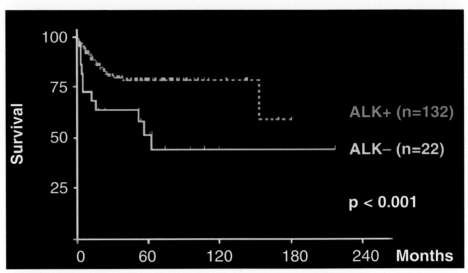

Fig. 7.79 Survival of 154 patients with ALCL based on the expression of ALK protein.

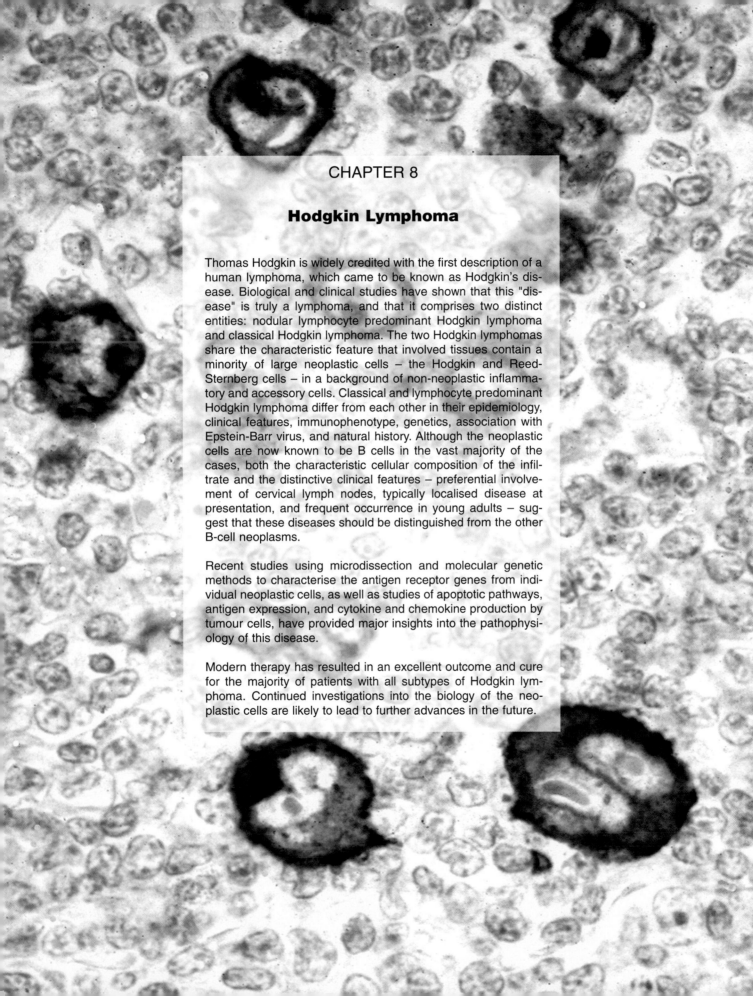

CHAPTER 8

Hodgkin Lymphoma

Thomas Hodgkin is widely credited with the first description of a human lymphoma, which came to be known as Hodgkin's disease. Biological and clinical studies have shown that this "disease" is truly a lymphoma, and that it comprises two distinct entities: nodular lymphocyte predominant Hodgkin lymphoma and classical Hodgkin lymphoma. The two Hodgkin lymphomas share the characteristic feature that involved tissues contain a minority of large neoplastic cells – the Hodgkin and Reed-Sternberg cells – in a background of non-neoplastic inflammatory and accessory cells. Classical and lymphocyte predominant Hodgkin lymphoma differ from each other in their epidemiology, clinical features, immunophenotype, genetics, association with Epstein-Barr virus, and natural history. Although the neoplastic cells are now known to be B cells in the vast majority of the cases, both the characteristic cellular composition of the infiltrate and the distinctive clinical features – preferential involvement of cervical lymph nodes, typically localised disease at presentation, and frequent occurrence in young adults – suggest that these diseases should be distinguished from the other B-cell neoplasms.

Recent studies using microdissection and molecular genetic methods to characterise the antigen receptor genes from individual neoplastic cells, as well as studies of apoptotic pathways, antigen expression, and cytokine and chemokine production by tumour cells, have provided major insights into the pathophysiology of this disease.

Modern therapy has resulted in an excellent outcome and cure for the majority of patients with all subtypes of Hodgkin lymphoma. Continued investigations into the biology of the neoplastic cells are likely to lead to further advances in the future.

WHO histological classification of Hodgkin lymphoma

Nodular lymphocyte predominant Hodgkin lymphoma   NLPHL   9659/3

Classical Hodgkin lymphoma   CHL   9650/3
  Nodular sclerosis classical Hodgkin lymphoma   NSHL   9663/3
  Mixed cellularity classical Hodgkin lymphoma   MCHL   9652/3
  Lymphocyte-rich classical Hodgkin lymphoma   LRCHL   9651/3
  Lymphocyte-depleted classical Hodgkin lymphoma   LDHL   9653/3

Hodgkin lymphomas: Introduction

H. Stein

Definition

Hodgkin lymphomas (HL) share the following characteristics: (1) they usually arise in lymph nodes, preferentially in the cervical region; (2) the majority of them manifest clinically in young adults; (3) neoplastic tissues usually contain a small number of scattered large mononucleated and multinucleated tumour cells (designated Hodgkin and Reed-Sternberg cells – HRS cells for short) residing in an abundant heterogeneous admixture of non-neoplastic inflammatory and accessory cells; (4) the tumour cells are usually ringed by T-lymphocytes in a rosette-like manner. Hodgkin lymphomas account for approximately 30% of all lymphomas. Their absolute incidence has not apparently changed, in contrast with non-Hodgkin lymphomas where there has been a steady increase in incidence.

Synonyms and historical annotation

This neoplasm was recognised in the first half of the 19th century by Thomas Hodgkin {528} and Samuel Wilks {1385, 1386}. The latter named it Hodgkin disease. The disease was also called lymphogranulomatosis, a term that is no longer in use. Since the origin of the Reed-Sternberg cell is known to be a lymphoid cell – most often of B cell type – the term Hodgkin lymphoma is preferred over Hodgkin's disease. The modern classification of Hodgkin lymphoma is based on the Lukes-Butler scheme {794, 793}.

Sub-classification

Biological and clinical studies in the last 20 years have shown that Hodgkin lymphomas are comprised of two disease entities {496}:

Nodular lymphocyte predominant Hodgkin lymphoma (NLPHL)
Classical Hodgkin lymphoma (CHL).

These two entities differ in their clinical features and behaviour, and in their morphology, immunophenotype and immunoglobulin transcription of the neoplastic cells, as well as in the composition of their cellular background. Within classical HL four subtypes have been distinguished: nodular sclerosis, mixed cellularity, lymphocyte rich and lymphocyte-depleted. These subtypes differ in their sites of involvement, clinical features, growth pattern, presence of fibrosis, composition of cellular background, number and/or degree of atypia of the tumour cells, and frequency of Epstein-Barr virus (EBV) infection, but not in the immunophenotype of the tumour cells, which is the same in all four variants.

A detailed account of the historical evolution of the subclassification of Hodgkin lymphoma is provided by Mauch et al {841} and by Anagnostopoulos et al {23}.

Staging

Treatment of HL is based on clinical, and occasionally on pathological staging of the disease. The modified (Cotswolds revision) Ann Arbor staging system is used (Table 8.01).

Table 8.01
Cotswold revision {777} of the Ann Arbor staging classification {179}.

Stage	Definition
I	Involvement of a single lymph node region or lymphoid structure (e.g., spleen, thymus, Waldeyer's ring)
II	Involvement of two or more lymph node regions on the same side of the diaphragm (the mediastinum is a single site; hilar lymph nodes are lateralized); the number of anatomic sites should be indicated by suffix (e.g., II_3)
III	Involvement of lymph node regions or structures on both sides of the diaphragm
III_1	With or without splenic, hilar, celiac, or portal nodes
III_2	With paraaortic, iliac, or mesenteric nodes
IV	Involvement of extranodal site(s) beyond those designated E

Annotation:
A – No symptoms
B – Fever, drenching sweats, or weight loss
X – Bulky disease: >1/3 widening of the mediastinum at T5-6, or maximum of nodal mass >10 cm
E – Involvement of a single extranodal site, or contiguous or proximal to known nodal site of disease
CS, Clinical stage
PS, Pathologic stage

Clinical data that have not been referenced were kindly provided by the German Hodgkin Lymphoma Study Group (GHSG) (V. Diehl and J. Franklin).

Nodular lymphocyte predominant Hodgkin lymphoma

H. Stein
G. Delsol
S. Pileri
J. Said

R. Mann
S. Poppema
S.H. Swerdlow
E.S. Jaffe

Definition

Nodular lymphocyte predominant Hodgkin lymphoma (NLPHL) is a monoclonal B-cell neoplasm characterised by a nodular, or a nodular and diffuse, polymorphous proliferation of scattered large neoplastic cells known as popcorn or L&H cells (lymphocytic and/or histiocytic Reed-Sternberg cell variants). These cells reside in large spherical meshworks of follicular dendritic cell processes that are filled with non-neoplastic lymphocytes.

It is currently not clear whether a purely diffuse form of LPHL exists. Most lesions diagnosed in the past as diffuse LPHL were probably either lymphocyte rich classical HL or more frequently T-cell rich large B-cell lymphoma. At present an overlap between NLPHL and T-cell rich large B-cell lymphoma cannot be excluded.

ICD-O code   9659/3

Synonyms

Jackson and Parker: Hodgkin's paragranuloma
Lukes and Butler: Lymphocytic and/or histiocytic (L&H) predominance Hodgkin's disease
Rye: Lymphocytic predominance Hodgkin's disease
REAL: Nodular lymphocyte predominance Hodgkin's disease

Epidemiology

NLPHL represents approximately 5% of all Hodgkin lymphomas. Patients are predominantly male and most frequently in the 30-50 year age group.

Sites of involvement

NLPHL usually involves cervical, axillary or inguinal lymph nodes. Mediastinal, spleen and bone marrow involvement are rare.

Clinical features

Most patients present with localised peripheral lymphadenopathy (stage I or II). 5-20% of patients present with advanced stage disease. The disease develops slowly, with fairly frequent relapses, and usually remains responsive to therapy and thus rarely being fatal.

Precursor lesions

In some patients, progressively transformed germinal centres (PTGC) may be seen simultaneously in the same lymph node with NLPHL, or in previous or subsequent lymph node biopsies that otherwise only show follicular hyperplasia. PTGC are large expanded follicles with a predominance of small mantle cell B-lymphocytes with resultant disruption and eventual replacement of the germinal centre. While PTGCs are often seen in association with NLPHL, it is uncertain whether these lesions are truly preneoplastic. Most patients with reactive hyperplasia and PTGC do not develop HL {981, 381}.

Table 8.02
Differential diagnosis of Hodgkin lymphoma: comparative tumour cell immunophenotypes.

Marker	NLPHL	TCRLBCL	CHL	DLBCL	ALCL
CD30	–[1]	–[1]	+	-/+[2]	+
CD15	–	–	+/-	-	–[3]
CD45	+	+	–	+	+/–
CD20	+	+	–/+[4]	+	–
CD79a	+	+	–/+[1]	+	–
BSAP	+	+	+[41]	+	–
J chain	+/–	+/–	–	–/+	–
Ig	+/–	+/–	–[5]	–/+	–
Oct2	S+	S+	–/+[6]	+	n.a.
BOB.1	+	+	–[7]	+	n.a.
CD3	–	–	–[1]	–	–/+
CD2	–	–	–[1]	–	+/–
perforin/Granzyme B	–	–	–[1]	–	+[8]
CD43	–	–	–	–/+	+/–
EMA	+/–	+/–	–[9]	–/+[10]	+/–
ALK	–	–	–	–	+/–

NLPHL, nodular lymphocyte prodominant Hodgkin lymphoma; TCRLBCL, T-cell rich large B-cell lymphoma; CHL, classical Hodgkin lymphoma; DLBCL, diffuse large cell B-cell lymphoma; ALCL, anaplastic large T-cell lymphoma

+ = all cases are positive; +/– = majority of cases positive; –/+ = minority of cases positive; – = all cases are negative; S = strong expression

[1] Positive in rare cases
[2] Prominent expression in anaplastic variant and variable expression in mediastinal large B-cell subtype
[3] Occasional cases may show focal positivity
[4] Present in 40% of the cases but usually expressed on a minority of tumour cells with variable intensity
[41] Up to 10% might be negative
[5] The common positivity for IgG and both Ig light chains reflects uptake of these proteins by the tumour cells rather than synthesis
[6] Strong expression in less than 5% of the cases
[7] Rare cases may show scattered weak positivity
[8] Only a small minority are negative
[9] Weak expression may be seen in tumour cells in 5% of the cases
[10] Most frequently seen in DLBCL with anaplastic morphology

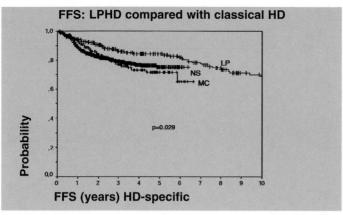

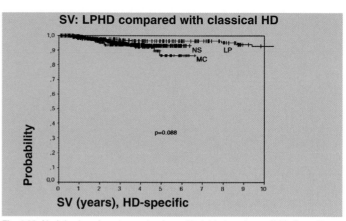

Fig. 8.01 Nodular lymphocyte predominant Hodgkin lymphoma (LP). Failure-free survival (FFS) (Hodgkin lymphoma specific) compared to nodular sclerosis (NS) and mixed cellularity (MC) subtypes of classical HL.

Fig. 8.02 Nodular lymphocyte predominant Hodgkin lymphoma (LP). Overall survival (SV) (Hodgkin lymphoma specific) compared to nodular sclerosis (NS) and mixed cellularity (MC) subtypes of classical HL.

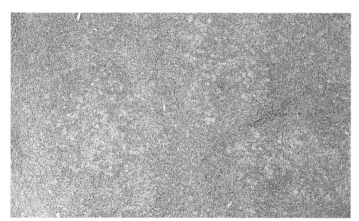

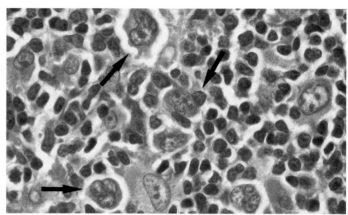

Fig. 8.03 Nodular lymphocyte predominant Hodgkin lymphoma (NLPHL). The nodules are usually larger than those present in follicular lymphoma and follicular hyperplasia, are closely packed and lack mantle zones..

Fig. 8.04 Nodular lymphocyte predominant Hodgkin lymphoma (NLPHL). Three popcorn cells (arrows) with the typically lobated nuclei are visible in a background of small lymphoid cells and a few histiocytes.

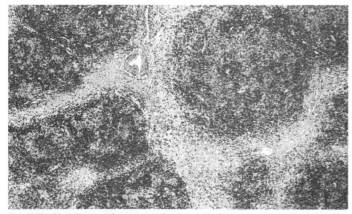

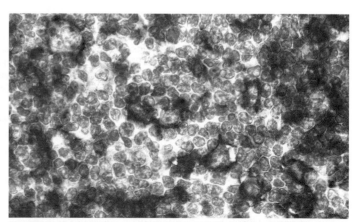

Fig. 8.05 Nodular lymphocyte predominant Hodgkin lymphoma (NLPHL). The CD20 staining reveals that the nodules of this lymphoma predominantly consist of B cells.

Fig. 8.06 Nodular lymphocyte predominant Hodgkin lymphoma (NLPHL). At higher magnification, the strong membrane staining of the popcorn cells for CD20 is visible.

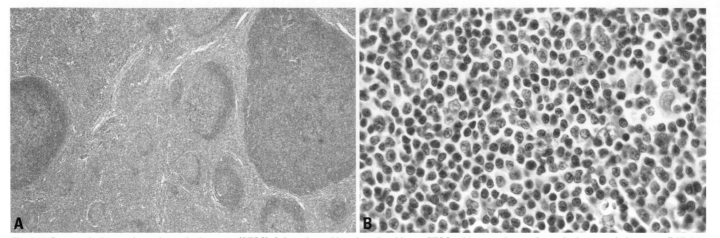

Fig. 8.07 Progressively transformed germinal centres (PTGC). **A** An enlarged lymph node with two PTGC, with several normal germinal centres in between. **B** Higher magnification shows a predominance of small lymphocytes with rare centroblasts and centrocytes.

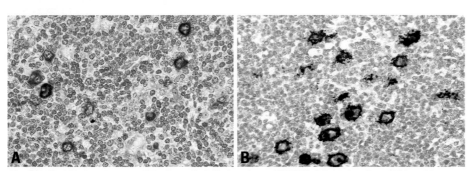

Fig. 8.08 Nodular lymphocyte predominant Hodgkin lymphoma (NLPHL). **A** Cytoplasmic positivity of the popcorn cells for J-chain is seen. **B** Membrane and dot-like staining in the Golgi region for epithelial membrane antigen (EMA) is visible in the popcorn cells.

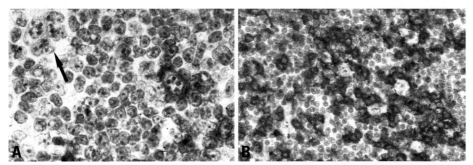

Fig. 8.09 Nodular lymphocyte predominant Hodgkin lymphoma (NLPHL). **A** Non-neoplastic bystander lymphoid blasts stain for CD30 whereas the neoplastic popcorn cell (arrow) remains unlabelled. **B** Many non-neoplastic bystander T-cells are labelled for CD57. These CD57+ cells may be involved in the rosette-like binding to the popcorn cells which is particularly pronounced in the case illustrated here.

Morphology

The lymph node architecture is totally or partially replaced by a nodular or a nodular and diffuse infiltrate, predominantly consisting of small lymphocytes, histiocytes, epithelioid histiocytes and intermingled L&H cells. The latter cells are large and usually have one large nucleus and scant cytoplasm. The nuclei are often folded or multilobated, often to such an extreme that they have also been termed "popcorn" cells. The chromatin is mostly vesicular with a thin nuclear membrane. The nucleoli are usually multiple, basophilic and smaller than those seen in classical HRS cells. However, some L&H cells may contain prominent nucleoli or have more than one nucleus, and thus may resemble classical HRS cells. Histiocytes and some polyclonal plasma cells can be found at the margin of the nodules. The diffuse areas are mainly composed of small lymphocytes with admixed histiocytes which are either single or in clusters. Variable numbers of L&H cells are also present. The process is rarely predominantly diffuse. According to current criteria the detection of one nodule showing the typical features of NLPHL in an otherwise diffuse growth pattern is sufficient to exclude the diagnosis of a primary T-cell-rich large B-cell lymphoma. Neutrophils and eosinophils are absent in both the nodular and diffuse regions. Occasionally, there is reactive follicular hyperplasia with progressive transformation of germinal centres adjacent to the lesion {23, 496}.

Immunophenotype

L&H cells are positive for CD20 {238, 1040, 1041}, CD79a, BCL6 and CD45 in nearly all cases, J chain {1051, 1231} and CD75 in most instances, and epithelial membrane antigen (EMA) in approximately 50% of cases {23} (Table 8.02). Labelling for immunoglobulin light and/or heavy chains is frequently strongly positive {1159, 1233, 1160}.

The labelling probably represents a synthesis product rather than uptake if the labelling includes the nuclear space {1233}. L&H cells lack CD15 and CD30 in nearly all instances; however CD30 positivity may occasionally be seen. This is in most instances due to the presence of reactive CD30+ lymphoid blasts unrelated to the L&H cells {23}. Infrequently the L&H cells show weak expression of CD30. As revealed by their nuclear positivity for Ki-67, most L&H cells are in cycle. Most of the L&H cells are ringed by CD3+ T cells, and to a lesser extent by CD57+ T cells.

Immunolabelling for Oct2 selectively highlights L&H cells and may become a useful means of identifying these cells {1233}. Oct2 is a transcription factor that induces immunoglobulin synthesis by activating the promoter of the immunoglobulin genes in conjunction with its co-activator BOB.1 {734}. Oct2 and BOB.1 may also be useful in the differential diagnosis between NLPHL and classical HL because both molecules are consistently present in L&H cells, whereas either one (20% of cases) or both (80% of cases) of the molecules are usually absent from HRS cells of classical HL. Classical HL cases in which the tumour cells express both Oct2 and BOB.1 have not been observed yet.

The architectural background in NLPHL is composed of large spherical meshworks of follicular dendritic cells, which are predominantly filled with small B-cells, and numerous CD57+ T-cells. CD10+ germinal centre cells are generally absent in affected areas. Immunostaining for a B-cell antigen like CD20 is most helpful in detecting nodules in lesions that appear to be totally diffuse in H&E stains. T cells are numerous in the diffuse areas and tend to increase over time even within the nodules {23}.

Genetics

L&H cells in any given case harbour identical, i.e. monoclonally rearranged immunoglobulin (Ig) genes {813, 134, 966}. The monoclonal rearrangements are usually not detectable in whole tissue DNA but only in the DNA of isolated single L&H cells. The variable region of the Ig heavy chain genes (VH) carries a high load of somatic mutations, and also shows signs of ongoing mutations. The rearrangements are usually functional and Ig mRNA transcripts are detectable in the L&H cells of most cases {813, 134, 966, 1288}. Latent EBV infection is consistently absent from L&H cells, but may be present in bystander lymphocytes {23}.

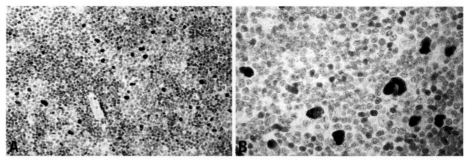

Fig. 8.10 Nodular lymphocyte predominant Hodgkin lymphoma (NLPHL). **A** Immunostaining for the transcription factor Oct2 which is involved in the regulation of immunoglobulin expression produces a strong nuclear staining of the popcorn cells and a weaker labelling of the bystander B cells and thus Oct2 often highlights the presence and the nuclear atypia of popcorn cells. **B** Higher magnification of A.

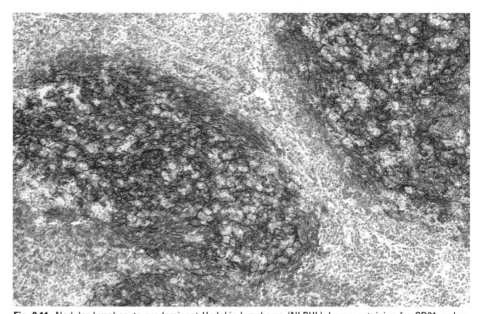

Fig. 8.11 Nodular lymphocyte predominant Hodgkin lymphoma (NLPHL). Immunostaining for CD21 makes the expanded meshwork of the follicular dendritic cells in the nodules of this lymphoma type visible.

Postulated cell of origin

Germinal centre B cell at the centroblastic stage of differentiation.

Prognosis and predictive factors

The prognosis of patients with stage I and stage II disease is very good; with 10 year overall survival in more than 80% of cases {299}. It is not clear yet whether immediate therapy is necessary to achieve this favourable prognosis. Therefore in some countries (e.g. France) stage I disease is not treated after the resection of the affected lymph node.

Advanced stages have an unfavourable prognosis {300}. Progression to large B-cell lymphoma has been reported in approximately 3-5% of cases {484, 875}. The large B-cell lymphomas associated with NLPHL, if localised, generally have a good prognosis {484}. A clonal relationship between NLPHL and the associated DLBCL has been demonstrated {1384, 453}.

Classical Hodgkin lymphoma

H. Stein
G. Delsol
S. Pileri
J. Said

R. Mann
S. Poppema
E.S. Jaffe
S.H. Swerdlow

Definition

Classical Hodgkin lymphoma (CHL) is a monoclonal lymphoid neoplasm composed of mononuclear Hodgkin cells and multinucleated Reed-Sternberg (HRS) cells residing in an infiltrate containing a variable mixture of non-neoplastic small lymphocytes, eosinophils, neutrophils, histiocytes, plasma cells, fibroblasts and collagen fibres. Based on the characteristics of the reactive infiltrate and the morphology of the HRS cells, four histological subtypes have been distinguished: lymphocyte rich CHL (LRCHL), nodular sclerosis Hodgkin lymphoma (NSHL), mixed cellularity Hodgkin lymphoma (MCHL) and lymphocyte depleted Hodgkin lymphoma (LDHL). The immunophenotypic and genetic features of the mononuclear and multinucleated cells are identical in these histological subtypes, whereas their clinical features and association with Epstein Barr virus (EBV) show differences (reviewed by Stein et al {1228}).

ICD-O code   9650/3

Epidemiology

Classical HL accounts for 95% of all Hodgkin lymphomas with a bimodal age curve showing a peak at 15-35 years of age and a second peak in late life.

Patients with a history of infectious mononucleosis have a higher incidence of HL {901}. Both familial and geographical clustering have been described {901}.

Sites of involvement

Classical Hodgkin lymphoma most often involves lymph nodes of the cervical region (75% of cases) followed by the mediastinal, axillary and paraaortic regions. Non-axial lymph node groups such as mesenteric or epitrochlear lymph nodes are rarely involved. Primary extranodal involvement is rare. 55% of patients have localised disease (stage I and II). Approximately 60% of patients, the majority of them with nodular sclerosis Hodgkin lymphoma, have mediastinal involvement. Splenic involvement is not uncommon (20%) and is associated with an increased risk of extranodal dissemination. Bone marrow involvement is much less common (5%). As the bone marrow lacks lymphatics, bone marrow infiltration indicates vascular dissemination of the disease (stage IV). The anatomic distribution varies among the histological subtypes of classical HL.

Clinical features

Patients usually present with peripheral lymphadenopathy, localised to 1 or 2 node-bearing areas. Mediastinal involve-

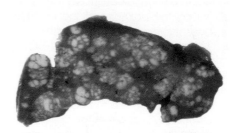

Fig. 8.12 Classical Hodgkin lymphoma. Spleen.

ment is most frequently seen in the nodular sclerosis subtype, while abdominal and splenic involvement are more common in mixed celluarity. Systemic symptoms consisting of fever, drenching night sweats, and significant body weight loss are present in approximately 40% of patients.

Aetiology

EBV has been postulated to play a role in the pathogenesis of classical HL. EBV is only found in a proportion of cases but a search for other viruses has been unsuccessful. Loss of immunosurveillance in immunodeficiency states such as HIV infection may predispose to the development of EBV-associated HL.

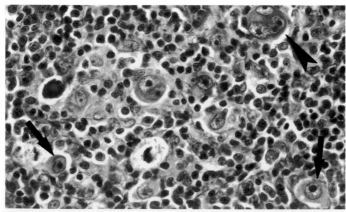

Fig. 8.13 Classical Hodgkin lymphoma. Uninucleated Hodgkin cells (arrows) and a multinucleated Reed-Sternberg cell (arrow head) are seen in a cellular background rich in eosinophils.

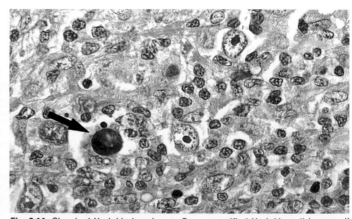

Fig. 8.14 Classical Hodgkin lymphoma. One mummified Hodgkin cell (arrowed) and four vital Hodgkin cells can be seen.

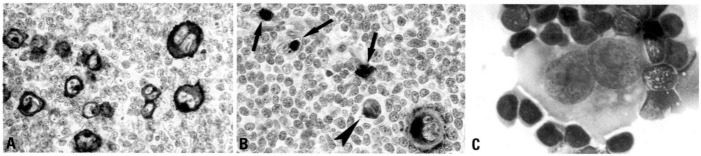

Fig. 8.15 Classical Hodgkin lymphoma. **A** The cytokine receptor CD30 is selectively expressed by the HRS cells. **B** The typical membrane and paranuclear dot-like staining of a large Reed-Sternberg cell for CD15 is seen; the small binucleated Reed-Sternberg cell (arrow head) shows only a very faint labelling. In addition, three neutrophil granulocytes (arrowed) are strongly labelled. **C** Touch imprint of a binucleated Reed-Sternberg cell ringed by lymphocytes.

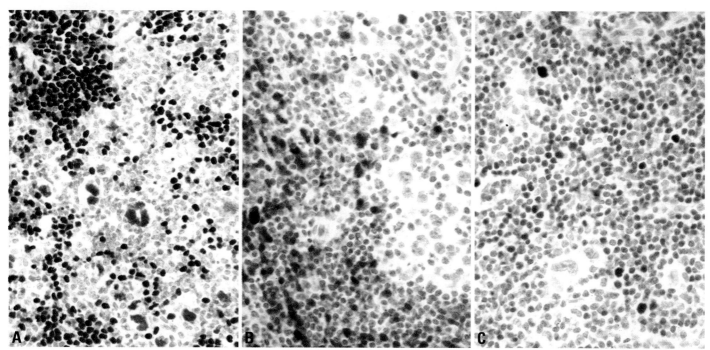

Fig. 8.16 Classical Hodgkin lymphoma. **A** The immunostaining for BSAP (B-cell-specific activator protein) encoded by the *PAX-5* gene labelled the nuclei of the HRS cells weakly and those of the non-neoplastic bystander B-cells strongly. **B** Immunostaining for BOB.1 (being the co-activator of the octamer-binding transcription factors Oct1 and Oct2) fails to stain the HRS cells in most instances. This is in difference to the non-neoplastic bystander B cells and plasma cells which show a moderately strong to strong labelling of their nuclei and in part of their cytoplasm. **C** Immunostaining for the octamer-binding transcription factor Oct2 is negative in the HRS cells whereas the non-neoplastic bystander B cells show a nuclear positivity.

Macroscopy

Lymph nodes are enlarged, encapsulated and on cut section show a fish flesh tumour. In the nodular sclerosis subtype there is prominent nodularity, dense fibrotic bands and a thickened capsule. Splenic involvement usually shows scattered nodules within the white pulp. Sometimes very large masses are seen, these can demonstrate fibrous bands in the nodular sclerosis subtype. HL in the thymus can be associated with cystic degeneration {770}.

Morphology

The lymph node architecture is effaced by variable numbers of HRS cells admixed with a rich inflammatory background. Classical diagnostic Reed-Sternberg cells are large, have abundant slightly basophilic cytoplasm and have at least two nuclear lobes or nuclei. The nuclei are large and often rounded in contour with a prominent nuclear membrane, pale chromatin and usually one prominent eosinophilic nucleolus. Diagnostic RS cells must have at least

two nucleoli in two separate nuclear lobes. Mononuclear variants are termed Hodgkin cells. Some HRS cells may have condensed cytoplasm and pyknotic nuclei. These variants are known as mummified cells. Many of the neoplastic cells are not prototypic HRS cells. The lacunar RS variant is characteristic of nodular sclerosis HL (see below). The neoplastic cells represent only a minority of the cellular infiltrate with a frequency typically ranging from 0.1-10%. The composition of the reactive cellular infiltrate varies according to the histological subtype (see below). Involvement of secondary sites (bone marrow and liver) is based on the identification of CD15-positve and/or CD30-positive atypical mononuclear cells in the appropriate inflammatory background; however, prototypic multinuclear RS cells are not required in a patient with classical HL diagnosed at another site.

Immunophenotype

HRS cells are positive for CD30 in nearly all cases {1234, 1230}, and for CD15 {1234, 1235, 546} in the majority (approximately 75-85%) of cases and are usually negative for CD45 and consistently negative for J chain, CD75 and macrophage specific markers such as the PG-M1-epitope of the CD68 molecule {224} (Table 8.02). CD15 may be expressed by only a minority of the neoplastic cells. In approximately 40% of cases CD20 may be detectable but is usually of varied intensity and present only on a minority of the neoplastic cells {1159, 1448}. The B-cell associated antigen CD79a is less often present. The B-cell nature of HRS cells is further demonstrated by their immunolabelling for the B-cell specific activator protein BSAP in approximately 90% of cases {391}. The immunostaining of HRS cells for BSAP is weaker than that of reactive B cells, a feature which makes the BSAP-positive HRS cells easily identifiable. BSAP is a B-cell specific transcription factor and a product of the *PAX5* gene. The EBV encoded latent membrane protein

(LMP1) is variably expressed dependent upon histological subtype and epidemiologic factors. An expression (usually weak) of one or more T-cell antigen(s) by a minority of HRS cells may be encountered in some cases {261}. This is, however, often difficult to assess because of the T cells that usually surround the HRS cells. Most of the T-cell antigen-positive classical HL cases do not show T-cell receptor rearrangement but Ig gene rearrangement in the HRS cells instead, so that the expression of T-cell antigens is frequently aberrant {1170}. Expression of epithelial membrane antigen (EMA) is rare (less than 5% of cases) and usually weak. A further characteristic finding is the absence of the transcription factor Oct2 and/or its co-activator BOB.1. The latter is critical for the induction of immunoglobulin transcription {734}. Most HRS cells express the proliferation-associated nuclear antigen Ki-67.

Classical HL cases rich in neoplastic cells may resemble anaplastic large cell lymphoma (ALCL). Their identification as classical HL is facilitated by demonstrating positivity for the B-cell specific activator protein BSAP (encoded by the *PAX5* gene) on the neoplastic cells, because it is consistently negative in ALCL. Negativity for EMA and ALK kinase protein is also helpful {391, 1229}. The detection of EBV encoded LMP1 also favours classical HL. The most difficult differential diagnosis is with large B-cell lymphoma displaying anaplastic morphology. There may be a true biologic overlap between such cases and CHL.

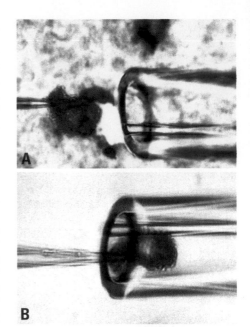

Fig. 8.17 Classical Hodgkin lymphoma. Isolation of a single Reed-Sternberg cell from a frozen section immunostained for CD30. **A** Extraction of a CD30-positive Reed-Sternberg cell from the frozen section by means of a hydraulically driven thin manipulation capillary. **B** Transfer of the picked CD30-positive Reed-Sternberg cell into a reception capillary.

Cytokines and chemokines

Classical Hodgkin lymphoma is associated with overexpression and an abnormal pattern of cytokines and chemokines and/or their receptors in HRS cells. These cells can express a variety of cytokines and chemokines including interleukin-2 (IL-2), IL-5, IL-6, IL-7, IL-9, I-10, IL-13 and IL13 receptor, granulocyte-macrophage colony-stimulating factor, lymphotoxin-a, transforming growth factor-β (TGF-β), eotaxin and CC chemokine TARC {617, 1138, 512, 615, 634, 1199, 1328, 1275, 601}. The abnormal cytokine and chemokine expression probably accounts for the abundant admixture of inflammatory cells present in CHL. Overexpression of eotaxin correlates with the extent of eosinophilia within the infiltrate {1275, 601}. Expression of TGF-β may account for the fibrosis {615}. The CC chemokine TARC may be responsible for the predominance of Th2 cells in the infiltrating T-cell population {1328}.

Genetics

Antigen-receptor-genes

HRS cells contain monoclonal immunoglobulin (Ig) gene rearrangements in greater than 98% of cases and mono-

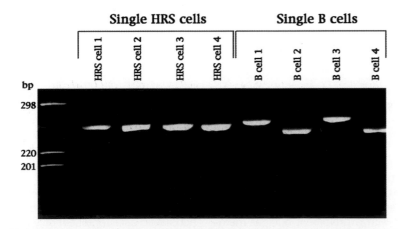

Fig. 8.18 IgH rearrangements in a case of classical Hodgkin lymphoma. Gel electrophoresis of the PCR products obtained from single cell HRS cells are identical sizes indicating monoclonality. The PCR products of the normal B cells differ in size, consistent with a polyclonal origin of these cells.

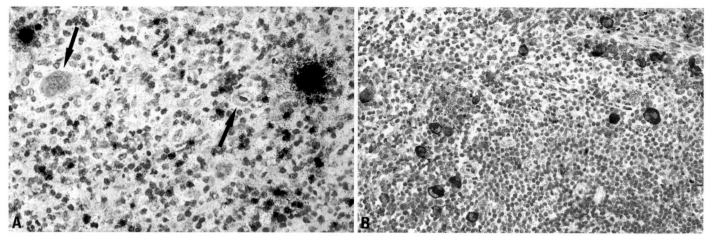

Fig. 8.19 Classical Hodgkin lymphoma. **A** Radioactive *in situ* hybridisation for Igµ mRNA is negative in the HRS cells (arrowed) while the two non-neoplastic plasma cells in the upper edges are strongly positive and the non-neoplastic bystander small B cells are moderately strongly positive. **B** Immunostaining for the antiapoptotic TRAF1 protein. The HRS cells strongly overexpress TRAF1.

clonal T-cell receptor gene rearrangements in rare cases {814, 631, 1170}. Only four cases with a T-cell genotype (three cases have been revealed by single cell polymerase chain reaction) have been described {267, 1170, 913}. The monoclonal rearrangements are usually not detectable in whole tissue DNA but only in the DNA of isolated single HRS cells. The detection of a T-cell form of CHL is complicated by the fact that peripheral T-cell lymphoma may simulate CHL {267}. However, in T-cell lymphomas a monoclonal rearrangement of the T-cell receptor genes is usually demonstrable in whole tissue DNA.

Somatic mutations of immunoglobulin genes

The rearranged Ig genes of the tumour cells harbour a high load of somatic mutations in the variable region of the Ig heavy chain genes (*VH*), usually without signs of ongoing mutations. These findings indicate a derivation of HRS cells from germinal centre B cells or their progeny, since somatic *VH* gene mutations are introduced when B cells participate in the germinal centre reaction. The study of composite lymphomas consisting of classical HL and follicular non-Hodgkin lymphoma has led to the identification of a common precursor cell. This precursor cell was shown to carry somatic mutations in its *VH* genes and thus corresponds to a germinal centre B cell {814, 135}. This finding supports the view that HRS cells of B-cell lineage are derived from a germinal centre B cell rather than from a post-germinal centre B cell.

Inactivation of immunoglobulin transcription

Initial single cell studies of classical HL led to the conclusion that HRS cells are incapable of producing functional immunoglobulin molecules due to the acquisition of replacement mutations generating stop codons or interfering with antigen binding, or heavy– and light chain pairing {631, 705, 608}.

In situ hybridisation studies {511, 736, 814} and more recent single cell investigations {814} have, however, revealed lack of immunoglobulin mRNA transcripts in HRS cells in all cases, regardless of the presence (25%) or absence (75%) of crippling immunoglobulin gene mutations {814, 1282}. Further studies have provided evidence that the absence of immunoglobulin transcription is caused by the inactivation of the immunoglobulin promoter {814} which appears to be the consequence of a lack of the octamer dependent transcription factor Oct2 and/or its coactivator BOB.1 {1233}. Absence of Oct2 and/or BOB.1 is usually

not seen in other B-cell lymphomas including NLPHL {1233}.

Blockage of apoptosis

B cells that have lost the capacity to express immunoglobulin rapidly undergo apoptosis {724}. Since HRS cells that are incapable of producing immunoglobulins do not die of apoptosis, it follows that the apoptotic pathway is blocked in these cells. The mechanism preventing apoptosis in classical HL has not yet been clarified. There are, however, studies suggesting that the nuclear transcription factor NFkB is involved because it was found to be constitutively activated in HRS cells {73}. Its involvement in the hindrance of apoptosis is supported by the in-vitro finding that inactivation of NFkB restores the sensitivity of HRS cells to apoptosis {72}. The persistent activation of NFκB in HRS cells might be caused by defects (e.g. mutations) of members of the IκB family which are the natural inhibitors of NFκB {72, 613, 345,

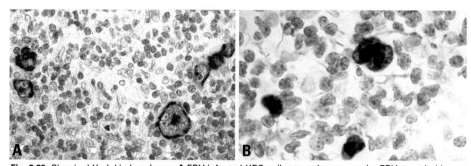

Fig. 8.20 Classical Hodgkin lymphoma. **A** EBV infected HRS cells strongly express the EBV encoded latent membrane protein 1 (LMP1). **B** EBV infected HRS cells consistently show a strong expression of EBER in their nuclei (revealed by non-radioactive *in situ* hybridisation).

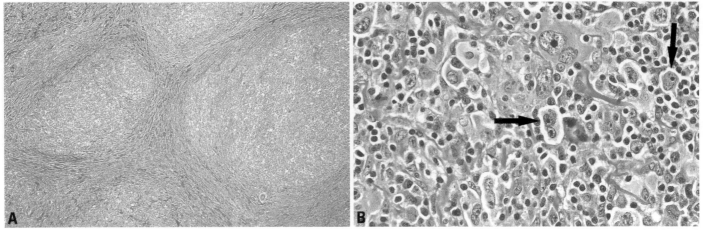

Fig. 8.21 Nodular sclerosis subtype of classical Hodgkin lymphoma. **A** Fibrous collagen bands divide the lymph node into nodules. **B** Nodular sclerosis subtype of CHL. Several lacunar cells (arrowed) are present.

167} or by aberrant activation of IκB kinase (IKK) {690}. Another molecule that mediates NFκB activation and prevents apoptosis and that is strongly over-expressed in HRS cells is the TNF Receptor associated factor (TRAF) 1 molecule {334}.

Other genes possibly involved in the pathogenesis of classical HL are EBV-encoded LMP1 and p53. EBV infection induces regular expression of LMP1 in classical HL (LMP1 possesses transforming and antiapoptotic potential). EBV infection is, however, present only in a proportion of cases and therefore cannot be the sole cause for prevention of apoptosis. It might however be a co-factor. Despite the frequent over-expression of p53, mutations of *TP53* have not been identified at the single cell level {893}.

Epstein-Barr-Virus infection
The prevalence of EBV in HRS cells varies according to the histological subtype and epidemiologic factors. The highest frequency (approximately 75%) is found in mixed cellularity HL, and the lowest incidence (10-40%) in nodular sclerosis HL. In developing regions and in patients infected with the human immune deficiency virus, EBV infection is much more prevalent, approaching 100%. The type of EBV strain also varies between different geographical areas. In developed countries strain 1 prevails, in developing countries strain 2. A dual infection by both strains is more common in developing countries {1365, 1364}. Hodgkin lymphoma that is positive for EBV at diagnosis is usually also positive at relapse with persistence of the same EBV strain {148}. EBV infected HRS cells express LMP1 and EBNA-1 without

EBNA-2. This expression pattern is characteristic of latency type II EBV infection {1117}.

Cytogenetics
Conventional cytogenetic and FISH studies show aneuploidy and hypertetraploidy consistent with the multinuclearity of the neoplastic cells; however, these techniques fail to demonstrate recurrent and specific chromosomal changes in classical HL {1157, 1145}. Comparative genomic hybridisation, however, reveals recurrent gains of the chromosomal sub-regions on chromosomal arms 2p, 9p, and 12q and distinct high-level amplifications on chromosomal bands 4p16, 4q23-q24 and 9p23-p24 {603}. The translocations t(14;18) and t(2;5) are absent from HRS cells {450, 1352, 1062, 726}.

Postulated cell of origin
In more than 98% of classical HL the neoplastic cells are derived from mature B cells at the germinal centre stage of differentiation {631, 814}. In rare cases, they are derived from peripheral (post-thymic) T cells {913, 1170}.

Prognosis and predictive factors
The introduction of modern radiation and chemotherapy has made HL curable in the majority of cases. Combined pathological and clinical stage determines the mode of therapy. Before the advent of modern therapy, there was a strong association between histological type and overall survival. Today, stage and the presence of systemic symptoms are much more important than histololgic

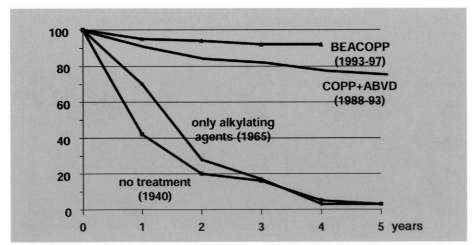

Fig. 8.22 Hodgkin lymphoma. Progress of the treatment of advanced stages since 1940.

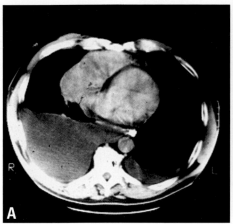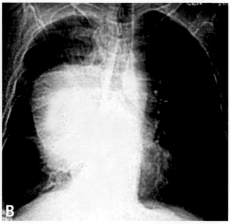

Fig. 8.23 Hodgkin lymphoma, nodular sclerosis. **A** CT scan shows a large anterior mediastinal mass. **B** Chest x-ray of the same patient shows mediastinal mass exceeding one-third of the chest diameter.

subtype as a predictive factor {607}. Clinical and laboratory parameters are also relevant to prognosis {500}.

Nodular sclerosis Hodgkin lymphoma

Definition
Nodular sclerosis Hodgkin lymphoma (NSHL) is a subtype of classical HL with collagen bands that surround at least one nodule and lacunar type HRS cells.

ICD-O code 9663/3

Epidemiology
NSHL accounts for approximately 70% of classical HL. The median age is 28 years. NSHL is the one type of HL without a male predominance; The male: female ratio is approximately 1:1.

Sites of involvement
Mediastinal involvement occurs in 80% of cases, bulky disease in 54%, spleen and/or lung involvement in 10%, and bone marrow involvement in 3% {299, 237}.

Clinical features
Most patients present with stage II disease. B-symptoms are encountered in approximately 40% of cases {1333, 801 and unpublished data of the German Hodgkin lymphoma study group}.

Morphology
Lymph nodes show classical HL with a nodular growth pattern, collagen bands and lacunar cells. The broad fibroblast-poor collagen bands surround at least one nodule. This fibrosing process is usually associated with a thickened lymph node capsule. The lymphoma contains a highly variable number of HRS cells, small lymphocytes and other non-neoplastic inflammatory cells. The HRS cells of this subtype tend to have more lobated nuclei with smaller lobes, and less prominent nucleoli than in other types of CHL. In formalin fixed tissues the cytoplasm of the HRS cells frequently shows retraction of the cytoplasmic membrane so that the cells seem to be sitting in lacunae. These cells have therefore been designated lacunar cells. Lacunar cells may form cellular aggregates which are occasionally associated with necrotic areas in the nodules. When aggregates are very prominent, the term syncitial variant has been used. Eosinophils, and to a lesser extent neutrophils, are often numerous.

Grading
The British National Lymphomas Investigation (BNLI) has established a grading system for NSHL. In Grade 1, 75% or more of the nodules contain scattered RS cells in a lymphocyte rich, mixed cellular, or fibrohistiocytic background. In Grade 2, at least 25% of the nodules contain increased numbers of RS cells (defined as a sheet of cells filling a 40x hpf) {95, 801}. Grading is not required for routine clinical purposes {518, 1333} but may serve a research purpose in protocol studies. Grade 2 NSHL corresponds to what had been termed nodular sclerosis with lymphocyte depletion in some studies {291}.

Immunophenotype
The malignant cells exhibit the CHL phenotype (see above); however, the EBV

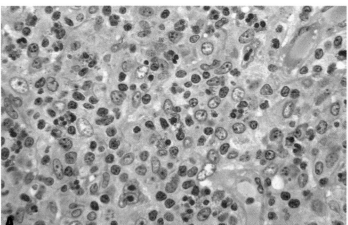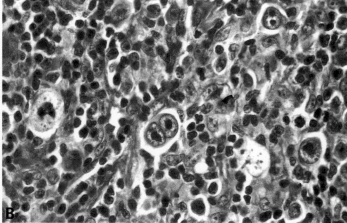

Fig. 8.24 Mixed cellularity subtype of classical Hodgkin lymphoma. **A** Low magnification showing that the mixed cellular infiltrate does not contain fibrotic bands. **B** A typical binucleated Reed-Sternberg cell in a mixed cellular infiltrate with lymphocytes, macrophages and eosinophils visible.

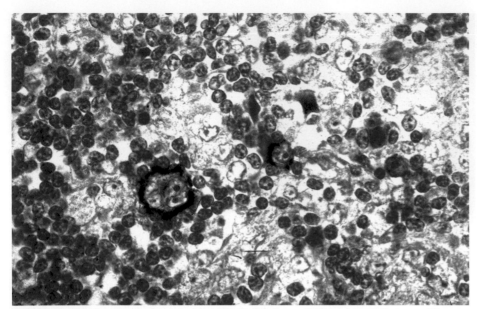

Fig. 8.25 Mixed cellularity subtype of classical Hodgkin lymphoma. CD30-negative histiocytes, with a pronounced epithelioid differentiation forming clusters, predominate. The CD30 immunostaining highlights the presence of a large Reed-Sternberg cell and a small Hodgkin cell.

encoded LMP1 is less frequently expressed (10-40%) than in other subtypes.

Prognosis and predictive factors

The prognosis of NSHL is slightly better than that of mixed cellularity or lymphocyte depleted subtype, in part based on its tendency to present with low stage disease. Massive mediastinal disease is an adverse risk factor {1213}.

Mixed cellularity Hodgkin lymphoma

Definition

Mixed cellularity Hodgkin lymphoma (MCHL) is a subtype of CHL with scattered classical HRS cells in a diffuse or vaguely nodular mixed inflammatory background without nodular sclerosing fibrosis. In contrast to the Rye classification MCHL is now regarded as a true subtype and not as a wastebasket of unclassifiable cases.

ICD-O code   9652/3

Epidemiology

The mixed cellularity subtype comprises approximately 20-25% of classical HL. MCHL is more frequent in patients with HIV infection and in developing countries. A bimodal age distribution is not seen. The median age is 37 years and approximately 70% are male.

Sites of involvement and clinical features

MCHL often presents with stage III or IV disease. B symptoms are frequent. Peripheral lymph nodes are frequently involved and mediastinal involvement uncommon. The spleen is involved in 30%, bone marrow in 10%, liver in 3%, and other organs in 1-3%.

Morphology

The lymph node architecture is usually obliterated, although an interfollicular growth pattern may be seen. Interstitial fibrosis may be present, but the lymph node capsule is not thickened and there are no broad bands of fibrosis as seen in nodular sclerosis HL. The HRS cells are typical in appearance. The background cells consist of a mixture of cell types, the composition of which varies greatly. Eosinophils, neutrophils, histiocytes and plasma cells are usually present. One of these cell types may predominate. The histiocytes may show pronounced epithelioid differentiation and may form granuloma-like clusters.

Immunophenotype

The malignant cells exhibit the CHL phenotype (see above); however, the EBV encoded LMP1 is expressed much more frequently (approximately 75% of cases) than in nodular sclerosis and lymphocyte rich CHL.

Prognosis

Before the introduction of modern therapy, MCHL had a worse prognosis than nodular sclerosis and a better prognosis than lymphocyte depleted HL. With current regimens, these differences have largely vanished.

Lymphocyte rich classical Hodgkin lymphoma

Definition

Lymphocyte rich CHL (LRCHL) is a subtype of CHL with scattered HRS cells and a nodular (most common) or diffuse cellular background characterised by an abundance of small lymphocytes, and with an absence of neutrophils and eosinophils {496, 23, 52}.

ICD-O code   9651/3

Epidemiology

LRCHL comprises approx. 5% of all HL, in similar frequency to NLPHL. The median age is higher than in other subtypes of CHL and NLPHL. Approximately 70% of the patients are male.

Sites of involvement

Peripheral lymph nodes are typically involved. Mediastinal involvement (15%) and bulky disease (11%) are uncommon {300}.

Clinical features

Most patients present with stage I or II disease. B symptoms are rare. The clinical features are similar to those of NLPHL with the exception that multiple relapses seem to occur less frequently {300}.

Morphology

There are two growth patterns: a common nodular one {52} and a rare diffuse one {23}. The nodules of the nodular variant encompass most of the involved tissue so that the T-zone is attenuated or absent between the nodules. The nodules are composed of small lymphocytes and may harbour germinal centres that are usually eccentrically located and relatively small or regressed. The HRS cells

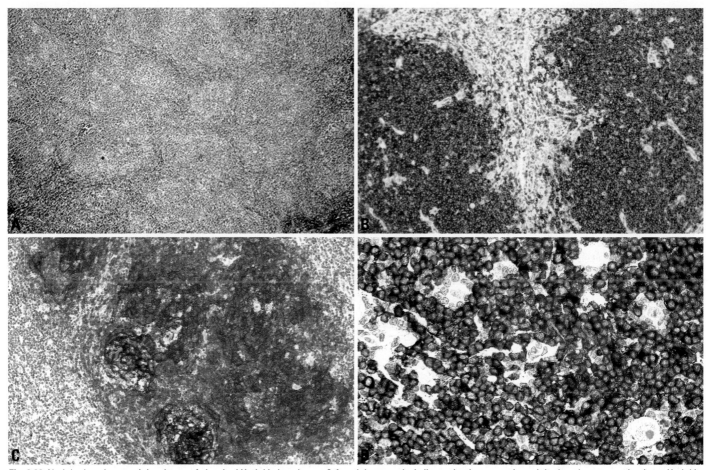

Fig. 8.26 Nodular lymphocyte rich subtype of classical Hodgkin lymphoma. **A** A nodular growth similar to that is present in nodular lymphocyte-predominant Hodgkin lymphoma. **B** Immunostaining for CD20 shows that the nodules predominantly consist of small B cells. The holes contain HRS cells. **C** Immunostaining for CD21 reveals that the nodules contain a meshwork of follicular dendritic cells and demonstrates that they predominantly represent follicular mantles with occasional, usually regressed germinal centres; the follicular dendritic cell meshwork is denser and more sharply defined in the germinal centres. **D** A higher magnification of one of the nodules stained for CD20 reveals a background of CD20+ B cells and CD20- HRS cells ringed by CD20-negative T cells.

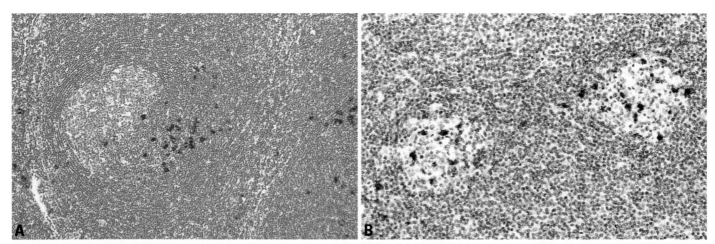

Fig. 8.27 Nodular lymphocyte rich subtype of classical Hodgkin lymphoma. **A** The CD30 staining highlights the presence of HRS cells. They are located within or at the peripheral margin of the follicular mantles but not within the germinal centres. **B** CD57+ T cells are seen but not surrounding the neoplastic cell in the mantle zones.

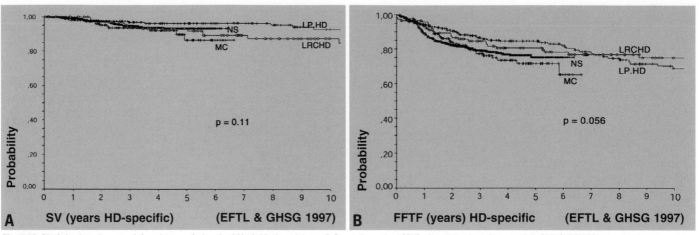

Fig. 8.28 Nodular lymphocyte rich subtype of classical Hodgkin lymphoma. **A** Overall survival (SV) of nodular lymphocyte rich CHL (LRCHD)in comparison to nodular lymphocyte-predominant Hodgkin lymphoma (LPHD) and other types of CHL. **B** Failure free survival of nodular lymphocyte rich CHL in comparison to nodular lymphocyte-predominant Hodgkin lymphoma and other types of CHL.

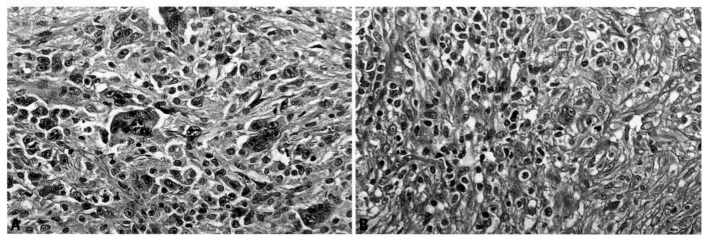

Fig. 8.29 Lymphocyte depleted subtype of classical Hodgkin lymphoma. **A** Many bizarre large and small HRS cells are present in a cellular background rich in fibrillary matrix. **B** Scattered HRS cells in a predominant fibrillary matrix with fibroblastic proliferation.

are generally found within the expanded mantle zone. A proportion of the HRS cells may resemble L&H cells or mononuclear lacunar cells. This subtype can easily be confused with the NLPHL. Recently approximately 30% of cases initially diagnosed as NLPHL were found to be LRCHL {23}. The demonstration of an immunophenotype typical for classical HRS cells (see below) is essential in making this distinction. Eosinophils and/or neutrophils are usually absent but may be present in small numbers. In diffuse cases the small lymphocytes of the cellular background may be admixed with a large number of histiocytes with or without epithelioid features.

Immunophenotype

The HRS cells show the same immunophenotype (CD30+, CD15+/-, CD20-/+, J

chain-) as in the other forms of classical HL. The small lymphocytes present in the nodules display the features of mantle cells (IgM+D+). Thus the nodules predominantly represent expanded mantle zones. At least some of them contain eccentrically located, usually small, germinal centres which are highlighted by a dense meshwork of CD21+ follicular dendritic cells. As intact germinal centres are rare in NLPL, this feature is helpful in differential diagnosis. In the diffuse subtype the lymphocytes are nearly all of T-cell type.

Prognosis and predictive factors

With modern risk-adjusted treatment, survival and progression free survival are slightly better than in the other subtypes of CHL and similar to that of NLPHL {300, 23}.

Patients with LRCHL who relapse have a less favourable prognosis than those with relapsed NLPHL {300, 23}.

Lymphocyte depleted Hodgkin lymphoma

Definition

Lymphocyte depleted Hodgkin lymphoma (LDHL) is a diffuse form of CHL rich in HRS cells and/or depleted in non-neoplastic lymphocytes.

The definition of LDHL has undergone several changes in the past few decades with the result that the body of reliable clinical data on this subtype is limited. Many cases previously diagnosed as lymphocyte depleted HL are now recognised as non-Hodgkin lymphomas, often

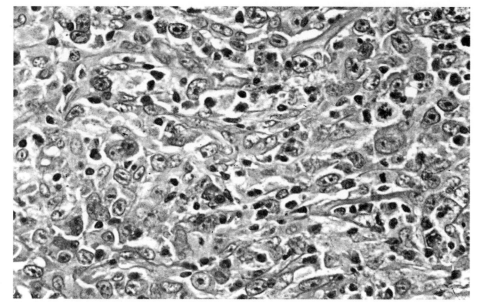

Fig. 8.30 Lymphocyte depleted subtype of classical Hodgkin lymphoma. Many Hodgkin cells with relatively few admixed lymphocytes are visible.

with anaplastic or pleomorphic large cell morphology {627}. It is likely that others represent lymphocyte depleted variants of NSHL.

ICD-O code   9653/3

Synonyms
Jackson and Parker: Hodgkin's sarcoma
Lukes and Butler: Lymphocytic depletion; Diffuse fibrosis and reticular types
Rye: Lymphocytic depletion
*REAL:*Lymphocyte depletion

Epidemiology
This is the rarest subtype of HL, accounting for less than 5% of cases. As current-ly defined, the median age is similar to other subtypes of CHL. The median age is 37 years, with 75% male {627}. This subtype is often associated with HIV infection and seen more often in developing countries {1299}.

Sites of involvement
Abdominal organs, retroperitoneal lymph nodes, and bone marrow are often selectively involved with relative sparing of peripheral lymph nodes.

Clinical features
LDHL is frequently associated with advanced stage (approximately 70%) and B symptoms (approximately 80%) {940}.

Morphology
Although the appearance of LDHL is highly variable, a unifying feature is the relative predominance of HRS cells to the background lymphocytes. One pattern may resemble mixed cellularity but compared with increased numbers of prototypic HRS cells. In some cases pleomorphic HRS cells may predominate, producing a sarcomatous appearance. These cases may be difficult to differentiate from anaplastic forms of large cell non-Hodgkin lymphoma. Another pattern is characterised by diffuse fibrosis with or without a proliferation of fibroblasts and only a few HRS cells. If a nodular sclerosing fibrosis is present, the disease should be assigned to nodular sclerosis Hodgkin lymphoma.

Immunophenotype
The HRS cells show the same immunophenotype as in the other forms of classical HL. Most HIV+ cases are EBV infected and stain positively for LMP1 {1316, 1193, 516}.

Prognosis and predictive factors
Historically the clinical course of LDHL was aggressive {940}. With modern therapy, the course is comparable to patients with other subtypes of CHL of similar stage {627}. Aggressive courses are still relatively frequent in HIV-positive patients.

CHAPTER 9

Immunodeficiency Associated Lymphoproliferative Disorders

The WHO classification recognises four broad clinical settings of immunodeficiency associated with an increased incidence of lymphoma and other lymphoproliferative disorders (LPDs). These are: 1) primary immunodeficiency syndromes and other primary immune disorders; 2) infection with the human immunodeficiency virus (HIV); 3) iatrogenic immunosuppression in patients who have received solid organ or bone marrow allografts; and 4) iatrogenic immunosuppression associated with methotrexate treatment, most commonly for autoimmune disease. The prevalence and types of LPD encountered varies in each of the above situations. Most cases are similar to sporadically-occurring the T-cell and B-cell neoplasms, the one exception being post-transplant lymphoproliferative disease (PTLD)

The LPDs associated with primary immunodeficiency and other primary immune disorders are particularly heterogeneous, as the nature of the immune defect is highly variable. In some situations the increased risk can be attributed mainly to defective immune surveillance, as in X-linked LPD. In other settings, the risk is due to defective DNA repair (ataxia telangiectasia), or defective apoptosis (autoimmune lymphoproliferative syndrome, ALPS). Each primary immune disorder must be considered independently.

The lymphoid neoplasms associated with HIV infection have been attributed to deficient immune surveillance of oncogenic viruses such as EBV and HHV8/KSHV, as well as chronic antigenic stimulation and defective immune regulation. The development of lymphoma in this setting is multifactorial, and is associated with antecedent lymphoid hyperplasia in most patients.

The risk of PTLD in organ transplant recipients has been linked to both defective immune surveillance and chronic antigenic stimulation from the engrafted organ. The spectrum of LPDs encountered suggests a multistep pathway of lymphomagenesis. Finally, the risk of LPD in patients treated with methotrexate is related to both immune suppression induced by the drug, as well as the inherent increased risk for the development of lymphoma in patients with autoimmune diseases.

Lymphoproliferative diseases associated with primary immune disorders

B. Borisch
M. Raphael
S.H. Swerdlow
E.S. Jaffe

Definition

A lymphoproliferative disease (LPD) arising in the setting of a primary immunodeficiency or a primary immunoregulatory disorder. Because the pathology and pathogenesis of the primary immune disorders (PID) are heterogeneous, the lymphoproliferative diseases occurring in the setting of PID are highly variable. The PIDs most commonly associated with lymphoproliferative disorders are ataxia telangiectasia (AT), Wiskott-Aldrich syndrome (WAS), common variable immunodeficiency (CVID), severe combined immunodeficiency (SCID), X-linked lymphoproliferative disorder (XLP), Nijmegen breakage syndrome (NBS), hyper-IgM syndrome, and autoimmune lymphoproliferative syndrome (ALPS) {9, 340}.

Epidemiology

The risk of developing lymphoma is highly related to the type of underlying PID. Age-specific mortality rates for all neoplasms in patients with PID are greater than 10-200 times the expected rates for the general population. However, given that PIDs are rare disorders, the overall occurrence of PID-associated lymphoproliferative diseases is low. These diseases present primarily in the paediatric age group. CVID is more common in adults. They are more common in males than females, primarily because many of the primary genetic abnormalities are X-linked, e.g., Duncan syndrome, XLP, SCID, and hyper-IgM syndrome {599}.

Sites of involvement

Most cases present in extranodal sites, most commonly the gastrointestinal tract and central nervous system (CNS). The lung and kidney are frequently involved in lymphomatoid granulomatosis.

Clinical features

Patients often present with symptoms resembling those of infection or neoplasia (i.e. fever, fatigue, infectious mononucleosis-like-syndromes). The nature of the clinical presentation will be influenced by the nature of the primary immune disorder. Rarely the occurrence of lymphoma or lymphoproliferative disease is the first sign of the underlying immune defect, such as in X-linked lymphoproliferative disorder.

Aetiology

The cause of the LPD is related to the underlying primary immune defect. Epstein-Barr virus (EBV) is involved in the majority of PID-associated lymphoid proliferations. In these cases defective immune surveillance to EBV is the primary mechanism {1065}. The absence of T-cell control may be complete, as in fatal infectious mononucleosis, or partial, as in lymphomatoid granulomatosis {590}. Hyper IgM syndrome results from mutations in CD40 ligand, which affects T-cell/B-cell interactions, and effective differentiation of B-cells into class-switched plasma cells {562}.

In ALPS the presence of *FAS* gene mutations may contribute directly to the LPD through the accumulation of lymphoid cells {1203, 768}. FAS blocks apoptosis, and in ALPS the severity of the apoptotic defect is an important risk factor for the development of lymphoma {589}. The importance of *FAS* gene mutations as an aetiologic factor is supported by the fact that sporadic mutations of *FAS* are associated with lymphomas in the absence of immune abnormalities {466}.

In AT an abnormal DNA repair mechanism secondary to mutations of the *ATM* gene can contribute to the development of lymphoma, leukaemia, as well as other neoplasms {340}. Defects in DNA repair also are identified in NBS. However, in patients with NBS lymphoma is much more common than other neoplasms. The causal relationship between PID and cancer is exemplified by the fact that treatment of AT or WAS by bone marrow transplantation leads to reduction in the susceptibility to malignancy {383}.

Chronic antigenic stimulation may predispose to the development of lymphoma in some patients. In patients with CVID chronic antigenic stimulation leads to marked lymphoid hyperplasia in the

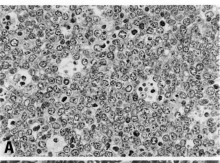
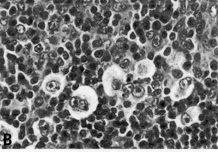
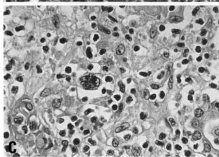

Fig. 9.01 Lymphomas in ALPS. **A** Burkitt lymphoma. **B** Hodgkin lymphoma, mixed cellularity subtype. **C** T-cell-rich/ histiocyte-rich large B-cell lymphoma. Histological features of these lymphoma subtypes resemble those occurring sporadically, without predisposing immune abnormalities.

lung and gastrointestinal tract {1140}. This benign lymphoid proliferation may simulate lymphoma, and may predispose to the development of lymphoid malignancies. However, a direct causal relationship has not been shown.

Intestinal lymphangiectasia and protein losing enteropathy lead to hypogammaglobulinemia and late-occurring lym-

The authors acknowledge the contributions of N. Brousse, D. Canioni and A. Fischer, Paris.

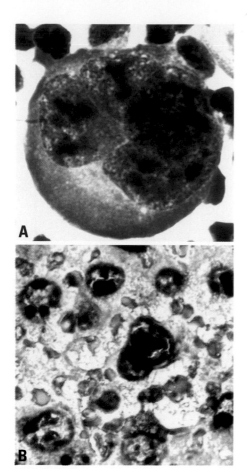

Fig. 9.02 Diffuse large B-cell lymphoma in a patient with long-standing common variable immunodeficiency syndrome. **A** Lymphoma cells are seen in ascites fluid and show marked pleomorphism. **B** Lymphoma cells are EBV-positive by EBER *in situ* hybridisation.

phomas {124}. In some instances treatment of lymphoma has resulted in cure of the primary intestinal defect {144}.

Precursor lesions

The underlying primary immune disorder is the principal precursor lesion leading to the development of LPD. Lymphoid hyperplasia may precede the development of LPD in some diseases, such as ALPS and WAS. Patients with WAS often have serum monoclonal gammopathy {253}. The lymph nodes may contain a marked plasmacytosis, which is monoclonal in some cases. However, monoclonal expansions, particularly if they are minor clones, do not necessarily progress to lymphoma. For example in CVID, VJ-PCR may detect clonal B-cell populations that are self-limited {733}. Hyper IgM syndrome is characterised by peripheral blood B-cells that bear only

IgM and IgD. Germinal centres are absent in lymph nodes. The patients often develop extensive proliferations of IgM-producing plasma cells, most commonly in extranodal sites, such as the gastrointestinal tract, liver and gallbladder. These lesions may be so extensive as to be fatal, without progression to overt lymphoma.

Morphology

In PID patients diverse types of lymphoma and LPD may occur. Some are the same lymphomas and leukaemias as in immunocompetent patients. Diffuse large B-cell lymphoma (DLBCL) is by far the most common LPD in the setting of PID (see Chapter 6). Hodgkin lymphoma and polymorphic lymphoproliferations resembling post-transplant associated lymphoproliferative disorders (PTLD) may also occur {1298}. The histological appearance of the lymphoma may be influenced by the nature of the underlying immune abnormality, which will also affect the histopathology of the lymphoid organs. Lymphomas composed of small B-lymphocytes do not appear increased in frequency.

B-cell neoplasms

Fatal infectious mononucleosis (FIM)
FIM is characterised by a highly polymorphous proliferation of lymphoid cells showing evidence of plasmacytoid and immunoblastic differentiation. Reed-Sternberg-like cells may be seen. This condition is primarily seen in patients with XLP (Duncan syndrome) and SCID {1065}. FIM results from the proliferation of EBV-positive B-cells in the absence of effective immune surveillance. The abnormal B-cell proliferation is systemic, involving both lymphoid and non-lymphoid organs, most commonly the terminal ileum. Haemophagocytosis is commonly seen, and is most readily identified in the bone marrow. A haemophagocytic syndrome may be the primary cause of death, usually associated with marked pancytopenia and further infectious complications.

Diffuse large B-cell lymphoma (see chapter 6)
DLBCL is the most common LPD in patients with PID. DLBCL are increased in patients with AT, WAS, Job syndrome,

CVID, and NBS. Both centroblastic and immunoblastic variants may be seen, although immunoblastic variants predominate.

Lymphomatoid granulomatosis (LYG) (see Chapter 6)
LYG is an EBV-driven proliferation of B-cells associated with a marked T-cell infiltration {470}. It is increased in frequency in patients with WAS {556}. WAS is a complex immune disorder, with defects in function of T cells, B cells, neutrophils, and macrophages. However, T-cell dysfunction is significant, and tends to increase in severity during the course of the disease. LYG is characterised by an angiocentric and angiodestructive infiltrate, often with extensive necrosis. The most common sites of involvement are lung, skin, brain, and kidney. LYG is not considered a lymphoma, since the EBV-driven B-cell expansion is often not autonomous, and may respond to immunoregulatory therapy using interferon alfa-2b {1397}. Variations in histological grade are seen, and tend to correlate with prognosis. Moreover, LYG may progress to DLBCL {471, 775}.

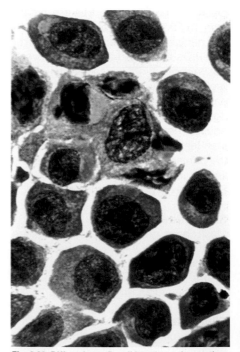

Fig. 9.03 Diffuse large B-cell lymphoma in a patient with intestinal lymphangiectasia and protein losing enteropathy. Cells appear plasmacytoid. Patient presented with a malignant pleural effusion. However, cells were negative for HHV-8/KSHV.

Burkitt lymphoma (see chapter 6)
This type of lymphoma may occur in XLP and AT-patients.

T-cell neoplasms

Ataxia telangiectasia is the one PID in which T-cell lymphomas and leukaemias are more common than B-cell neoplasms {1270}. Both precursor T-lymphoblastic lymphoma/leukaemia (pre-T ALL/LBL) and T-cell prolymphocytic leukaemia (T-PLL) have been reported. Rare cases of peripheral T-cell lymphoma have been seen in patients with ALPS {1028}. However, benign T-cell expansions of double-negative (CD4-/CD8-) alpha beta T-cells are much more common than T-cell lymphomas. Because the T-cell expansion is very marked, caution is warranted in the diagnosis of T-cell lymphoma in patients with ALPS. Clonal T-cell expansions and rare cases of T-cell lymphoma also have been reported in CVID.

Hodgkin lymphoma

Classical Hodgkin lymphoma has been reported in patients with WAS, ALPS, and AT {340}. Hodgkin-like lymphoproliferations resembling those seen in the setting of methotrexate therapy also may be seen {623}. Nodular lymphocyte predominant HL has been reported in association with ALPS {768}.

Immunophenotype
Most of the LPDs in patients with PID are of B-cell lineage, and thus carry the specific B-cell markers corresponding to their differentiation stage. EBV infection of B-cells often leads to down-regulation of B-cell antigens. Thus, CD20, CD19, and CD79a may be negative or expressed on only some of the neoplastic cells in EBV-positive LPDs. Similarly, EBV leads to the expression of CD30 in most cases. In patients with EBV-positive LPD resulting from defective immune surveillance, the latency genes including LMP1 may be expressed.

In cases showing evidence of plasmacytoid differentiation, monoclonal cytoplasmic immunoglobulin (Ig) may be identified.

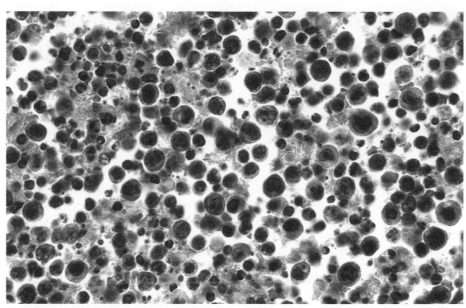

Fig. 9.04 Lymphoproliferative disease occurring in XLP with features of fatal infectious mononucleosis. There is a proliferation of B-cells with plasmacytoid and immunoblastic features. Prominent apoptosis is seen in the background, and a T-cell response is absent. The lymphoid cells are universally EBV-positive (not shown).

Genetics
FIM may be polyclonal at the genetic level. However, B-cell lymphomas are monoclonal as evidenced by Ig gene rearrangement studies. Because many PIDs are associated with atypical lymphoid hyperplasia, the absence of clonality at the genetic level is helpful in ruling out progression to lymphoma {1140}. Monoclonal Ig heavy chain gene rearrangement may be seen rarely in the absence of lymphoma, such as in WAS and CVID {340, 733}.

Because a majority of LPDs in patients with PID are linked to EBV, EBV terminal repeat analysis may be used as another marker of clonality. Other genetic lesions may be directly related to the primary immune defect, such as *FAS* gene mutation in patients with ALPS, or mutations of *SAP/SLAM* in XLP {437, 1266}.

In AT, in addition to mutations of the *ATM* gene, inversions and transpositions of the T-cell receptor genes on chromosomes 7 and 14 are common. These often show breakpoints at 14q11-12, 7q32-35, and 7p15. These translocations may involve the *TCL1* gene, leading to T-cell lymphoproliferative disease including both pre T-ALL/LBL as well as T-cell PLL. Other chromosomal rearrangements/translocations include inv(7)(p13q35), t(7;7)(p13q35), t(7;14)(p13;q11), and t(14;14)(q11;q32). The immunoglobulin gene loci also may be involved {1270}.

Prognosis and predictive factors
The prognosis is related to both the underlying primary immune disorder as well as the type of lymphoma. The immunological status of the host is an important risk factor {176}. Most of the lymphomas and leukaemias in patients with PID are aggressive. However, given the wide variety of underlying conditions and ensuing lymphoproliferative disorders, the prognosis must be evaluated in each case individually. Treatment is based both on the nature of the neoplastic process, as well as the underlying genetic defect. Allogeneic bone marrow transplantation has been used in patients WAS, SCID, and hyper IgM syndrome {327, 477}.

Lymphomas associated with infection by the human immune deficiency virus (HIV)

M. Raphael
B. Borisch
E.S. Jaffe

Definition

Lymphomas that develop in HIV-positive patients are predominantly aggressive B-cell lymphomas. In a proportion of cases they are considered acquired immuno-deficiency syndrome (AIDS)-defining conditions and are the initial manifestation of AIDS {757}. These disorders are heterogeneous, and include lymphomas usually diagnosed in immunocompetent patients, as well as those seen much more often in the setting of HIV infection. The most common HIV-associated lymphomas include: Burkitt lymphoma (BL), diffuse large B-cell lymphoma (DLBCL) (often involving the central nervous system [CNS]), primary effusion lymphoma (PEL), and plasmablastic lymphoma of the oral cavity. Hodgkin lymphoma is also increased in the setting of HIV.

Epidemiology

The incidence of all subtypes of non-Hodgkin lymphoma (NHL) is increased 60-200 fold in HIV-positive patients. Before highly active antiretroviral therapy (HAART) was available, primary central nervous system (CNS) lymphoma and BL were increased approximately 1000 fold in comparison with the general population {96}. The incidence of Hodgkin lymphoma may be increased up to 8 fold {443}. Lymphoma is the first AIDS defining illness in three to five per cent of patients. Since the introduction of HAART, some studies have indicated a decrease in the incidence of lymphoma in AIDS patients and they contribute to a greater percentage of first AIDS-defining illness {832}. However, large datasets are needed to evaluate the impact of HAART on HIV-related lymphoma {467}.

Aetiology

The lymphomas in HIV patients are heterogeneous, reflecting several pathogenetic mechanisms: chronic antigen stimulation, genetic abnormalities, cytokine disregulation and the role of the herpes viruses: Epstein-Barr virus (EBV) and Kaposi Sarcoma Human Virus (KSHV/

HHV8) {412, 64}. HIV-related lymphomas are consistently monoclonal, and are characterised by a number of common genetic abnormalities of oncogenes involving the *MYC* and *BCL-6* oncogenes, as well as tumour suppressor genes. {69, 412, 413, 414} The recognition of a polyclonal or oligoclonal nature of some HIV-related lymphoid proliferations suggests a multistep process in the pathogenesis of lymphoma {1018}. B-cell stimulation, hypergammaglogulinemia and persistent generalised lymphadenopathy preceding the development of these lymphomas probably reflect the role of chronic antigen stimulation {468}.

Disruption of the cytokine network leading to high serum levels of IL6 and IL10 is a feature of HIV-related lymphomas associated with EBV or KSHV/HHV8 {1005}. EBV is identified in the neoplastic cells of approximately 60% of HIV-related lymphomas, but the detection of EBV varies considerably with the site of presentation and histological subtype. EBV infection occurs in almost all of the cases of primary CNS lymphoma {172} and PEL, 80% of DLBCL with immunoblastic features, and 30 to 50% of BL {482}. Nearly all cases of Hodgkin lymphoma in

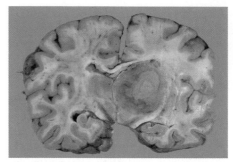

Fig. 9.05 Diffuse large B-cell lymphoma, HIV-associated. A large tumour involves the basal ganglia.

the setting of HIV infection are associated with EBV {54, 758, 1219}. KSHV/HHV8 is specifically associated with PEL, which often occurs in late stages of the disease in the setting of profound immunosuppression {198}.

Sites of involvement

These lymphomas display a marked propensity to involve extranodal sites, in particular the gastrointestinal tract, CNS (less frequent since HAART), liver, and bone marrow. The peripheral blood is rarely involved except in occasional cases of BL presenting as acute leukaemia. Unusual sites such as the oral cavity,

Table 9.01
Categories of HIV-associated lymphomas

1. Lymphomas also occurring in immunocompetent patients
Burkitt lymphoma
Classical
With plasmacytoid differentiation
Atypical
Diffuse large B-cell lymphoma
Centroblastic
Immunoblastic
Extranodal marginal zone B-cell lymphoma of mucosa-associated lymphoid tissue type (MALT lymphoma) (rare)
Peripheral T- cell lymphoma (rare)
Classical Hodgkin lymphoma
2. Lymphomas occurring more specifically in HIV+ patients
Primary effusion lymphoma
Plasmablastic lymphoma of the oral cavity
3. Lymphomas also occurring in other immunodeficiency states
Polymorphic B-cell lymphoma (PTLD-like)

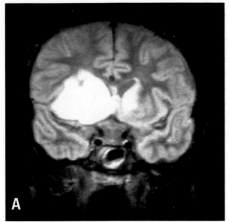

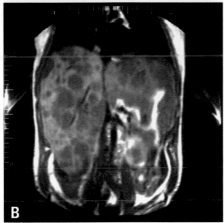

Fig. 9.06 Radiological findings in HIV-associated lymphoma. **A** Nuclear magnetic resonance (NMR) imaging scan of the brain shows a large tumour mass in the basal ganglia. **B** Multiple filling defects are seen in liver.

jaw, and body cavities are often involved. Many other extranodal sites, e.g., lung, skin, testis, heart, breast can be involved. Lymph nodes are involved in about one-third of patients at presentation {106, 671, 1087}

Clinical features
Most patients present with advanced clinical stage; bulky disease with a high tumour burden is frequent. LDH is usually markedly elevated. There is a significant relationship between the subtype of lymphoma and the HIV disease status. DLBCL more often occurs in the setting of long-standing AIDS before the diagnosis of lymphoma, and a trend towards a higher rate of opportunistic infections and lower CD4+ T-cell counts with a mean below 100 x 10⁶/L. In contrast, BL occurs in less immunodeficient patients, with a shorter mean interval between the diagnosis of HIV seropositivity and lym-

phoma, and patients have significantly higher CD4+ T-cell counts (more than 200 x 10⁶/L) {133, 177}.

Morphology
In HIV positive patients, diverse types of lymphoma can occur. Some are the same aggressive B-cell lymphomas that occur sporadically in the absence of HIV infection. Some polymorphic lymphoproliferations and unusual lymphomas occur more specifically in AIDS patients.

Lymphomas also occurring in immunocompetent patients

These should be classified according to usual criteria for these diseases.

Burkitt lymphoma (see chapter 6)
Classical
This variant shows morphological features of classical BL with a monomorphous, medium sized cell proliferation. It represents 30% of all HIV-associated lymphomas. EBV is positive in about 30% of cases {1087, 1088}.

Burkitt lymphoma with plasmacytoid differentiation
This morphological variant is relatively unique to AIDS patients and represents about 20% of non-Hodgkin lymphoma (NHL) cases. It is characterised by medium-sized cells with abundant basophilic cytoplasm, and an eccentric nucleus, often with one centrally located prominent nucleolus. The cells often contain cytoplasmic immunoglobulin. EBV is positive in about 50-70% of cases {265}.

Atypical Burkitt/Burkitt-like
These tumours are less frequent than the two other morphological variants. They have nuclear features similar to those of classical BL, but exhibit greater pleomorphism in the size and shape of cells. The nuclei may contain more prominent nucleoli. EBV is present in 30-50% of cases.

Diffuse large B-cell lymphoma
The majority of these lymphomas contain numerous centroblasts admixed with a variable component of immunoblasts, consistent the centroblastic variant. This type represents about 25% of HIV-associated lymphomas; EBV is present in

30% of cases. Cases containing more than 90% immunoblasts and usually exhibiting plasmacytoid features are classified as the immunoblastic variant. They represent about 10% of HIV-associated lymphomas, are associated with EBV in 90%, and often occur late in the course of HIV disease. Primary central nervous system lymphomas are usually of the immunoblastic type {172, 671}.

Hodgkin lymphoma
Most cases correspond to either the mixed cellularity or lymphocyte depleted forms of classical Hodgkin lymphoma. Some cases of nodular sclerosis Hodgkin

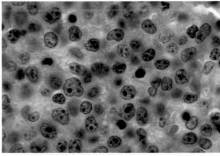

Fig. 9.07 Primary CNS lymphoma, classified as diffuse large B-cell lymphoma in an HIV-positive patient.

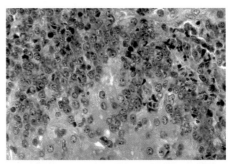

Fig. 9.08 HIV-associated Burkitt lymphoma involving the liver.

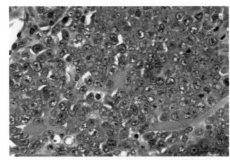

Fig. 9.09 "Primary effusion lymphoma", KSHV/HHV8-associated, presenting as a soft tissue mass. The tumour cells are monomorphic with an immunoblastic appearance.

lymphoma are also seen. HIV-related Hodgkin lymphoma is associated with EBV in nearly all cases; the cells express latent membrane protein (LMP1) and are EBER-positive {54, 758, 1219}.

Other lymphomas (rare)
Rare cases of MALT lymphoma have been described in both paediatric and adult patients with HIV infection {846, 1277}. Rare cases of peripheral T-cell and natural killer lymphoma can also occur {38, 106, 160, 175, 472, 529, 598}.

Lymphomas occurring more specifically in HIV positive patients

Primary effusion lymphoma (PEL) (see chapter 6)

Synonym Body cavity-based lymphoma
This rare lymphoma (representing less than 5% of cases of NHL), which was not fully characterised until after the discovery of the virus KSHV/HHV8, usually presents with lymphomatous effusions. It represents a distinct clinicopathological entity, based on characteristic morphologic, immunophenotypic, molecular, and viral features. While typically presenting with either pleural or peritoneal effusion, it can present as a solid tumour mass, most commonly affecting the gastrointestinal tract or soft tissue {81, 287}. PEL is associated with both Kaposi sarcoma and multicentric Castleman disease in HIV-positive patients.
With Wright or May Grunwald Giemsa staining performed on cytocentrifuge preparations, the cells exhibit a range of appearances, from large immunoblastic or plasmablastic cells to cells with more anaplastic morphology. Nuclei are large, round to more irregular in shape, with prominent nucleoli. The cytoplasm can be very abundant and is deeply basophilic with the presence of vacuoles in occasional cells. A perinuclear hof consistent with plasmacytoid differentiation may be seen. Some cells can resemble Reed-Sternberg cells. The cells often appear more uniform in histological sections than in cytospin preparations.
However, the cells are generally large, with some pleomorphism, ranging from large cells with round or ovoid nuclei to very large cells having irregular nuclei and abundant cytoplasm {287, 914, 1356, 198}.

Plasmablastic lymphoma of the oral cavity
These tumours, localised in the oral cavity or the jaw, are rapidly growing with a high mitotic index. The tumours display a diffuse pattern of growth interspersed by macrophages. The tumour cells are large with eccentrically located nuclei, and usually single, centrally located, prominent nucleoli. The cytoplasm is deeply basophilic with a paranuclear hof. Some cells display cytoplasmic immunoglobulins. EBV is present in more than 50% of cases, but no association with KSHV/HHV8 has been detected {279}.

Lymphomas occurring in other immunodeficient states

Polymorphic lymphoid proliferations resembling post-transplant associated lymphoproliferative disease (PTLD) may be seen in adults and also in children but are much less common than in the post-transplant setting, comprising less than 5% of HIV-associated lymphomas. These conform to the criteria of polymorphic B-cell PTLD. The infiltrates contain a range of lymphoid cells from small cells, often with plasmacytoid features, to large cells having the features of immunoblasts, with scattered large bizarre cells expressing CD30. EBV is often present, but some cases may be EBV negative {656, 817, 915, 1268}.

Immunophenotype
The immunophenotype varies according to the histological subtype of the lymphoma. The vast majority of HIV-related lymphomas are of B-cell origin. CD19, CD20 and CD79a and CD10 are expressed in virtually all the tumours

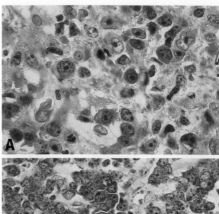
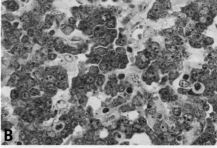
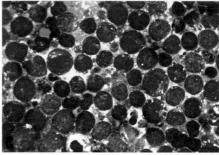

Fig. 9.10 A Plasmablastic lymphoma of the oral cavity in an HIV-positive patient. Tumour cells have prominent central nucleoli. **B** Classical Burkitt lymphoma. Cell population is uniform. **C** Atypical Burkitt lymphoma, HIV-associated. Touch imprint shows deeply basophilic cytoplasm and cytoplasmic vacuoles. Variability in nuclear size and shape is evident.

cells in BL; DLBCL have a more variable immunophenotype. Tumour cells lose the expression of CD20 in immunoblastic lymphomas with plasmacytic differentiation, plasmablastic lymphoma of the oral

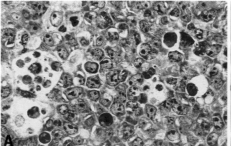
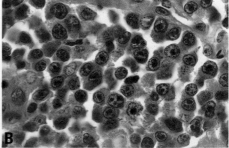

Fig. 9.11 A Atypical Burkitt lymphoma. Cells show much greater variation in size and shape, than seen in classical Burkitt lymphoma. **B** Burkitt lymphoma with plasmacytoid differentiation. Cells have an eccentric rim of deeply stained cytoplasm. This variant is often EBV-positive.

cavity and PEL {671, 914, 1088}.
Cytoplasmic immunoglobulins are detectable in some cells of Burkitt lymphoma with plasmacytoid differentiation, in immunoblastic lymphomas with plasmacytoid features, in plasmablastic lymphomas of the oral cavity, and in about 20% of cases of PEL.

In PEL and plasmablastic lymphomas, other markers of plasmacytic differentiation are also present such as CD138, and the molecules recognised by the monoclonal antibody VS38c. CD45 is expressed in most cases of PEL, despite a null cell or aberrant phenotype with other markers {177, 178, 1088}.

Activation-associated antigens expressed in some diffuse large cell lymphomas, especially those of immunoblastic subtype, and PEL include epithelial membrane antigen (EMA), CD30, CD38 and CD71 {177, 287, 671, 914, 1088, 178, 1356}. PEL may aberrantly express cytoplasmic CD3 {529, 265, 81}. However, true T-cell lymphomas are infrequent. Mature T-cell lymphomas, when they exist, express T-cell-associated antigens, such as CD2, CD3, CD5, CD4 or CD8, CD16 or CD56. The loss of one or more antigens can be observed {106, 160, 175}.

Genetic features

Antigen receptor genes
Most of the lymphomas diagnosed in HIV positive patients are monoclonal B-cell neoplasms, with clonal rearrangement of immunoglobulins genes detected by Southern blot or PCR techniques {671, 1088, 1356}. Most cases have somatically mutated immunoglobulin genes {280, 336}. T-cell cases have clonal rearrangement of T-cell receptor genes {106, 160, 529}.

Oncogenes and tumour suppressor genes
Cases of HIV-associated BL, like other cases of BL, have genetic abnormalities affecting band 8q24, the location of *MYC* locus. The classical translocation t(8 ; 14) (q24 ; q32) or its variants affecting the light chain genes at 2p11 and 22q11 have been described. Besides the truncation within or around the *MYC* locus,

point mutations in the first intron-first exon regulatory regions and amino acid substitution in the second exon are also detected and contribute to the deregulation of *MYC* {265, 412, 287}. Trans-locations of the 8q24 band are also detected in about 20% of diffuse large B-cell lymphomas in HIV-positive patients, while in PEL no *MYC* abnormalities have been found {178, 914}.

Rearrangement of *BCL6*, a proto-oncogene located at band 3q27 and belonging to the family of transcription factors containing zinc finger domains, is confined to diffuse large B-cell lymphomas and is absent in BL. Frequent mutations of the 5' noncoding region of the *BCL6* gene occurring independently of *BCL6* rearrangements are detected in BL and DLBCL and represent the most common genetic alteration in HIV–related lymphomas {69, 413, 414}.

Mutations of the Ras family proto-oncogenes are present, although in a small number of cases (15%). *RAS* mutation appears to be peculiar to HIV related lymphomas, as there is no significant

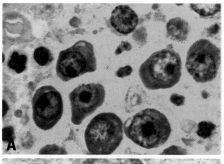

Fig. 9.12 Diffuse large B-cell lymphoma, immunoblastic variant. **A** The cells have prominent nucleoli and abundant amphophilic cytoplasm. **B** Cells exhibit marked plasmacytoid differentiation.

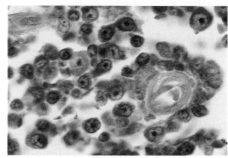

Fig. 9.13 Diffuse large B-cell lymphoma, immunoblastic variant, presenting in the central nervous system. The cells have prominent central nucleoli.

detection of *RAS* abnormalities in lymphoma occurring in immunocompetent hosts {69}.

Point mutations and deletions of the *TP53* tumour suppressor gene are detected in 50-60% of BL and in 40% of DLBCL, leading to the inactivation of this gene and overexpression of p53 protein {817}. Deletions of the long arm of chromosome 6 clustering to 6q27, and other recurrent genetic abnormalities occurring in 25% of cases may implicate other tumour suppressor genes {412}.

Prognosis and predictive factors
The rate of complete remission is about 50%, in most of the histological subtypes. However, the 2-year survival was significantly lower in DLBCL than in BL in an univariate analysis {439}. The International Prognostic Index (IPI) appears to be a reliable indicator. The degree of immunodeficiency also correlates positively with the IPI score {1114}. Some other adverse prognostic factors have been identified, such as age greater than 35 years, intravenous drug use, stage III/IV and CD4 counts less than 100×10^6/L. Despite dose adjustment, the outcome of patients with lymphoma and HIV infection is most closely related to the severity of immunodeficiency {439}. Long term survival can be achieved in approximately one third of patients with HIV-associated lymphoma with favourable prognostic characteristics {1240}. PEL usually has a very poor prognosis with a low complete remission rate.

Post-transplant lymphoproliferative disorders

N.L. Harris
S. H. Swerdlow
G. Frizzera
D. M. Knowles

Definition

Post-transplant lymphoproliferative disorder (PTLD) is a lymphoid proliferation or lymphoma that develops as a consequence of immunosuppression in a recipient of a solid organ or bone marrow allograft. PTLDs comprise a spectrum ranging from early, Epstein-Barr virus (EBV)-driven polyclonal proliferations resembling infectious mononucleosis to EBV-positive or EBV-negative lymphomas of predominantly B-cell or less often T-cell type.

Epidemiology

The characteristics of PTLD appear to differ somewhat from one institution to another, probably as a result of different patient populations, allograft types, and immunosuppressive regimens. The risk of lymphoma varies depending on the type of allograft and the immunosuppressive regimen. Among solid organ recipients, patients receiving renal allografts have the lowest frequency of PTLD (<1%). Those with hepatic and cardiac allografts have an intermediate risk (1-2%), and those receiving heart-lung or liver-bowel allografts develop PTLD at the highest frequency (5%).

The overall incidence of PTLD for solid organ transplant recipients is <2% {931}. This risk is estimated to be 20 times that of the normal population for renal allograft recipients and 120 times normal for cardiac allograft recipients {977}. Marrow allograft recipients in general have a low risk of PTLD (1%), but those who receive HLA-mismatched or T-cell depleted bone marrow and those who receive immunosuppressive therapy for graft vs host disease (GVHD) are at the highest risk for development of lymphoma – up to 20% for patients with more than one of these risk factors {258}.

Aetiology

The majority of PTLD are associated with EBV infection, and appear to represent EBV-induced monoclonal or, less often, polyclonal B-cell or rarely T-cell proliferations that occur in a setting of decreased T-cell immune surveillance {931, 232, 380, 670, 200}.

About 20% of PTLD are EBV-negative; among renal allograft recipients up to 50% may be EBV-negative {380, 742, 941}. EBV-negative cases tend to occur later than EBV-positive cases, and the majority of cases occurring >5 years after transplant are EBV-negative. The aetiology of EBV-negative PTLD is not known. Although these occur less frequently than EBV-positive cases, their frequency is still higher than would be expected in the normal population; in addition, some cases respond to decreased immunosuppression. Thus, it is likely that they are also in some way related to decreased immune competence.

The majority of PTLD in solid organ recipients are of host origin, reflecting escape of host EBV-positive cells from immune surveillance. A minority (<10% of the cases) are of donor origin, indicating that lymphoid cells transplanted with the allograft can survive and undergo malignant transformation in some cases. Donor origin PTLD appear to be most common in liver and lung allograft recipients, and frequently involve the allograft {1220, 44, 732, 1249, 1373, 201}. In contrast, the majority of PTLD in marrow allograft recipients are of donor origin, as would be expected, since successful allografting results in an immune system that is exclusively of donor origin {1451}.

Sites of involvement

In solid organ recipients immunosuppressed with azathioprine-based regimens, PTLDs tend to involve extranodal sites, including the allograft and the central nervous system (CNS). Patients treated with cyclosporine-based or Tacrolimus-based regimens develop PTLDs that tend to involve lymph nodes and the gastrointestinal tract, but less frequently involve the CNS {931, 380, 1021}. The bone marrow, liver, and lungs are often involved, but peripheral blood is rarely involved. The allograft is involved in approximately 25% of the cases overall, and on biopsy specimens this may give rise to a differential diagnosis of rejection vs PTLD. Bone marrow allograft recipients tend to present with widespread disease involving nodal and extranodal sites, including liver, spleen, gastrointestinal tract and lungs {1451, 1021, 1181}.

Clinical features

The clinical features of PTLD at presentation are variable, and correlate with the

Table 9.02
Categories of post-transplant lymphoproliferative disease (PTLD).

1. Early lesions
    Reactive plasmacytic hyperplasia
    Infectious mononucleosis-like

2. Polymorphic PTLD

3. Monomorphic PTLD (classify according to lymphoma classification)
    B-cell neoplasms
        Diffuse large B-cell lymphoma (immunoblastic, centroblastic, anaplastic)
        Burkitt/Burkitt-like lymphoma
        Plasma cell myeloma
        Plasmacytoma-like lesions
 	
    T-cell neoplasms
        Peripheral T-cell lymphoma, not otherwise specified
        Other types

4. Hodgkin lymphoma (HL) and Hodgkin lymphoma-like PTLD

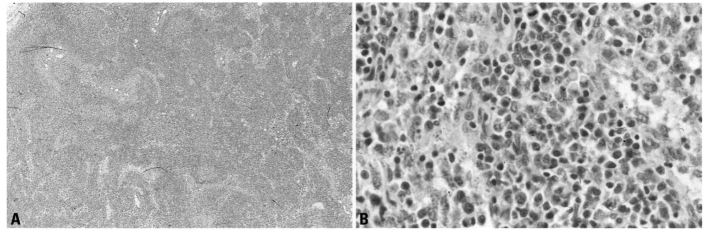

Fig. 9.14 Plasmacytic hyperplasia. **A** The normal architecture of the lymph node is intact. **B** Numerous plasma cells are present.

type of immunosuppression, type of allograft, and to some extent with morphologically defined categories (see below). In solid organ recipients treated with azathioprine the mean interval to PTLD following transplanation is 48 months, while in those treated with cyclosporine A it is 15 months {1021}. The majority of PTLD in bone marrow allograft recipients develop within the first 5 months {258}. EBV-positive cases tend to occur earlier than EBV-negative cases, with a median interval of 6-10 months compared with 4-5 years for EBV-negative cases {742, 941}.

Plasmacytic hyperplasia (PH) and infectious-mononucleosis like (IM-like) lesions may arise at any time, most often within the first 2 years after transplantation, but some as late as 5 years {931, 200, 780}. The majority of both polymorphic and monomorphic PTLDs occur in the first year after transplantation; patients may present with lymphadenopathy in one or multiple sites, or with organ dysfunction, including the allograft, related to extranodal infiltrates. Monomorphic PTLD overlap clinically with polymorphic cases; however, late-occurring, EBV-negative cases are more likely to be monomorphic {742, 941}.

Morphologic categories of PTLD

"Early" lesions: Plasmacytic hyperplasia (PH) and infectious-mononucleosis-like PTLD

These lesions are defined as a lymphoid proliferation in an allograft recipient, characterised by some degree of architectural preservation of the involved tissue, with preservation of the nodal sinuses or tonsillar crypts, and residual reactive follicles in some cases. Plasmacytic hyperplasia is characterised by numerous plasma cells and rare immunoblasts, while the IM-like lesion has the typical morphologic features of IM, with paracortical expansion and numerous immunoblasts in a background of T cells and plasma cells.

These are two possibly overlapping lymphoid proliferations that differ from typical reactive follicular hyperplasia in having a diffuse prolifcration of plasma cells and immunoblasts, but do not completely efface the architecture of the involved tissue. The term "reactive plasmacytic hyperplasia" was used by Nalesnik and colleagues for a reactive lesion that was occasionally seen in lymph nodes in patients who had PTLD in concurrent or subsequent biopsies {931}; they did not consider this a form of PTLD. Knowles and colleagues also used this term, and found that 3/8 cases they diagnosed as PH involved lymph nodes, while 4/8

Table 9.03
Pathologic evaluation of specimens for the diagnosis of PTLD.

Technique	Necessity	Purpose
Routine morphology	Essential	Architecture (preserved vs effaced) Cytology (polymorphic vs monomorphic)
Immunophenotyping	Essential	Lineage Clonality (flow cytometry or frozen section immunohistochemistry more useful than paraffin section immunohistochemistry)
Molecular genetic studies of antigen receptor genes	Useful	Clonality
EBER *in situ* hybridisation	Useful	Detection of EBV as an aid in diagnosis; PTLD vs rejection in allograft
EBV clonality	Not required	Identification of minor clones

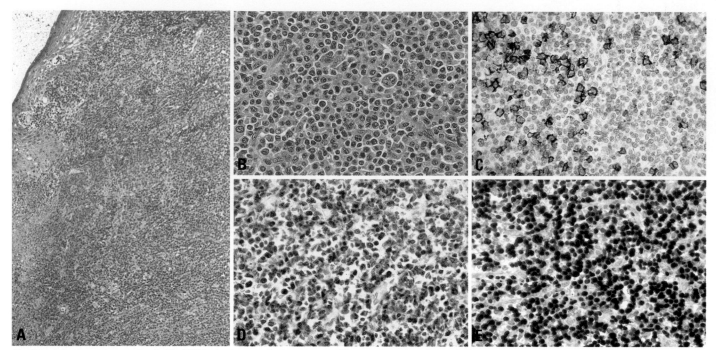

Fig. 9.15 Infectious mononucleosis-like (IM) lesion in a tonsil of an 11-year-old renal allograft recipient. **A** There is preservation of overlying epithelium and crypts, but normal follicles are absent, and there is a diffuse lymphoid proliferation. **B** There is a polymorphous proliferation of immunoblasts, small lymphoid cells and plasma cells. **C** A stain for CD20 shows scattered B cells. **D** In contrast, a stain for CD79a shows more numerous positive cells, indicating plasmacytoid differentiation. **E** *In situ* hybridisation (ISH) for Epstein-Barr virus latency-associated RNA (EBER) shows staining of the majority of the cells. This lesion regressed with reduction in immunosuppression.

involved Waldeyer's ring and one involved the lung; the latter cases may correspond to what others have called infectious mononucleosis-like (IM-like) lesions {1424}.

PH and IM-like lesions occur at a younger age than the other PTLDs and are often seen in children or in adult solid organ recipients who have not had prior EBV infection {200, 780}. They involve lymph nodes (PH) or tonsils and adenoids (IM-like) more often than true extranodal sites, and often regress spontaneously or with reduction in immunosuppression {780}. However, IM-like lesions can be fatal, as can infectious mononucleosis in other settings. They may be followed by polymorphic or monomorphic PTLD in some cases {931, 1424}.

Polymorphic PTLD

ICD-O code   9970/1

Synonyms Polymorphic B-cell hyperplasia, polymorphic B-cell lymphoma

Polymorphic PTLD are defined as destructive lesions composed of immuno-

blasts, plasma cells, and intermediate-sized lymphoid cells, that efface the architecture of lymph nodes or form destructive extranodal masses.

In contrast to early IM-like lesions, the tissue architecture is effaced {407, 488}, but in contrast to most lymphomas, they show the full range of B-cell maturation, from immunoblasts to plasma cells, with small and medium-sized lymphocytes and cells with irregular nuclei resembling centrocytes. Overall the impression is often that of "mixed small and large cell" lymphoma, resembling the "polymorphic immunocytoma" of the original Kiel classification. There may be areas of necrosis and scattered large, bizarre cells (atypical immunoblasts); numerous mitoses may be present. This category was at one time subdivided into "polymorphic B-cell hyperplasia" and "polymorphic B-cell lymphoma" based on the presence of atypical immunoblasts and necrosis, but it is now felt that attempting to distinguish between these is not practical or necessary, since both are typically monoclonal and have similar clinical features {670, 200, 1424}. Some cases have areas that appear more monomorphic in the same or other tissues; thus, there may be a continuous spectrum between these lesions

and the monomorphic PTLD.

The frequency of polymorphic PTLD varies from one institution to another, ranging from 20% to over 80% of the cases {931, 232, 380, 670, 941, 407, 632}. Reduction in immunosuppression leads to regression in a variable number of the cases; others may progress and require treatment for lymphoma {931, 670, 1227}.

Monomorphic PTLD

Monomorphic B-cell PTLD

Monomorphic B-PTLD have sufficient architectural and cytologic atypia to be diagnosed as lymphoma on morphologic grounds, and have expression of B-cell-associated antigens. These tumours should be classified as B-cell lymphomas, according to the classification scheme for B-cell lymphomas, but the term, PTLD, should also appear in the diagnosis. The infiltrates are characterised by nodal architectural effacement and/or invasive, tumoural growth in extranodal sites, with confluent sheets of transformed cells. All or most cells in the infiltrate are large, transformed, blastic

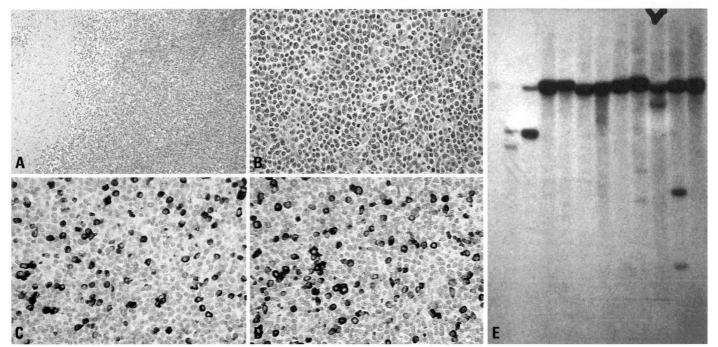

Fig. 9.16 Polymorphic PTLD. **A** There is diffuse effacement of the nodal architecture. There is a large, geographic area of necrosis present. **B** There is a mixed proliferation of immunoblasts, plasma cells and medium-sized lymphoid cells with irregular nuclei (Giemsa stain). Immunoperoxidase stains on paraffin sections with antibodies to kappa (**C**) and (**D**) lambda immunoglobulin light chains show polyclonal staining (**C** = kappa, **D** = lambda). **E** Southern blot probed for immunoglobulin heavy chain joining region shows a single rearranged (clonal) band.

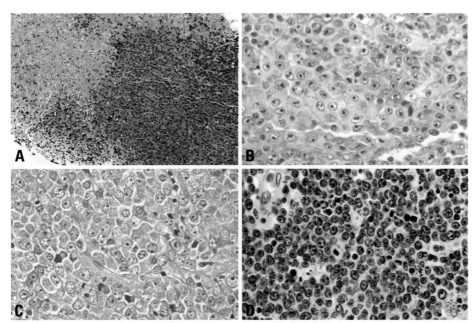

Fig. 9.17 Monomorphic B-PTLD. **A** Liver biopsy showing partial replacement by diffuse large B-cell lymphoma, immunoblastic variant. **B** Diffuse large B-cell lymphoma, immunoblastic variant, EBV-positive, showing a monotonous proliferation of large immunoblast-like cells with prominent central nucleoli and basophilic cytoplasm (Giemsa stain). **C** Diffuse large B-cell lymphoma, centroblastic variant, EBV-negative, showing large transformed cells, many of which have peripheral nucleoli, consistent with centroblasts. **D** Atypical variant of Burkitt lymphoma showing monontonous, medium-sized cells with multiple nucleoli, basophilic cytoplasm, and numerous mitoses.

cells with prominent nucleoli and basophilic cytoplasm, in contrast to the full range of maturation seen in lesions characterised as polymorphic PTLD. It is important to recognise, however, that there may be pleomorphism of the transformed cells – some may be bizarre and multinucleated – and there may be plasmacytoid or plasmacytic differentiation. Thus, the term, monomorphic, does not mean complete cellular monotony, only that most of the cells appear to be transformed.

Diffuse large B-cell lymphoma and Burkitt lymphoma

The majority of monomorphic B-PTLDs fall into the category of diffuse large B-cell lymphoma. Most would be subclassified as the immunoblastic variant, although some are centroblastic. Some cases show features of the anaplastic variant {232, 632}. A minority of the cases have morphologic features of Burkitt lymphoma {632}.

Plasma cell myeloma

Rare transplant patients develop plasma

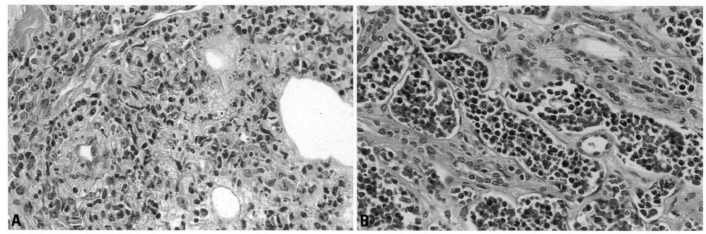

Fig. 9.18 Monomorphic T-PTLDs. **A** Subcutaneous panniculitis-like T-cell lymphoma in an adult female renal allograft recipient, showing diffuse involvement of subcutaneous tissue. This case was EBV-negative. **B** Hepatosplenic gamma-delta T-cell lymphoma (EBV-negative) in a 29 year-old male renal allograft recipient. There is infiltration of small blood vessels in the allograft.

cell myeloma. These may be EBV-positive or EBV-negative; most reported cases have failed to regress with decreased immunosuppression {670, 228}.

Plasmacytoma-like PTLD
Rare extramedullary plasmacytic neoplasms, which appear to be similar to extramedullary plasmacytoma in the non-immunocompromised host, have been reported in the post-transplant setting {606, 494}. They may occur in the gastrointestinal tract, lymph nodes, or other extranodal sites. Their clinical behaviour is not well studied.

Monomorphic T-cell PTLD

Similarly to the monomorphic B-PTLDs, monomorphic T-PTLDs have sufficient atypia and monomorphism to be recognised as neoplastic, and should be classified according to the classification of T-cell neoplasms. Numerous single case reports and small series of T-cell lymphomas in allograft recipients have been reported. Penn {1021} reported 14% of the cases in his registry to be of T-cell origin, but two more recent series report 12.5% (4 of 32) {742} and 4% (3 of 80) {941}.
T-PTLDs appear to span the spectrum of T-cell neoplasms, including subcutaneous panniculitis-like T-cell lymphoma {633}, hepatosplenic gamma-delta T-cell lymphoma {691, 47, 1113, 398}, NK/T-cell lymphomas {487, 937, 545}, T-cell large granular lymphocyte leukaemia {426}, and peripheral T-cell lymphoma,

unspecified. Some cases may be CD30+ {1187, 703, 1330}. The interval to lymphoma development is typically longer for the T-PTLDs than for the B-cell cases, and patients are less likely to respond to decreased immunosuppression. Many reported cases of T-PTLD are EBV-negative, but some are EBV-positive. Leblond and colleagues reported 3/11 EBV-negative PTLDs to be of T-cell type, compared with only 1/21 EBV-positive cases {742}.

Hodgkin lymphoma (HL) and HD-like PTLD

Both classical HL and cases of HL-like PTDL have been reported in allograft recipients. Because Reed-Sternberg-like cells may be seen in polymorphic PTLD, the diagnosis of HL should be based on both classical morphologic and immunophenotypic features. An increased incidence of classical HL has been reported after allogeneic bone marrow transplantation, with an observed-to-expected incidence ratio of 6.2 {1120}. Rarely, allograft recipients develop polymorphic, HL-like lesions in nodal or extranodal sites {932, 318, 449}, similar to those that develop in patients treated with methotrexate for rheumatoid arthritis or psoriasis.
HL-like PTLD are similar to both methotrexate-related HL and HL in HIV infection in that they are virtually always EBV-positive. Some cases have responded to therapy for HL, while others have

been clinically aggressive. Given the small number of reported cases, further study is required to determine their spectrum of clinical behaviour.

Immunophenotype
Plasmacytic hyperplasia and infectious-mononucleosis-like lesions
Immunophenotypic studies show an admixture of polyclonal B cells, plasma cells, and T cells. Immunoblasts are typically EBV-LMP+ {780}.

Polymorphic PTLD
Immunophenotyping on paraffin or frozen sections typically shows a mixture of B and T cells; surface and cytoplasmic Ig may be either polytypic or monotypic. EBV-LMP1 and EBNA2 are detectable in the immunoblasts in the majority of the cases

Monomorphic B-cell PTLD
Immunophenotyping studies show B-cell-associated antigen expression (CD19, CD20, CD79a), with monotypic immunoglobulin (often with expression of gamma or alpha heavy chain) in 50% of the cases. EBV-associated antigens EBNA2 and LMP1 are expressed in the majority of the cases. Many express antigens usually associated with T-cells, specifically, CD43 and CD45RO, which are upregulated in EBV-infected B cells, and are expressed by some conventional B-cell lymphomas. Therefore, these antigens alone cannot be used to determine T lineage, particularly in EBV-positive lymphomas. Many cases are CD30+, with or without anaplastic morphology.

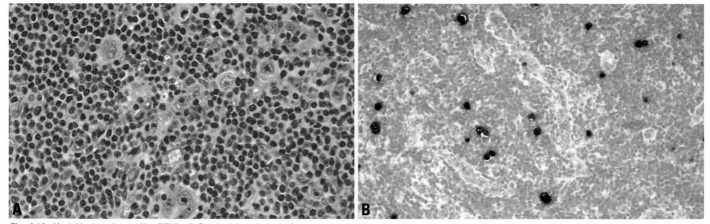

Fig. 9.19 Hodgkin lymphoma-like PTLD. **A** Cervical lymph node from a 30-year-old man with a renal allograft, who developed psoriasis and was treated with methotrexate; there is effacement of the architecture and mononuclear and diagnostic Reed-Sternberg cells in a lymphocyte-rich background. **B** EBER-ISH shows the RS cells as well as small bystander lymphocytes to be positive for EBV RNA.

sion of pan-T cell antigens, and depending on the specific type, may express CD4 or CD8, CD56, or CD30, and either αβ or γδ T-cell receptors. They are variable with respect to EBV positivity.

HL and HL-like PTLD
Classical HL cases have expressed CD15 and CD30 {932, 1120}. Cases diagnosed as HL-like PTLD more often have an atypical immunophenotype with B-cell antigen expression {494}; virtually all cases are EBV-positive.

Genetic features

Antigen receptor genes and EBV
Plasmacytic hyperplasia and infectious-mononucleosis-like lesions
Immunoglobulin genes are polyclonally rearranged. EBV is present in many but not all of the cases of nodal PH {670}. EBV-negative PH may represent nonspecific lymphoid hyperplasia or a reaction to an infection other than EBV, and should not be considered PTLD. Extranodal and nodal IM-like cases are typically EBV-positive and may have small monoclonal or oligoclonal bands on Southern blots probed for episomal EBV genomes. The significance of oligoclonality or a small clonal band in these cases is unknown {670, 1424}.

Polymorphic PTLD
Molecular genetic studies virtually always show clonal rearrangements of immunoglobulin genes and/or EBV genomes, but cytogenetic analysis and studies of oncogenes such as MYC,

RAS, and TP53 typically show no mutations {670, 200}. Early studies reporting a high frequency of polyclonal lesions were based on detection of immunoglobulin light chains in paraffin sections {407, 488}; subsequent studies using molecular genetic analysis have confirmed that the majority of both polymorphic and monomorphic lesions are in fact monoclonal. In some reported cases, tumours at different sites in the same patient may be clonally distinct {199}. In most cases that lack Ig gene rearrangements, clonal episomal EBV genomes can be detected {632, 231}. EBV in PTLD is reported to be exclusively of type A {401}.

Detection of EBV by EBER in situ hybridisation is a useful tool in the differential diagnosis of PTLD versus rejection in allografts. Most cases of polymorphic PTLD contain numerous EBER positive cells. The detection of only rare EBV positive cells should not be considered diagnostic of a PTLD.

Monomorphic B-PTLD
Genetic studies show clonal Ig gene rearrangement in virtually all cases, and the majority contain EBV genomes, which, if present, are in clonal episomal form {232, 632, 231}.

Monomorphic T-PTLD
Most reported cases show clonal T-cell receptor gene rearrangement; about 25% are have clonal episomal EBV genomes {703, 1334}.

Oncogenes
In the polymorphic PTLD, one study showed no mutations of the RAS or TP53

genes, and no rearrangements of the MYC gene, while, monomorphic B-PTLD frequently showed such abnormalities, similarly to de novo DLBCL {670}. Mutations of the BCL6 gene were described in 40% of polymorphic cases and 90% of monomorphic cases, and were associated with failure to respond to decreased immunosuppression; this finding awaits confirmation {197}.

Prognosis and predictive factors
Early and infectious mononucleosis-like lesions tend to regress with reduction in immune suppression, and if this can be accomplished without graft rejection, the prognosis is excellent, particularly in children {780}. Polymorphic and less often monomorphic PTLD may regress with reduction in immune suppression; a proportion of cases of both types fail to regress, and require cytotoxic chemotherapy {931, 670, 1227}. Overall, the mortality of PTLD in solid organ allograft recipients is approximately 60%, while that of marrow allograft recipients with PTLD is 80%. Administration of antibody to CD20 antigen has been useful in abrogating PTLD development in some cases, particularly in the marrow allograft setting. Monitoring for evidence of reactivation of EBV infection may provide an early warning of PTLD development {258}. With early diagnosis, prompt reduction of immune suppression, and careful administration of chemotherapy or radiation therapy, the prognosis for all types of PTLD has improved.

Methotrexate-associated lymphoproliferative disorders

N.L. Harris
S.H. Swerdlow

Definition
A lymphoid proliferation or lymphoma in a patient immunosuppressed with methotrexate, typically for treatment of autoimmune disease (rheumatoid arthritis, psoriasis, dermatomyositis), which may resemble large B-cell lymphoma, Hodgkin lymphoma, or polymorphous post-transplant lymphoproliferative disorders. These LPDs are often Epstein-Barr-virus related, and may regress with cessation of methotrexate therapy.

Epidemiology
The frequency of these disorders is not known. Slightly over 100 cases have been reported in the literature {58, 622, 621, 623, 991, 1010, 1135, 1191, 1257, 1296, 864}. 85% of the cases have been seen in patients with rheumatoid arthritis (RA), 6% in dermatomyositis, and 6% in psoriasis. Patients with RA are estimated to have a 2-20-fold increased risk of lymphoma in the absence of methotrexate therapy {573, 1256}. It remains debated whether methotrexate *per se* increases the risk of lymphoma development {428, 60}. A case control study of lymphoma developing in patients with and without RA demonstrated no increased frequency of EBV-positivity in the RA patients, suggesting that most lymphomas developing in RA patients are not immunosuppression-related {620}. The interval from the diagnosis of connective tissue disease to the development of lymphoma is approximately 15 years, which is not significantly different from that in patients not treated with methotrexate; the mean duration of therapy with methotrexate is 3 years, with a range of 0.5-5.5 years {621, 864}; the median cumulative dose of methotrexate in one study was 0.8 g (0.01-2.9g) {864}.

Sites of involvement
Overall approximately 40% of reported cases have been extranodal, including the gastrointestinal tract, skin, lung, kidney, and soft tissue {1135, 864}. The frequency of extranodal involvement differs among histological types, with 50% of diffuse large B-cell lymphomas (DLBCL),

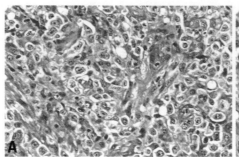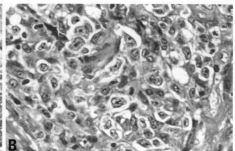

Fig. 9.20 A Polymorphous EBV-positive lymphoproliferation in a patient with rheumatoid arthritis treated with methotrexate. This lesion regressed following cessation of therapy. **B** Diffuse large B-cell lymphoma, EBV-positive, involving soft tissue in a patient with rheumatoid arthritis treated with methotrexate.

20% of Hodgkin lymphomas (HL), 100% of lymphoplasmacytic lymphomas and atypical lymphoplasmacytic infiltrates, and 40% of follicular lymphomas being extranodal.

Clinical features
These do not appear to differ from those of non-immunosuppressed patients with lymphomas of similar histological types.

Aetiology
Approximately 50% of the lymphoproliferative disorders are EBV+ {1135}. The frequency of EBV infection differs among the histological types, with EBV detected in approximately 50% of DLBCL, 75% of Hodgkin lymphoma and Hodgkin-like lesions, 50% of lymphoplasmacytic infiltrates, and 40% of cases reported as follicular lymphoma.

Morphology
The reported cases are most commonly diffuse large B-cell lymphoma (35%) and Hodgkin lymphoma (HL) (25%) or HL-like lesions (8%), with less frequent cases of follicular lymphoma (10%), Burkitt lymphoma (4%), and peripheral T-cell lymphomas (4%). Polymorphous, small lym-

Table 9.04
Characteristics of methotrexate–associated lymphoproliferative disorders (63 cases with details reported).

Type	Total	EBV+	Extranodal	Regress
DLBCL	23	9/17	7/15	4/10
Lymphoplasmacytic infiltrates	9	3/6	6/6	1/3
Burkitt lymphoma	3	1/3	0/1	0/3
Follicular lymphoma	6	2/5	2/5	1/4
Peripheral T-cell lymphoma	3	–	–	2/2
Hodgkin lymphoma	15	10/14	1/12	2/9
Hodgkin-like lesions	4	4/4	2/4	4/4
Total	63	30/51	18/45	13/34

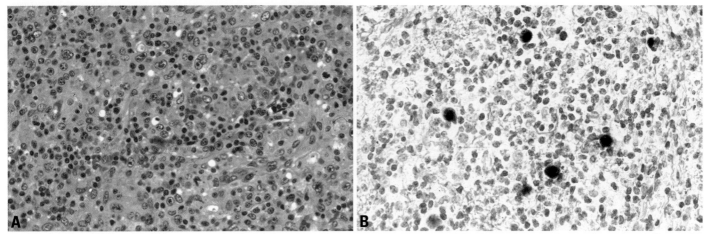

Fig. 9.21 Hodgkin lymphoma-like lesion in a patient with rheumatoid arthritis, treated with methotrexate. **A** Routine sections showing a polymorphous infiltrate with lymphocytes, histiocytes, and Reed-Sternberg-like cells. **B** In situ hybridisation for Epstein-Barr RNA (EBER) showing numerous positive large cells as well as many positive small lymphocytes.

phocytic or lymphoplasmacytic infiltrates have been described in approximately 14% of the cases.

Immunophenotype
The immunophenotypes of the lymphomas do not appear to differ from those of similar histological types not associated with methotrexate therapy. In cases classified as Hodgkin-like, the large cells were CD20+ and CD30+ but CD15-, while in cases classified as Hodgkin lymphoma, the large cells were CD15+.

Genetic features
The genetic features of these cases do not appear to differ from those of similar histological types not associated with methotrexate therapy. Only a few cases of follicular lymphoma have been reported; however, these have not been studied for the BCL2 translocation (t14;18).

Prognosis and predictive factors
Overall, approximately 60% of the reported cases have shown at least partial regression in response to withdrawal of methotrexate; the majority of responses have occurred in EBV-positive cases {1135}. In DLBCL, approximately 40% have regressed, while 60% require cytotoxic therapy; overall survival is approximately 50%. In HL about 30% regress, while of the HL-like lesions, 100% regressed; the overall survival for HL cases is about 75% {622, 621, 623}. Cases classified as lymphoplasmacytic infiltrates or lymphoplasmacytic lymphoma typically regress with withdrawal of methotrexate therapy and survival is about 75%.

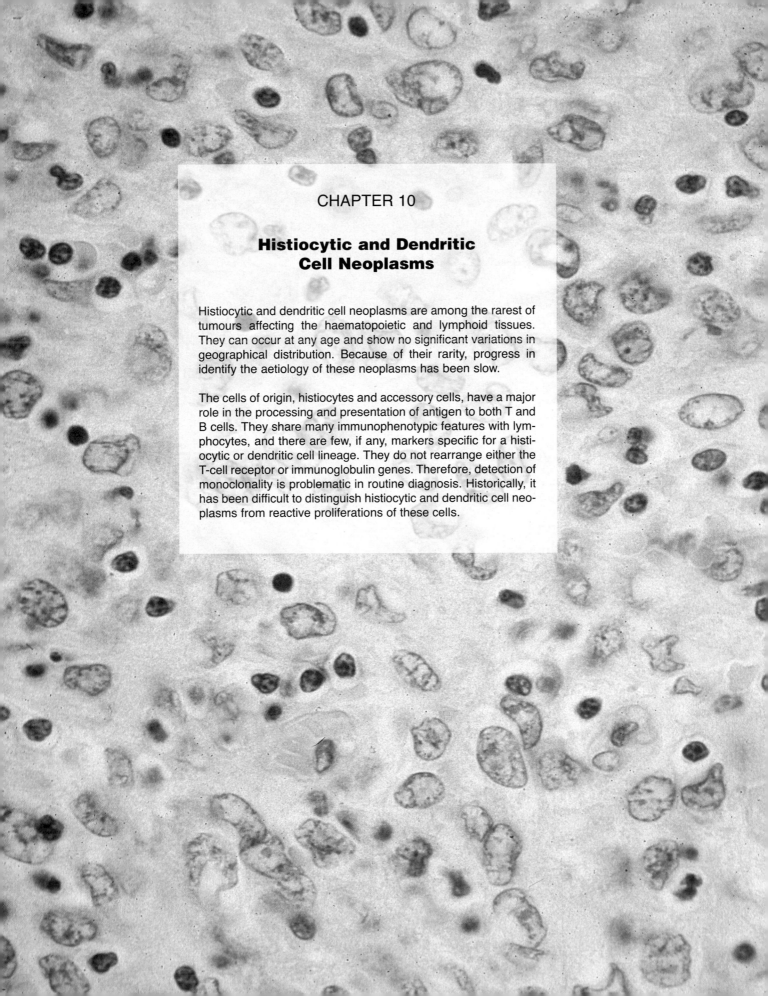

CHAPTER 10

Histiocytic and Dendritic
Cell Neoplasms

Histiocytic and dendritic cell neoplasms are among the rarest of
tumours affecting the haematopoietic and lymphoid tissues.
They can occur at any age and show no significant variations in
geographical distribution. Because of their rarity, progress in
identify the aetiology of these neoplasms has been slow.

The cells of origin, histiocytes and accessory cells, have a major
role in the processing and presentation of antigen to both T and
B cells. They share many immunophenotypic features with lymphocytes, and there are few, if any, markers specific for a histiocytic or dendritic cell lineage. They do not rearrange either the
T-cell receptor or immunoglobulin genes. Therefore, detection of
monoclonality is problematic in routine diagnosis. Historically, it
has been difficult to distinguish histiocytic and dendritic cell neoplasms from reactive proliferations of these cells.

WHO histological classification of histiocytic and dendritic cell neoplasms

Histiocytic sarcoma	9755/3
Langerhans cell histiocytosis	9751/1
Langerhans cell sarcoma	9756/3
Interdigitating dendritic cell sarcoma[1] / tumour[2]	9757/3[1]
	9757/1[2]
Follicular dendritic cell sarcoma[1] / tumour[2]	9758/3[1]
	9758/1[2]
Dendritic cell sarcoma, not otherwise specified	9757/3

Histiocytic and dendritic cell neoplasms: Introduction

E.S. Jaffe

Definition

Histiocytic and dendritic cell neoplasms are derived from phagocytes and accessory cells, which have major roles in the processing and presentation of antigens to lymphocytes.

Incidence

Tumours of histiocytes and dendritic cells are among the rarest of tumours affecting lymphoid tissues. They represent less than 1% of tumours presenting in lymph nodes. At one point many tumours of lymph nodes were felt to be of histiocytic or reticulum cell origin, based on a morphologic resemblance to normal cells {415, 1089}. Subsequently, most of these tumours were shown to be of B-cell or T-cell derivation. Thus, the incidence of histiocytic or dendritic cell sarcoma is less than once was thought. In some respects, histiocytic sarcoma is a "vanishing diagnosis". These tumours do not appear to be changing in their true incidence. Due to their rarity and infrequent reporting, it is difficult to obtain detailed epidemiological data. However, there are no significant geographical differences in incidence, and they have been reported from all continents and in all races.

Pathophysiology

The normal cellular counterparts of this group of neoplasms consist of two major subsets: the antigen-presenting cells, or dendritic cells, and the antigen-processing cells, or phagocytic cells {577}. Most of these cells are derived from a bone marrow stem cell, and share a common cellular origin. However, phagocytes and antigen presenting cells are generally considered to represent two parallel and independent lines of differentiation {32}. Histiocytes or mononuclear phagocytes have as their primary role the removal of particulate antigens. They are felt to be derived from the circulating blood monocyte pool that migrate through the blood vessel wall to enter lymphoid organs. Therefore, it is not surprising that the distinction between a leukaemia of monocytic origin and a histiocytic sarcoma can sometimes be ambiguous. However, histiocytes or macrophages are not recirculating cells, and therefore, most histiocytic sarcomas present as localised tumour masses without a leukaemic phase {577}. Metchnikoff is considered the father of the macrophage. In 1883 he coined the term phagocytosis, and postulated that phagocytosis was the main defense against infection. He named two types of circulating phagocytes, the macrophages and "microphages", polymorphonuclear leukocytes {1109}.

All of the macrophages of lymph nodes share many enzyme histochemical and immunophenotypic characteristics. CD68 is the most useful antigen for detection of macrophages in routine paraffin sections {359}. Histiocytes have abundant and diffuse activity for lysosomal enzymes, including acid phosphatase and nonspecific esterases. These cells also can demonstrate phagocytosis under appropriate conditions. However, phagocytic activity is usually not a prominent feature of histiocytic malignancies, and is more common in benign proliferations of histiocytes, such as the haemophagocytic syndrome. Activity for lysozyme and alpha-1-antitrypsin is a feature of most mononuclear phagocytes, but is most prominent in epithelioid histiocytes. Activity for lysozyme decreases abruptly with phagocytosis, presumably because of its loss into lysosomal vacuoles.

A variety of monoclonal antibodies that react with monocytes and macrophages have been derived. These include antibodies to cell surface receptors for the Fc portion of IgG (CD64, CD32, and CD16) and receptors for complement (CD21 and CD35) {797}. Other antigens found on macrophages are molecules involved in adhesion and cellular activation, such as CD11a, CD11b, CD11c, CD14, and CD18. Unfortunately, most of these antigens lack specificity for the mononuclear phagocytic system, and many react with other haematopoietic cells as well: myeloid cells, T cells, or B cells. For example, CD11c is present on monocytes and macrophages, and is weak or absent on normal T and B-lymphocytes. However, this antigen is found on the cells of hairy cell leukaemia (a B-cell lymphoproliferative disorder) and in some cases of chronic lymphocytic leukaemia / small lymphocytic lymphoma {1164}. Cross-reactivities with T cells are present as well. For example, CD4, a T-cell associated antigen, is found in normal monocytes

Table 10.01
True histiocytic malignancy – a vanishing diagnosis.

Original diagnosis	Currently considered
Histiocytic lymphoma, nodular and diffuse	Diffuse large B-cell lymphoma, Follicular lymphoma Grade 3 Peripheral T-cell lymphomas
Histiocytic medullary reticulosis or malignant histiocytosis	Haemophagocytic syndrome (HPS)
Malignant histiocytosis	Anaplastic large cell lymphoma (ALCL)
Regressing atypical histiocytosis	Primary cutaneous ALCL
Malignant histiocytosis of the intestine	Enteropathy type T-cell lymphoma
Histiocytic cytophagic panniculitis	Subcutaneous panniculitis-like T-cell lymphoma with HPS

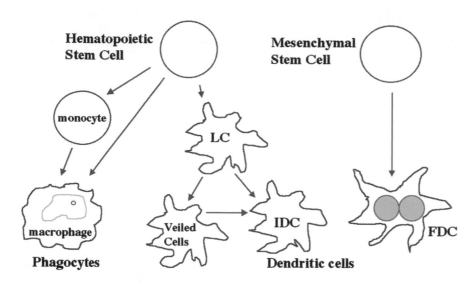

Fig. 10.01 Schematic diagram of the origin and differentiation of macrophages and dendritic cells. Both macrophages and dendritic cells (antigen presenting cells) are derived from a common bone marrow precursor. In contrast, follicular dendritic cells are thought to be of non-haematopoietic origin.

and macrophages. CD25, in addition to being found on activated T lymphocytes, also is positive on histiocytic cells. CD68, one of the better markers for histiocytes in paraffin sections, also reacts with granulocytic precursors {1063, 1064}.

The interdigitating dendritic cells (IDC) and Langerhans cells (LC) are bone marrow derived cells that present antigen to T lymphocytes. LC are found primarily in the skin but also in other organs. First

identified by their characteristic Birbeck granules, they are phenotypically distinct from IDC and are positive for CD1a and CD4 {797, 946}. IDC are found in lymph nodes and other lymphoid organs. Both LC and IDC are strongly S-100-protein positive and also express high levels of MHC Class II antigens. LC can migrate from the skin to enter the peripheral blood, where they have been described as veiled cells. The enter lymph nodes via

the afferent lymphatics where they take up residence in the paracortex as interdigitating dendritic cells.

Follicular dendritic cells (FDC) are found in follicles and present antigen to B lymphocytes, but most likely are not of haematopoietic origin. They are positive for CD21, CD23, and CD35, but are CD45 negative. They are a non-migrating population which form a stable meshwork within lymphoid follicles via cell-to-cell attachments or desmosomes. They trap and store antigen-antibody complexes in organelles termed iccosomes {1279}. Antigens may be stored in this fashion for many years. B-cell activation in the follicle cannot take place without FDC, which provide important stimuli to B-cells.

Fibroblastic reticular cells (FRC) are involved in transport of cytokines and other mediators {457}. In lymph nodes they ensheathe the post-capillary venules. They are of mesenchymal rather than haematopoietic origin, and express smooth muscle actin {31}. Because these cells are not of haematopoietic or lymphoid origin, neoplasms of FRC are not included in the WHO classification of haematopoietic and lymphoid tumours. However, tumours of FRC arise in lymph nodes, where they should be considered in the differential diagnosis of neoplasms of IDC and FDC origin {31}. The neoplastic cells are positive for vimentin, smooth muscle actin, and usually positive for desmin. Factor XIII also is positive. However, in contrast to neoplasms of FDC or IDC origin, they are negative for CD21, CD35 and S-100-protein. The cells have features of myofibroblasts, and myofibroblastic tumours of lymph nodes may be closely related neoplasms {1249, 1372}.

The subsequent sections discuss the features of neoplasms of histiocytic and dendritic cell origin. Because there are few if any markers with absolute specificity for macrophages or dendritic cells, the investigator must rigorously exclude other cell lineages (T-cell, B-cell) with both immmunophenotypic and molecular means {446, 1396, 735}.

Another disorder, the haemophagocytic syndrome (HPS) is an important nonneoplastic proliferative disorder that should be kept in mind in the differential diagnosis of histiocytic neoplasms. The HPS is the most common and clinically significant of the proliferative disorders of macrophages, and in fact is more common than histiocytic neoplasms. First

Table 10.02
Immunophenotypic markers of macrophages and dendritic cells.

Marker	LC	IDC	FDC	MP	B-cells	T-cells
MHC II	++	+	–	+	+	–
FCR	+	–	–	+	+/–	–
CD21	–	–	++	+	+	–
CD35	–	–	++	+	+	–
CD2	–	–	–	–	–	+
CD4	+	–	–	+	–	+
CD1a	+	–	–	–	–	(+)*
CD68	–	–	–	+	–	–
S-100-protein	+	+	–	+/–	–	–/+
CD3	–	–	–	–	–	+
CD20	–	–	–	–	+	–
Lysozyme	–	–	–	+	–	–
Phagocytosis	–	–	–	+	–	–
NSE	–	–	–	+	–	–

FCR, Fc IgG receptors (includes CD32, CD64, and CD16 on some cells); NSE, non-specific esterases (α-napthyl acetate esterase and α-naphthyl butyrate esterase); LC, Langerhans cell;
IDC, interdigitating dendritic cell; FDC, follicular dendritic cell; MP, macrophage
* CD1a is expressed on cortical thymocytes, but is absent on mature T-cells

recognised as a clinical syndrome by Scott and Robb-Smith {1167}, Rappaport subsequently interpreted the disorder as a malignancy of histiocytic derivation {1089}. While the HPS has a fulminant and often fatal clinical course, it is not a clonal or neoplastic proliferation of histiocytes. The HPS usually is seen in association with immunodeficiency or another haematopoietic malignancy {1108, 585, 360, 447}.

This syndrome is pathogenetically related to an excessive production of cytokines and chemokines capable of stimulating mononuclear phagocytes {737, 1276}. Infection with Epstein-Barr virus, or another virus, is a frequent precipitating event {1097, 643, 1070}. A cytokine storm ensues, leading to profound and uncontrolled macrophage activation with marked phagocytosis. The enhanced phagocytic activity leads to pancytopenia. Because phagocytosis is usually inconspicuous in most histiocytic tumours, a process showing both pathological and clinical evidence of florid phagocytosis is most likely a haemophagocytic syndrome and not a neoplasm of macrophages.

Survival

The clinical behaviour of histiocytic and dendritic cell tumours varies widely. Both histiocytic and interdigitating dendritic cell

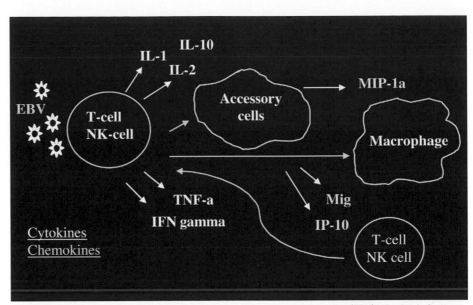

Fig. 10.02 Pathogenesis of the haemophagocytic syndrome. Epstein-Barr virus (EBV) infection is frequently a precipitating event. EBV stimulates T-cells and NK-cells to release cytokines, interleukins IL-1, IL-2, and IL-10, and tumour necrosis factor-α and interferon-γ. Accessory cells are stimulated by cytokines to release chemokines including MIP-1 α, Mig, and IP-10, which activate both macrophages and T-cells and NK-cells. The stimulation of T-cells and NK-cells, results in further cytokine release, producing an autocrine loop with profound and persistent macrophage activation. The haemophagocytic syndrome has been likened to a cytokine storm.

sarcomas tend to have an aggressive clinical course, with the potential for systemic spread. In contrast, follicular dendritic cell tumours are generally localised, with a potential for local invasion and recurrence, but infrequent distant metastases. Langerhans cell histiocytosis exhibits a wide spectrum of clinical behaviours that correlate with the extent of organ system involvement and the age of the patient.

Histiocytic sarcoma

L.M. Weiss
T.M. Grogan
H.-K. Müller-Hermelink
H. Stein

T. Dura
B. Favara
M. Paulli
A.C. Feller

Definition

Histiocytic sarcoma is a malignant proliferation of cells showing morphologic and immunophenotypic features similar to those of mature tissue histiocytes. There is expression of one or more histiocytic markers without accessory/ dendritic cell markers. Neoplastic proliferations associated with acute monocytic leukaemia are excluded.

ICD-O code   9755/3

Synonyms and historical annotation

Lymphoid neoplasms have long been mistaken for histiocytic proliferations. Virtually all cases previously regarded as diffuse histiocytic lymphoma are now recognised as diffuse large B-cell lymphomas. Similarly, most cases formerly regarded as histiocytic medullary reticulosis and malignant histiocytosis are now recognised to represent systemic anaplastic large cell lymphomas {1396}. Other cases of histiocytic medullary reticulosis and malignant histiocytosis have been identified to represent haemophagocytic syndromes.

Epidemiology

Histiocytic sarcoma is a rare neoplasm with only a few series of bone fide neoplasms reported {244, 1035, 396, 619, 188, 486, 1209, 982}. There is a wide age range, including infants, children, and adults; however, most cases occur in adults (median age 46 years) {1209}. Male predilection is found in some studies {1209}.

A subset of cases occurs in patients with a prior mediastinal germ cell tumour, and particularly a malignant teratoma, with or without yolk sac tumour differentiation {286}. Since teratocarcinoma cells have been shown to differentiate along haematopoietic lines in vitro {256}, it has, therefore, been suggested that these histiocytic neoplasms arise from pluripotential germ cells. Other cases may be associated with malignant lymphoma, either preceding or subsequent, or with myelodysplasia.

Sites of involvement

About one-third of cases present in lymph nodes, about one-third in skin (solitary or multiple lesions), and about one-third in a variety of other extranodal sites, most commonly in the intestinal tract. Some patients have a "systemic" presentation, with multiple sites of involvement, sometimes referred to as "malignant histiocytosis".

Clinical features

Patients may present with a solitary mass, but systemic symptoms are relatively common, e.g. fever and weight loss. Skin manifestations may range from a benign-appearing rash to solitary lesions to innumerable tumours on the trunk and extremities. Patients with intestinal lesions may present with intestinal obstruction. Hepatosplenomegaly is relatively common. The bone may show lytic lesions, and pancytopenia is not an uncommon feature in the bone marrow.

Aetiology

The aetiology is unknown.

Precursor lesions

No precursor lesions are recognised with the possible exception of mediastinal germ cell tumours {1035, 286}.

Morphology

The normal architecture is effaced by a diffuse non-cohesive proliferation of neoplastic cells. When visceral organs are involved, a sinusoidal pattern may be seen. The proliferating cells may be monomorphic or, more commonly, polymorphic. The individual neoplastic cells are usually large and round to oval in shape; however, focal areas of spindling may be observed. The cytoplasm is usually abundant and eosinophilic. On occasion, the cytoplasm may be foamy. Haemophagocytosis occurs occasionally in the neoplastic cells. The nuclei are generally large, round to oval, and often eccentrically placed; large multinucleated forms are commonly seen. The chromatin pattern is usually vesicular, and atypia varies from mild to pleomorphic, with highly irregular nuclear outlines. A vari-

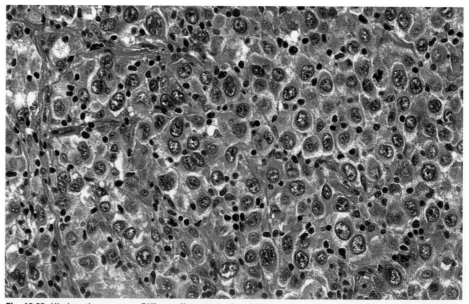

Fig. 10.03 Histiocytic sarcoma. Diffuse effacement of architecture is seen by a large cell proliferation that is indistinguishable from a diffuse large B-cell lymphoma by conventional histopathology.

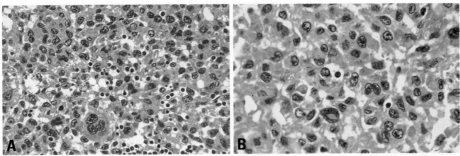

Fig. 10.04 Histiocytic sarcoma. **A** Note the multinucleated tumour cell. **B** The cytoplasm is relatively abundant, but the neoplasm would still be quite difficult to distinguish from a large B-cell lymphoma without a battery of immunohistochemical studies.

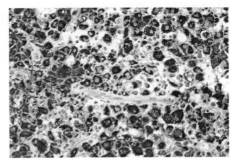

Fig. 10.05 Histiocytic sarcoma. There is strong and diffuse staining for the lysosomal marker CD68.

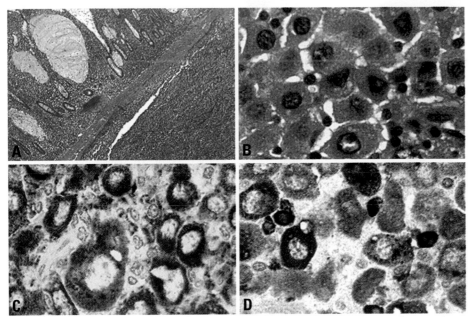

Fig. 10.06 Histiocytic sarcoma. **A** Histiocytic sarcoma involving the bowel. **B** Note the abundant cytoplasm, which stains strongly for the histiocyte markers CD68 (**C**) and lysozyme (**D**).

able number of reactive cells may be seen, including small lymphocytes, plasma cells, benign histiocytes, and eosinophils. The overall appearance may be indistinguishable from a diffuse large B-cell lymphoma or an anaplastic large cell lymphoma, although the cytoplasm is often more abundant and cell size overall is often larger. Markers are usually necessary to make a certain lineage distinction.

Ultrastructure
The neoplastic cells show abundant cytoplasm with numerous lysosomes. Birbeck granules and cellular junctions are not seen.

Immunophenotype
By definition, there is expression of one or more "histiocytic markers," including CD68 (KP1, and more specifically, PG-M1), lysozyme, CD11c, and CD14. Given that many of the above listed "histiocytic" markers may overlap with the myeloid lineage, the mature histiocytic phenotype has to be established as well by the absence of specific myeloid markers (e.g. myeloperoxidase, CD33 and CD34) {1209}. The lysozyme staining is usually granular with accentuation in the Golgi region, in distinction to the diffuse staining that may occur in other neoplasms. In addition, CD45, CD45RO, and HLA-DR

are usually positive. There may be expression of S-100-protein, but if positive, it is usually weak or focal. There is no positivity for specific B-cell and T-cell markers. CD4 is present, reflecting the physiologic pattern of expression of this T-helper antigen by histiocytes. These tumours are devoid of accessory/dendritic cell markers (CD1a, CD21, CD35), as well as CD30, HMB-45, epithelial membrane antigen, or keratin. The Ki-67 index is variable, from 10 to 90% with a mean of approximately 20% {1209}.

Genetics
While the historical literature suggests the possibility of antigen receptor gene rearrangements being present in histiocytic sarcoma {1080, 486}, the more recent precise phenotypic definition of histiocytic sarcoma requires the absence of clonal immunoglobulin and T-cell receptor genes for the definition of this neoplastic disease {244}.

Postulated cell of origin
The mature tissue histiocyte is the putative normal counterpart of histiocytic sarcoma.

Prognosis and predictive factors
Histiocytic sarcoma is usually an aggressive neoplasm, with a poor response to therapy, although some exceptions have been reported. Most patients (60%) die of progressive disease reflecting the high clinical stage at presentation (stage III/IV) in the majority (70%) of patients {1209}.

Langerhans cell histiocytosis

L.M. Weiss
T.M. Grogan
H.-K. Müller-Hermelink
H. Stein
T. Dura
B. Favara
M. Paulli
A.C. Feller

Definition

Langerhans cell histiocytosis (LCH) is a neoplastic proliferation of Langerhans cells, with expression of CD1a, S-100-protein, and the presence of Birbeck granules by ultrastructural examination.

ICD-O code   9751/1

Synonyms and historical annotation

Langerhans cell histiocytosis has been usually referred to in the past as histiocytosis X and less commonly as Langerhans cell granulomatosis. Clinical variants have been referred to as Letterer-Siwe disease, Hand-Schüller-Christian disease, and solitary eosinophilic granuloma.

Epidemiology

The incidence is about 5 per million, with most cases occurring in childhood {951}. There is a predilection for males (male:female ratio 3.7:1) {1035}. It is more common in Whites of northern European descent and rare in Blacks. There is an association between disseminated LCH and acute lymphoblastic leukaemia. There may be an association with a history of neonatal infection, solvent exposure, and lack of childhood vaccination. Langerhans cell histiocytosis is also associated with malignant lymphoma, either

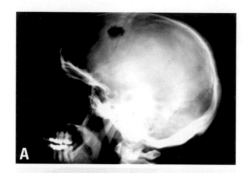

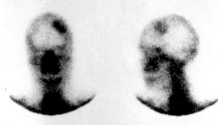

Fig. 10.07 Langerhans cell histiocytosis. **A** Radiograph from a patient with eosinophilic granuloma of bone illustrates a discrete punched-out lesion. **B** A gallium scan shows high uptake in lytic bone lesion.

non-Hodgkin or Hodgkin lymphoma {944}. Langerhans cell histiocytosis of the lung in adults is nearly always associated with smokers (of tobacco or marijuana) and probably represents a separate, perhaps reactive, disease entity {1337}.

Sites of involvement

Three major overlapping syndromes are recognised {766}. There is unifocal disease in a majority of cases (solitary eosinophilic granuloma), usually involving the bone (particularly the skull, femur, pelvic bones or the ribs), or less commonly, the lymph node, skin or lung. In multifocal, unisystem disease (Hand-Schüller-Christian disease), there is involvement of several sites in one organ system, almost always the bone. In multifocal, multisystem disease (Letterer-Siwe disease), multiple organ systems are involved, including the bones, skin, liver, spleen, and lymph nodes.

Clinical features

Patients with unifocal disease are usually older children or adults, who usually present with a lytic lesion of bone involving the diaphysis, with erosion of the adjacent cortical bone or in other extranodal sites (e.g. skin). Patients with multifocal, unisystem disease are usually young children who present with multiple destructive bone lesions, often associated with adjacent soft tissue masses. There is frequent involvement of the skull with exophthalmos, diabetes insipidus, and tooth loss. Patients with multifocal, multisystem disease are usually infants, who present with fever, skin manifestations, hepato-

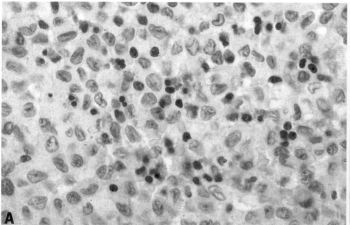

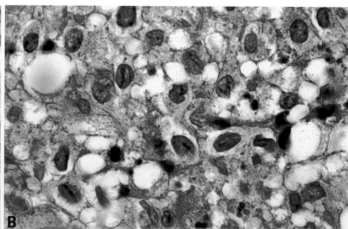

Fig. 10.08 Langerhans cell histiocytosis. **A** Numerous Langerhans cells are seen, with scattered eosinophils and small lymphocytes. **B** Note the typical cytologic features of Langerhans cells, with many nuclei containing linear grooves.

splenomegaly, lymphadenopathy, bone lesions, and pancytopenia. Langerhans cell histiocytosis of the lung in adults generally presents as innumerable bilateral nodules, usually less than 2.0 cm in diameter.

Aetiology
Aetiology is unknown. There is specifically no convincing evidence for involvement of viruses including: Human herpes virus-6, Epstein-Barr virus, herpes simplex virus, adenovirus, cytomegalovirus, parvovirus, human T-cell leukaemia viruses types 1 and 2, or human immunodeficiency virus {845}.

Morphology
The key feature is the identification of Langerhans cells in the appropriate milieu. Langerhans cells are about 10-15 µm, and are recognised histologically by their characteristic grooved, folded, indented, or lobulated nuclei, with fine chromatin, inconspicuous nucleoli and thin nuclear membranes. Some nuclear atypia may occur, but the presence of frankly malignant cytological features would prompt consideration of Langerhans cell sarcoma, discussed below. Mitotic activity is very variable. The cytoplasm is usually moderately abundant and slightly eosinophilic. The characteristic milieu usually includes variable numbers of eosinophils, histiocytes (including multinucleated forms, often appearing similar to osteoclasts), neutrophils, and small lymphocytes. Occasionally, eosinophilic abscesses with central necrosis may be found. In early lesions, there is usually a large number of Langerhans

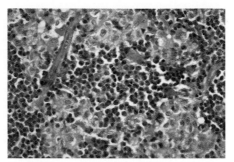

Fig. 10.09 Langerhans cell histiocytosis. An eosinophilic microabscess is seen.

cells, eosinophils and neutrophils, while later lesions show a greater degree of fibrosis, and often contain foamy macrophages. Involved lymph nodes show preferential involvement of the sinuses with secondary infiltration of the paracortical regions, while the spleen shows preferential involvement of the red pulp. When Langerhans cell histiocytosis is associated with malignant lymphoma, it is usually present as a small focus within or adjacent to the lymphoma. Involvement of the bone marrow is more easily seen in biopsies rather than in smears, and usually consists of a focal lesion which may be associated with fibrosis.

Grading
Although attempts at grading have been made, it is generally believed that, with the exception of the presence of frank neoplastic features, the degree of atypia does not correspond well with clinical outcome.

Ultrastructure
The hallmark of the Langerhans cell is the cytoplasmic Birbeck granule, which

is present in variable numbers. Birbeck granules usually have a characteristic shape (tennis racket form). Birbeck granules are about 200-400 nanometers with a consistent width of 33 nanometers. They are present in 1-75% of the Langerhans cells in a given lesion, with earlier lesions usually containing a greater number of Birbeck granules. Langerhans cells have nuclei with irregular nuclear outlines, while their cytoplasm have variable numbers of lysosomes. No cell junctions are seen.

Immunophenotype
The neoplastic Langerhans cells are similar to normal normal Langerhans cells in their consistent expression of CD1a and S-100-protein {693, 478}. They are usually positive for vimentin, HLA-DR, peanut agglutinin lectin and placental alkaline phosphatase. They are variably and weakly positive for CD45, CD68, and lysozyme. They are negative for most B-cell and T-cell lineage markers (with the exception of CD4); CD30, myeloperoxidase, CD34, and epithelial membrane are also negative. They are almost always negative for specific markers of follicular dendritic cell lineage, such as CD21 and CD35. CD15 is usually negative, unless sialic acid residues have been removed by pretreatment. Ki-67 usually stains between 2 and 25% of the Langerhans cells with a mean of approximately 10% {1035}.

Enzyme cytochemistry
The neoplastic Langerhans cells are positive for adenosine triphosphase, α-D-mannosidase, α-naphthyl acetate

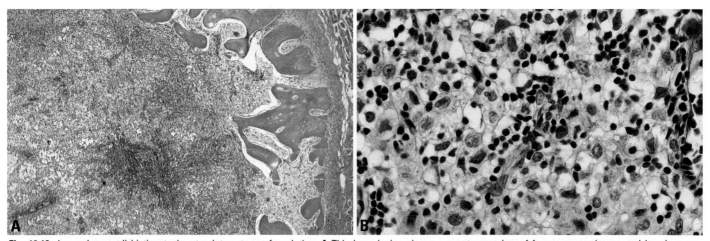

Fig. 10.10 Langerhans cell histiocytosis, at a later stage of evolution. **A** This bony lesion shows a greater number of foamy macrophages and lymphocytes. **B** A greater number of foamy macrophages and lymphocytes are present, although nuclei with typical grooves are still discernable.

esterase (with variable inhibition by sodium fluoride), α-naphthyl butyrate esterase, and acid phosphatase. They are negative for tartrate-resistant acid phosphatase, 5'-nucleotidase, peroxidase, chloroactetate esterase, and β-glucuronidase.

Genetics
Studies of the X-linked androgen receptor gene have demonstrated a monoclonal proliferation of Langerhans cells in all major clinical syndromes {1395, 1436}. The immunoglobulin heavy chain gene and β, δ and γ chain genes of the T-cell receptor are in a germline state {1435}.

Postulated cell of origin
Neoplastic Langerhans cells are morphologically and immunophenotypically very similar to non-neoplastic Langerhans cells, the antigen-processing cells of epithelia. However, they are not identical {270}. For example, normal Langerhans cells are negative for placental alkaline phosphatase, and have a different pattern of expression of cellular adhesion molecules.

Prognosis and predictive factors
The clinical course is generally related to the number of organs affected at presentation {452}, as underlined by the staging system proposed by the Histiocyte Society. However, exceptions occur. For example, the absence of bone lesions in the presence of multiorgan involvement is a poor prognostic sign, while the presence of multiple bone lesions in the same circumstance is a marker of good prognosis. There is progression of unifocal lesions into multisystem disease in about 10% of patients, and spontaneous regression of multisystem disease may occur in rare instances. The overall survival of patients with unifocal disease is higher than 95%; this figure, however, drops to 75% in subjects with two organs involved and continues to drop with increasing number of affected sites. Age is a less important prognostic factor than

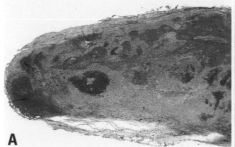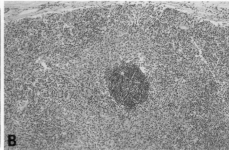

Fig. 10.11 Langerhans cell histiocytosis. **A** and **B** This lymph node biopsy shows extensive involvement of the sinuses and paracortical regions.

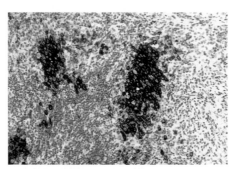

Fig. 10.12 Langerhans cell histiocytosis, CD1a stain. Strong membrane positivity is seen in the Langerhans cells.

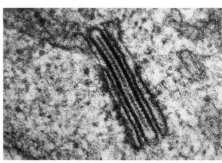

Fig. 10.13 Langerhans cell histiocytosis, ultrastructure. A typical Birbeck granule is seen.

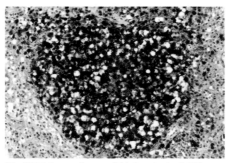

Fig. 10.14 Langerhans cell histiocytosis, S-100-protein stain. Strong nuclear positivity is seen in the Langerhans cells.

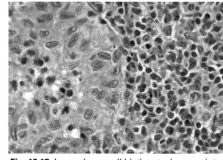

Fig. 10.15 Langerhans cell histiocytosis associated with malignant lymphoma. A focus of Langerhans cell histiocytosis is seen within a focus of follicular lymphoma.

the number of involved organs. In the absence of frankly malignant cytological features, the presence of cytological atypia or an increased mitotic rate does not correlate with prognosis {1107}. In patients with multifocal multisystem disease, a prompt response to chemotherapy usually heralds an increased survival.

Adults with isolated Langerhans cell histiocytosis of the lung usually undergo spontaneous regression or stabilisation upon cessation of smoking, with only a small subset progressing to irreversible interstitial and honeycomb fibrosis.

Langerhans cell sarcoma

L.M. Weiss
T.M. Grogan
S.A. Pileri
B. Favara
T. Dura
M. Paulli
A.C. Feller

Definition

Langerhans cell sarcoma (LCS) is a neoplastic proliferation of Langerhans cells with overtly malignant cytologic features. It can be considered a higher grade variant of Langerhans cell histiocytosis (LCH), and can present *de novo* or progress from antecedent LCH.

ICD-O code   9756/3

Epidemiology

Langerhans cell sarcoma is exceedingly rare {1408, 88, 1035}. In the few reported cases, there is a wide age range, including adults and children (median age 41 years) {88}. In contrast with Langerhans cell histiocytosis a female predominance has been described {88}.

Sites of involvement

Langerhans cell sarcoma is characterised by multiorgan involvement including: lymph nodes, liver, spleen, lung, and bone.

Morphology

The most prominent feature is the presence of large cells with overtly malignant cytologic features. Chromatin abnormalities are conspicuous, and nucleoli are prominent. Some of the atypical cells show occasional nuclear grooves reminiscent of Langerhans cell histiocytosis, a key feature to suggest the diagnosis. The mitotic rate is high, usually greater than 50 per 10 high power fields. Rare eosinophils can be identified, but the polymorphic infiltrate typical of Langerhans cell histiocytosis is usually absent. In involved lymph nodes a sinusoidal pattern of involvement is usual.

Ultrastructure

Birbeck granules have been identified in all but one case {88}, and theoretically should be present in all cases in which adequate examination can be carried out. Variable numbers of lysosomes may also be present.

Immunophenotype

Use of phenotypic markers is often critical, as the frank cytologic atypia and rarity of characteristic Langerhans cell feature (e.g. nuclear grooves) make histiopathological diagnosis problematic. The phenotype is identical to that of Langerhans cell histiocytosis, with consistent expression of S-100-protein and CD1a. However, the CD1a positivity is often focal. There is also usually some expression of CD68, lysozyme, and CD45, The Ki-67 index ranges from 10 to 60% with a median of 22% {88}.

Postulated cell of origin

Similar to Langerhans cell histiocytosis, the postulated normal counterpart of Langerhans cell sarcoma is the normal Langerhans cell of the skin and other epithelial sites.

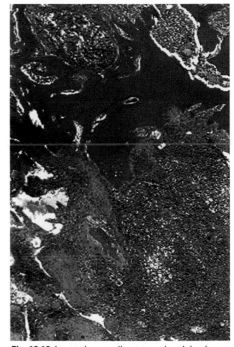

Fig. 10.16 Langerhans cell sarcoma involving bone.

Prognosis and predictive factors

Langerhans cell sarcoma behaves in a very aggressive fashion. Overall survival is approximately 50% {88}.

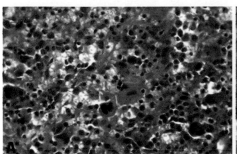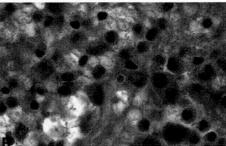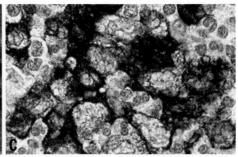

Fig. 10.17 Langerhans cell sarcoma. **A** This bony lesion contains a pleomorphic infiltrate of cells vaguely resembling Langerhans cells. **B** The cells have malignant cytologic features. **C** The CD1a stain is strongly positive, consistent with Langerhans cell sarcoma. The identification of Birbeck granules by electron microscopic examination would provide helpful confirmation.

Interdigitating dendritic cell sarcoma / tumour

L.M. Weiss
T.M. Grogan
H.-K. Müller-Hermelink
H. Stein

T. Dura
B. Favara
M. Paulli
A.C. Feller

Definition

Interdigitating dendritic cell (IDC) sarcoma/tumour is a neoplastic proliferation of spindle to ovoid cells with phenotypic features similar to those of interdigitating dendritic cells. The designation sarcoma/tumour is used because of the variable cytological grade and clinical behaviour encountered in these neoplasms.

ICD-O code

Interdigitating dendritic cell sarcoma
9757/3
Interdigitating dendritic cell tumour
9757/1

Synonyms

Reticulum cell sarcoma/tumour
Interdigitating cell sarcoma/tumour

Epidemiology

Interdigitating dendritic cell sarcoma / tumour is an extremely rare neoplasm, with most studies representing single case reports or very small series {1035, 1367, 792, 925, 874, 1116, 371, 923, 31}. The largest series to date has consisted of four cases {1035}. The reported cases have all occurred in adults, with a median age of 71 years {371}. There has been no sex predilection.

Sites of involvement

The presentation has shown wide variation. Solitary lymph node involvement is most common, but extranodal presentations, particularly the the skin, have been reported. Intestinal, soft tissue and hepatosplenomegaly have also been reported.

Clinical features

Patients usually present with an asymptomatic mass, although systemic symptoms, such as fatigue, fever, and night sweats, have been reported. Complete remissions are described following localised treatment {371}.

Aetiology

Aetiology is unknown.

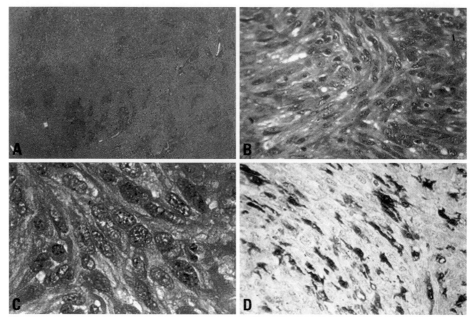

Fig. 10.18 Interdigitating dendritic cell sarcoma/tumour. **A** The tumour infiltrates the paracortex. Note the residual lymphoid tissue in one corner. **B** Sheets of spindled cells with a whorled pattern are seen. **C** The cells show marked cytologic atypia. **D** The stain for S-100-protein is focally positive.

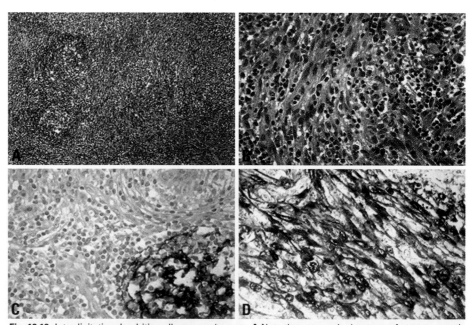

Fig. 10.19 Interdigitating dendritic cell sarcoma/tumour. **A** Note the paracortical pattern of tumour growth in the lymph node. **B** There are scattered small lymphocytes throughout the lesion. **C** The CD21 stain is negative on the tumour cells, but labels follicular dendritic cells in residual follicles. **D** In contrast, the stain for S-100-protein is strongly positive in the tumour cells.

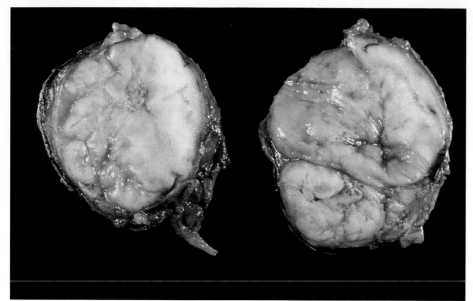

Fig. 10.20 Interdigitating dendritic cell sarcoma/tumour. Tumour is vaguely lobulated in lymph node, and firm in consistency.

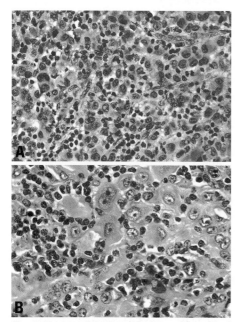

Fig. 10.21 Interdigitating dendritic cell sarcoma/tumour. **A** The cells are rounded, and the nuclei are relatively bland. **B** The nuclei are relatively bland, but have a vesicular chromatin pattern and a single medium-sized nucleolus.

Macroscopy
The tumours usually have a grossly lobulated appearance and are firm in consistency. On cut sections they appear tan, sometimes with focal areas of necrosis or haemorrhage.

Morphology
The lesional tissue in lymph nodes is present in a paracortical distribution with residual follicles. The neoplastic proliferation usually forms fascicles, a storiform pattern, and whorls of spindled to ovoid cells. Sheets of round cells are occasionally found. The cytoplasm of the neoplastic cells is usually abundant, slightly eosinophilic, and often has an indistinct border. The nuclei also appear spindled to ovoid. The chromatin is often vesicular, with a small to large, distinct nucleoli. Cytologic atypia varies from case to case, although the mitotic rate is usually low – less than 5 per 10 high power fields. Necrosis is usually not present. There are often numerous admixed lymphocytes, and less commonly, plasma cells. The histological appearance is sometimes indistinguishable from a follicular dendritic cell sarcoma/tumour and phenotyping may be necessary for precise diagnosis.

Ultrastructure
The neoplastic cells show complex interdigitating cell processes; however, well-formed desmosomes are not present. Scattered lysosomes may be present, but Birbeck granules are not seen.

Immunophenotype
The neoplastic cells generally demonstrate the phenotype of non-neoplastic interdigitating dendritic cells. They consistently express S-100-protein and vimentin with CD1a being negative. They are variably, weakly positive for CD68, lysozyme, and CD45. They are negative for markers of follicular dendritic cells (CD21, CD35), myeloperoxidase, CD34, specific B-cell and T-cell associated antigens, CD30, epithelial membrane antigen, and cytokeratins. The Ki-67 index usually ranges between 10 and 20% (median 11%) {371}. The admixed small lymphocytes are almost always of T-cell lineage, with a near-absence of B cells.

Genetics
The immunoglobulin heavy chain gene and the β, δ and γ chain genes of the T-cell receptor are in a germline configuration {1367}.

Postulated cell of origin
The interdigitating dendritic cell of the paracortical region of the lymph node is the putative normal counterpart

Prognosis and predictive factors
The clinical course appears to be variable ranging from benign localised disease to widespread lethal disease {371}. Visceral organs that are commonly affected include the bone marrow, spleen, skin, liver, kidney, and lung.

Follicular dendritic cell sarcoma / tumour

L.M. Weiss
T.M. Grogan
H.-K. Müller-Hermelink
H. Stein

T. Dura
B. Favara
M. Paulli
A.C. Feller

Definition
Follicular dendritic cell (FDC) sarcoma / tumour is a neoplastic proliferation of spindled to ovoid cells showing morphologic and phenotypic features of follicular dendritic cells. The designation sarcoma/tumour is used because of the variable cytologic grade and indeterminate clinical behaviour in many cases.

ICD-O code
Follicular dendritic cell sarcoma
9758/3
Follicular dendritic cell tumour
9758/1

Synonyms and historical annotation
This neoplasm has also been designated reticulum cell sarcoma/tumour and dendritic reticulum cell sarcoma/tumour.

Epidemiology
Follicular dendritic cell sarcoma/tumour is a rare neoplasm, with most studies representing single case reports or small series {31, 891, 206, 1023, 1035, 1367, 949}. The largest series to date have consisted of 17 cases {206} and 13 cases {949}. There is a wide age range, with an adult predominance {1035, 949}. The sex distribution is about even.
Follicular dendritic cell sarcoma/tumour may occur in association with Castleman disease in about 10-20% of cases, usually the hyaline vascular type {209}. In these cases, either the Castleman disase precedes the follicular dendritic cell sarcoma/tumour or the two lesions may occur simultaneously. There also may be an increased incidence in patients who have been treated for longstanding schizophrenia {1035}.

Sites of involvement
Follicular dendritic cell sarcoma/tumour presents in lymph nodes in between one-half to two-thirds of cases. The cervical lymph nodes are most often affected, although the involvement of axillary, mediastinal, mesenteric and retroperitoneal lymph nodes is also relatively common. A wide variety of extranodal sites may be affected, including the tonsil, spleen, oral cavity, gastrointestinal tract, liver, soft tissue, skin and even the breast {211, 530}. Common sites for metastasis include the lymph nodes, lung, and liver.

Clinical features
Patients most often present with a slow-growing, painless mass, although patients with abdominal disease may present with abdominal pain. Systemic symptoms are unusual.

Aetiology
There is no known aetiology for most cases of follicular dendritic cell sarcoma/tumour. However, a high proportion of cases of putative follicular dendritic cell sarcoma/tumour showing features of inflammatory pseudotumour have been associated with the Epstein-Barr virus {41}. In these cases, Epstein-Barr virus encoded RNA (EBER) has been found in all or virtually all the spindle cells, and Southern blot studies have demonstrated that the virus is present in a monoclonal episomal form {1175}.

Precursor lesions
In rare cases of Castleman disease, there is a proliferation of follicular dendritic cells outside of the follicles forming clusters and small sheets {1123}. The neoplasm therefore may evolve via intermediate steps of hyperplasia and dysplasia of follicular dendritic cells.

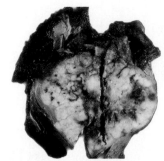

Fig. 10.22 Follicular dendritic cell sarcoma/tumour. This mass occurred in the soft tissues, and has the appearance of a sarcoma.

Macroscopy
Follicular dendritic cell sarcoma/tumour range from 1-20 cm, with a median size of about 5 cm. The smallest tumours occur in the cervical lymph nodes, while largest tumours are found in the retroperitoneum. Most are well-circumscribed masses, and are solid tan-grey on cut section, although necrosis or gross haemorrhage may be seen on occasion, particularly in the larger tumours.

Morphology
A spindle to ovoid cell proliferation is seen. The neoplasm forms fascicles, storiform patterns, and whorls – at times reminiscent of the 360° pattern observed in meningioma. Uncommonly, there may be fluid-filled cystic spaces, some in a perivascular location resembling thymoma, or amyloid change. The individual

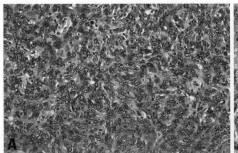 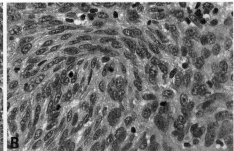

Fig. 10.23 Follicular dendritic cell sarcoma/tumour. **A** A spindle cell proliferation is seen. **B** A 360° whorl is seen. Note the occasional multinucleated cells.

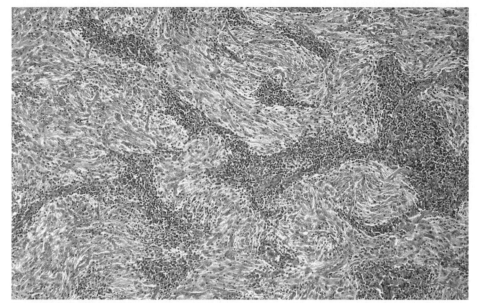

Fig. 10.24 Follicular dendritic cell sarcoma/tumour. Residual small lymphocytes are seen, particularly in a perivascular location.

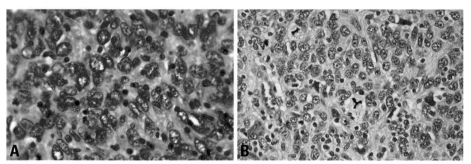

Fig. 10.25 Follicular dendritic cell sarcoma/tumour. **A** These ovoid cells have indistinct cytoplasmic outlines. **B** A greater than usual degree of cytologic atypia is present. Note the atypical mitotic figure.

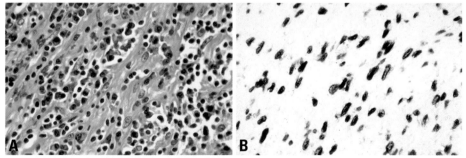

Fig. 10.26 Putative follicular dendritic cell sarcoma/tumour of the liver showing histological features of inflammatory pseudotumour. **A** This lesion showed focal expression of CD21. Positivity for EBER was also seen. **B** This lesion showed positivity for EBER in almost all of the proliferating spindle cells.

neoplastic cells generally have plump, slightly eosinophilic cytoplasm with indistinct cell borders. The nuclei are elongated, with vesicular or granular finely dispersed chromatin, small but distinct nucleoli, and a delicate nuclear membrane. Occasional multinucleated cells may be seen, occasionally resembling Warthin-Finkeldy giant cells. In addition, pseudo-nuclear inclusions may be seen. Although the cytologic features are usually bland, significant cytologic atypia may be found in a subset of cases. The mitotic rate is usually between 0 and 10 per 10 high power fields, although cases with cytologic atypia may have much higher mitotic rates, greater than 30 per 10 high power fields, as well as easily found atypical mitoses.

Uninvolved residual lymphoid tissue is often present. This may take the form of residual germinal centres or clusters of small lymphocytes (or more rarely plasma cells), particularly in a perivascular location. In the lesional tissue there is a scattering of small lymphocytes. These tumours may also contain foci of necrosis. Very rarely, epithelioid cells may be seen {205}.

Putative cases of follicular dendritic cell sarcoma/tumour of the liver and spleen often have histological features more consistent with inflammatory pseudotumour. In these benign inflammatory pseudotumours the spindle cells are not as cohesive as typically seen in other cases of follicular dendritic cell sarcoma/tumour, and are often scattered and obscured by a prominent lymphoplasmacytic reaction. The spindle cell nuclei usually have a vesicular chromatin pattern, with varying degrees of nuclear atypia and may contain prominent nucleoli, occasionally resembling Reed-Sternberg cells {1175}.

Ultrastructure

The neoplastic cells of follicular dendritic cell sarcoma/tumour have elongated nuclei, often with cytoplasmic invagination. The cytoplasm often contains numerous polysomes. The most distinctive feature is the presence of numerous long, slender cytoplasmic processes, often connected by scattered, mature desmosomes. Birbeck granules and numerous lysosomes are not seen.

Immunophenotype

The neoplastic cells generally demonstrate the phenotype of non-neoplastic follicular dendritic cells {949, 993}. Thus, they are positive for one or more of the follicular dendritic markers, including CD21, CD35 and CD23. In addition, they are usually positive for desmoplakin, vimentin, fascin, HLA-DR, and often positive for epithelial membrane antigen. They are variably positive for S-100-protein, and CD68. CD45, CD20 are occasionally expressed. Staining for CD1a, lysozyme, myeloperoxidase, CD34, CD3, CD79a, CD30, HMB-45, and cytokeratins are consistently negative. Ki-67 labelling ranges from 1 to 25% with a mean value of 13% {949}. The small lymphocytes

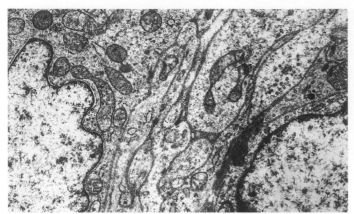

Fig. 10.27 Follicular dendritic cell sarcoma/tumour. This electron micrograph shows numerous cytoplasmic processes, with one well-formed desmosome present in the centre.

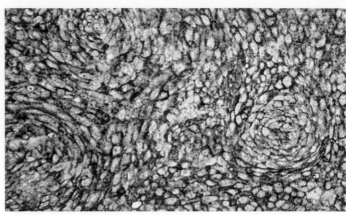

Fig. 10.28 Follicular dendritic cell sarcoma/tumour, CD21 stain. Strong positivity is seen in this case. Often, the staining is more focal.

show in some cases a B-cell phenotype, while T cells predominate in others. Muscle specific actin expression is controversial. While the historic literature may associate muscle specific actin with FDC tumours, in the modern era with more FDC specific markers (e.g. CD21, CD35) muscle specific actin is less associated with FDC and more associated with fibroblastic reticular cell tumours with myofibroblastic features {31}.

In cases of putative follicular dendritic cell sarcoma/tumour of the liver and spleen showing histological features of inflammatory pseudotumour, the expression of follicular dendritic cell markers is often weak and focal.

Genetics

The immunoglobulin heavy chain gene and β, δ and γ chain genes of the T-cell receptor are in a germline configuration {1367}.

Postulated cell of origin

The follicular dendritic cell of the follicle is the putative normal counterpart

Prognosis and predictive factors

The behaviour is typically indolent; much like a low grade tissue sarcoma {206}. Most patients are treated by complete surgical excision, without or without adjuvant radiotherapy or chemotherapy. Local recurrences occur in about 40-50%

of cases, and metastases occur in about 25% of patients, often after local recurrence {1024}. Cases with an intra-abdominal presentation, significant cytologic atypia, extensive coagulative necrosis, a high proliferative index, larger tumour size greater than 6 cm., and lack of adjuvant therapy have a poorer prognosis. At least 10-20% of patients ultimately die of their disease, often after a long period of time {1035, 949}.

Dendritic cell sarcoma, not otherwise specified

L.M. Weiss
T.M. Grogan
H.-K. Müller-Hermelink
H. Stein

T. Dura
B. Favara
M. Paulli
A.C. Feller

Definition
Occasional dendritic cell neoplasms do not fall into well-defined categories, as defined in the previous sections.

ICD-O code   9757/3

General comments
These tumours have been called indeterminate cell sarcoma/tumour. Only extremely rare cases have been reported, generally as single case reports {116, 104, 682, 215, 1410, 1336, 1423, 31}. This is a diagnosis of exclusion, not well characterised morphologically and immunophenotypically. Tumours with CD1a and S-100-protein but without Birbeck granules have been called indeterminate neoplasm said to derive from a cell in transition between the Langerhans cell and interdigitating dendritic cell. In a recent large series with multiple markers and electron microscopy no cases of this indeterminate category were found {1035}.

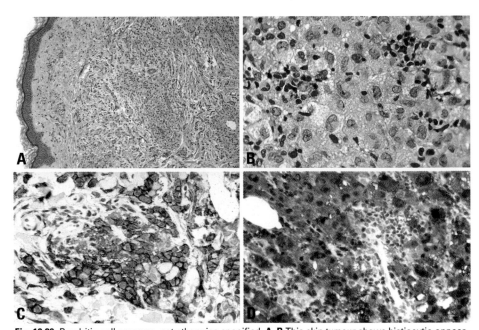

Fig. 10.29 Dendritic cell sarcoma, not otherwise specified. **A, B** This skin tumour shows histiocytic appearing cells. Although the characteristic grooves of the nuclei of Langerhans cell histiocytosis are not present, the lesion was positive for CD1a **(C)** and S-100-protein **(D)**. Birbeck granules were not identified on ultrastructural examination.

CHAPTER 11

Mastocytosis (Mast Cell Disease)

The term mastocytosis denotes a heterogeneous group of disorders characterised by the abnormal growth and accumulation of mast cells in one or more organ system. The disease manifestations of mastocytosis range from skin lesions that may spontaneously regress, to highly aggressive neoplasms with multisystem involvement and short survival times. Recent data suggest that most variants of mastocytosis (at least those with systemic involvement) are clonal disorders; the mast cells from these patients demonstrate a somatic mutation in *KIT*, the proto-oncogene that encodes a receptor tyrosine kinase, the receptor for stem cell factor. This mutation undoubtedly plays a role in the pathogenesis of mastocytosis, and also offers a target for the development of more specific therapy.

Over the past several years, there have been several proposals for the classification of mast cell disease, but none has been universally accepted. The proposal adopted by the WHO is a consensus classification system developed at the Year 2000 Working Conference, held in Vienna in September, 2000. At that meeting, experts working in the field of mast cell disease, including many authorities who had proposed previous classification schemes, agreed that the classification of mast cell disease must include not only morphologic but also clinical parameters, and be flexible enough to incorporate new molecular data that is emerging for this group of diseases. The consensus classification agreed upon at the Vienna conference meets those criteria.

WHO histological classification of mastocytosis

Cutaneous mastocytosis	
Indolent systemic mastocytosis (ISM)	9741/1
Systemic mastocytosis with associated clonal, haematological non-mast-cell lineage disease (SM-AHNMD)	9741/3
Aggressive systemic mastocytosis (ASM)	9741/3
Mast cell leukaemia (MCL)	9742/3
Mast cell sarcoma (MCS)	9740/3
Extracutaneous mastocytoma	9740/1

Mastocytosis

P. Valent*
H.-P. Horny
C.Y. Li
B.J. Longley

D.D. Metcalfe
R.M. Parwaresch
J.M. Bennett

Definition

Mastocytosis is a proliferation of mast cells and their subsequent accumulation in one or more organ systems. Mast cells are derived from haematopoietic progenitors, thus mastocytosis is a haematopoietic disorder. The manifestations of mastocytosis are heterogeneous, ranging from skin lesions that may spontaneously regress to highly aggressive neoplasms associated with multisystem involvement and short survival times. In cutaneous mastocytosis (CM), the mast cell proliferation is confined to the skin; systemic mastocytosis (SM) is characterised by involvement of at least one extracutaneous organ, with or without evidence of skin infiltration. Tables 11.01-11.04 outline the classification of mastocytosis, as well as criteria for recognition of its subtypes.

ICD-O codes

Urticaria pigmentosa	
Diffuse cutaneous mastocytosis	
Solitary mastocytoma of skin	9740/1
Indolent systemic mastocytosis	9741/1
Systemic mastocytosis with AHNMD	9741/3
Aggressive systemic mastocytosis	9741/3
Mast cell leukaemia	9742/3
Mast cell sarcoma	9740/3
Extracutaneous mastocytoma	9740/1

Table 11.01
Classification of mastocytosis.

> **Cutaneous mastocytosis (CM)**
>
> **Indolent systemic mastocytosis (ISM)**
>
> **Systemic mastocytosis with associated clonal, haematological non-mast-cell lineage disease (SM-AHNMD)**
>
> **Aggressive systemic mastocytosis (ASM)**
>
> **Mast cell leukaemia (MCL)**
>
> **Mast cell sarcoma (MCS)**
>
> **Extracutaneous mastocytoma**

Synonyms

Mast cell disease
Mast cell proliferative disease

Epidemiology

Mastocytosis may occur at any age. Cutaneous mast cell disease is most common in children. It may be present at birth, and 80% of afflicted children demonstrate lesions by 6 months of age. In adults, CM usually appears in the third and fourth decade of life {1211}. There is no sex predilection reported for CM. Systemic mastocytosis is generally diagnosed after the third decade of life; the male to female ratio has been reported to vary from 1 to 1:3 {1308, 155, 1363, 532}.

Sites of involvement

In approximately 80% of patients with mastocytosis, only the skin is clinically involved. In the remaining 10-20% of patients who have SM, bone marrow involvement is almost always morphologically apparent, and a bone marrow biopsy is the usual specimen from which the diagnosis of SM is established {1308, 155, 1363, 532, 1211}. The peripheral blood rarely shows circulating mast cells {153}. Other organs frequently involved include the spleen, lymph nodes, liver or gastrointestinal tract, but any tissue may show deposits of abnormal mast cells. Skin lesions occur in 50% or more of the

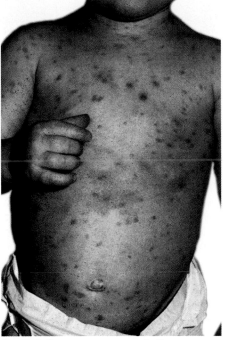

Fig. 11.01 Cutaneous mastocytosis. Numerous typical macular and maculopapular pigmented lesions of urticaria pigmentosa in a young child.

patients with SM, and when present they usually imply an indolent course {1308, 750, 1002, 57}.

Clinical findings

Cutaneous mastocytosis includes several distinct clinico-histopathological entities (see below). The lesions of all forms of CM may urticate when stroked (Darier's sign) and most may show pigment which is epidermal in location. The term "urticaria pigmentosa" describes these two clinical features (urticaria and hyperpigmentation) and has been used as a general term for all forms of cutaneous mastocytosis. Blistering or bullous mastocytosis represents an exaggerated Darier's sign, usually in very young

*For the participants of the Year 2000 Working Conference on Mastocytosis: L. Escribano, L.B. Schwartz, G. Marone, R. Nunez, C. Akin, K. Sotlar, W.R. Sperr, K. Wolff, R.D. Brunning, K.F. Austen, K. Lennert, J.W. Vardiman.
Text excerpted from {1148} by J.W. Vardiman

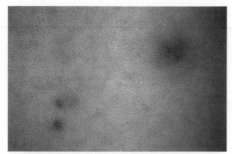

Fig. 11.02 Cutaneous mastocytosis; Darier's sign. The skin lesions of all forms of cutaneous mastocytosis may urticate when stroked. A palpable wheal appears a few moments after the physical stimulation, due to the release of histamine from the mast cells.

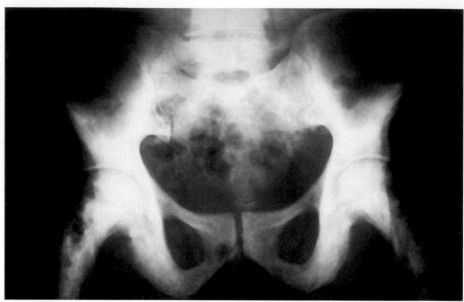

Fig. 11.03 Systemic mastocytosis. Skeletal lesions are common in systemic mastocytosis. This X-ray shows patchy osteosclerosis, osteoporosis, as well as multiple lytic lesions in the femur.

patients, and can occur in any form of paediatric mastocytosis {1211, 785, 784}.

In *systemic mastocytosis*, organ dysfunction may be due to infiltration by mast cells or to the release of various biochemical mediators, such as histamine, eicosanoids, proteases or heparin. For example, gastrointestinal complaints, such as peptic ulcer disease and diarrhoea, are more commonly due to release of biologically active mediators than to infiltration of the gastrointestinal tract by abnormal mast cells {1308, 57, 483, 646, 596}.

Systemic mastocytosis has signs and symptoms at presentation that can generally be grouped into the following categories: 1) constitutional symptoms (fatigue, weight loss, fever, sweats), 2) skin manifestations (pruritus, urticaria, dermatographism, 3) mediator-related events (abdominal pain, gastrointestinal distress, flushing, syncope, hypertension, headache, hypotension, tachycardia, respiratory symptoms), and 4) bone-related complaints (bone pain, fractures, arthralgia) {1308}. Physical findings at the time of diagnosis may include splenomegaly; lymphadenopathy and hepatomegaly are found less frequently {1308, 155, 1363, 537, 540, 869}. Symptoms are mild in many patients, but in others the mediator-related events or organ impairment may be life threatening.

Haematological abnormalities occur in a significant number of patients with SM. Anaemia, leukocytosis or leukopenia, and thrombocytopenia or thrombocytosis may occur; bone marrow failure can be seen in patients with marked marrow infiltration {153}. Eosinophilia may be observed, and

is sometimes so marked that it mimics the hypereosinophilic syndrome {153, 880, 406}. Circulating mast cells are infrequently observed, except in rare cases of mast cell leukaemia {153, 1309}. In up to 20-30% of cases of SM, an associated, clonal haematopoietic, non-mast cell lineage disorder (AHNMD) may be discovered simultaneously or after the diagnosis of mastocytosis. In such cases, symptoms may be related to the associated haematological disorder as well as to the SM {1308, 155, 750, 1310}.

Serum total tryptase is a useful test in the evaluation of patients with mastocytosis. In the absence of other myeloid disorders, the finding of serum total tryptase levels >20 ng/mL is indicative of SM. In contrast, serum total tryptase levels are normal (<1 to 15 ng/mL) or only slightly elevated in patients with pure CM {1165}.

Aetiology

The cause of mast cell disease is unknown. Rare familial cases are reported {1211}.

Morphology

The diagnosis of mast cell disease requires the demonstration of multi-focal clusters or aggregates of mast cells in an adequate biopsy specimen; staining of tissue sections with Giemsa or for mast cell tryptase are strongly recommended for confirmation of the diagnosis. The histological pattern of the mast cell infiltrate

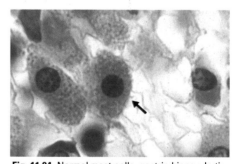

Fig. 11.04 Normal mast cells, gastric biopsy. In tissue sections, normal mast cells (arrow) have round or oval nuclei with a coarse chromatin pattern. Nucleoli are not observed or are small and inconspicuous. The cells have variable amounts of cytoplasm with faintly eosinophilic granular cytoplasm.

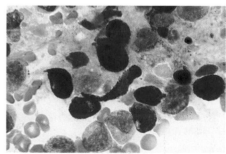

Fig. 11.05 Mast cell hyperplasia. Reactive mast cells from a bone marrow aspirate smear of a patient treated with stem cell factor for severe aplastic anaemia. In the Wright-Giemsa stained smear, mast cells have round to oval nuclei and cytoplasm that is densely packed with small basophilic granules that often obscure the nucleus. Occasional cells are elongated.

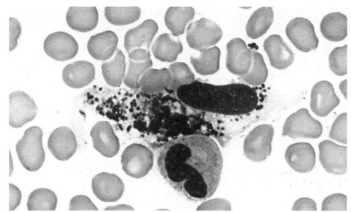

Fig. 11.06 Mast cell in systemic mastocytosis. Bone marrow smear of a patient with indolent systemic mast cell disease. The cell is atypical, with an indented nucleus in an eccentric location, and cytoplasm that shows an elongated extrusion with irregular distribution of granules.

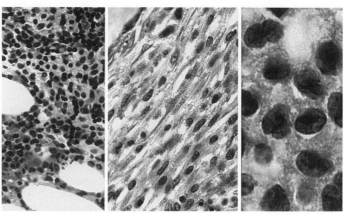

Fig. 11.07 Systemic mastocytosis. The cells may have bland nuclei with moderate amounts of pale cytoplasm, spindled shapes that resemble fibroblasts, or lobulated nuclei with abundant clear cytoplasm. The latter cells may resemble monocytes or histiocytes, and are more commonly seen in aggressive mast cell lesions.

may vary according to the tissue sampled. If the mast cells are loosely scattered without forming aggregates, it may be impossible to establish the diagnosis without additional studies, such as demonstration of an aberrant phenotype, detection of point mutations of *KIT*, or additional biopsies {916, 782, 14, 979, 348, 1216, 783}.

In tissue sections stained with haematoxylin and eosin (H&E), normal mast cells usually display a round to oval nucleus with clumped chromatin, low N/C ratio, and no or indistinct nucleoli. They have moderately abundant oval or polygonal-shaped cytoplasm filled with small, faintly visible, slightly eosinophilic granules, and they are usually sprinkled diffusely in tissues without forming clusters {750, 1002}. In smear preparations, mast cells are readily visible in Romanowsky stains as, round, oval or polygonal cells with cytoplasm densely packed with small, deeply basophilic granules, and round or oval nuclei. In

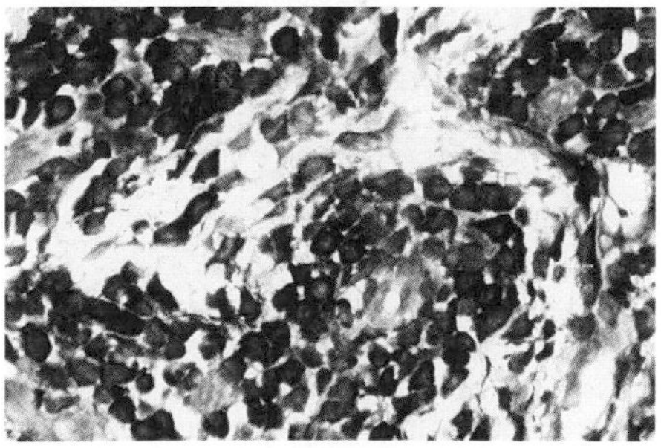

mastocytosis, the cytology of mast cells is variable (for a detailed discussion of the various forms of mast cells in mast cell disease see {1322}). In some cases they may closely resemble normal mast cells, but more frequently at least a proportion of the cells have abnormal cytologic features, in that they are more spindled-shaped, and have reniform or indented nuclei. In some cases, neoplastic mast cells have abundant cytoplasm with sparse granules. This feature may be appreciated in tissue sections as pale, almost clear cytoplasm, in which case the mast cells may resemble histiocytes, or the cells of hairy cell leukaemia, monocytoid B cell lymphoma, or other disorders characterised by "clear" cells. In smear preparations, mast cells may demonstrate so few granules that their mast cell origin may not be readily appreciated even in the Romanowsky stains. This is particularly true of immature mast cells ("nonmetachromatic" and "metachromatic" blasts) seen in the high grade lesions, such as mast cell leukaemia {155, 750, 1310, 1322}. The finding of mast cells with bi- or multi-lobated nuclei usually indicates an aggressive mast cell proliferation, and although they are commonly observed in mast cell leukaemia, they may be seen in other subtypes of the disease as well {155, 750, 1310, 1322}. Mitotic figures are generally scarce, even in the aggressive variants.

All mast cell proliferations should be confirmed by special stains. Metachromatic stains (Giemsa, toluidine blue) are strongly recommended as routine stains for mast cells. Fixation methods common-

ly employed for bone marrow biopsies, however, may result in no or diminished toludine blue staining. The most specific method for identification of mast cells in all tissues is immunohistochemical staining for mast cell tryptase {541, 1319}. Napthol ASD chloroacetate esterase and

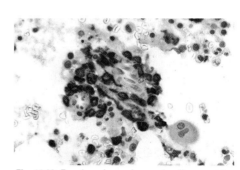

Fig. 11.09 Focal, perivascular mast cell accumulation. Immunohistochemical stain for mast cell tryptase identifies a focal collection of mast cells in the bone marrow biopsy of a patient with systemic mast cell disease. Although this small focus is not sufficient by itself for a diagnosis of mastocytosis by itself, it is suspicious.

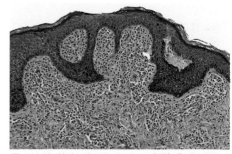

Fig. 11.10 Urticaria pigmentosa (UP). Typical skin lesion of a child with UP. Aggregates of mast cells fill the papillary dermis and extend as sheets into the reticular dermis.

Fig. 11.08 Systemic mastocytosis. Mast cells usually demonstrate metachromatic granules that are stained with Giemsa, or as in this case, with toluidine blue.

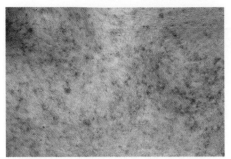

Fig. 11.11 Telangiectasia macularis eruptive perstans (TMEP). Skin lesions of a patient with the TMEP variant of urticaria pigmentosa/maculopapular cutaneous mastocytosis. The skin lesions are usually flat, and variably pigmented.

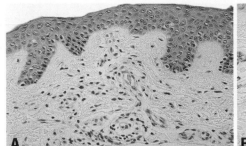

Fig. 11.12 Telangiectasia macularis eruptive perstans (TMEP). Often, the number of mast cells is minimally increased in this variant, and may overlap with the upper range seen in normal and inflamed skin. **A** The mast cells may be difficult to appreciate on H&E stained slides. **B** In the toluidine blue stain, the increase in the number of mast cells is more readily appreciated.

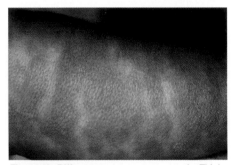

Fig. 11.13 Diffuse cutaneous mastocytosis. Thickened, reddish "peau chagrine" lesions characteristic of diffuse cutaneous mastocytosis. This variant occurs almost exclusively in children.

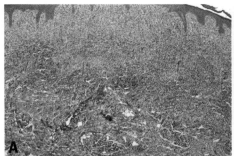

Fig. 11.14 Mastocytoma of skin. An isolated lesion from the wrist of an infant. **A** The papillary and reticular dermis are filled with mast cells. **B** At higher magnification, the bland appearance of the mast cell infiltrate can be appreciated.

CD117 are also characteristic markers of mast cells, but they are not specific. In contrast to normal mast cells, CD2 and CD25 are reportedly expressed on the surface of neoplastic mast cells {979, 348, 1216, 1321, 936}.

Cutaneous mastocytosis (CM)

The diagnosis of cutaneous mastocytosis (CM) requires the demonstration of typical clinical findings and histological evidence of infiltration of the skin by mast cells. In cases of pure cutaneous mastocytosis, there is no evidence for any systemic involvement, such as elevated levels of total serum tryptase or organomegaly. Three major variants of CM are recognised:

1. Urticaria pigmentosa (UP) / Maculopapular Cutaneous Mastocytosis (MPCM). This is the most frequent form of CM. In children, the lesions of UP tend to be papular, and are characterised by aggregates of elongated or spindle-shaped mast cells which typically fill the papillary dermis and extend as sheets and aggregates into the reticular dermis, often following the vasculature {1211}. A subvariant is a non-pigmented, plaque-forming lesion that most often occurs in infants. In adults the lesions tend to be macular, more darkly pigmented, and sometimes associated with telangiectasia. Some authorities refer to the small hyperpigmented macular lesions of adult-type UP as the telangiectasia macularis eruptiva perstans subvariant (TMEP). Others reserve TMEP for a more rare form characterised by a small number of larger lesions (>1cm) which are lightly pigmented, telangiectatic macules with minimal or no increase in the number of mast cells {1302, 86}. Adult UP tends to have fewer mast cells than the

Table 11.02
Subclassification of cutaneous mastocytosis.

Urticaria pigmentosa (UP) / maculopapular cutaneous mastocytosis (MPCM)
Typical UP
Plaque form
Nodular form
Telangiectasia macularis eruptiva perstans
Diffuse cutaneous mastocytosis
Solitary mastocytoma of skin

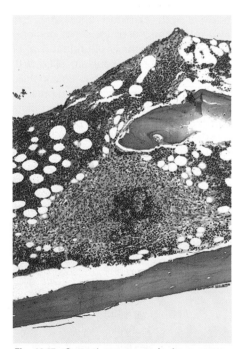

Fig. 11.15 Systemic mastocytosis, bone marrow biopsy. The bone marrow biopsy is the most frequent specimen from which a diagnosis of systemic mastocytosis is made. The lesions are often well-circumscribed, and may occur in paratrabecular or paravascular locations, but may be randomly distributed in the intertrabecular regions as well.

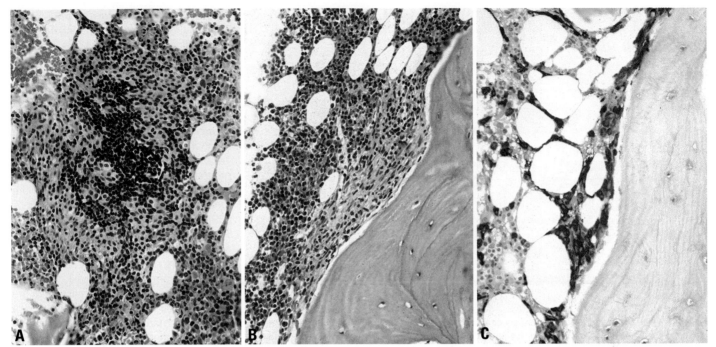

Fig. 11.16 Systemic mastocytosis, bone marrow biopsy. **A** The focal lesions of mast cells often consist of a central core of lymphocytes, surrounded by polygonal-shaped mast cells with pale, faintly granular cytoplasm, with reactive eosinophils at the outer margin of the lesion. **B** Focal paratrabecular aggregates of spindled mast cells sometimes resemble collections of fibroblasts or histiocytes. **C** An immunohistochemical stain for mast cell tryptase confirms that the cells are mast cells.

lesions in children, and in some macular lesions the number of mast cells may overlap with the upper range seen in normal or inflamed skin. In such cases, examination of multiple sections for aggregates of mast cells or biopsies of multiple lesions may be necessary to establish the diagnosis.

2. Diffuse cutaneous mastocytosis. This lesion is less frequent than UP, and is seen almost exclusively in children. Patients lack the typical maculopapular lesions of UP, and may have relatively smooth skin, red skin, or skin which is greatly thickened (peau chagrine, grain leather skin). Histologically, in patients with less clinically obvious infiltration of the skin, the biopsy may show a band like infiltrate of mast cells in the papillary and upper reticular dermis. In nodular, plaque-like or greatly infiltrated skin lesions, the histological picture may be identical to that seen in solitary mastocytoma {1388, 1099, 1340}.

3. Mastocytoma of skin. This occurs as a single lesion, usually in infants, with a predilection for the trunk and wrist. Sheets of mast cells with abundant cytoplasm fill the papillary and reticular dermis, and may extend into the deep dermis and subcutaneous tissues. There is no cytologic atypia {1154}.

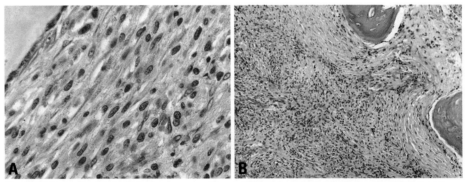

Fig. 11.17 Systemic mastocytosis, bone marrow biopsy. **A** Densely packed, spindled mast cells along a bony trabeculum. **B** Often, the monomorphic, spindled mast cells are accompanied by fibrosis, and may replace large areas of the bone marrow biopsy specimen. Osteosclerosis often accompanies such lesions.

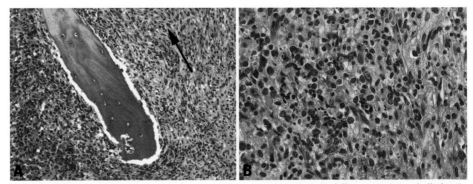

Fig. 11.18 Systemic mastocytosis with associated acute myeloid leukaemia. **A** The streaming, spindled cells of a large mast cell aggregate can be seen on one side of the bony trabeculum (arrow), whereas a monotonous population of blast cells is seen on the opposite side. **B** The spindled cells of mast cell disease abut next to a large aggregate of blasts.

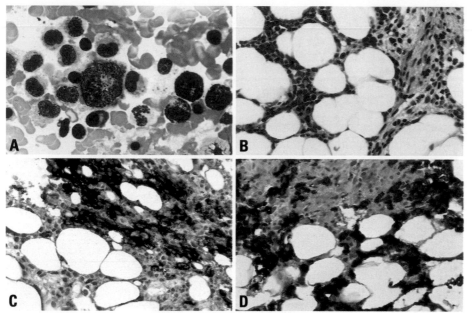

Fig. 11.19 Systemic mastocytosis with associated hairy cell leukaemia. **A** illustrates a bone marrow aspirate smear with hairy cells and atypical mast cells. **B** The spindled mast cells are present adjacent to the hairy cell infiltrate in the interstitial regions of the marrow. Although hairy cell leukaemia may occasionally assume a spindled morphology, in this case the mast cell tryptase illustrated in **C** clearly demonstrates the mast cell origin of the spindled cells, and an immunostain for CD20 identifies the hairy cells in **D**.

Table 11.03
Criteria for cutaneous and systemic mastocytosis.

Cutaneous mastocytosis (CM)
Typical skin lesions demonstrating the typical clinical findings of UP/MPCM, diffuse cutaneous mastocytosis or solitary mastocytoma, and typical infiltrates of mast cells in a multi-focal or diffuse pattern in an adequate skin biopsy.
Systemic mastocytosis (SM)

Major criteria
   Multifocal, dense infiltrates of mast cells (15 or more mast cells in aggregates) detected in sections of bone marrow and/or other extracutaneous organ(s), and confirmed by tryptase immunohistochemistry or other special stains
 	
Minor criteria
   a. In biopsy sections of bone marrow or other extracutaneous organs, more than 25% of the mast cells in the infiltrate are spindle-shaped or have atypical morphology, or, of all mast cells in bone marrow aspirate smears, more than 25% are immature or atypical mast cells
 	
   b. Detection of *KIT* point mutation at codon 816 in bone marrow, blood or other extracutaneous organ(s)
 	
   c. Mast cells in bone marrow, blood or other extracutaneous organs that co-express CD117 with CD2 and/or CD25
 	
   d. Serum total tryptase persistently >20 ng/ml (unless there is an associated clonal myeloid disorder, in which case this parameter is not valid).
 	
The diagnosis of SM may be made if one major and one minor criterion are present, or, if three minor criteria are fulfilled.

Systemic mastocytosis (SM)

The requirements for the diagnosis of SM are outlined in Table 11.03. In most cases, aggregates of neoplastic cells are readily appreciated in tissue sections, although their mast cell lineage must be confirmed by the use of special stains.

Bone marrow

In most cases, multifocal, sharply demarcated deposits of mast cells are found in peritrabecular or perivascular locations in bone marrow biopsy specimens, or are randomly distributed {1308, 155, 1363, 539}. The focal lesions are comprised of varying proportions of mast cells, lymphocytes, eosinophils and fibroblasts. Often, these show a central core of lymphocytes, surrounded by mast cells, with reactive eosinophilia at the margins of the lesion. In other cases, the lesions are more monomorphic, and are comprised of spindled mast cells that abut against or stream along the bony trabeculae. Significant fibrosis and thickening of the adjacent bone are frequently observed. Sometimes the marrow space is diffusely replaced by mast cells, which may be so spindled that they resemble fibroblasts. Marked reticulin or collagen fibrosis is usual in such cases.

Careful inspection of the marrow apart from the mast cell proliferation is important. The marrow may be hypercellular due to the proliferation of neutrophils, eosinophils, or both. In other cases, the marrow may show evidence of a coexisting haematopoietic neoplasm, such as acute myeloid leukaemia, a chronic myeloproliferative or myelodysplastic disorder, or a lymphoproliferative disease {1308, 155, 1363, 750, 1310, 539}. In such cases, the associated haematologic disease should be classified according to the WHO criteria. It is important to note whether there is increased cellularity of the marrow or disturbed maturation in the haematopoietic cells, because even if criteria for a coexisting myeloid neoplasm are not present, hypercellularity or abnormal myeloid maturation patterns have been associated with an unfavourable outcome {750, 539}. Reactive, non-clonal mast cell hyperplasia may accompany a number of haematological disorders, including myeloid and lymphoid neoplasms in the marrow. In such cases, the mast cells lack cytologic atypia, and are sprinkled interstitially throughout the marrow, in contrast to the aggregates of neoplastic mast cells found in mastocytosis. The diagnosis of bone marrow involvement by SM is usually established by a bone marrow biopsy specimen, but examination of marrow aspirate smears may also provide useful information. In some cases, the mast cells will not be easily aspirated because of accompanying fibrosis, or they may be found only in the thick regions of the aspirated spicules. Still, their morphology can easily be assessed in such preparations with Romanowsky stains. Although an increase in mast cell numbers can sometimes be suspected from the aspirate smear, their number may be underrepresented in the aspirated specimen, so correlation with the biopsy is essential.

Rarely, the blood and bone marrow may show mast cell leukaemia. In this aggressive form of mastocytosis, the marrow space is diffusely infiltrated in an interstitial pattern by atypical mast cells that often are poorly granulated and have irregularly lobated or bilobated nuclei {1309}. Sometimes, nucleoli may be prominent. Most often in mast cell leukaemia, the marrow aspirate smears will show sheets of abnormal mast cells. When mast cells account for 20% or more of the cells on the bone marrow aspirate, the diagnosis of mast cell leukaemia can be suspected. The final diagnosis of mast cell leukaemia, however, should be established on the basis of the criteria for SM, together with the findings in the bone marrow biopsy sections and aspirate smear. In typical mast cell leukaemia, mast cells account for 10% or more of the peripheral blood white cells. If there are fewer than 10% mast cells in the blood, and the morphology of the marrow biopsy and aspirate is that of mast cell leukaemia, the diagnosis of the "aleukaemic" variant is appropriate.

Lymph node

In lymph nodes, the abnormal mast cell infiltrates may be observed in any compartment. The infiltrate may be focal, and tends to involve the paracortical areas, but can also be diffuse and totally obliterate the lymph node architecture. Hyperplasia of germinal centres, small blood vessel hyperplasia, eosinophilia, plasmacytosis and collagen fibrosis often accompany the mast cell infiltration {537, 869, 539}. In some patients, lymphadenopathy may be progressive, and if accompanied by peripheral blood or

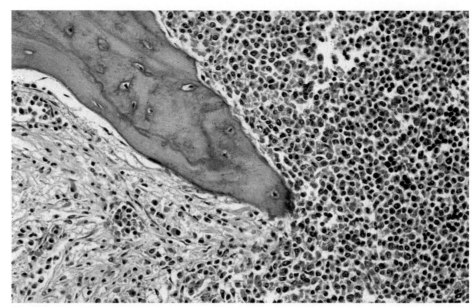

Fig. 11.20 Systemic mastocytosis, bone marrow biopsy. One region of the marrow is occupied by mast cells with fibrosis, whereas the adjacent area is hypercellular, with panmyelosis. Even though there may be insufficient criteria for the diagnosis of an associated clonal myeloid disorder, hypercellularity and abnormal myeloid maturation have been associated with a less favourable outcome, and constitute one of the criteria for the provisional subvariant, "smouldering systemic mastocytosis".

marked tissue eosinophilia, may identify a subset of patients with aggressive mastocytosis {406}.

Spleen

Any compartment of the spleen may be involved by mastocytosis. Mast cell accumulations may be found as focal lesions in the paratrabecular or parafollicular areas or in the lymphoid follicles, or they may be diffusely distributed in the red pulp. Eosinophilia, fibrosis, and plasmacytosis are frequently observed in the areas of mast cell infiltration. In some

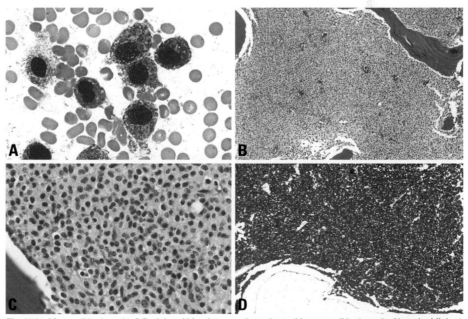

Fig. 11.21 Mast cell leukaemia. **A** Peripheral blood smear of a patient with mast cell leukaemia. Note the bilobed nuclei and relatively poorly-granulated cytoplasm which are often seen in this aggressive form of mastocytosis. **B** The bone marrow biopsy is diffusely infiltrated by the neoplastic mast cells. **C** demonstrates the "clear cell" appearance that is due to the poor granulation of the cytoplasm that is typical of immature mast cells of mast cell leukaemia. **D** The immunohistochemical stain for mast cell tryptase in the cases of mast cell leukaemia.

Table 11.04
Criteria for variants for systemic mastocytosis

Indolent systemic mastocytosis (ISM)
Meets criteria for SM
No "B" or "C" findings (see below)
No evidence of an associated clonal haematological malignancy/disorder
(In this variant, the mast cell burden is low, skin lesions are almost invariably present)
*Bone marrow mastocytosis** – as above with bone marrow involvement, but no skin lesions
*Smouldering systemic mastocytosis** – as above, but with 2 or more "B" findings but no "C" finding.

Systemic mastocytosis with associated clonal haematological non-mast cell lineage disease (SM-AHNMD)
Meets criteria for SM *and*
Associated, clonal haematological non-mast cell lineage disorder (MDS, CMPD, AML, lymphoma, or other haematological neoplasm that meets the criteria for a distinct entity in the WHO classification).

Aggressive systemic mastocytosis (ASM)
Meets criteria for SM
One or more "C" findings
No associated clonal haematological malignancy/disorder
No evidence of mast cell leukaemia
*Lymphadenopathic mastocytosis with eosinophilia** – (progressive lymphadenopathy with peripheral blood eosinophilia, often with extensive bony involvement, and hepatosplenomegaly, but usually without skin lesions).

Mast cell leukaemia
Meets criteria for SM
Biopsy shows diffuse infiltration, usually interstitial pattern, by atypical, immature mast cells
Bone marrow aspirate smears show 20% or more mast cells
Mast cells account for 10% or more of peripheral blood white cells
Variant: Aleukaemic mast cell leukaemia – as above, but <10% of WBCs are mast cells.

Mast cell sarcoma
Unifocal mast cell tumour
No evidence of SM
No skin lesions
Destructive growth pattern
High grade cytology

Extracutaneous mastocytoma
Unifocal mast cell tumour
No evidence of SM
No skin lesions
Non-destructive growth pattern
Low-grade cytology

"B" findings
1. Bone marrow biopsy showing >30% infiltration by mast cells (focal, dense aggregates) and/or serum total tryptase level >200ng/ml
2. Signs of dysplasia or myeloproliferation, in non-mast cell lineage, but insufficient criteria for definitive diagnosis of a haematopoietic neoplasm by WHO, with normal or only slightly abnormal blood counts
3. Hepatomegaly without impairment of liver function, and/or palpable splenomegaly without hypersplenism, and/or palpable or visceral lymphadenopathy

"C" findings
1. Bone marrow dysfunction manifested by one or more cytopenia (ANC < 1.0 x 10⁹/L, Hb <10g/dl, or platelets <100 x 10⁹/L), but no frank non-mast cell haematopoietic malignancy.
2. Palpable hepatomegaly with impairment of liver function, ascites, and/or portal hypertension
3. Skeletal involvement with large-sized osteolysis and/or pathological fractures
4. Palpable splenomegaly with hypersplenism
5. Malabsorption with weight loss due to GI mast cell infiltrates

*Provisional subvariants

cases, an associated haematological disorder may be apparent in the splenic tissue {155, 540, 869, 1307}.

Liver
Small foci of atypical mast cells may be found in the sinuses, periportal areas, or both {535}. Fibrosis is present in 20% of the cases, but fully developed cirrhosis is only occasionally observed.

Skeletal lesions
Osteosclerosis is the most common bony change associated with mast cell infiltration, but lytic lesions and concurrent osteosclerotic and osteolytic lesion may occur concurrently {1308}.

Mast cell sarcoma
Mast cell sarcoma is an exceedingly rare entity characterised by localised but destructive growth of a tumour consisting of highly atypical, immature mast cells . Although initially localised, distant spread is possible. The cells may resemble those of mast cell leukaemia, and a leukaemic phase may occur {538, 681}.

Extracutaneous mastocytoma
The morphology of this localised tumour is that of an accumulation of mature mast cells, in contrast to the atypical mast cells observed in mast cell sarcoma. Extracutaneous mastocytoma is very rare, and most reported cases have been localised in the lung {217}.

Cytochemistry / immunophenotype
Normal mast cells lack myeloperoxidase, but demonstrate napthol ASD chloroacetate esterase. They express CD45, CD33, CD68, and CD117, and lack CD14, CD15, and CD16, as well as T- and B-cell related antigens {1319, 764}. All mast cells demonstrate mast cell tryptase, whereas chymase is demonstrated in a subpopulation {1319}. Neoplastic mast cells show a similar antigenic profile, but in contrast to normal mast cells, have been reported to demonstrate CD2 and CD25 {979, 348, 1216}. In some cases, neoplastic mast cells may lack napthol ASD chloroacetate esterase, particularly if they are poorly granulated.

Genetics
Somatic point mutations of *KIT*, a proto-oncogene that encodes the tyrosine kinase receptor for stem cell factor (SCF,

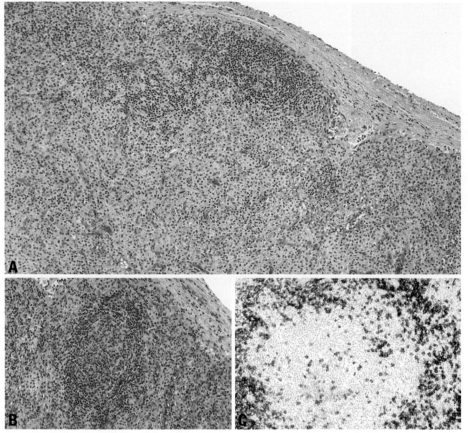

Fig. 11.22 Systemic mastocytosis, lymph node biopsy. **A** Lymph node biopsy that is diffusely infiltrated by neoplastic mast cells, leaving only a remnant of a normal follicle. **B** The infiltrate often is parafollicular in distribution. **C** An immunohistochemical stain for mast cell tryptase illustrates the parafollicular distribution of the mast cell infiltrate in the same biopsy.

or mast cell growth factor), are recurring genetic abnormalities in mastocytosis {916, 782, 14, 1413, 781, 783}. The most commonly observed mutation substitutes Val for Asp at codon 816, which results in spontaneous activation of the kit protein (SCF receptor). This mutation is seen in the mast cells of the vast majority of adults with SM. It may be found in the mast cells of rare cases of paediatric CM in which case the presentation and course are atypical, but most cases of typical paediatric CM lack the codon 816 mutation. Variant mutations have been reported {781, 783}.

Postulated cell of origin

Mast cells are derived from haematopoietic progenitor cells {1319, 1115, 661}.

Prognosis and predictive factors

Cutaneous mastocytosis in children usually has a favourable outcome and regresses spontaneously before or during puberty {869, 1320}. In adults, CM rarely regresses, and is often associated with SM {1302}. Currently, there is no cure for SM, and the prognosis is variable, depending on the disease category into which the patient belongs. Patients with aggressive disease, such as mast cell leukaemia, may survive only weeks to months, whereas those with indolent SM usually experience no impact of the disease on their survival {1412}. A major prognostic feature in SM is the presence or absence of skin involvement. Patients with SM and cutaneous involvement often experience an indolent course, whereas those with no detectable skin lesions usually have more aggressive and progressive disease {1308, 750}. Mast cell leukaemia and mast cell sarcoma are high grade disorders {1309, 538, 681}. If there is an associated haematological malignancy, the clinical course usually follows the course of the related haematological disease {1310}.

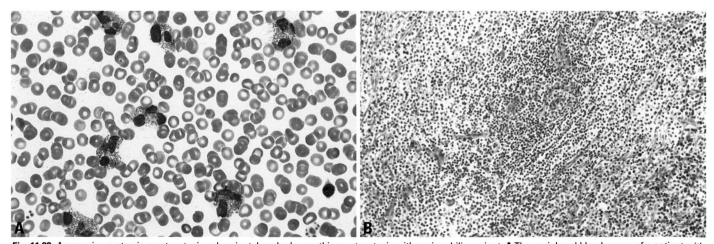

Fig. 11.23 Aggressive systemic mastocytosis subvariant, lymphadenopathic mastocytosis with eosinophilia variant. **A** The peripheral blood smear of a patient with systemic mastocytosis. The peripheral blood smear shows eosinophilia. **B** Lymph node biopsy. The lymph node is infiltrated by mast cells with a significant infiltrate by eosinophils. The patient expired of heart failure, secondary to eosinophilic infiltration and myocardial fibrosis.

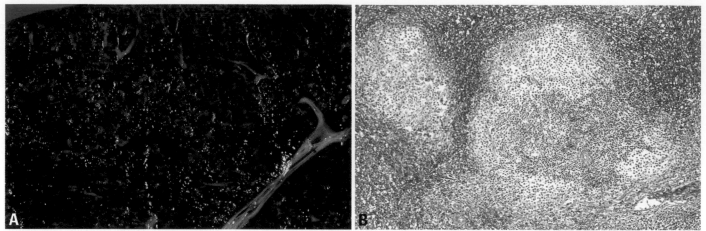

Fig. 11.24 Systemic mastocytosis, spleen. **A** Spleen from a patient with systemic mastocytosis. **B** Aggregates of mast cells may be seen in the red or white pulp, or both. In this case, mast cells are seen in a parafollicular location.

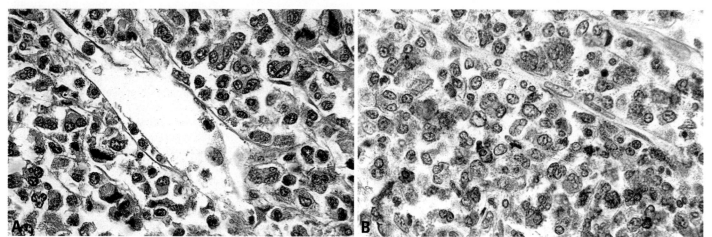

Fig. 11.25 Mast cell sarcoma. **A** This tumour is comprised of poorly differentiated neoplastic cells that show no evidence of mast cell differentiation in the H &E stained section. A Giemsa stain failed to demonstrate metachromatic granules, and α napthol ASD chloroacetate esterase reaction failed to showed positivity in the tumour cells. **B** The immunohistochemical detection of mast cell tryptase confirms the mast cell origin of the tumour.

Contributors

Dr John ANASTASI
Department of Pathology
University of Chicago Medical Center
5841 South Maryland Avenue, MC0008
Chicago, IL 60637-1470
USA
Tel. +1 773 702 6196
Fax +1 773 702 1200
anastasi@uchicago.edu

Dr James ANDERSON
Preventive & Societal Medicine
University of Nebraska Medical Center
984350 Nebraska Medical Center
Omaha, NE 68198-4350
Tel. +1 402 559 4112
USA
janderson@unmc.edu

Dr Barbara J. BAIN
Department of Haematology
St. Mary's Hospital
Praed Street
London W2 1NY
UNITED KINGDOM
Tel. +44 207 886 6806
Fax +44 207 886 6809
b.bain@ic.ac.uk

Dr Peter M. BANKS
Department of Pathology & Lab Medicine
Carolinas Medical Center
1000 Blythe Blvd.
Charlotte, NC 28203
USA
Tel. +1 704 355 2251
Fax +1 704 355 2156
drpeterbanks.com

---

* The asterisk indicates participation in the Working Group Meeting on the WHO Classification of Tumours of Haematopoietic and Lymphoid Tissues that was held in Lyon, France, Nov 8-11, 2000.

Members of the Clinical Advisory Committee are listed on page 310.

Dr John BENNETT
James P Wilmot Cancer Center, Box 704
University of Rochester Medical Center
601 Elmwood Avenue
Rochester, NY 14642
USA
Tel. +1 716 275 4915
Fax +1 716 442 0039
John_Bennett@urmc.rochester.edu

Dr Costan W. BERARD
471 Porpoise Circle
Fripp Island, SC 29920
USA
Tel. +1 803 838 5564
Fax +1 803 838 2480
cosberard@palm.net

Dr Francoise BERGER
Service d'Anatomie Pathologique
Centre Hospitalier Lyon-Sud
69495 Pierre-Benite
FRANCE
Tel. +33 4 78 86 1187
Fax +33 4 78 86 5713
francoise.berger@chu-lyon.fr

Dr Bettina BORISCH
Division of Pathologie Clinique
Hopitaux Universitaires de Geneve, CMU
1 rue Michel Servet
1211 Geneve 4
SWITZERLAND
Tel. +41 22 372 4901
Fax +41 22 372 4944
Bettina.Borisch@dim.hcuge.ch

Dr Michael J. BOROWITZ
Johns Hopkins Medical Institutions
Weinberg 2335
401 N. Broadway
Baltimore, MD 21232
USA
Tel. +1 410 614 2889
Fax +1 410 502 1493
mborowit@jhmi.edu

Dr Richard D. BRUNNING *
Department of Laboratory Medicine and Pathology
University of Minnesota Hospital
420 Delaware Street S.E., Box 609
Minneapolis, MN 55455-0385
USA
Tel. +1 612 626 5704
Fax +1 612 625 0617
brunn001@maroon.tc.umn.edu

Dr Daniel CATOVSKY
Academic Dept. of Haematology and Cytogenetics
Royal Marsden Hospital
Fulham Road
London SW3 6JJ
UNITED KINGDOM
Tel. +44 207 808 2880
Fax +44 207 351 6420
d.catovsky@icr.ac.uk

Dr John K.C. CHAN
Department of Pathology
Queen Elizabeth Hospital
Wylie Road
Kowloon
HONG KONG
Tel. +852 2958 6830
Fax +852 2385 2455
jkcchan@ha.org.hk

Dr Wing C. CHAN
Department of Pathology
University of Nebraska Medical Center
983135 Nebraska Medical Center
Omaha, NE 68198
USA
Tel. +1 402 559 7689
Fax +1 402 559 6018
jchan@unmc.edu

Dr Georges DELSOL
Laboratoire D'Anatomie Pathologique
C.H.U. Purpan
Place du Docteur Baylac
31059 Toulouse Cedex
FRANCE
Tel. +33 5 6177 7525
Fax +33 5 6177 7603
delsol.g@chu-toulouse.fr

Dr. Jacques DIEBOLD *
Serv. Central D'Anatomie et de Cytologie
Pathologiques, Hotel Dieu de Paris
1, Place du Parvis Notre Dame
75181 Paris, Cedex 04
FRANCE
Tel. +33 1 4234 8282
Fax +33 1 4234 8641
anapath.hd@htd.ap-hop-paris.fr

Dr Wieslaw T. DURA
Department of Pathology
Children's Memorial Health Center
Al Dzieci Polskich 20
04-737 Warsaw
POLAND
Tel. +48 22 815 1965
Fax +48 22 608 7231
dura@pfeso.edu.pl

Dr Blaise FAVARA
Laboratory for Persistent Viral Diseases
National Institutes of Health
1114 W. Main Street
Hamilton, MT 59840
USA
Tel. +1 406 363 5013
Fax +1 406 375 0907
Blaise@svpeds.net

Dr Alfred C. FELLER
Institut für Pathologie
Universitätsklinikum Lübeck (UKL)
Ratzeburger Allee 160
23538 Lübeck
GERMANY
Tel. +49 451 500 2705
Fax +49 451 500 3328
feller@patho.mu-luebeck.de

Dr Georges FLANDRIN *
Lab Central d'Hematologie
Hopital Necker
149 Rue de Sevres
75743 Paris Cedex 15
FRANCE
Tel. +33 1 4449 4932
Fax +33 1 4438 1620
georges.flandrin@nck.ap-hop-paris.fr

Dr Kathryn M. FOUCAR
Department of Pathology
University of New Mexico Hospital 2W
2211 Lomas Blvd., NE
Albuquerque, NM 87106
USA
Tel. +1 505 272 2201
Fax +1 505 272 2235
Kfoucar@salud.unm.edu

Dr Glauco FRIZZERA
Department of Pathology
Weill Medical College of Cornell University
525 East 68th Street
New York, NY 10021-4885
USA
Tel. +1 212 746 6401
Fax +1 212 746 8945
gfrizzer@mail.med.cornell.edu

Dr Kevin GATTER
Nuffield Dept. of Clinical Laboratory Sciences
John Radcliffe Hospital, University of Oxford
Level 4, Academic Block
Headington, Oxford OX3 9DU
UNITED KINGDOM
Tel. +44 186 522 0559
Fax +44 186 522 2916
kevin.gatter@ndcls.ox.ac.uk

Dr Thomas M. GROGAN *
Department of Pathology
University of Arizona School of Medicine
1501 N. Campbell Avenue
Tucson, AZ 85724
USA
Tel. +1 520 626 2212
Fax +1 520 626 6081
tmgrogan@email.arizona edu

Dr Nancy Lee HARRIS *
Department of Pathology, Warren 2
Massachusetts General Hospital
Fruit Street
Boston, MA 02114
USA
Tel. +1 617 726 5155
Fax +1 617 726 7474
nlharris@partners.org

Dr David R. HEAD
Department of Pathology/Lab Administration
Vanderbilt University Medical Center, 4605-TVC
1161 21st Avenue South
Nashville,TN 37232-5310
USA
Tel. +1 615 343 3867
Fax +1 615 343 8976
david.head@mcmail.vanderbilt.edu

Dr Betsy HIRSCH
Dept. of Laboratory Medicine and Pathology
University of Minnesota School of Medicine
420 Delaware St. SE
Minneapolis, MN 55455
USA
Tel. +1 612 273 4952
Fax +1 612 273 4689
hirsc003@tc.umn.edu

Dr Hans-P. HORNY
Institut für Pathologie
Universitätsklinikum Lübeck (UKL)
Ratzeburger Allee 160
23538 Lübeck
GERMANY
Tel. +49 451 500 2712
Fax +49 451 500 3328
horny@patho.mu-luebeck.de

Dr A. HUSAIN
Dept. of Pathology
Lyola University Medical Center
2160 S. 1st Ave.
Maywood, Illinois 60153
USA
Tel. +1 708 327 2614
Fax +1 708 327 2620

Dr Michele IMBERT
Service d'Hematologie-Biologique
Hopital Henri Mondor
51 Avenue du Mal de Lattre de Tassigny
94010 Creteil
FRANCE
Tel. +33 1 4981 2887
Fax +33 1 4981 2878
michele.imbert@hmn.ap-hop-paris.fr

Dr Peter G. ISAACSON
Department of Histopathology
Royal Free and University College Medical School
University College London, University Street
London WC1E 6JJ
UNITED KINGDOM
Tel. +44 20 6769 6045
Fax +44 20 7387 3674
p.isaacson@ucl.ac.uk

Dr Elaine S. JAFFE *
Laboratory of Pathology
NIH, Building 10, Room 2N-202
10 Center Drive MSC-1500
Bethesda, MD 20892-1500
USA
Tel. +1 301 496 0183
Fax +1 301 402 2415
ejaffe@mail.nih.gov

Dr Masahiro KIKUCHI
First Department of Pathology
Fukuoka University School of Medicine
7-45-1 Nanakuma, Jonan-ku
814-08 Fukuoka
JAPAN
Tel. +81 092 801 1011
Fax +81 092 861 7300
masakiku@fukuoka-u.ac.jp

Dr Daniel M. KNOWLES
Department of Pathology
Weill Medical College of Cornell University
525 East 68th Street
New York, NY 10021-4885
USA
Tel. +1 212 746 6464
Fax +1 212 746 8192
dknowles@med.cornell.edu

Dr Robert A. KYLE
Department of Hematology and Internal Medicine
Mayo Clinic
20 First Street, S.W.
Rochester, MN 55905
USA
Tel. +1 507 284 3039
Fax +1 507 266 4088
kyle.robert@mayo.edu

Dr Michelle LE BEAU
Department of Medicine
University of Chicago
5841 S. Maryland Avenue
Chicago, IL 60657
USA
Tel. +1 773 702 0795
Fax +1 773 702 3163
mmlebeau@mcis.bsd.uchicago.edu

Dr Karl LENNERT
Center of Pathology and Applied Cancer Research
University of Kiel
Niemannsweg 11
24105 Kiel
GERMANY
Tel. +49 431 597 3445
Fax +49 431 597 3426

Dr Chin Yang Li
Hilton 1020/Hematopathology
Mayo Clinic
200 First St., S.W.
Rochester, MN 55905
USA
Tel. +1 507 284 3038
Fax +1 507 284 5115
li.chinyang@mayo.edu

Dr Jack B. LONGLEY
Department of Dermatology and Pathology
College of Physicians and Surgeons of Columbia Univ.
630 W. 168th Street, VC15-207
New York, NY 10030
USA
Tel. +1 212 305 2155
Fax +1 212 927 9704
jl691@columbia.edu

Dr Risa MANN
Department of Pathology
Johns Hopkins Hospital
401 N. Broadway, Wenberg Bldg., Room 2242
Baltimore, MD 21231
USA
Tel. +1 410 614 6330
Fax +1 410 955 0115
rmann@jhmi.edu

Dr Estelle MATUTES
Academic Department of Haematology
Royal Marsden Hospital
Fulham Road
London SW3 6JJ
UNITED KINGDOM
Tel. +44 207 808 2876
Fax +44 207 351 6420
estella@icr.ac.uk

Dr Maria MEDENICA
Department of Medicine
University of Chicago
5841 S. Maryland Avenue
Chicago, IL 60657
USA
Tel. +1 773 528 0223
Fax +1 773 702 8398

Dr Junia MELO
Department of Haematology ISCM
Hammersmith Hospital
Ducane Road
London W12 0NN
UNITED KINGDOM
Tel. +44 20 8383 2167
Fax +44 20 8742 9335
j.melo@ic.ac.uk

Dr Dean D. METCALFE
Laboratory of Allergic Diseases
NIH, Building 10, Room 11C205
10 Center Drive MSC 1881
Bethesda, MD 20892 1881
USA
Tel. +1 301 496 2165
Fax +1 301 480 8384
dean_metcalfe@nih.gov

Dr Emili MONTSERRAT
Department of Hematology
Hospital Clinic, IDIBAPS, University of Barcelona
Villarroel, 170
08036 Barcelona
SPAIN
Tel. +34 93 227 5475
Fax+ 34 93 227 5475
emontse@clinic.ub.es

Dr Hans-Konrad MÜLLER-HERMELINK *
Department of Pathology
Universität Würzburg
Josef-Schneider-Str. 2
8700 Würzburg
GERMANY
Tel. +49 931 201 3776
Fax +49 931 201 3440
path062@mail.uni-wuerzburg.de

Dr Bharat N. NATHWANI
Department of Hematopathology
LA County-Univ. of Southern California Medical Ctr.
1200 North State Street #2422
Los Angeles, CA 90033
USA
Tel. +1 323 226 7064
Fax +1 323 226 7119
nathwani@usc.edu

Dr Beverly P. NELSON
Dept. of Pathology
Northwestern University Memorial Hospital
251 E. huron St., Feinberg pavilion
Chicago, IL 60611-2908
USA
Tel. +1 312 926 9045
Fax +1 312 926 0560
bpnelson@northwestern.edu

Dr Reza M. PARWARESCH
Institute of Hematopathology & Lymphnode
Registry Kiel, Christian-Albrechts-Universität
Michaelis-Str. 11
24105 Kiel
GERMANY
Tel. +49 431 597 3390
Fax +49 431 597 4052
rparwaresch@path.uni-kiel.de

Dr Marco PAULLI
Department of Pathology
IRCCS Policlinico S. Matteo and University of Pavia
Via Forlanini 14
27100 Pavia
ITALY
Tel. +39 038 252 8474
Fax +39 038 252 5866
m.paulli@smatteo.pv.it

Dr Robert V. PIERRE
Mayo Clinic
Impath, 5300 McConnell Ave.
Los Angeles, CA 90066
USA
Tel. +1 818 552 2239
Fax +1 818 242 4476
rpierre@earthlink.net

Dr Stefano PILERI
Unità di Anatomia Patologica ed Ematopatologia
Istituto di Ematologia e Oncologia Medica
Policlinico S. Orsola, Università di Bologna
Via G. Massarenti, 9
40138 Bologna, ITALY
Tel. +39 051 636 3044
Fax +39 051 39 8973
pileri@almadns.unibo.it

Dr Miguel PIRIS
Programa de Patologia Molecular
Centro Nacional de Investigaciones Oncolεgicas
Ctra. Majadahonda-Pozuelo, Km 2
28220 Majadahonda - Madrid
SPAIN
Tel. +34 915 097 055
Fax +34 915 097 054
mapiris@cnio.es

Dr Stefania PITTALUGA
Laboratory of Pathology
NIH, Building 10, Room 2N-109
10 Center Drive MSC-1500
Bethesda, MD 20892-1500
USA
Tel. +1 301 402 0297
Fax +1 301 402 2415
stefpitt@box-s.nih.gov

Dr Sibrand POPPEMA
Department of Pathology
University Hospital of Groningen
POB 30.001
9700 RB Groningen
THE NETHERLANDS
Tel. +31 50 363 2876
Fax +31 50 363 2510
s.poppema@med.rug.nl

Dr Elisabeth RALFKIAER *
Department of Pathology 5444
Rigshospitalet, University of Copenhagen
11 Frederik V's vej
2100 Copenhagen O
DENMARK
Tel. +45 3545 5346
Fax +45 3545 5346
e.ralfkiaer@rh.dk-work

Dr Martine RAPHAEL *
Service Biologique d'Hematologie
Hopital Avicenne
125 Route de Stalingrad
93009 Bobigny
FRANCE
Tel. +33 1 4895 5640
Fax +33 1 4895 5648
martine.raphael@avc.ap-hop-paris.fr

Dr Jonathan SAID
Department of Pathology and Laboratory Medicine
Center for the Health Sciences, 13-226, UCLA
10833 Le Conte Avenue
Los Angeles, CA 90095-1732
USA
Tel. +1 310 825 1149
Fax +1 310 794 4161
jsaid@mednet.ucla.edu

Dr Christian SANDER
Institut für Dermatologie
Ludwig-Maximilians-Universität
Frauenlobstr. 9-11
80337 München
GERMANY
Tel. +49 89 5160 6217
Fax +49 89 5160 6182
Christian.Sander@lrz.uni-muenchen.de

Dr Leslie H. SOBIN *
Division of Gastrointestinal Pathology
Armed Forces Institute of Pathology
Washington, DC 20306-6000
USA
Tel. +1 202 782 2880
Fax +1 202 782 9020
sobin@afip.osd.mil

Dr Harald STEIN *
Institut für Pathologie, Freie Universität Berlin
Universitätsklinikum Steglitz
Hindenburgdamm 30
12200 Berlin
GERMANY
Tel. +49 30 84 45 2295
Fax +49 30 84 45 4473
stein@medizin.fu-berlin.de

Dr Steven H. SWERDLOW *
Division of Hematopathology
UPMC- Presbyterian, Room PUH-C606
200 Lothrop Street
Pittsburgh, PA 15213
USA
Tel. +1 412 647 5191
Fax +1 412 647 4008
swerdlowsh@msx.upmc.edu

Dr Jürgen THIELE
Institute of Pathology
Universität Köln
Joseph-Stelzmann-Str. 9
D-50924 Köln
GERMANY
Tel. +49 221 478 5008
Fax +49 221 478 6360
j.thiele@uni-koeln.de

Dr Peter VALENT
Department of Internal Medicine I
University of Vienna – General Hospital
Waehringer Gürtel 18-20
1090 Wien
AUSTRIA
Tel. +43 1 40 400 6085
Fax +43 1 402 6930
peter.valent@akh-wien.ac.at

Dr Benjamin VAN CAMP
Department of Medical Oncology and Hematology
Academic Hospital-Free University of Brussels
Laarbeeklaan #101
1090 Brussels
BELGIUM
Tel. +1 322 477 6211
Fax +1 322 477 6210
Benjamin.Vancamp@az.vub.ac.be

Dr James W. VARDIMAN *
Department of Pathology
University of Chicago Medical Center
5841 South Maryland Ave., MC0008 Room TW-055
Chicago, IL 60637-1470
USA
Tel. +1 773 702 6196
Fax +1 773 702 1200
jvardima@mcis.bsd.uchicago.edu

Dr Mohammed VASEF
University of Iowa Hospital
Department of Pathology
University of Iowa Hospitals and Clinics
Iowa City, IA 52242
USA
Tel. +1 319 356 3981
Fax +1 319 384 8053
mohammad-vasef@uiowa.edu

Dr Peter VOGT
Department of Pathology
University Hospital USZ
Schmelzbergstr. 12
8091 Zürich
SWITZERLAND
Tel. +41 1 255 2524
Fax +41 1 255 4551
peter.vogt@pty.usz.ch

Dr Roger A. WARNKE
Department of Pathology
Stanford University Medical Center
300 Pasteur Drive
Stanford, CA 94305-5324
USA
Tel. +1 650 725 5167
Fax +1 650 725 6902
rwarnke@stanford.edu

Dr Dennis D. WEISENBURGER
Department of Pathology & Microbiology
University of Nebraska Medical Center
983135 Nebraska Medical Center
Omaha, NE 68198-3135
USA
Tel. +1 402 559 7688
Fax +1 402 559 6018
dweisenb@unmc.edu

Dr Lawrence M. WEISS
Division of Pathology
City of Hope National Medical Center
1500 E. Duarte Road
Duarte, CA 91010-0269
USA
Tel. +1 626 359 8111
Fax +1 626 301 8145
lweiss@coh.org

Dr Rein WILLEMZE
Department of Dermatology, B1-Q-93
Leiden University Medical Center
PO Box 9600
2300 RC Leiden
THE NETHERLANDS
Tel.+31 71 526 2421
Fax +31 71 524 8106
willemze.dermatology@lumc.nl

Dr. Wyndham H. WILSON
National Institutes of Health
Bldg. 10, Rm. 12N226
10 Center Drive
Bethesda, MD 20892
USA
Tel. +1 301 435 2415
Fax +1 301 402 2359
wilsonw@mail.nih.gov

Dr K.F. WONG
Department of Pathology
Queen Elisabeth Hospital
Wylie Road
Kowloon
HONG KONG
Tel. +85 229 586 791
Fax +85 223 852 455
kfwong@ha.org.hk

Dr Dennis H. WRIGHT
Brae House
31 Chilbolton Avenue
Winchester
Hampshire SO22 5HE
UNITED KINGDOM
Tel. +44 196 286 3778
Fax +44 196 286 9530
denniswright@totalise.co.net

Dr Kazunari YAMAGUCHI
Blood Transfusion Service
Kumamoto University School of Medicine
Honjo 1-1-1
860-8556 Kumamoto
JAPAN
Tel. +81 96 373 5811
Fax +81 96 373 5813
kyama@gpo.kumamoto-u.ac.jp

Clinical Advisory Committee

Dr James O. ARMITAGE
College of Medicine
University of Nebraska Medical Center
986545 Nebraska Medical Center
Omaha, NE 68198-3332
USA
Tel. +1 402 559 7290
Fax +1 402 559 6114
Joarmita@unmc.edu

Dr Clara D. BLOOMFIELD (co-chair)
Arthur G. James Cancer Hospital and Research
Institute
300 W. 10th Ave., Suite A455
Columbus, OH 43210
USA
Tel. +1 614 293 7518
Fax +1 614 293 7520
bloomfield-1@medctr.osu.edu

Dr Günter BRITTINGER
Department of Internal Medicine
Division of Haematology
Hufelandstr. 55
45122 Essen
GERMANY
Tel. +49 201 723 2417
Fax +49 201 723 5928
guenter.brittinger@uni-essen.de

Dr Alan K. BURNETT
Department of Hematology
College of Medicine, University of Wales
Health Park
Cardiff CF4 4XN
UNITED KINGDOM
Tel. +44 122 274 7747
Fax +44 122 274 4655
burnettak@cardiff.ac.uk

Dr Fernando CABANILLAS
Department of Lymphoma/Myeloma
M.D. Anderson Cancer Center
1515 Holcombe Boulevard, Box 429 FCC.2001
Houston, TX 77030
USA
Tel. +1 713 792 2863
Fax +1 713 794 5656
fcabanil@mdanderson.org

Dr George P. CANELLOS
Dana Farber Cancer Institute
Harvard Medical School
44 Binney Street
Boston, MA 02115
USA
Tel. +1 617 632 3470
Fax +1 617 632 3477
george_canellos@dfci.harvard.edu

Dr Franco CAVALLI
Division of Oncology
Oncology Institute of Southern Switzerland
Ospedale Regionale Bellinzona e Valli
6500 Bellinzona
SWITZERLAND
Tel. +41 91 820 8666
Fax +41 91 820 9044
oncosg@siak.ch

Dr Bertrand COIFFIER
Department of Hematology
Centre Hospitaslier Lyon-Sud
Hospices Civils de Lyon
69495 Pierre Benite
FRANCE
Tel. +33 4 7886 1194
Fax +33 4 7886 6566
bertrand.coiffier@chu-lyon.Fr

Dr Joseph CONNORS
B.C. Cancer Agency
Vancouver Clinic
600 W. 10 Avenue
Vancouver, BC V5Z 4E6
CANADA
Tel. +1 604 877 6000
Fax +1 604 877 0585
jconnors@bccancer.bc.ca

Dr Christine DE WOLF-PEETERS
Departement Morfologie en Medische Beeldvorming
Pathologische Ontleedkunde
Minderbroedersstraat 12
3000 Leuven
BELGIUM
Tel. +32 1633 6582
Fax +32 1633 6548
christiane.peeters@uz.kuleuven.ac.be

Dr Vincent T. DEVITA, jr.
Yale Cancer Center
Yale University School of Medicine
333 Cedar Street, WWW 205, PO Box 208028
New Haven, CT 06520-8028
USA
Tel. +1 203 785 4371
Fax +1 203 785 4116
vincent.devita@yale.edu

Dr Volker DIEHL
Klinik 1 für Innere Medizin
University of Köln
Joseph-Stelzmann-Str. 9
50924 Köln
GERMANY
Tel. +49 221 478 4400
Fax +49 221 478 5455
v.diehl@uni-koeln.de

Dr Elibu ESTEY
M.D. Anderson Cancer Center
1515 Holcombe Blvd.
Box 61
Houston, TX 77030
USA
Tel. +1 713 792 7544
Fax +1 713 794 4297
eestey@notes.mdacc.tmc.edu

Dr Brunangelo FALINI
Institute of Haematology
University of Perugia
Policlinico, Monteluce
06122 Perugia
ITALY
Tel. +39 075 578 3190
Fax +39 075 578 3834
faliniem@unipg.it

Dr Richard I. FISHER
Cardinal Bernardin Cancer Center
2160 S. First Ave.
Maywood, IL 60153
USA
Tel. +1 708 327 3300
Fax +1 708 327 3319
rfisher@lumc.edu

Dr Helmut GADNER
St. Anna Children's Hospital
Kinderspitalgasse 6
1090 Wien
AUSTRIA
Tel. +43 1 401 70 250
Fax +43 1 401 70 70
gadner@ccri.univie.ac.at

Dr Axel GEORGII
Institut für Pathologie
Medizinsche Hochschule Hannover
Carl-Neuberg-Str. 1
30623 Hannover
GERMANY
Tel. +49 511 532 4500
Fax +49 511 532 5799

Dr Christian GISSELBRECHT
St. Louis Hospital
1 Rue Claude Vellefaux
75010 Paris
FRANCE
Tel. +33 1 42 49 9296
Fax +33 1 42 49 9641
christian.gisselbrecht@sls.ap-hop-paris.fr

Dr John M. GOLDMAN
Department of Haematology
ICSM at Hammersmith Hospital
Du Cane Road
London W12 0NN
UNITED KINGDOM
Tel. +44 208 383 3234
Fax +44 208 742 9335
j.goldman@ic.ac.uk

Dr Wolfgang HIDDEMANN
Ludwig-Maximilians-Universität
Klinikum Grosshadern, Medizinische Klinik III
Marchioninistr. 23
37075 Göttingen
GERMANY
Tel. +49 551 39 8535
Fax +49 551 39 8587

Dr Dieter F. HOELZER
Hematology Department
Universität Frankfurt
Theodor-Stern-Kai 7
60590 Frankfurt
GERMANY
Tel. +49 696 301 5194
Fax +49 696 301 7326
hoelzer@em.uni-frankfurt.de

Dr Richard T. HOPPE
Department of Radiation Oncology
Stanford University Medical Center
Stanford, CA 94305
USA
Tel. +1 650 723 5510
Fax +1 650 498 6922
Hoppe@reyes.stanford.edu

Dr Sandra J. HORNING
Stanford University Medical Center
1000 Welch Road, Suite 202
Palo Alto, CA 94304-1808
USA
Tel. +1 650 725 6456
Fax +1 650 725 8222

Dr Philip M. KLUIN
Department of Pathology and Laboratory Medicine
Academic Hospital Groningen, Room U1-109
PO Box 30001
9700 RB Groningen
THE NETHERLANDS
Tel. +31 50 361 1766
Fax +31 50 363 2510
p.m.kluin@path.azg.nl

Dr J.C. KLUIN-NELEMANS
Deptartment of Hematology
University Hospital Groningen
PO Box 30.001
9700 RB Groningen
THE NETHERLANDS
Tel. +31 50 361 2354
Fax +31 50 360 4862
j.c.kluin.nelemans@int.azg.nl

Dr Alexandra LEVINE
USC/Norris Cancer Hospital
USC School of Medicine
1441 Eastlake Ave., Room 3468
Los Angeles CA 90033
USA
Tel. +1 323 865 3913
Fax +1 213 764 0060
hornor@hsc.usc.edu

Dr T. Andrew LISTER (co-chair)
Department of Medical Oncology
St. Bartholomew's Hospital
West Smithfield
London EC1A 7BE
UNITED KINGDOM
Tel. +44 171 601 7462
Fax +44 171 796 3979
a.lister@icrg.icnet.uk

Dr Dan L. LONGO
National Institute on Aging
Gerontology Research Center
5600 Nathan Shock Drive, Box 09
Baltimore, MD 21224-6825
USA
Tel. +1 410 558 8110
Fax +1 410 558 8137
LongoD@grc.nia.nih.gov

Dr Ian MAGRATH
International Network for Cancer Treatment and
Research, Institut Pasteur
Rue Engeland 642
B-1180 Brussels
BELGIUM
Tel. +32 2 373 9323
Fax +32 2 373 9313
imagrath@inctr.be

Dr Franco MANDELLI
Dipartmento di Biotecnologie Cellulari ed
Ematologia, Universita degli studi "La Sapienza"
Via Benevento 6
00161 Roma
ITALY
Tel. +39 685 7951
Fax +39 685 795 293
mandelli@bce.med.uniroma1.it

Dr David Y. MASON
Haematology Department
John Radcliffe Hospital
Oxford OX3 9DU
UNITED KINGDOM
Tel. +44 186 522 0356
Fax +44 186 576 3272
david.mason@ndcls.ox.ac.uk

Dr Sharon B. MURPHY
Division of Hematology/Oncology
Children's Memorial Hospital
2300 Children's Plaza, Box #30
Chicago, IL 60614
USA
Tel. +1 773 880 4562
Fax +1 773 880 3223
sbmurphy@northwestern.edu

Dr Ryuzo OHNO
Department of Medicine III
School of Medicine, Hamamatsu University
3600 Handacho
Hamammatsu 431-31
JAPAN
Tel. +81 52 762 6111
Fax +81 52 765 6948

Dr Ching-Hon PUI
St. Jude Children's Medical Center
332 N Lauderdale
Box 318
Memphis, TN 38101
USA
Tel. +1 901 495 3335
Fax +1 901 521 9005
ching-hon.pui@stjude.org

Dr John A. RADFORD
Department of Medical Oncology
Christie Hospital
Wilmslow Road, Withington
Manchester M20 4BX
UNITED KINGDOM
Tel. +44 161 446 3753
Fax +44 161 446 3109
lorraine.campbell@christie-tr.nwest.nhs.uk

Dr Kanti R. RAI
Long Island Jewish Medical Center
Division of Hematology-Oncology
Long Island Jewish Medical Center
New Hyde Park, NY 11040
USA
Tel. +1 718 470 7135
Fax. +1 718 470 0169
rai@aecom.yu.edu

Dr Saul ROSENBERG
Stanford University
Stanford University Medical Center
Room M-211
Stanford, CA 94305-5306
USA
Tel. +1 415 725 6455
Fax +1 415 725 1420
ml.sar@forsythe

Dr Jacob M. ROWE
Dept. of Hematology and Bone Marrow Trans.
Rambam Medical Center and Technion
Israel Institute of Technology
Haifa 31096
ISRAEL
Tel. +00972 4 854 2541
Fax +00972 4 854 2343
rowe@jimmy.harvard.edu

Dr Andreas H. SARRIS
Department of Lymphoma and Myeloma
M.D. Anderson Cancer Center
1515 Holcombe Boulevard, Box 429 FCC.2001
Houston, TX 77030
USA
Tel. +1 713 792 2860
Fax +1 713 794 5656
asarris@mdanderson.org

Dr Margaret A. SHIPP
Dana Farber Cancer Institute
Harvard Medical School
44 Binney Street
Boston, MA 02115
USA
Tel. +1 617 632 3874
Fax +1 617 632 4734
margaret_shipp@macmailgw.dfci.harvard.edu

Dr John E. ULTMANN †
Department of Hematology/Oncology
University of Chicago School of Medicine
Chicago
USA

Dr Cheryl WILLMAN
UNM Cancer Research Facility
2325 Camino de Salud NE
Albuquerque, NM 87131
USA
Tel. +1 505 272 5622
Fax +1 505 272 3049
cwillman@unm.edu

Dr Robert A. ZITTOUN
Department of Hematology
Hotel Dieu de Paris
1, Place du Parvis Notre Dame
75181 Paris cedex 04
FRANCE
Tel. +33 1 4234 8413
Fax +33 1 4234 8406
vekhoff-a@ap-hop-paris.fr

Dr Emanuele ZUCCA
Department of Medical Oncology
Ospedale Regionale "La Carita"
Via all'ospedale 1
6601 Locarno
SWITZERLAND
Tel. +41 91 756 7111
Fax +41 91 752 2726
oncosg.@siak.ch

Source of charts and photographs

1.

1.01	J.W. Vardiman
1.02	J.W. Vardiman
1.03	J.W. Vardiman
1.04	J.W. Vardiman
1.05 A, B	J.W. Vardiman
1.06 A, B	J.W. Vardiman
1.07 A, B	J.W. Vardiman
1.07 C	J.W. Vardiman
1.08 A-C	J.W. Vardiman
1.09 A-D	J.W. Vardiman
1.10	J.W. Vardiman
1.11 A-D	J.W. Vardiman
1.12 A-C	J.W. Vardiman
1.13 A-C	J.W. Vardiman
1.14 A-C	R.D. Brunning
1.15	J. Melo
1.16	M. Le Beau
1.17 A, B	M. LeBeau
1.18 A, B	J. Anastasi
1.19 A, B	J.W. Vardiman
1.20	J.W. Vardiman
1.21	J.W. Vardiman
1.22	B.J. Bain
1.23 A, B	J.W. Vardiman
1.24 A, B	B.J. Bain
1.25	J.W. Vardiman
1.26 A	J. Thiele
1.26 B-D	J.W. Vardiman
1.27 A	J.W. Vardiman
1.27 B-D	J. Thiele
1.28	J.W. Vardiman
1.29	J.W. Vardiman
1.30	J. Thiele
1.31	J. Thiele
1.32	J. Thiele
1.33	J. Thiele
1.34	J. Thiele
1.35	J.W. Vardiman
1.36	J.W. Vardiman
1.37	J. Thiele
1.38	J. Thiele
1.39	J. Thiele
1.40	J.W. Vardiman
1.41	J.W. Vardiman
1.42	J. Thiele
1.43	J.W. Vardiman
1.44 A, B	J.W. Vardiman
1.45	J.W. Vardiman
1.46 A, B	J.W. Vardiman
1.47 A, B	J.W. Vardiman
1.48 A, B	J.W. Vardiman
1.49	J.W. Vardiman
1.50 A, B	J. Thiele

2.

2.01 A, B	J.W. Vardiman
2.02 A, B	J.W. Vardiman
2.03 A, B	J.W. Vardiman
2.04 A, B	J.W. Vardiman
2.05 A-C	J.W. Vardiman
2.06 A, B	J.W. Vardiman
2.07 A-C	J.W. Vardiman
2.08 A-C	J.W. Vardiman
2.09	J.W. Vardiman
2.10 A, B	J.W. Vardiman
2.11 A, B	J.W. Vardiman
2.12 A, B	A. Husain
2.13 A, B	J.W. Vardiman
2.14 A-E	J.W. Vardiman

3.

3.01	R.D. Brunning
3.02	R.D. Brunning
3.03	R.D. Brunning
3.04	R.D. Brunning
3.05 A, B	R.D. Brunning
3.06	R.D. Brunning
3.07 A, B	R.D. Brunning
3.08	R.D. Brunning
3.09	R.D. Brunning
3.10	R.D. Brunning
3.11 A-C	R.D. Brunning
3.12	R.D. Brunning
3.13 A, B	R.D. Brunning
3.14	R.D. Brunning
3.15	R.D. Brunning

4.

4.01	D. Grimwade et al. {1163}
4.02 A, B	G. Flandrin
4.03	R.D. Brunning
4.04 A, B	R.D. Brunning
4.05	B. Hirsch
4.06 A, B	R.D. Brunning
4.07	R.D. Brunning
4.08 A, B	B. Hirsch
4.09	G.Flandrin
4.10 A, B	B. Hirsch
4.11 A	G. Flandrin
4.11 B	R.D. Brunning
4.12	R.D. Brunning
4.13 A, B	R.D. Brunning
4.14 A, B	R.D. Brunning
4.15	D. Grimwade et al. {1163}
4.16 A, B	R.D. Brunning
4.17	D. Grimwade et al. {1163}
4.18	R.D. Brunning
4.19	R.D. Brunning
4.20	G. Flandrin
4.21	G. Flandrin
4.22	G. Flandrin
4.23	R.D. Brunning
4.24 A-C	R.D. Brunning
4.25 A-C	G. Flandrin
4.26 A, B	R.D. Brunning
4.27 A, B	R.D. Brunning
4.28 A, B	R.D. Brunning
4.29	R.D. Brunning
4.30 A, B	G. Flandrin
4.31	R.D. Brunning
4.32 A, B	R.D. Brunning
4.33 A, B	G. Flandrin
4.34 A, B	R.D. Brunning
4.35	R.D. Brunning
4.36 A-C	R.D. Brunning
4.37	R.D. Brunning
4.38	R.D. Brunning
4.39	R.D. Brunning
4.40	G. Flandrin
4.41 A-D	R.D. Brunning
4.42	E. Matutes
4.43	R.D. Brunning

5.

5.01	R.D. Brunning
5.02	G. Flandrin
5.03 A	R.D. Brunning
5.03 B	E.S. Jaffe
5.04 A, B	E.S. Jaffe
5.05	R.D. Brunning
5.06	R.D. Brunning
5.07	R.D. Brunning
5.08 A. B	R.D. Brunning
5.09 A, B	R.D. Brunning

7.61 A	E.S. Jaffe
7.61 B, C	E. Ralfkiaer
7.62 A, B	E.S. Jaffe
7.63 A-D	E.S. Jaffe
7.64 A, B	E.S. Jaffe
7.65	J. Toro
7.66 A, B	E. Ralfkiaer
7.67 A, B	E.S. Jaffe
7.68 A, B	E. Ralfkiaer
7.69 A, B	E. Ralfkiaer
7.70	E. Ralfkiaer
7.71 A	E.S. Jaffe
7.71 B	E. Ralfkiaer
7.71 C	E.S. Jaffe
7.72	G. Delsol
7.73 A-E	G. Delsol
7.74 A	E. Ralfkiaer
7.74 B	G. Delsol
7.75 A-C	G. Delsol
7.76 A-D	G. Delsol
7.77 A-C	G. Delsol
7.78	G. Delsol
7.79	G. Delsol

8.

8.01	H. Stein
8.02	H. Stein
8.03	H. Stein
8.04	H. Stein
8.05	H. Stein
8.06	H. Stein
8.07 A, B	N.L. Harris
8.08 A, B	H. Stein
8.09 A, B	H. Stein
8.10 A, B	H. Stein
8.11	H. Stein
8.12	H. Stein
8.13	H. Stein
8.14	H. Stein
8.15 A-C	H. Stein
8.16 A-C	H. Stein
8.17 A, B	H. Stein
8.18	H. Stein
8.19 A, B	H. Stein
8.20 A, B	H. Stein
8.21 A, B	H. Stein
8.22	H. Stein
8.23 A, B	E.S. Jaffe
8.24 A, B	H. Stein
8.25	H. Stein
8.26 A-D	H. Stein
8.27 A, B	H. Stein
8.28 A, B	H. Stein
8.29 A, B	H. Stein
8.30	H. Stein

9.

9.01 A-C	E.S. Jaffe
9.02 A, B	E.S. Jaffe
9.03	E.S. Jaffe
9.04	S. Pittaluga
9.05	E.S. Jaffe

9.06 A, B	E.S. Jaffe
9.07	E.S. Jaffe
9.08	E.S. Jaffe
9.09	E.S. Jaffe
9.10 A-C	M. Raphael
9.11 A, B	M. Raphael
9.12 A, B	M. Raphael
9.13	M. Raphael
9.14 A, B	S.H. Swerdlow, B.P. Nelson
9.15 A-E	N.L. Harris
9.16 A	S.H. Swerdlow, B.P. Nelson
9.16 B-E	N.L. Harris
9.17 A, B	N.L. Harris
9.17 C	S.H. Swerdlow
9.17 D	N.L. Harris
9.18 A, B	N.L. Harris
9.19 A, B	N.L. Harris
9.20 A, B	N.L. Harris
9.21 A, B	N.L. Harris

10.

10.01	E.S. Jaffe
10.02	E.S. Jaffe
10.03	T.M. Grogan
10.04 A, B	L.M. Weiss
10.05	T.M. Grogan
10.06 A-D	T.M. Grogan
10.07 A, B	E.S. Jaffe
10.08 A, B	L.M. Weiss
10.09	L.M. Weiss
10.10 A, B	L.M. Weiss
10.11 A	T.M. Grogan
10.11 B	L.M. Weiss
10.12	L.M. Weiss
10.13	L.M. Weiss
10.14	L.M. Weiss
10.15	L.M. Weiss
10.16	L.M. Weiss
10.17 A-C	L.M. Weiss
10.18 A-D	T.M. Grogan
10.19 A-D	T.M. Grogan
10.20	E.S. Jaffe
10.21 A, B	L.M. Weiss
10.22	L.M. Weiss
10.23 A, B	L.M. Weiss
10.24	L.M. Weiss
10.25 A, B	L.M. Weiss
10.26 A, B	L.M. Weiss
10.27	L.M. Weiss
10.28	L.M. Weiss
10.29 A-D	L.M. Weiss

11.

11.01	M. Medenica
11.02	M. Medenica
11.03	R.D. Brunning
11.04	J.W. Vardiman
11.05	P. Valent
11.06	P. Valent
11.07	J.W. Vardiman
11.08	J.W. Vardiman
11.09	J.W. Vardiman

11.10	B.J. Longley
11.11	M. Medenica
11.12 A, B	B.J. Longley
11.13	B.J. Longley
11.14 A, B	B.J. Longley
11.15	J.W. Vardiman
11.16 A-C	J.W. Vardiman
11.17 A, B	J.W. Vardiman
11.18 A, B	J.W. Vardiman
11.19 A-D	J.W. Vardiman
11.20	J.W. Vardiman
11.21 A-D	J.W. Vardiman
11.22 A-C	J.W. Vardiman
11.23 A, B	R.D. Brunning
11.24 A	E.S. Jaffe
11.24 B	J.W. Vardiman
11.25 A, B	H.-P. Horny

References

1. Anon. (1969). Histopathological definition of Burkitt's tumour. *Bull World Health Organ* 40: 601-607.

2. Anon. (1981). Report on essential thrombocythemia. *Cancer Genet Cytogenet* 4: 138-142.

3. Anon. (1982). National Cancer Institute sponsored study of classifications of non-Hodgkin's lymphomas: summary and description of a working formulation for clinical usage. The Non-Hodgkin's Lymphoma Pathologic Classification Project. *Cancer* 49: 2112-2135.

4. Anon. (1988). Recommendations for a morphologic, immunologic, and cytogenetic (MIC) working classification of the primary and therapy-related myelodysplastic disorders. Report of the workshop held in Scottsdale, Arizona, USA, on February 23-25, 1987. Third MIC Cooperative Study Group. *Cancer Genet Cytogenet* 32: 1-10.

5. Anon. (1991). Chronic myelomonocytic leukemia: single entity or heterogeneous disorder? A prospective multicenter study of 100 patients. Groupe Francais de Cytogenetique Hematologique. *Cancer Genet Cytogenet* 55: 57-65.

6. Anon. (1992). Case records of the Massachusetts General Hospital. Weekly clinicopathological exercises. Case 17-1992. Repeated bouts of hematochezia in an 80-year-old hypertensive man. *N Engl J Med* 326: 1137-1146.

7. Anon. (1993). A predictive model for aggressive non-Hodgkin's lymphoma. The International Non-Hodgkin's Lymphoma Prognostic Factors Project. *N Engl J Med* 329: 987-994.

8. Anon. (1997). A clinical evaluation of the International Lymphoma Study Group classification of non-Hodgkin's lymphoma. The Non-Hodgkin's Lymphoma Classification Project. *Blood* 89: 3909-3918.

9. Anon. (1997). Primary immunodeficiency diseases. Report of a WHO scientific group. *Clin Exp Immunol* 109 Suppl 1:1-28: 1-28.

10. Anon. (1998). The value of c-kit in the diagnosis of biphenotypic acute leukemia. EGIL (European Group for the Immunological Classification of Leukaemias). *Leukemia* 12: 2038.

11. Abruzzo LV, Jaffe ES, Cotelingam JD, Whang-Peng J, Del DV, Jr., Medeiros LJ (1992). T-cell lymphoblastic lymphoma with eosinophilia associated with subsequent myeloid malignancy. *Am J Surg Pathol* 16: 236-245.

12. Abruzzo LV, Schmidt K, Weiss LM, Jaffe ES, Medeiros LJ, Sander CA, Raffeld M (1993). B-cell lymphoma after angioimmunoblastic lymphadenopathy: a case with oligoclonal gene rearrangements associated with Epstein-Barr virus. *Blood* 82: 241-246.

13. Agnello V, Chung RT, Kaplan LM (1992). A role for hepatitis C virus infection in type II cryoglobulinemia. *N Engl J Med* 327: 1490-1495.

14. Akin C, Kirshenbaum AS, Semere T, Worobec AS, Scott LM, Metcalfe DD (2000). Analysis of the surface expression of c-kit and occurrence of the c-kit Asp816Val activating mutation in T cells, B cells, and myelomonocytic cells in patients with mastocytosis. *Exp Hematol* 28: 140-147.

15. Albitar M, Freireich EJ (2000). Molecular defects in chronic myeloproliferative disorders. *Mol Med* 6: 555-567.

16. Alexander A, Anicito I, Buxbaum J (1988). Gamma heavy chain disease in man. Genomic sequence reveals two non-contiguous deletions in a single gene. *J Clin Invest* 82: 1244-1252.

17. Alexanian R (1980). Localized and indolent myeloma. *Blood* 56: 521-525.

18. Alexiou C, Kau RJ, Dietzfelbinger H, Kremer M, Spiess JC, Schratzenstaller B, Arnold W (1999). Extramedullary plasmacytoma: tumor occurrence and therapeutic concepts. *Cancer* 85: 2305-2314.

19. Alizadeh AA, Eisen MB, Davis RE, Ma C, Lossos IS, Rosenwald A, Boldrick JC, Sabet H, Tran T, Yu X, Powell JI, Yang L, Marti GE, Moore T, Hudson J, Jr., Lu L, Lewis DB, Tibshirani R, Sherlock G, Chan WC, Greiner TC, Weisenburger DD, Armitage JO, Warnke R, Staudt LM (2000). Distinct types of diffuse large B-cell lymphoma identified by gene expression profiling. *Nature* 403: 503-511.

20. Alonsozana EL, Stamberg J, Kumar D, Jaffe ES, Medeiros LJ, Frantz C, Schiffer CA, O'Connell BA, Kerman S, Stass SA, Abruzzo LV (1997). Isochromosome 7q: the primary cytogenetic abnormality in hepatosplenic gammadelta T cell lymphoma. *Leukemia* 11: 1367-1372.

21. Altman AJ, Palmer CG, Baehner RL (1974). Juvenile "chronic granulocytic" leukemia: a panmyelopathy with prominent monocytic involvement and circulating monocyte colony-forming cells. *Blood* 43: 341-350.

22. Amenomori T, Tomonaga M, Yoshida Y, Kuriyama K, Matsuo T, Jinnai I, Ichimaru M, Omiya A, Tsuji Y (1986). Cytogenetic evidence for partially committed myeloid progenitor cell origin of chronic myelomonocytic leukaemia and juvenile chronic myeloid leukaemia: both granulocyte-macrophage precursors and erythroid precursors carry identical marker chromosome. *Br J Haematol* 64: 539-546.

23. Anagnostopoulos I, Hansmann ML, Franssila K, Harris M, Harris NL, Jaffe ES, Han J, van Krieken JM, Poppema S, Marafioti T, Franklin J, Sextro M, Diehl V, Stein H (2000). European Task Force on Lymphoma project on lymphocyte predominance Hodgkin disease: histologic and immunohistologic analysis of submitted cases reveals 2 types of Hodgkin disease with a nodular growth pattern and abundant lymphocytes. *Blood* 96: 1889-1899.

24. Anagnostopoulos I, Hummel M, Finn T, Tiemann M, Korbjuhn P, Dimmler C, Gatter K, Dallenbach F, Parwaresch MR, Stein H (1992). Heterogeneous Epstein-Barr virus infection patterns in peripheral T-cell lymphoma of angioimmunoblastic lymphadenopathy type. *Blood* 80: 1804-1812.

25. Anastasi J, Feng J, Dickstein JI, Le Beau MM, Rubin CM, Larson RA, Rowley JD, Vardiman JW (1996). Lineage involvement by BCR/ABL in Ph+ lymphoblastic leukemias: chronic myelogenous leukemia presenting in lymphoid blast vs Ph+ acute lymphoblastic leukemia. *Leukemia* 10: 795-802.

26. Anastasi J, Musvee T, Roulston D, Domer PH, Larson RA, Vardiman JW (1998). Pseudo-Gaucher histiocytes identified up to 1 year after transplantation for CML are BCR/ABL-positive. *Leukemia* 12: 233-237.

27. Anderson JR, Armitage JO, Weisenburger DD (1998). Epidemiology of the non-Hodgkin's lymphomas: distributions of the major subtypes differ by geographic locations. Non-Hodgkin's Lymphoma Classification Project. *Ann Oncol* 9: 717-720.

28. Anderson JR, Vose JM, Bierman PJ, Weisenburger DD, Sanger WG, Pierson J, Bast M, Armitage JO (1993). Clinical features and prognosis of follicular large-cell lymphoma: a report from the Nebraska Lymphoma Study Group. *J Clin Oncol* 11: 218-224.

29. Anderson RE, Hoshino T, Yamamoto T (1964). Myelofibrosis with myeloid metaplasia in survivors of the atomic bomb in Hiroshima. *Ann Intern Med* 1: 1-17.

30. Anderson T, Bender RA, Fisher RI, DeVita VT, Chabner BA, Berard CW, Norton L, Young RC (1977). Combination chemotherapy in non-Hodgkin's lymphoma: results of long-term followup. *Cancer Treat Rep* 61: 1057-1066.

31. Andriko JW, Kaldjian EP, Tsokos M, Abbondanzo SL, Jaffe ES (1998). Reticulum cell neoplasms of lymph nodes: a clinico-pathologic study of 11 cases with recognition of a new subtype derived from fibroblastic reticular cells. *Am J Surg Pathol* 22: 1048-1058.

32. Anjuere F, del Hoyo GM, Martin P, Ardavin C (2000). Langerhans cells develop from a lymphoid-committed precursor. *Blood* 96: 1633-1637.

33. Annaloro C, Lambertenghi DG, Oriani A, Pozzoli E, Lambertenghi DD, Radaelli F, Faccini P (1999). Prognostic significance of bone marrow biopsy in essential thrombocythemia. *Haematologica* 84: 17-21.

34. Ansari MQ, Dawson DB, Nador R, Rutherford C, Schneider NR, Latimer MJ, Picker L, Knowles DM, McKenna RW (1996). Primary body cavity-based AIDS-related lymphomas. *Am J Clin Pathol* 105: 221-229.

35. Anwar N, Kingma DW, Bloch AR, Mourad M, Raffeld M, Franklin J, Magrath I, el Bolkainy N, Jaffe ES (1995). The investigation of Epstein-Barr viral sequences in 41 cases of Burkitt's lymphoma from Egypt: epidemiologic correlations. *Cancer* 76: 1245-1252.

36. Aoki Y, Yarchoan R, Braun J, Iwamoto A, Tosato G (2000). Viral and cellular cytokines in AIDS-related malignant lymphomatous effusions. *Blood* 96: 1599-1601.

37. Aozasa K (1990). Hashimoto's thyroiditis as a risk factor of thyroid lymphoma. *Acta Pathol Jpn* 40: 459-468.

38. Arber DA, Chang KL, Weiss LM (1999). Peripheral T-cell lymphoma with Touton-like tumor giant cells associated with HIV infection: report of two cases. *Am J Surg Pathol* 23: 519-522.

39. Arber DA, Jenkins KA (1996). Paraffin section immunophenotyping of acute leukemias in bone marrow specimens. *Am J Clin Pathol* 106: 462-468.

40. Arber DA, Weiss LM, Albujar PF, Chen YY, Jaffe ES (1993). Nasal lymphomas in Peru. High incidence of T-cell immunophenotype and Epstein-Barr virus infection. *Am J Surg Pathol* 17: 392-399.

41. Arber DA, Weiss LM, Chang KL (1998). Detection of Epstein-Barr Virus in inflammatory pseudotumor. *Semin Diagn Pathol* 15: 155-160.

42. Argatoff LH, Connors JM, Klasa RJ, Horsman DE, Gascoyne RD (1997). Mantle cell lymphoma: a clinicopathological study of 80 cases. *Blood* 89: 2067-2078.

43. Arico M, Biondi A, Pui CH (1997). Juvenile myelomonocytic leukemia. *Blood* 90: 479-488.

44. Armes JE, Angus P, Southey MC, Battaglia SE, Ross BC, Jones RM, Venter DJ (1994). Lymphoproliferative disease of donor origin arising in patients after orthotopic liver transplantation. *Cancer* 74: 2436-2441.

45. Armitage JO, Dick FR, Corder MP (1981). Diffuse histiocytic lymphoma after histologic conversion: a poor prognostic variant. *Cancer Treat Rep* 65: 413-418.

46. Armitage JO, Weisenburger DD (1998). New approach to classifying non-Hodgkin's lymphomas: clinical features of the major histologic subtypes. Non-Hodgkin's Lymphoma Classification Project. *J Clin Oncol* 16: 2780-2795.

47. Arnulf B, Copie-Bergman C, Delfau-Larue MH, Lavergne-Slove A, Bosq J, Wechsler J, Wassef M, Matuchansky C, Epardeau B, Stern M, Bagot M, Reyes F, Gaulard P (1998). Nonhepatosplenic gammadelta T-cell lymphoma: a subset of cytotoxic lymphomas with mucosal or skin localization. *Blood* 91: 1723-1731.

48. Arvanitakis L, Mesri EA, Nador RG, Said JW, Asch AS, Knowles DM, Cesarman E (1996). Establishment and characterization of a primary effusion (body cavity-based) lymphoma cell line (BC-3) harboring kaposi's sarcoma-associated herpesvirus (KSHV/HHV-8) in the absence of Epstein-Barr virus. *Blood* 88: 2648-2654.

49. Ascani S, Zinzani PL, Gherlinzoni F, Sabattini E, Briskomatis A, de Vivo A, Piccioli M, Fraternali OG, Pieri F, Goldoni A, Piccaluga PP, Zallocco D, Burnelli R, Leoncini L, Falini B, Tura S, Pileri SA (1997). Peripheral T-cell lymphomas. Clinicopathologic study of 168 cases diagnosed according to the R.E.A.L. Classification. *Ann Oncol* 8: 583-592.

50. Ascoli V, Lo CF, Artini M, Levrero M, Martelli M, Negro F (1998). Extranodal lymphomas associated with hepatitis C virus infection. *Am J Clin Pathol* 109: 600-609.

51. Ashton-Key M, Diss TC, Pan L, Du MQ, Isaacson PG (1997). Molecular analysis of T-cell clonality in ulcerative jejunitis and enteropathy-associated T-cell lymphoma. *Am J Pathol* 151: 493-498.

52. Ashton-Key M, Thorpe PA, Allen JP, Isaacson PG (1995). Follicular Hodgkin's disease. *Am J Surg Pathol* 19: 1294-1299.

53. Aucouturier P, Khamlichi AA, Touchard G, Justrabo E, Cogne M, Chauffert B, Martin F, Preud'Homme JL (1993). Brief report: heavy-chain deposition disease. *N Engl J Med* 329: 1389-1393.

54. Audouin J, Diebold J, Pallesen G (1992). Frequent expression of Epstein-Barr virus latent membrane protein-1 in tumour cells of Hodgkin's disease in HIV-positive patients. *J Pathol* 167: 381-384.

55. Aul C, Bowen DT, Yoshida Y (1998). Pathogenesis, etiology and epidemiology of myelodysplastic syndromes. *Haematologica* 83: 71-86.

56. Aul C, Gattermann N, Schneider W (1992). Age-related incidence and other epidemiological aspects of myelodysplastic syndromes. *Br J Haematol* 82: 358-367.

57. Austen KF (1992). Systemic mastocytosis. *N Engl J Med* 326: 639-640.

58. Bachman TR, Sawitzke AD, Perkins SL, Ward JH, Cannon GW (1996). Methotrexate-associated lymphoma in patients with rheumatoid arthritis: report of two cases. *Arthritis Rheum* 39: 325-329.

59. Baddoura FK, Hanson C, Chan WC (1992). Plasmacytoid monocyte proliferation associated with myeloproliferative disorders. *Cancer* 69: 1457-1467.

60. Baecklund E, Ekbom A, Sparen P, Feltelius N, Klareskog L (1998). Disease activity and risk of lymphoma in patients with rheumatoid arthritis: nested case-control study. *BMJ* 317: 180-181.

61. Baer MR, Stewart CC, Lawrence D, Arthur DC, Byrd JC, Davey FR, Schiffer CA, Bloomfield CD (1997). Expression of the neural cell adhesion molecule CD56 is associated with short remission duration and survival in acute myeloid leukemia with t(8;21)(q22;q22). *Blood* 90: 1643-1648.

62. Bagdi E, Diss TC, Munson P, Isaacson PG (1999). Mucosal intra-epithelial lymphocytes in enteropathy-associated T-cell lymphoma, ulcerative jejunitis, and refractory celiac disease constitute a neoplastic population. *Blood* 94: 260-264.

63. Bain BJ (1996). Eosinophilic leukaemias and the idiopathic hypereosinophilic syndrome. *Br J Haematol* 95: 2-9.

64. Bain BJ (1997). The haematological features of HIV infection. *Br J Haematol* 99: 1-8.

65. Bain BJ (1999). The relationship between the myelodysplastic syndromes and the myeloproliferative disorders. *Leuk Lymphoma* 34: 443-449.

66. Bakels V, Van Oostveen JW, Geerts ML, Gordijn RL, Walboomers JM, Scheffer E, Meijer CJ, Willemze R (1993). Diagnostic and prognostic significance of clonal T-cell receptor beta gene rearrangements in lymph nodes of patients with mycosis fungoides. *J Pathol* 170: 249-255.

67. Bakkus MH, Heirman C, Van R, I, Van Camp B, Thielemans K (1992). Evidence that multiple myeloma Ig heavy chain VDJ genes contain somatic mutations but show no intraclonal variation. *Blood* 80: 2326-2335.

68. Ballard HS, Hamilton LM, Marcus AJ, Illes CH (1970). A new variant of heavy-chain disease (mu-chain disease). *N Engl J Med* 282: 1060-1062.

69. Ballerini P, Gaidano G, Gong JZ, Tassi V, Saglio G, Knowles DM, Dalla-Favera R (1993). Multiple genetic lesions in acquired immunodeficiency syndrome-related non-Hodgkin's lymphoma. *Blood* 81: 166-176.

70. Banks PM, Chan J, Cleary ML, Delsol G, Wolf-Peeters C, Gatter K, Grogan TM, Harris NL, Isaacson PG, Jaffe ES (1992). Mantle cell lymphoma. A proposal for unification of morphologic, immunologic, and molecular data. *Am J Surg Pathol* 16: 637-640.

71. Baranger L, Szapiro N, Gardais J, Hillion J, Derre J, Francois S, Blanchet O, Boasson M, Berger R (1994). Translocation t(5;12)(q31-q33;p12-p13): a non-random translocation associated with a myeloid disorder with eosinophilia. *Br J Haematol* 88: 343-347.

72. Bargou RC, Emmerich F, Krappmann D, Bommert K, Mapara MY, Arnold W, Royer HD, Grinstein E, Greiner A, Scheidereit C, Dorken B (1997). Constitutive nuclear factor-kappaB-RelA activation is required for proliferation and survival of Hodgkin's disease tumor cells. *J Clin Invest* 100: 2961-2969.

73. Bargou RC, Leng C, Krappmann D, Emmerich F, Mapara MY, Bommert K, Royer HD, Scheidereit C, Dorken B (1996). High-level nuclear NF-kappa B and Oct-2 is a common feature of cultured Hodgkin/Reed-Sternberg cells. *Blood* 87: 4340-4347.

74. Barlogie B, Epstein J, Selvanayagam P, Alexanian R (1989). Plasma cell myeloma – new biological insights and advances in therapy. *Blood* 73: 865-879.

75. Barosi G (1999). Myelofibrosis with myeloid metaplasia: diagnostic definition and prognostic classification for clinical studies and treatment guidelines. *J Clin Oncol* 17: 2954-2970.

76. Bartl R, Frisch B, Burkhardt R, Fateh-Moghadam A, Mahl G, Gierster P, Sund M, Kettner G (1982). Bone marrow histology in myeloma: its importance in diagnosis, prognosis, classification and staging. *Br J Haematol* 51: 361-375.

77. Bartl R, Frisch B, Wilmanns W (1993). Potential of bone marrow biopsy in chronic myeloproliferative disorders (MPD). *Eur J Haematol* 50: 41-52.

78. Bartlett NL, Rizeq M, Dorfman RF, Halpern J, Horning SJ (1994). Follicular large-cell lymphoma: intermediate or low grade? *J Clin Oncol* 12: 1349-1357.

79. Bartram CR, de Klein A, Hagemeijer A, van Agthoven T, Geurts vK, Bootsma D, Grosveld G, Ferguson-Smith MA, Davies T, Stone M (1983). Translocation of c-abl oncogene correlates with the presence of a Philadelphia chromosome in chronic myelocytic leukaemia. *Nature* 306: 277-280.

80. Bea S, Ribas M, Hernandez JM, Bosch F, Pinyol M, Hernandez L, Garcia JL, Flores T, Gonzalez M, Lopez-Guillermo A, Piris MA, Cardesa A, Montserrat E, Miro R, Campo E (1999). Increased number of chromosomal imbalances and high-level DNA amplifications in mantle cell lymphoma are associated with blastoid variants. *Blood* 93: 4365-4374.

81. Beaty MW, Kumar S, Sorbara L, Miller K, Raffeld M, Jaffe ES (1999). A biophenotypic human herpesvirus 8 – associated primary bowel lymphoma. *Am J Surg Pathol* 23: 992-994.

82. Bekkenk MW, Geelen FA, Voorst Vader PC, Heule F, Geerts ML, van Vloten WA, Meijer CJ, Willemze R (2000). Primary and secondary cutaneous CD30(+) lymphoproliferative disorders: a report from the Dutch Cutaneous Lymphoma Group on the long-term follow-up data of 219 patients and guidelines for diagnosis and treatment. *Blood* 95: 3653-3661.

83. Belec L, Mohamed AS, Authier FJ, Hallouin MC, Soe AM, Cotigny S, Gaulard P, Gherardi RK (1999). Human herpesvirus 8 infection in patients with POEMS syndrome-associated multicentric Castleman's disease. *Blood* 93: 3643-3653.

84. Bellamy WT, Richter L, Sirjani D, Roxas C, Glinsmann-Gibson B, Frutiger Y, Grogan TM, List AF (2001). Vascular endothelial cell growth factor is an autocrine promoter of abnormal localized immature myeloid precursors and leukemia progenitor formation in myelodysplastic syndromes. *Blood* 97: 1427-1434.

85. Bellucci S, Janvier M, Tobelem G, Flandrin G, Charpak Y, Berger R, Boiron M (1986). Essential thrombocythemias. Clinical evolutionary and biological data. *Cancer* 58: 2440-2447.

86. Beltrani G, Carlesimo OA (1966). [Telangiectasia macularis eruptiva perstans with mastocytosis]. *Minerva Dermatol* 41: 436-442.

87. Ben Ayed F, Halphen M, Najjar T, Boussene H, Jaafoura H, Bouguerra A, Ben Salah N, Mourali N, Ayed K, Ben Khalifa H (1989). Treatment of alpha chain disease. Results of a prospective study in 21 Tunisian patients by the Tunisian-French intestinal Lymphoma Study Group. *Cancer* 63: 1251-1256.

88. Ben Ezra J, Bailey A, Azumi N, Delsol G, Stroup R, Sheibani K, Rappaport H (1991). Malignant histiocytosis X. A distinct clinicopathologic entity. *Cancer* 68: 1050-1060.

89. Ben Ezra J, Burke JS, Swartz WG, Brownell MD, Brynes RK, Hill LR, Nathwani BN, Oken MM, Wolf BC, Woodruff R (1989). Small lymphocytic lymphoma: a clinicopathologic analysis of 268 cases. *Blood* 73: 579-587.

90. Benharroch D, Meguerian-Bedoyan Z, Lamant L, Amin C, Brugieres L, Terrier-Lacombe MJ, Haralambieva E, Pulford K, Pileri S, Morris SW, Mason DY, Delsol G (1998). ALK-positive lymphoma: a single disease with a broad spectrum of morphology. *Blood* 91: 2076-2084.

91. Bennett JM, Catovsky D, Daniel MT, Flandrin G, Galton DA, Gralnick H, Sultan C, Cox C (1994). The chronic myeloid leukaemias: guidelines for distinguishing chronic granulocytic, atypical chronic myeloid, and chronic myelomonocytic leukaemia. Proposals by the French-American-British Cooperative Leukaemia Group. *Br J Haematol* 87: 746-754.

92. Bennett JM, Catovsky D, Daniel MT, Flandrin G, Galton DA, Gralnick HR, Sultan C (1982). Proposals for the classification of the myelodysplastic syndromes. *Br J Haematol* 51: 189-199.

93. Bennett JM, Catovsky D, Daniel MT, Flandrin G, Galton DA, Gralnick HR, Sultan C (1985). Proposed revised criteria for the classification of acute myeloid leukemia. A report of the French-American-British Cooperative Group. *Ann Intern Med* 103: 620-625.

94. Bennett JM, Catovsky D, Daniel MT, Flandrin G, Galton DA, Gralnick HR, Sultan C (1989). Proposals for the classification of chronic (mature) B and T lymphoid leukaemias. French-American-British (FAB) Cooperative Group. *J Clin Pathol* 42: 567-584.

95. Bennett MH, MacLennan KA, Easterling MJ, Vaughan HB, Jelliffe AM, Vaughan HG (1983). The prognostic significance of cellular subtypes in nodular sclerosing Hodgkin's disease: an analysis of 271 non-laparotomised cases (BNLI report no. 22). *Clin Radiol* 34: 497-501.

96. Beral V, Peterman T, Berkelman R, Jaffe H (1991). AIDS-associated non-Hodgkin lymphoma. *Lancet* 337: 805-809.

97. Berger F, Felman P, Sonet A, Salles G, Bastion Y, Bryon PA, Coiffier B (1994). Nonfollicular small B-cell lymphomas: a heterogeneous group of patients with distinct clinical features and outcome. *Blood* 83: 2829-2835.

98. Berger F, Felman P, Thieblemont C, Pradier T, Baseggio L, Bryon PA, Salles G, Callet-Bauchu E, Coiffier B (2000). Non-MALT marginal zone B-cell lymphomas: a description of clinical presentation and outcome in 124 patients. *Blood* 95: 1950-1956.

99. Bergman R (1999). How useful are T-cell receptor gene rearrangement studies as an adjunct to the histopathologic diagnosis of mycosis fungoides? *Am J Dermatopathol* 21: 498-502.

100. Berkowicz M, Rosner E, Rechavi G, Mamon Z, Neuman Y, Ben Bassat I, Ramot B (1991). Atypical chronic myelomonocytic leukemia with eosinophilia and translocation (5;12). A new association. *Cancer Genet Cytogenet* 51: 277-278.

101. Berlin NI (1975). Diagnosis and classification of the polycythemias. *Semin Hematol* 12: 339-351.

102. Bernard A, Murphy SB, Melvin S, Bowman WP, Caillaud J, Lemerle J, Boumsell L (1982). Non-T, non-B lymphomas are rare in childhood and associated with cutaneous tumor. *Blood* 59: 549-554.

103. Bernstein J, Dastugue N, Haas OA, Harbott J, Heerema NA, Huret JL, Landman-Parker J, LeBeau MM, Leonard C, Mann G, Pages MP, Perot C, Pirc-Danoewinata H, Roitzheim B, Rubin CM, Slociak M, Viguie F (2000). Nineteen cases of the t(1;22)(p13;q13) acute megakaryoblastic leukaemia of infants/children and a review of 39 cases: report from a t(1;22) study group. *Leukemia* 14: 216-218.

104. Berti E, Gianotti R, Alessi E (1988). Unusual cutaneous histiocytosis expressing an intermediate immunophenotype between Langerhans' cells and dermal macrophages. *Arch Dermatol* 124: 1250-1253.

105. Beylot-Barry M, Groppi A, Vergier B, Pulford K, Merlio JP (1998). Characterization of t(2;5) reciprocal transcripts and genomic breakpoints in CD30+ cutaneous lymphoproliferations. *Blood* 91: 4668-4676.

106. Beylot-Barry M, Vergier B, Masquelier B, Bagot M, Joly P, Souteyrand P, Vaillant L, Avril MF, Franck N, Fraitag S, Delaunay M, Laroche L, Esteve E, Courville P, Dechelotte P, Beylot C, de Mascarel A, Wechsler J, Merlio JP (1999). The Spectrum of Cutaneous Lymphomas in HIV infection: a study of 21 cases. *Am J Surg Pathol* 23: 1208-1216.

107. Bhatia KG, Gutierrez MI, Huppi K, Siwarski D, Magrath IT (1992). The pattern of p53 mutations in Burkitt's lymphoma differs from that of solid tumors. *Cancer Res* 52: 4273-4276.

108. Bilgrami S, Greenberg BR (1995). Polycythemia rubra vera. *Semin Oncol* 22: 307-326.

109. Binet JL, Auquier A, Dighiero G, Chastang C, Piguet H, Goasguen J, Vaugier G, Potron G, Colona P, Oberling F, Thomas M, Tchernia G, Jacquillat C, Boivin P, Lesty C, Duault MT, Monconduit M, Belabbes S, Gremy F (1981). A new prognostic classification of chronic lymphocytic leukemia derived from a multivariate survival analysis. *Cancer* 48: 198-206.

110. Bischof D, Pulford K, Mason DY, Morris SW (1997). Role of the nucleophosmin (NPM) portion of the non-Hodgkin's lymphoma-associated NPM-anaplastic lymphoma kinase fusion protein in oncogenesis. *Mol Cell Biol* 17: 2312-2325.

111. Bishop PC, Wilson WH, Pearson D, Janik J, Jaffe ES, Elwood PC (1999). CNS involvement in primary mediastinal large B-cell lymphoma. *J Clin Oncol* 17: 2479-2485.

112. Bizzozero OJ, Jr., Johnson KG, Ciocco A (1966). Radiation-related leukemia in Hiroshima and Nagasaki, 1946-1964. I. Distribution, incidence and appearance time. *N Engl J Med* 274: 1095-1101.

113. Blayney DW, Jaffe ES, Blattner WA, Cossman J, Robert-Guroff M, Longo DL, Bunn PA, Jr., Gallo RC (1983). The human T-cell leukemia/lymphoma virus associated with American adult T-cell leukemia/lymphoma. *Blood* 62: 401-405.

114. Bloomfield CD, Lawrence D, Byrd JC, Carroll A, Pettenati MJ, Tantravahi R, Patil SR, Davey FR, Berg DT, Schiffer CA, Arthur DC, Mayer RJ (1998). Frequency of prolonged remission duration after high-dose cytarabine intensification in acute myeloid leukemia varies by cytogenetic subtype. *Cancer Res* 58: 4173-4179.

115. Bonato M, Pittaluga S, Tierens A, Criel A, Verhoef G, Wlodarska I, Vanutysel L, Michaux L, Vandekerckhove P, Van den BH, Wolf-Peeters C (1998). Lymph node histology in typical and atypical chronic lymphocytic leukemia. *Am J Surg Pathol* 22: 49-56.

116. Bonetti F, Knowles DM, Chilosi M, Pisa R, Fiaccavento S, Rizzuto N, Zamboni G, Menestrina F, Fiore-Donati L (1985). A distinctive cutaneous malignant neoplasm expressing the Langerhans cell phenotype. Synchronous occurrence with B-chronic lymphocytic leukemia. *Cancer* 55: 2417-2425.

117. Boni R, Davis-Daneshfar A, Burg G, Fuchs D, Wood GS (1996). No detection of HTLV-I proviral DNA in lesional skin biopsies from Swiss and German patients with cutaneous T-cell lymphoma. *Br J Dermatol* 134: 282-284.

118. Borowitz MJ, Croker BP, Metzgar RS (1983). Lymphoblastic lymphoma with the phenotype of common acute lymphoblastic leukemia. *Am J Clin Pathol* 79: 387-391.

119. Borowitz MJ, Guenther KL, Shults KE, Stelzer GT (1993). Immunophenotyping of acute leukemia by flow cytometric analysis. Use of CD45 and right-angle light scatter to gate on leukemic blasts in three-color analysis. *Am J Clin Pathol* 100: 534-540.

120. Borowitz MJ, Rubnitz J, Nash M, Pullen DJ, Camitta B (1998). Surface antigen phenotype can predict TEL-AML1 rearrangement in childhood B-precursor ALL: a Pediatric Oncology Group study. *Leukemia* 12: 1764-1770.

121. Bosch F, Campo E, Jares P, Pittaluga S, Munoz J, Nayach I, Piris MA, Dewolf-Peeters C, Jaffe ES, Rozman C (1995). Increased expression of the PRAD-1/CCND1 gene in hairy cell leukaemia. *Br J Haematol* 91: 1025-1030.

122. Bosch F, Lopez-Guillermo A, Campo E, Ribera JM, Conde E, Piris MA, Vallespi T, Woessner S, Montserrat E (1998). Mantle cell lymphoma: presenting features, response to therapy, and prognostic factors. *Cancer* 82: 567-575.

123. Bosman C, Fusilli S, Bisceglia M, Musto P, Corsi A (1996). Oncocytic nonsecretory multiple myeloma. A clinicopathologic study of a case and review of the literature. *Acta Haematol* 96: 50-56.

124. Bouhnik Y, Etienney I, Nemeth J, Thevenot T, Lavergne-Slove A, Matuchansky C (2000). Very late onset small intestinal B cell lymphoma associated with primary intestinal lymphangiectasia and diffuse cutaneous warts. *Gut* 47: 296-300.

125. Boulland ML, Kanavaros P, Wechsler J, Casiraghi O, Gaulard P (1997). Cytotoxic protein expression in natural killer cell lymphomas and in alpha beta and gamma delta peripheral T-cell lymphomas. *J Pathol* 183: 432-439.

126. Boulland ML, Wechsler J, Bagot M, Pulford K, Kanavaros P, Gaulard P (2000). Primary CD30-positive cutaneous T-cell lymphomas and lymphomatoid papulosis frequently express cytotoxic proteins. *Histopathology* 36: 136-144.

127. Boultwood J, Lewis S, Wainscoat JS (1994). The 5q-syndrome. *Blood* 84: 3253-3260.

128. Bourantas K (1996). Nonsecretory multiple myeloma. *Eur J Haematol* 56: 109-111.

129. Bouroncle BA (1994). Thirty-five years in the progress of hairy cell leukemia. *Leuk Lymphoma* 14 Suppl 1:1-12: 1-12.

130. Bouroncle BA, Wiseman BK, Doan CA (1958). Leukaemic reticuloendotheliosis. *Blood* 13: 609-630.

131. Bower CP, Standen GR, Pawade J, Knechtli CJ, Kennedy CT (2000). Cutaneous presentation of steroid responsive blastoid natural killer cell lymphoma. *Br J Dermatol* 142: 1017-1020.

132. Boyd MT, Maclean N, Oscier DG (1989). Detection of retrovirus in patients with myeloproliferative disease. *Lancet* 1: 814-817.

133. Boyle MJ, Swanson CE, Turner JJ, Thompson IL, Roberts J, Penny R, Cooper DA (1990). Definition of two distinct types of AIDS-associated non-Hodgkin lymphoma. *Br J Haematol* 76: 506-512.

134. Braeuninger A, Kuppers R, Strickler JG, Wacker HH, Rajewsky K, Hansmann ML (1997). Hodgkin and Reed-Sternberg cells in lymphocyte predominant Hodgkin disease represent clonal populations of germinal center-derived tumor B cells. *Proc Natl Acad Sci U S A* 94: 9337-9342.

135. Brauninger A, Hansmann ML, Strickler JG, Dummer R, Burg G, Rajewsky K, Kuppers R (1999). Identification of common germinal-center B-cell precursors in two patients with both Hodgkin's disease and non-Hodgkin's lymphoma. *N Engl J Med* 340: 1239-1247.

136. Brecher M, Banks PM (1990). Hodgkin's disease variant of Richter's syndrome. Report of eight cases. *Am J Clin Pathol* 93: 333-339.

137. Brinkman K, van Dongen JJ, van Lom K, Groeneveld K, Misere JF, van der HC (1998). Induction of clinical remission in T-large granular lymphocyte leukemia with cyclosporin A, monitored by use of immunophenotyping with Vbeta antibodies. *Leukemia* 12: 150-154.

138. Brito-Babapulle V, Catovsky D (1991). Inversions and tandem translocations involving chromosome 14q11 and 14q32 in T-prolymphocytic leukemia and T-cell leukemias in patients with ataxia telangiectasia. *Cancer Genet Cytogenet* 55: 1-9.

139. Brito-Babapulle V, Garcia-Marco J, Maljaie SH, Hiorns L, Coignet L, Conchon M, Catovsky D (1997). The impact of molecular cytogenetics on chronic lymphoid leukaemia. *Acta Haematol* 98: 175-186.

140. Brito-Babapulle V, Maljaie SH, Matutes E, Hedges M, Yuille M, Catovsky D (1997). Relationship of T leukaemias with cerebriform nuclei to T-prolymphocytic leukaemia: a cytogenetic analysis with in situ hybridization. *Br J Haematol* 96: 724-732.

141. Brito-Babapulle V, Pittman S, Melo JV, Pomfret M, Catovsky D (1987). Cytogenetic studies on prolymphocytic leukemia. 1. B-cell prolymphocytic leukemia. *Hematol Pathol* 1: 27-33.

142. Brittinger G, Bartels H, Common H, Duhmke E, Fulle HH, Gunzer U, Gyenes T, Heinz R, Konig E, Meusers P (1984). Clinical and prognostic relevance of the Kiel classification of non-Hodgkin lymphomas results of a prospective multicenter study by the Kiel Lymphoma Study Group. *Hematol Oncol* 2: 269-306.

143. Brizard A, Huret JL, Lamotte F, Guilhot F, Benz-Lemoine E, Giraud C, Desmarest MC, Tanzer J (1989). Three cases of myelodysplastic-myeloproliferative disorder with abnormal chromatin clumping in granulocytes. *Br J Haematol* 72: 294-295.

144. Broder S, Callihan TR, Jaffe ES, DeVita VT, Strober W, Bartter FC, Waldmann TA (1981). Resolution of longstanding protein-losing enteropathy in a patient with intestinal lymphangiectasia after treatment for malignant lymphoma. *Gastroenterology* 80: 166-168.

145. Brody JP, Allen S, Schulman P, Sun T, Chan WC, Friedman HD, Teichberg S, Koduru P, Cone RW, Loughran TP, Jr. (1995). Acute agranular CD4-positive natural killer cell leukemia. Comprehensive clinicopathologic studies including virologic and in vitro culture with inducing agents. *Cancer* 75: 2474-2483.

146. Brouet JC, Sasportes M, Flandrin G, Preud'Homme JL, Seligmann M (1975). Chronic lymphocytic leukaemia of T-cell origin. Immunological and clinical evaluation in eleven patients. *Lancet* 2: 890-893.

147. Brousset P, Rochaix P, Chittal S, Rubie H, Robert A, Delsol G (1993). High incidence of Epstein-Barr virus detection in Hodgkin's disease and absence of detection in anaplastic large-cell lymphoma in children. *Histopathology* 23: 189-191.

148. Brousset P, Schlaifer D, Meggetto F, Bachmann E, Rothenberger S, Pris J, Delsol G, Knecht H (1994). Persistence of the same viral strain in early and late relapses of Epstein-Barr virus-associated Hodgkin's disease. *Blood* 84: 2447-2451.

149. Brown RS, Campbell C, Lishman SC, Spittle MF, Miller RF (1998). Plasmablastic lymphoma: a new subcategory of human immunodeficiency virus-related non-Hodgkin's lymphoma. *Clin Oncol (R Coll Radiol)* 10: 327-329.

150. Brubaker LH, Wasserman LR, Goldberg JD, Pisciotta AV, McIntyre OR, Kaplan ME, Modan B, Flannery J, Harp R (1984). Increased prevalence of polycythemia vera in parents of patients on polycythemia vera study group protocols. *Am J Hematol* 16: 367-373.

151. Brugieres L, Deley MC, Pacquement H, Meguerian-Bedoyan Z, Terrier-Lacombe MJ, Robert A, Pondarre C, Leverger G, Devalck C, Rodary C, Delsol G, Hartmann O (1998). CD30(+) anaplastic large-cell lymphoma in children: analysis of 82 patients enrolled in two consecutive studies of the French Society of Pediatric Oncology. *Blood* 92: 3591-3598.

152. Brugnoni D, Airo P, Rossi G, Bettinardi A, Simon HU, Garza L, Tosoni C, Cattaneo R, Blaser K, Tucci A (1996). A case of hypereosinophilic syndrome is associated with the expansion of a CD3-CD4+ T-cell population able to secrete large amounts of interleukin-5. *Blood* 87: 1416-1422.

153. Brunning RD, McKenna RW (1994). Mast cell disease. In: *Atlas of tumor pathology. Tumors of the bone marrow*, Atlas of tumor pathology. Tumors of the bone marrow Armed Forces Institute of Pathology: Washington, D.C.: 419-434.

154. Brunning RD, McKenna RW (1994). *Tumors of the bone marrow.* Armed Forces Institute of Pathology: Washington, D.C.

155. Brunning RD, McKenna RW, Rosai J, Parkin JL, Risdall R (1983). Systemic mastocytosis. Extracutaneous manifestations. *Am J Surg Pathol* 7: 425-438.

156. Brynes RK, Almaguer PD, Leathery KE, McCourty A, Arber DA, Medeiros LJ, Nathwani BN (1996). Numerical cytogenetic abnormalities of chromosomes 3, 7, and 12 in marginal zone B-cell lymphomas. *Mod Pathol* 9: 995-1000.

157. Buhr T, Georgii A, Choritz H (1993). Myelofibrosis in chronic myeloproliferative disorders. Incidence among subtypes according to the Hannover Classification. *Pathol Res Pract* 189: 121-132.

158. Buhr T, Georgii A, Schuppan O, Amor A, Kaloutsi V (1992). Histologic findings in bone marrow biopsies of patients with thrombocythemic cell counts. *Ann Hematol* 64: 286-291.

159. Bunn PA, Jr., Schechter GP, Jaffe E, Blayney D, Young RC, Matthews MJ, Blattner W, Broder S, Robert-Guroff M, Gallo RC (1983). Clinical course of retrovirus-associated adult T-cell lymphoma in the United States. *N Engl J Med* 309: 257-264.

160. Burke AP, Andriko JA, Virmani R (2000). Anaplastic large cell lymphoma (CD 30+), T-phenotype, in the heart of an HIV-positive man. *Cardiovasc Pathol* 9: 49-52.

161. Burkhardt R, Bartl R, Jager K, Frisch B, Kettner G, Mahl G, Sund M (1984). Chronic myeloproliferative disorders (CMPD). *Pathol Res Pract* 179: 131-186.

162. Burkitt DP (1958). A sarcoma involving the jaws in African children. Br J Surg 1958; 46: 218. *Br J Surg* 46: 218.

163. Burkitt DP (1970). General features and facial tumours. In: *Burkitt's lymphoma.*, Burkitt DP, Wright DH, eds. Livingstone: Edinburgh and London

164. Busque L, Gilliland DG, Prchal JT, Sieff CA, Weinstein HJ, Sokol JM, Belickova M, Wayne AS, Zuckerman KS, Sokol L (1995). Clonality in juvenile chronic myelogenous leukemia. *Blood* 85: 21-30.

165. Butcher EC (1990). Cellular and molecular mechanisms that direct leukocyte traffic. *Am J Pathol* 136: 3-11.

166. Buxbaum J (1992). Mechanisms of disease: monoclonal immunoglobulin deposition. Amyloidosis, light chain deposition disease, and light and heavy chain deposition disease. *Hematol Oncol Clin North Am* 6: 323-346.

167. Cabannes E, Khan G, Aillet F, Jarrett RF, Hay RT (1999). Mutations in the IkBa gene in Hodgkin's disease suggest a tumour suppressor role for IkappaBalpha. *Oncogene* 18: 3063-3070.

168. Caldwell GG, Kelley DB, Heath CW, Jr., Zack M (1984). Polycythemia vera among participants of a nuclear weapons test. *JAMA* 252: 662-664.

169. Caligaris-Cappio F (1996). B-chronic lymphocytic leukemia: a malignancy of anti-self B cells. *Blood* 87: 2615-2620.

170. Caligaris-Cappio F, Hamblin TJ (1999). B-cell chronic lymphocytic leukemia: a bird of a different feather. *J Clin Oncol* 17: 399-408.

171. Caligiuri MA, Strout MP, Gilliland DG (1997). Molecular biology of acute myeloid leukemia. *Semin Oncol* 24: 32-44.

172. Camilleri-Broet S, Davi F, Feuillard J, Seilhean D, Michiels JF, Brousset P, Epardeau B, Navratil E, Mokhtari K, Bourgeois C, Marelle L, Raphael M, Hauw JJ (1997). AIDS-related primary brain lymphomas: histopathologic and immunohistochemical study of 51 cases. The French Study Group for HIV-Associated Tumors. *Hum Pathol* 28: 367-374.

173. Campo E, Miquel R, Krenacs L, Sorbara L, Raffeld M, Jaffe ES (1999). Primary nodal marginal zone lymphomas of splenic and MALT type. *Am J Surg Pathol* 23: 59-68.

174. Campo E, Raffeld M, Jaffe ES (1999). Mantle-cell lymphoma. *Semin Hematol* 36: 115-127.

175. Canioni D, Arnulf B, Asso-Bonnet M, Raphael M, Brousse N (2000). Nasal natural killer lymphoma associated with Epstein-Barr virus in a patient infected with human immunodeficiency virus. *Arch Pathol Lab Med* (in press).

176. Canioni D, Jabado N, Macintyre E, Patey N, Emile JF, Brousse N (2001). Lymphoproliferative disorders in children with primary immunodeficiencies: immunological status may be more predictive of the outcome than other criteria. *Histopathology* 38: 146-159.

177. Carbone A (1997). The spectrum of AIDS-related lymphoproliferative disorders. *Adv Clin Path* 1: 13-19.

178. Carbone A, Gaidano G (1997). HHV-8-positive body-cavity-based lymphoma: a novel lymphoma entity. *Br J Haematol* 97: 515-522.

179. Carbone PP, Kaplan HS, Musshoff K, Smithers DW, Tubiana M (1971). Report of the Committee on Hodgkin's Disease Staging Classification. *Cancer Res* 31: 1860-1861.

180. Carbonell F, Swansbury J, Min T, Matutes E, Farahat N, Buccheri V, Morilla R, Secker-Walker L, Catovsky D (1996). Cytogenetic findings in acute biphenotypic leukaemia. *Leukemia* 10: 1283-1287.

181. Cario G, Stadt UZ, Reiter A, Welte K, Sykora KW (2000). Variant translocations in sporadic Burkitt's lymphoma detected in fresh tumour material: analysis of three cases. *Br J Haematol* 110: 537-546.

182. Carroll A, Civin C, Schneider N, Dahl G, Pappo A, Bowman P, Emami A, Gross S, Alvarado C, Phillips C (1991). The t(1;22)(p13;q13) is nonrandom and restricted to infants with acute megakaryoblastic leukemia: a Pediatric Oncology Group Study. *Blood* 78: 748-752.

183. Carroll AJ, Poon MC, Robinson NC, Crist WM (1986). Sideroblastic anemia associated with thrombocytosis and a chromosome 3 abnormality. *Cancer Genet Cytogenet* 22: 183-187.

184. Cashell AW, Buss DH (1992). The frequency and significance of megakaryocytic emperipolesis in myeloproliferative and reactive states. *Ann Hematol* 64: 273-276.

185. Castaigne S, Chomienne C, Daniel MT, Ballerini P, Berger R, Fenaux P, Degos L (1990). All-trans retinoic acid as a differentiation therapy for acute promyelocytic leukemia. I. Clinical results. *Blood* 76: 1704-1709.

186. Castro-Malaspina H, Schaison G, Passe S, Pasquier A, Berger R, Bayle-Weisgerber C, Miller D, Seligmann M, Bernard J (1984). Subacute and chronic myelomonocytic leukemia in children (juvenile CML). Clinical and hematologic observations, and identification of prognostic factors. *Cancer* 54: 675-686.

187. Cattoretti G, Chang CC, Cechova K, Zhang J, Ye BH, Falini B, Louie DC, Offit K, Chaganti RS, Dalla-Favera R (1995). BCL-6 protein is expressed in germinal-center B cells. *Blood* 86: 45-53.

188. Cattoretti G, Villa A, Vezzoni P, Giardini R, Lombardi L, Rilke F (1990). Malignant histiocytosis. A phenotypic and genotypic investigation. *Am J Pathol* 136: 1009-1019.

189. Cazals-Hatem D, Lepage E, Brice P, Ferrant A, d'Agay MF, Baumelou E, Briere J, Blanc M, Gaulard P, Biron P, Schlaifer D, Diebold J, Audouin J (1996). Primary mediastinal large B-cell lymphoma. A clinicopathologic study of 141 cases compared with 916 nonmediastinal large B-cell lymphomas, a GELA ("Groupe d'Etude des Lymphomes de l'Adulte") study. *Am J Surg Pathol* 20: 877-888.

190. Cehreli C, Undar B, Akkoc N, Onvural B, Altungoz O (1994). Coexistence of chronic neutrophilic leukemia with light chain myeloma. *Acta Haematol* 91: 32-34.

191. Cellier C, Patey N, Mauvieux L, Jabri B, Delabesse E, Cervoni JP, Burtin ML, Guy-Grand D, Bouhnik Y, Modigliani R, Barbier JP, Macintyre E, Brousse N, Cerf-Bensussan N (1998). Abnormal intestinal intraepithelial lymphocytes in refractory sprue. *Gastroenterology* 114: 471-481.

192. Cerroni L, Zochling N, Putz B, Kerl H (1997). Infection by Borrelia burgdorferi and cutaneous B-cell lymphoma. *J Cutan Pathol* 24: 457-461.

193. Cervantes F, Barosi G, Demory JL, Reilly J, Guarnone R, Dupriez B, Pereira A, Montserrat E (1998). Myelofibrosis with myeloid metaplasia in young individuals: disease characteristics, prognostic factors and identification of risk groups. *Br J Haematol* 102: 684-690.

194. Cervantes F, Lopez-Guillermo A, Bosch F, Terol MJ, Rozman C, Montserrat E (1996). An assessment of the clinicohematological criteria for the accelerated phase of chronic myeloid leukemia. *Eur J Haematol* 57: 286-291.

195. Cervantes F, Pereira A, Esteve J, Cobo F, Rozman C, Montserrat E (1998). The changing profile of idiopathic myelofibrosis: a comparison of the presenting features of patients diagnosed in two different decades. *Eur J Haematol* 60: 101-105.

196. Cervantes F, Pereira A, Esteve J, Rafel M, Cobo F, Rozman C, Montserrat E (1997). Identification of 'short-lived' and 'long-lived' patients at presentation of idiopathic myelofibrosis. *Br J Haematol* 97: 635-640.

197. Cesarman E, Chadburn A, Liu YF, Migliazza A, Dalla-Favera R, Knowles DM (1998). BCL-6 gene mutations in posttransplantation lymphoproliferative disorders predict response to therapy and clinical outcome. *Blood* 92: 2294-2302.

198. Cesarman E, Chang Y, Moore PS, Said JW, Knowles DM (1995). Kaposi's sarcoma-associated herpesvirus-like DNA sequences in AIDS-related body-cavity-based lymphomas. *N Engl J Med* 332: 1186-1191.

199. Chadburn A, Cesarman E, Liu YF, Addonizio L, Hsu D, Michler RE, Knowles DM (1995). Molecular genetic analysis demonstrates that multiple posttransplantation lymphoproliferative disorders occurring in one anatomic site in a single patient represent distinct primary lymphoid neoplasms. *Cancer* 75: 2747-2756.

200. Chadburn A, Chen JM, Hsu DT, Frizzera G, Cesarman E, Garrett TJ, Mears JG, Zangwill SD, Addonizio LJ, Michler RE, Knowles DM (1998). The morphologic and molecular genetic categories of posttransplantation lymphoproliferative disorders are clinically relevant. *Cancer* 82: 1978-1987.

201. Chadburn A, Suciu-Foca N, Cesarman E, Reed E, Michler RE, Knowles DM (1995). Post-transplantation lymphoproliferative disorders arising in solid organ transplant recipients are usually of recipient origin. *Am J Pathol* 147: 1862-1870.

202. Chan AC, Ho JW, Chiang AK, Srivastava G (1999). Phenotypic and cytotoxic characteristics of peripheral T-cell and NK-cell lymphomas in relation to Epstein-Barr virus association. *Histopathology* 34: 16-24.

203. Chan JK (1998). Natural killer cell neoplasms. *Anat Pathol* 3: 77-145: 77-145.

204. Chan JK, Buchanan R, Fletcher CD (1990). Sarcomatoid variant of anaplastic large-cell Ki-1 lymphoma. *Am J Surg Pathol* 14: 983-988.

205. Chan JK, Chan JK (1997). Proliferative lesions of follicular dendritic cells: An overview, including a detailed account of follicular dendritic cell sarcoma, a neoplasm with many faces and uncommon etiologic associations. *Adv Anat Pathol* 4: 387-411.

206. Chan JK, Fletcher CD, Nayler SJ, Cooper K (1997). Follicular dendritic cell sarcoma. Clinicopathologic analysis of 17 cases suggesting a malignant potential higher than currently recognized. *Cancer* 79: 294-313.

207. Chan JK, Ng CS, Lau WH, Lo ST (1987). Most nasal/nasopharyngeal lymphomas are peripheral T-cell neoplasms. *Am J Surg Pathol* 11: 418-429.

208. Chan JK, Sin VC, Wong KF, Ng CS, Tsang WY, Chan CH, Cheung MM, Lau WH (1997). Nonnasal lymphoma expressing the natural killer cell marker CD56: a clinicopathologic study of 49 cases of an uncommon aggressive neoplasm. *Blood* 89: 4501-4513.

209. Chan JK, Tsang WY, Ng CS (1994). Follicular dendritic cell tumor and vascular neoplasm complicating hyaline-vascular Castleman's disease. *Am J Surg Pathol* 18: 517-525.

210. Chan JK, Tsang WY, Ng CS (1996). Clarification of CD3 immunoreactivity in nasal T/natural killer cell lymphomas: the neoplastic cells are often CD3 epsilon+. *Blood* 87: 839-841.

211. Chan JK, Tsang WY, Ng CS, Tang SK, Yu HC, Lee AW (1994). Follicular dendritic cell tumors of the oral cavity. *Am J Surg Pathol* 18: 148-157.

212. Chan JK, Yip TT, Tsang WY, Ng CS, Lau WH, Poon YF, Wong CC, Ma VW (1994). Detection of Epstein-Barr viral RNA in malignant lymphomas of the upper aerodigestive tract. *Am J Surg Pathol* 18: 938-946.

213. Chan WC, Gu LB, Masih A, Nicholson J, Vogler WR, Yu G, Nasr S (1992). Large granular lymphocyte proliferation with the natural killer-cell phenotype. *Am J Clin Pathol* 97: 353-358.

214. Chan WC, Link S, Mawle A, Check I, Brynes RK, Winton EF (1986). Heterogeneity of large granular lymphocyte proliferations: delineation of two major subtypes. *Blood* 68: 1142-1153.

215. Chan WC, Zaatari G (1986). Lymph node interdigitating reticulum cell sarcoma. *Am J Clin Pathol* 85: 739-744.

216. Chang A, Zic JA, Boyd AS (1998). Intravascular large cell lymphoma: a patient with asymptomatic purpuric patches and a chronic clinical course. *J Am Acad Dermatol* 39: 318-321.

217. Charrette EE, Mariano AV, Laforet EG (1966). Solitary mast cell "tumor" of lung. Its place in the spectrum of mast cell disease. *Arch Intern Med* 118: 358-362.

218. Chen SJ, Zelent A, Tong JH, Yu HQ, Wang ZY, Derre J, Berger R, Waxman S, Chen Z (1993). Rearrangements of the retinoic acid receptor alpha and promyelocytic leukemia zinc finger genes resulting from t(11;17)(q23;q21) in a patient with acute promyelocytic leukemia. *J Clin Invest* 91: 2260-2267.

219. Chesi M, Bergsagel PL, Brents LA, Smith CM, Gerhard DS, Kuehl WM (1996). Dysregulation of cyclin D1 by translocation into an IgH gamma switch region in two multiple myeloma cell lines. *Blood* 88: 674-681.

220. Cheson BD, Cassileth PA, Head DR, Schiffer CA, Bennett JM, Bloomfield CD, Brunning R, Gale RP, Grever MR, Keating MJ (1990). Report of the National Cancer Institute-sponsored workshop on definitions of diagnosis and response in acute myeloid leukemia. *J Clin Oncol* 8: 813-819.

221. Cheuk W, Hill RW, Bacchi C, Dias MA, Chan JK (2000). Hypocellular anaplastic large cell lymphoma mimicking inflammatory lesions of lymph nodes. *Am J Surg Pathol* 24: 1537-1543.

222. Cheung MM, Chan JK, Lau WH, Foo W, Chan PT, Ng CS, Ngan RK (1998). Primary non-Hodgkin's lymphoma of the nose and nasopharynx: clinical features, tumor immunophenotype, and treatment outcome in 113 patients. *J Clin Oncol* 16: 70-77.

223. Chittal SM, Brousset P, Voigt JJ, Delsol G (1991). Large B-cell lymphoma rich in T-cells and simulating Hodgkin's disease. *Histopathology* 19: 211-220.

224. Chittal SM, Caveriviere P, Schwarting R, Gerdes J, al Saati T, Rigal-Huguet F, Stein H, Delsol G (1988). Monoclonal antibodies in the diagnosis of Hodgkin's disease. The search for a rational panel. *Am J Surg Pathol* 12: 9-21.

225. Chott A, Haedicke W, Mosberger I, Fodinger M, Winkler K, Mannhalter C, Muller-Hermelink HK (1998). Most CD56+ intestinal lymphomas are CD8+CD5-T-cell lymphomas of monomorphic small to medium size histology. *Am J Pathol* 153: 1483-1490.

226. Chott A, Vesely M, Simonitsch I, Mosberger I, Hanak H (1999). Classification of intestinal T-cell neoplasms and their differential diagnosis. *Am J Clin Pathol* 111: S68-S74.

227. Chott A, Vonderheid EC, Olbricht S, Miao NN, Balk SP, Kadin ME (1996). The dominant T cell clone is present in multiple regressing skin lesions and associated T cell lymphomas of patients with lymphomatoid papulosis. *J Invest Dermatol* 106: 696-700.

228. Chucrallah AE, Crow MK, Rice LE, Rajagopalan S, Hudnall SD (1994). Multiple myeloma after cardiac transplantation: an unusual form of posttransplant lymphoproliferative disorder. *Hum Pathol* 25: 541-545.

229. Chusid MJ, Dale DC, West BC, Wolff SM (1975). The hypereosinophilic syndrome: analysis of fourteen cases with review of the literature. *Medicine (Baltimore)* 54: 1-27.

230. Cleary ML, Meeker TC, Levy S, Lee E, Trela M, Sklar J, Levy R (1986). Clustering of extensive somatic mutations in the variable region of an immunoglobulin heavy chain gene from a human B cell lymphoma. *Cell* 44: 97-106.

231. Cleary ML, Nalesnik MA, Shearer WT, Sklar J (1988). Clonal analysis of transplant-associated lymphoproliferations based on the structure of the genomic termini of the Epstein-Barr virus. *Blood* 72: 349-352.

232. Cleary ML, Warnke R, Sklar J (1984). Monoclonality of lymphoproliferative lesions in cardiac-transplant recipients. Clonal analysis based on immunoglobulin-gene rearrangements. *N Engl J Med* 310: 477-482.

233. Cobo F, Hernandez S, Hernandez L, Pinyol M, Bosch F, Esteve J, Lopez-Guillermo A, Palacin A, Raffeld M, Montserrat E, Jaffe ES, Campo E (1999). Expression of potentially oncogenic HHV-8 genes in an EBV-negative primary effusion lymphoma occurring in an HIV-seronegative patient. *J Pathol* 189: 288-293.

234. Cogswell PC, Morgan R, Dunn M, Neubauer A, Nelson P, Poland-Johnston NK, Sandberg AA, Liu E (1989). Mutations of the ras protooncogenes in chronic myelogenous leukemia: a high frequency of ras mutations in bcr/abl rearrangement-negative chronic myelogenous leukemia. *Blood* 74: 2629-2633.

235. Cohen LF, Balow JE, Magrath IT, Poplack DG, Ziegler JL (1980). Acute tumor lysis syndrome. A review of 37 patients with Burkitt's lymphoma. *Am J Med* 68: 486-491.

236. Colby TV, Burke JS, Hoppe RT (1981). Lymph node biopsy in mycosis fungoides. *Cancer* 47: 351-359.

237. Colby TV, Hoppe RT, Warnke RA (1982). Hodgkin's disease: a clinicopathologic study of 659 cases. *Cancer* 49: 1848-1858.

238. Coles FB, Cartun RW, Pastuszak WT (1988). Hodgkin's disease, lymphocyte-predominant type: immunoreactivity with B-cell antibodies. *Mod Pathol* 1: 274-278.

239. Colombi M, Radaelli F, Zocchi L, Maiolo AT (1991). Thrombotic and hemorrhagic complications in essential thrombocythemia. A retrospective study of 103 patients. *Cancer* 67: 2926-2930.

240. Colwill R, Dube I, Scott JG, Bailey D, Deharven E, Carstairs K, Pantalony D (1990). Isochromosome 7q as the sole abnormality in an unusual case of T-cell lineage malignancy. *Hematol Pathol* 4: 53-58.

241. Cooke CB, Krenacs L, Stetler-Stevenson M, Greiner TC, Raffeld M, Kingma DW, Abruzzo L, Frantz C, Kaviani M, Jaffe ES (1996). Hepatosplenic T-cell lymphoma: a distinct clinicopathologic entity of cytotoxic gamma delta T-cell origin. *Blood* 88: 4265-4274.

242. Copie-Bergman C, Gaulard P, Maouche-Chretien L, Briere J, Haioun C, Alonso MA, Romeo PH, Leroy K (1999). The MAL gene is expressed in primary mediastinal large B-cell lymphoma. *Blood* 94: 3567-3575.

243. Copie-Bergman C, Niedobitek G, Mangham DC, Selves J, Baloch K, Diss TC, Knowles DN, Delsol G, Isaacson PG (1997). Epstein-Barr virus in B-cell lymphomas associated with chronic suppurative inflammation. *J Pathol* 183: 287-292.

244. Copie-Bergman C, Wotherspoon AC, Norton AJ, Diss TC, Isaacson PG (1998). True histiocytic lymphoma: a morphologic, immunohistochemical, and molecular genetic study of 13 cases. *Am J Surg Pathol* 22: 1386-1392.

245. Corbellino M, Pizzuto M, Bestetti G, Corsico L, Piazza M, Pigozzi B, Galli M, Baldini L, Neri A, Parravicini C (1999). Absence of Kaposi's sarcoma-associated herpesvirus DNA sequences in multiple myeloma. *Blood* 93: 1110-1111.

246. Corcoran MM, Mould SJ, Orchard JA, Ibbotson RE, Chapman RM, Boright AP, Platt C, Tsui LC, Scherer SW, Oscier DG (1999). Dysregulation of cyclin dependent kinase 6 expression in splenic marginal zone lymphoma through chromosome 7q translocations. *Oncogene* 18: 6271-6277.

247. Cordone I, Masi S, Mauro FR, Soddu S, Morsilli O, Valentini T, Vegna ML, Guglielmi C, Mancini F, Giuliacci S, Sacchi A, Mandelli F, Foa R (1998). p53 expression in B-cell chronic lymphocytic leukemia: a marker of disease progression and poor prognosis. *Blood* 91: 4342-4349.

248. Corey SJ, Locker J, Oliveri DR, Shekhter-Levin S, Redner RL, Penchansky L, Gollin SM (1994). A non-classical translocation involving 17q12 (retinoic acid receptor alpha) in acute promyelocytic leukemia (APML) with atypical features. *Leukemia* 8: 1350-1353.

249. Correa PN, Eskinazi D, Axelrad AA (1994). Circulating erythroid progenitors in polycythemia vera are hypersensitive to insulin-like growth factor-1 in vitro: studies in an improved serum-free medium. *Blood* 83: 99-112.

250. Corso A, Lazzarino M, Morra E, Merante S, Astori C, Bernasconi P, Boni M, Bernasconi C (1995). Chronic myelogenous leukemia and exposure to ionizing radiation – a retrospective study of 443 patients. *Ann Hematol* 70: 79-82.

251. Cortes JE, Talpaz M, Kantarjian H (1996). Chronic myelogenous leukemia: a review. *Am J Med* 100: 555-570.

252. Costello R, Sainty D, Lafage-Pochitaloff M, Gabert J (1997). Clinical and biological aspects of Philadelphia-negative/BCR-negative chronic myeloid leukemia. *Leuk Lymphoma* 25: 225-232.

253. Cotelingam JD, Witebsky FG, Hsu SM, Blaese RM, Jaffe ES (1985). Malignant lymphoma in patients with the Wiskott-Aldrich syndrome. *Cancer Invest* 3: 515-522.

254. Criel A, Michaux L, Wolf-Peeters C (1999). The concept of typical and atypical chronic lymphocytic leukaemia. *Leuk Lymphoma* 33: 33-45.

255. Cuadra-Garcia I, Proulx GM, Wu CL, Wang CC, Pilch BZ, Harris NL, Ferry JA (1999). Sinonasal lymphoma: a clinicopathologic analysis of 58 cases from the Massachusetts General Hospital. *Am J Surg Pathol* 23: 1356-1369.

256. Cudennec CA, Johnson GR (1981). Presence of multipotential hemopoietic cells in teratocarcinoma cultures. *J Embryol Exp Morphol* 61:51-9: 51-59.

257. Cuneo A, Bigoni R, Rigolin GM, Roberti MG, Bardi A, Piva N, Milani R, Bullrich F, Veronese ML, Croce C, Birg F, Dohner H, Hagemeijer A, Castoldi G (1999). Cytogenetic profile of lymphoma of follicle mantle lineage: correlation with clinicobiologic features. *Blood* 93: 1372-1380.

258. Curtis RE, Travis LB, Rowlings PA, Socie G, Kingma DW, Banks PM, Jaffe ES, Sale GE, Horowitz MM, Witherspoon RP, Shriner DA, Weisdorf DJ, Kolb HJ, Sullivan KM, Sobocinski KA, Gale RP, Hoover RN, Fraumeni JF, Jr., Deeg HJ (1999). Risk of lymphoproliferative disorders after bone marrow transplantation: a multi-institutional study. *Blood* 94: 2208-2216.

259. Czuczman MS, Dodge RK, Stewart CC, Frankel SR, Davey FR, Powell BL, Szatrowski TP, Schiffer CA, Larson RA, Bloomfield CD (1999). Value of immunophenotype in intensively treated adult acute lymphoblastic leukemia: cancer and leukemia Group B study 8364. *Blood* 93: 3931-3939.

260. d'Amore F, Johansen P, Houmand A, Weisenburger DD, Mortensen LS (1996). Epstein-Barr virus genome in non-Hodgkin's lymphomas occurring in immunocompetent patients: highest prevalence in nonlymphoblastic T-cell lymphoma and correlation with a poor prognosis. Danish Lymphoma Study Group, LYFO. *Blood* 87: 1045-1055.

261. Dallenbach FE, Stein H (1989). Expression of T-cell-receptor beta chain in Reed-Sternberg cells. *Lancet* 2: 828-830.

262. Dalton WS, Grogan TM, Meltzer PS, Scheper RJ, Durie BG, Taylor CW, Miller TP, Salmon SE (1989). Drug-resistance in multiple myeloma and non-Hodgkin's lymphoma: detection of P-glycoprotein and potential circumvention by addition of verapamil to chemotherapy. *J Clin Oncol* 7: 415-424.

263. Damle RN, Wasil T, Fais F, Ghiotto F, Valeto A, Allen SL, Buchbinder A, Budman D, Dittmar K, Kolitz J, Lichtman SM, Schulman P, Vinciguerra VP, Rai KR, Ferrarini M, Chiorazzi N (1999). Ig V gene mutation status and CD38 expression as novel prognostic indicators in chronic lymphocytic leukemia. *Blood* 94: 1840-1847.

264. Danish EH, Rasch CA, Harris JW (1980). Polycythemia vera in childhood: case report and review of the literature. *Am J Hematol* 9: 421-428.

265. Davi F, Delecluse HJ, Guiet P, Gabarre J, Fayon A, Gentilhomme O, Felman P, Bayle C, Berger F, Audouin J, Bryon PA, Diebold J, Raphael M (1998). Burkitt-like lymphomas in AIDS patients: characterization within a series of 103 human immunodeficiency virus-associated non-Hodgkin's lymphomas. Burkitt's Lymphoma Study Group. *J Clin Oncol* 16: 3788-3795.

266. Davis RE, Dorfman RF, Warnke RA (1990). Primary large-cell lymphoma of the thymus: a diffuse B-cell neoplasm presenting as primary mediastinal lymphoma. *Hum Pathol* 21: 1262-1268.

267. Davis TH, Morton CC, Miller-Cassman R, Balk SP, Kadin ME (1992). Hodgkin's disease, lymphomatoid papulosis, and cutaneous T-cell lymphoma derived from a common T-cell clone. *N Engl J Med* 326: 1115-1122.

268. De Boer CJ, Schuuring E, Dreef E, Peters G, Bartek J, Kluin PM, Van Krieken JH (1995). Cyclin D1 protein analysis in the diagnosis of mantle cell lymphoma. *Blood* 86: 2715-2723.

269. De Boer CJ, Van Krieken JH, Kluin-Nelemans HC, Kluin PM, Schuuring E (1995). Cyclin D1 messenger RNA overexpression as a marker for mantle cell lymphoma. *Oncogene* 10: 1833-1840.

270. de Graaf JH, Tamminga RY, Dam-Meiring A, Kamps WA, Timens W (1996). The presence of cytokines in Langerhans' cell histiocytosis. *J Pathol* 180: 400-406.

271. De Jong D, Voetdijk BM, Beverstock GC, van Ommen GJ, Willemze R, Kluin PM (1988). Activation of the c-myc oncogene in a precursor-B-cell blast crisis of follicular lymphoma, presenting as composite lymphoma. *N Engl J Med* 318: 1373-1378.

272. de The H, Chomienne C, Lanotte M, Degos L, Dejean A (1990). The t(15;17) translocation of acute promyelocytic leukaemia fuses the retinoic acid receptor alpha gene to a novel transcribed locus. *Nature* 347: 558-561.

273. De Vita S, Sacco C, Sansonno D, Gloghini A, Dammacco F, Crovatto M, Santini G, Dolcetti R, Boiocchi M, Carbone A, Zagonel V (1997). Characterization of overt B-cell lymphomas in patients with hepatitis C virus infection. *Blood* 90: 776-782.

274. De Zen A, Orfao A, Cazzaniga G, Masiero L, Cocito MG, Spinelli M, Rivolta A, Biondi A, Zanesco L, Basso G (2000). Quantitative multiparametric immunophenotyping in acute lymphoblasticleukemia; correlation with specific genotype: I ETV6/AML1 ALL identification. *Leukemia* (in press).

275. Dearden CE, Matutes E, Hilditch BL, Swansbury GJ, Catovsky D (1999). Long-term follow-up of patients with hairy cell leukaemia after treatment with pentostatin or cladribine. *Br J Haematol* 106: 515-519.

276. DeCoteau JF, Butmarc JR, Kinney MC, Kadin ME (1996). The t(2;5) chromosomal translocation is not a common feature of primary cutaneous CD30+ lymphoproliferative disorders: comparison with anaplastic large-cell lymphoma of nodal origin. *Blood* 87: 3437-3441.

277. Dekmezian R, Kantarjian HM, Keating MJ, Talpaz M, McCredie KB, Freireich EJ (1987). The relevance of reticulin stain-measured fibrosis at diagnosis in chronic myelogenous leukemia. *Cancer* 59: 1739-1743.

278. Delabie J, Vandenberghe E, Kennes C, Verhoef G, Foschini MP, Stul M, Cassiman JJ, Wolf-Peeters C (1992). Histiocyte-rich B-cell lymphoma. A distinct clinicopathologic entity possibly related to lymphocyte predominant Hodgkin's disease, paragranuloma subtype. *Am J Surg Pathol* 16: 37-48.

279. Delecluse HJ, Anagnostopoulos I, Dallenbach F, Hummel M, Marafioti T, Schneider U, Huhn D, Schmidt-Westhausen A, Reichart PA, Gross U, Stein H (1997). Plasmablastic lymphomas of the oral cavity: a new entity associated with the human immunodeficiency virus infection. *Blood* 89: 1413-1420.

280. Delecluse HJ, Hummel M, Marafioti T, Anagnostopoulos I, Stein H (1999). Common and HIV-related diffuse large B-cell lymphomas differ in their immunoglobulin gene mutation pattern. *J Pathol* 188: 133-138.

281. Delsol G, al Saati T, Gatter KC, Gerdes J, Schwarting R, Caveriviere P, Rigal-Huguet F, Robert A, Stein H, Mason DY (1988). Coexpression of epithelial membrane antigen (EMA), Ki-1, and interleukin-2 receptor by anaplastic large cell lymphomas. Diagnostic value in so-called malignant histiocytosis. *Am J Pathol* 130: 59-70.

282. Delsol G, Blancher A, al Saati T, Ralfkiaer E, Lauritzen A, Bruigeres L, Brousset P, Rigal-Huguet F, Mazerolles C, Robert A (1991). Antibody BNH9 detects red blood cell-related antigens on anaplastic large cell (CD30+) lymphomas. *Br J Cancer* 64: 321-326.

283. Delsol G, Lamant L, Mariame B, Pulford K, Dastugue N, Brousset P, Rigal-Huguet F, al Saati T, Cerretti DP, Morris SW, Mason DY (1997). A new subtype of large B-cell lymphoma expressing the ALK kinase and lacking the 2; 5 translocation. *Blood* 89: 1483-1490.

284. Delves PJ, Roitt IM (2000). The immune system. First of two parts. *N Engl J Med* 343: 37-49.

285. Delves PJ, Roitt IM (2000). The immune system. Second of two parts. *N Engl J Med* 343: 108-117.

286. deMent SH (1990). Association between mediastinal germ cell tumors and hematologic malignancies: an update. *Hum Pathol* 21: 699-703.

287. DePond W, Said JW, Tasaka T, de Vos S, Kahn D, Cesarman E, Knowles DM, Koeffler HP (1997). Kaposi's sarcoma-associated herpesvirus and human herpesvirus 8 (KSHV/HHV8)-associated lymphoma of the bowel. Report of two cases in HIV-positive men with secondary effusion lymphomas. *Am J Surg Pathol* 21: 719-724.

288. Derderian PM, Kantarjian HM, Talpaz M, O'Brien S, Cork A, Estey E, Pierce S, Keating M (1993). Chronic myelogenous leukemia in the lymphoid blastic phase: characteristics, treatment response, and prognosis. *Am J Med* 94: 69-74.

289. Derringer GA, Thompson LD, Frommelt RA, Bijwaard KE, Heffess CS, Abbondanzo SL (2000). Malignant lymphoma of the thyroid gland: a clinicopathologic study of 108 cases. *Am J Surg Pathol* 24: 623-639.

290. Devesa SS, Silverman DT, Young JL, Jr., Pollack ES, Brown CC, Horm JW, Percy CL, Myers MH, McKay FW, Fraumeni JF, Jr. (1987). Cancer incidence and mortality trends among whites in the United States, 1947-84. *J Natl Cancer Inst* 79: 701-770.

291. DeVita VT, Simon RM, Hubbard SM, Young RC, Berard CW, Moxley JH, Frei E, Carbone PP, Canellos GP (1980). Curability of advanced Hodgkin's disease with chemotherapy. Long-term follow-up of MOPP-treated patients at the National Cancer Institute. *Ann Intern Med* 92: 587-595.

292. Dewald GW, Davis MP, Pierre RV, O'Fallon JR, Hoagland HC (1985). Clinical characteristics and prognosis of 50 patients with a myeloproliferative syndrome and deletion of part of the long arm of chromosome 5. *Blood* 66: 189-197.

293. Dewald GW, Kyle RA, Hicks GA, Greipp PR (1985). The clinical significance of cytogenetic studies in 100 patients with multiple myeloma, plasma cell leukemia, or amyloidosis. *Blood* 66: 380-390.

294. Dewald GW, Wright PI (1995). Chromosome abnormalities in the myeloproliferative disorders. *Semin Oncol* 22: 341-354.

295. Di Donato C, Croci G, Lazzari S, Scarduelli L, Vignoli R, Buia M, Tramaloni C, Maccari S, Plancher AC (1986). Chronic neutrophilic leukemia: description of a new case with karyotypic abnormalities. *Am J Clin Pathol* 85: 369-371.

296. Diamandidou E, Colome-Grimmer M, Fayad L, Duvic M, Kurzrock R (1998). Transformation of mycosis fungoides/ Sezary syndrome: clinical characteristics and prognosis. *Blood* 92: 1150-1159.

297. Diamandidou E, Colome M, Fayad L, Duvic M, Kurzrock R (1999). Prognostic factor analysis in mycosis fungoides/ Sezary syndrome. *J Am Acad Dermatol* 40: 914-924.

298. Dickstein JI, Vardiman JW (1995). Hematopathologic findings in the myeloproliferative disorders. *Semin Oncol* 22: 355-373.

299. Diehl V, Franklin J, Sextro M, Mauch P (1999). Clinical presentation and treatment of Lymphocyte Predominance Hodgkin's Disease. In: *Hodgkin's Disease*, Mauch P, Armitage JO, Diehl V, eds. Lippincott Williams & Wilkins: Philadelphia, 563.

300. Diehl V, Sextro M, Franklin J, Hansmann ML, Harris N, Jaffe E, Poppema S, Harris M, Franssila K, van Krieken J, Marafioti T, Anagnostopoulos I, Stein H (1999). Clinical presentation, course, and prognostic factors in lymphocyte-predominant Hodgkin's disease and lymphocyte-rich classical Hodgkin's disease: report from the European Task Force on Lymphoma Project on Lymphocyte-Predominant Hodgkin's Disease. *J Clin Oncol* 17: 776-783.

301. Dierlamm J, Baens M, Wlodarska I, Stefanova-Ouzounova M, Hernandez JM, Hossfeld DK, Wolf-Peeters C, Hagemeijer A, Van den BH, Marynen P (1999). The apoptosis inhibitor gene API2 and a novel 18q gene, MLT, are recurrently rearranged in the t(11;18)(q21;q21) p6ssociated with mucosa-associated lymphoid tissue lymphomas. *Blood* 93: 3601-3609.

302. Dierlamm J, Wlodarska I, Michaux L, Stefanova M, Hinz K, Van den BH, Hagemeijer A, Hossfeld DK (2000). Genetic abnormalities in marginal zone B-cell lymphoma. *Hematol Oncol* 18: 1-13.

303. DiGiuseppe JA, Louie DC, Williams JE, Miller DT, Griffin CA, Mann RB, Borowitz MJ (1997). Blastic natural killer cell leukemia/lymphoma: a clinicopathologic study. *Am J Surg Pathol* 21: 1223-1230.

304. DiGiuseppe JA, Nelson WG, Seifter EJ, Boitnott JK, Mann RB (1994). Intravascular lymphomatosis: a clinicopathologic study of 10 cases and assessment of response to chemotherapy. *J Clin Oncol* 12: 2573-2579.

305. Dimopoulos MA, Panayiotidis P, Moulopoulos LA, Sfikakis P, Dalakas M (2000). Waldenstrom's macroglobulinemia: clinical features, complications, and management. *J Clin Oncol* 18: 214-226.

306. Divine M, Casassus P, Koscielny S, Bosq J, Moullet I, Lemaignan C, Stamberg J, Dupriez B, Najman A, Pico J (1999). Small non-cleaved cell lymphoma. A prospective multicenter study of 51 adults treated with the LMB pediatric protocol. *Blood* 10 Suppl 1:523a: 523a.

307. Dogan A, Du MQ, Aiello A, Diss TC, Ye HT, Pan LX, Isaacson PG (1998). Follicular lymphomas contain a clonally linked but phenotypically distinct neoplastic B-cell population in the interfollicular zone. *Blood* 91: 4708-4714.

308. Doggett RS, Wood GS, Horning S, Levy R, Dorfman RF, Bindl J, Warnke RA (1984). The immunologic characterization of 95 nodal and extranodal diffuse large cell lymphomas in 89 patients. *Am J Pathol* 115: 245-252.

309. Doglioni C, Wotherspoon AC, Moschini A, de Boni M, Isaacson PG (1992). High incidence of primary gastric lymphoma in northeastern Italy. *Lancet* 339: 834-835.

310. Dohner H, Fischer K, Bentz M, Hansen K, Benner A, Cabot G, Diehl D, Schlenk R, Coy J, Stilgenbauer S (1995). p53 gene deletion predicts for poor survival and nonresponse to therapy with purine analogs in chronic B-cell leukemias. *Blood* 85: 1580-1589.

311. Dohner H, Stilgenbauer S, Dohner K, Bentz M, Lichter P (1999). Chromosome aberrations in B-cell chronic lymphocytic leukemia: reassessment based on molecular cytogenetic analysis. *J Mol Med* 77: 266-281.

312. Dohner H, Stilgenbauer S, Fischer K, Bentz M, Lichter P (1997). Cytogenetic and molecular cytogenetic analysis of B cell chronic lymphocytic leukemia: specific chromosome aberrations identify prognostic subgroups of patients and point to loci of candidate genes. *Leukemia* 11 Suppl 2: S19-S24.

313. Dohner H, Stilgenbauer S, James MR, Benner A, Weilguni T, Bentz M, Fischer K, Hunstein W, Lichter P (1997). 11q deletions identify a new subset of B-cell chronic lymphocytic leukemia characterized by extensive nodal involvement and inferior prognosis. *Blood* 89: 2516-2522.

314. Domizio P, Hall PA, Cotter F, Amiel S, Tucker J, Besser GM, Levison DA (1989). Angiotropic large cell lymphoma (ALCL): morphological, immunohistochemical and genotypic studies with analysis of previous reports. *Hematol Oncol* 7: 195-206.

315. Dorfman DM, Pinkus GS (1994). Distinction between small lymphocytic and mantle cell lymphoma by immunoreactivity for CD23. *Mod Pathol* 7: 326-331.

316. Downing JR (1999). *Molecular genetics of acute myeloid leukemia (in) childhood leukemias*. Cambridge University Press

317. Downing JR (1999). The AML1-ETO chimaeric transcription factor in acute myeloid leukaemia: biology and clinical significance. *Br J Haematol* 106: 296-308.

318. Doyle TJ, Venkatachalam KK, Maeda K, Saeed SM, Tilchen EJ (1983). Hodgkin's disease in renal transplant recipients. *Cancer* 51: 245-247.

319. Drach J, Ackermann J, Fritz E, Kromer E, Schuster R, Gisslinger H, DeSantis M, Zojer N, Fiegl M, Roka S, Schuster J, Heinz R, Ludwig H, Huber H (1998). Presence of a p53 gene deletion in patients with multiple myeloma predicts for short survival after conventional-dose chemotherapy. *Blood* 92: 802-809.

320. Drenou B, Lamy T, Amiot L, Fardel O, Caulet-Maugendre S, Sasportes M, Diebold J, Le Prise PY, Fauchet R (1997). CD3- CD56+ non-Hodgkin's lymphomas with an aggressive behavior related to multidrug resistance. *Blood* 89: 2966-2974.

321. Druker BJ, Lydon NB (2000). Lessons learned from the development of an abl tyrosine kinase inhibitor for chronic myelogenous leukemia. *J Clin Invest* 105: 3-7.

322. Du M, Diss TC, Xu C, Peng H, Isaacson PG, Pan L (1996). Ongoing mutation in MALT lymphoma immunoglobulin gene that antigen stimulation plays a role in the clonal expansion. *Leukemia* 10: 1190-1197.

323. Du MQ, Diss TC, Xu CF, Wotherspoon AC, Isaacson PG, Pan LX (1997). Ongoing immunoglobulin gene mutations in mantle cell lymphomas. *Br J Haematol* 96: 124-131.

324. Dunn-Walters DK, Boursier L, Spencer J, Isaacson PG (1998). Analysis of immunoglobulin genes in splenic marginal zone lymphoma suggests ongoing mutation. *Hum Pathol* 29: 585-593.

325. Dupin N, Diss TL, Kellam P, Tulliez M, Du MQ, Sicard D, Weiss RA, Isaacson PG, Boshoff C (2000). HHV-8 is associated with a plasmablastic variant of Castleman disease that is linked to HHV-8-positive plasmablastic lymphoma. *Blood* 95: 1406-1412.

326. Dupin N, Fisher C, Kellam P, Ariad S, Tulliez M, Franck N, van Marck E, Salmon D, Gorin I, Escande JP, Weiss RA, Alitalo K, Boshoff C (1999). Distribution of human herpesvirus-8 latently infected cells in Kaposi's sarcoma, multicentric Castleman's disease, and primary effusion lymphoma. *Proc Natl Acad Sci U S A* 96: 4546-4551.

327. Duplantier JE, Seyama K, Day NK, Hitchcock R, Nelson RP, Ochs HD, Haraguchi S, Klemperer MR, Good RA (2001). Immunologic reconstitution following bone marrow transplantation for X-linked hyper IgM syndrome. *Clin Immunol* 98: 313-318.

328. Dupriez B, Morel P, Demory JL, Lai JL, Simon M, Plantier I, Bauters F (1996). Prognostic factors in agnogenic myeloid metaplasia: a report on 195 cases with a new scoring system. *Blood* 88: 1013-1018.

329. Durie BG (1986). Staging and kinetics of multiple myeloma. *Semin Oncol* 13: 300-309.

330. Durie BG (1992). Cellular and molecular genetic features of myeloma and related disorders. *Hematol Oncol Clin North Am* 6: 463-477.

331. Durie BG, Persky B, Soehnlen BJ, Grogan TM, Salmon SE (1982). Amyloid production in human myeloma stem-cell culture, with morphologic evidence of amyloid secretion by associated macrophages. *N Engl J Med* 307: 1689-1692.

332. Durie BG, Salmon SE (1975). A clinical staging system for multiple myeloma. Correlation of measured myeloma cell mass with presenting clinical features, response to treatment, and survival. *Cancer* 36: 842-854.

333. Durie BG, Salmon SE (1977). Multiple myeloma, macroglobulinemia, and monoclonal gammopathies. In: *Recent Advances in Hematology*, Hoffbrand AV, Brain MC, Hirsch J, eds. Churchill-Livingstone: Edinburgh, 243.

334. Durkop H, Foss HD, Demel G, Klotzbach H, Hahn C, Stein H (1999). Tumor necrosis factor receptor-associated factor 1 is overexpressed in Reed-Sternberg cells of Hodgkin's disease and Epstein-Barr virus-transformed lymphoid cells. *Blood* 93: 617-623.

335. Eck M, Schmausser B, Greiner A, Muller-Hermelink HK (2000). Helicobacter pylori in gastric mucosa-associated lymphoid tissue type lymphoma. *Recent Results Cancer Res* 156:9-18: 9-18.

336. Eclache V, Magnac C, Pritsch O, Delecluse HJ, Davi F, Raphael M, Dighiero G (1996). Complete nucleotide sequence of Ig V genes in three cases of Burkitt lymphoma associated with AIDS. *Leuk Lymphoma* 20: 281-290.

337. Eichel BS, Harrison EG, Jr., Devine KD, Scanlon PW, Brown HA (1966). Primary lymphoma of the nose including a relationship to lethal midline granuloma. *Am J Surg* 112: 597-605.

338. el Kassar N, Hetet G, Briere J, Grandchamp B (1997). Clonality analysis of hematopoiesis in essential thrombocythemia: advantages of studying T lymphocytes and platelets. *Blood* 89: 128-134.

339. Elenitoba-Johnson KS, Gascoyne RD, Lim MS, Chhanabai M, Jaffe ES, Raffeld M (1998). Homozygous deletions at chromosome 9p21 involving p16 and p15 are associated with histologic progression in follicle center lymphoma. *Blood* 91: 4677-4685.

340. Elenitoba-Johnson KS, Jaffe ES (1997). Lymphoproliferative disorders associated with congenital immunodeficiencies. *Semin Diagn Pathol* 14: 35-47.

341. Elenitoba-Johnson KS, Zarate-Osorno A, Meneses A, Krenacs L, Kingma DW, Raffeld M, Jaffe ES (1998). Cytotoxic granular protein expression, Epstein-Barr virus strain type, and latent membrane protein-1 oncogene deletions in nasal T-lymphocyte/natural killer cell lymphomas from Mexico. *Mod Pathol* 11: 754-761.

342. Ellis JT, Peterson P, Geller SA, Rappaport H (1986). Studies of the bone marrow in polycythemia vera and the evolution of myelofibrosis and second hematologic malignancies. *Semin Hematol* 23: 144-155.

343. Ellis M, Ravid M, Lishner M (1993). A comparative analysis of alkylating agent and epipodophyllotoxin-related leukemias. *Leuk Lymphoma* 11: 9-13.

344. Emanuel PD, Bates LJ, Castleberry RP, Gualtieri RJ, Zuckerman KS (1991). Selective hypersensitivity to granulocyte-macrophage colony-stimulating factor by juvenile chronic myeloid leukemia hematopoietic progenitors. *Blood* 77: 925-929.

345. Emmerich F, Meiser M, Hummel M, Demel G, Foss HD, Jundt F, Mathas S, Krappmann D, Scheidereit C, Stein H, Dorken B (1999). Overexpression of I kappa B alpha without inhibition of NF-kappaB activity and mutations in the I kappa B alpha gene in Reed-Sternberg cells. *Blood* 94: 3129-3134.

346. Engelhard M, Brittinger G, Huhn D, Gerhartz HH, Meusers P, Siegert W, Thiel E, Wilmanns W, Aydemir U, Bierwolf S, Griesser H, Tiemann M, Lennert K (1997). Subclassification of diffuse large B-cell lymphomas according to the Kiel classification: distinction of centroblastic and immunoblastic lymphomas is a significant prognostic risk factor. *Blood* 89: 2291-2297.

347. Epstein MA, Achong BG, Barr YM (1964). Virus particles in cultured lymphoblasts from Burkitt's lymphoma. *Lancet* 1: 702.

348. Escribano L, Orfao A, Villarrubia J, Diaz-Agustin B, Cervero C, Rios A, Velasco JL, Ciudad J, Navarro JL, San Miguel JF (1998). Immunophenotypic characterization of human bone marrow mast cells. A flow cytometric study of normal and pathological bone marrow samples. *Anal Cell Pathol* 16: 151-159.

349. Estey E, Pierce S, Kantarjian H, O'Brien S, Beran M, Andreeff M, Escudier S, Koller C, Kornblau S, Robertson L (1993). Treatment of myelodysplastic syndromes with AML-type chemotherapy. *Leuk Lymphoma* 11 Suppl 2:59-63: 59-63.

350. Estey E, Thall P, Beran M, Kantarjian H, Pierce S, Keating M (1997). Effect of diagnosis (refractory anemia with excess blasts, refractory anemia with excess blasts in transformation, or acute myeloid leukemia [AML]) on outcome of AML-type chemotherapy. *Blood* 90: 2969-2977.

351. Eyster ME, Saletan SL, Rabellino EM, Karanas A, McDonald TP, Locke LA, Luderer JR (1986). Familial essential thrombocythemia. *Am J Med* 80: 497-502.

352. Ezdinli EZ, Costello WG, Kucuk O, Berard CW (1987). Effect of the degree of nodularity on the survival of patients with nodular lymphomas. *J Clin Oncol* 5: 413-418.

353. Facchetti F, Wolf-Peeters C, Kennes C, Rossi G, De Vos R, van den Oord JJ, Desmet VJ (1990). Leukemia-associated lymph node infiltrates of plasmacytoid monocytes (so-called plasmacytoid T-cells). Evidence for two distinct histological and immunophenotypical patterns. *Am J Surg Pathol* 14: 101-112.

354. Facer CA, Playfair JH (1989). Malaria, Epstein-Barr virus, and the genesis of lymphomas. *Adv Cancer Res* 53:33-72: 33-72.

355. Faderl S, Talpaz M, Estrov Z, Kantarjian HM (1999). Chronic myelogenous leukemia: biology and therapy. *Ann Intern Med* 131: 207-219.

356. Faguet GB, Barton BP, Smith LL, Garver FA (1977). Gamma heavy chain disease: clinical aspects and characterization of a deleted, noncovalently linked gamma1 heavy chain dimer (BAZ). *Blood* 49: 495-505.

357. Falini B, Bigerna B, Fizzotti M, Pulford K, Pileri SA, Delsol G, Carbone A, Paulli M, Magrini U, Menestrina F, Giardini R, Pilotti S, Mezzelani A, Ugolini B, Billi M, Pucciarini A, Pacini R, Pelicci PG, Flenghi L (1998). ALK expression defines a distinct group of T/null lymphomas ("ALK lymphomas") with a wide morphological spectrum. *Am J Pathol* 153: 875-886.

358. Falini B, Flenghi L, Fagioli M, Coco FL, Cordone I, Diverio D, Pasqualucci L, Biondi A, Riganelli D, Orleth A, Liso A, Martelli MF, Pelicci PG, Pileri S (1997). Immunocytochemical diagnosis of acute promyelocytic leukemia (M3) with the monoclonal antibody PG-M3 (anti-PML). *Blood* 90: 4046-4053.

359. Falini B, Flenghi L, Pileri S, Gambacorta M, Bigerna B, Durkop H, Eitelbach F, Thiele J, Pacini R, Cavaliere A (1993). PG-M1: a new monoclonal antibody directed against a fixative-resistant epitope on the macrophage-restricted form of the CD68 molecule. *Am J Pathol* 142: 1359-1372.

360. Falini B, Pileri S, De S, I, Martelli MF, Mason DY, Delsol G, Gatter KC, Fagioli M (1990). Peripheral T-cell lymphoma associated with hemophagocytic syndrome. *Blood* 75: 434-444.

361. Falini B, Pileri S, Zinzani PL, Carbone A, Zagonel V, Wolf-Peeters C, Verhoef G, Menestrina F, Todeschini G, Paulli M, Lazzarino M, Giardini R, Aiello A, Foss HD, Araujo I, Fizzotti M, Pelicci PG, Flenghi L, Martelli MF, Santucci A (1999). ALK+ lymphoma: clinico-pathological findings and outcome. *Blood* 93: 2697-2706.

362. Falini B, Pulford K, Pucciarini A, Carbone A, Wolf-Peeters C, Cordell J, Fizzotti M, Santucci A, Pelicci PG, Pileri S, Campo E, Ott G, Delsol G, Mason DY (1999). Lymphomas expressing ALK fusion protein(s) other than NPM-ALK. *Blood* 94: 3509-3515.

363. Falk S, Mix D, Stutte HJ (1990). The spleen in osteomyelofibrosis. A morphological and immunohistochemical study of 30 cases. *Virchows Arch A Pathol Anat Histopathol* 416: 437-442.

364. Farcet JP, Gaulard P, Marolleau JP, Le Couedic JP, Henni T, Gourdin MF, Divine M, Haioun C, Zafrani S, Goossens M (1990). Hepatosplenic T-cell lymphoma: sinusal/sinusoidal localization of malignant cells expressing the T-cell receptor gamma delta. *Blood* 75: 2213-2219.

365. Fauci AS, Haynes BF, Costa J, Katz P, Wolff SM (1982). Lymphomatoid granulomatosis. Prospective clinical and therapeutic experience over 10 years. *N Engl J Med* 306: 68-74.

366. Felgar RE, Macon WR, Kinney MC, Roberts S, Pasha T, Salhany KE (1997). TIA-1 expression in lymphoid neoplasms. Identification of subsets with cytotoxic T lymphocyte or natural killer cell differentiation. *Am J Pathol* 150: 1893-1900.

367. Felix CA (2000). Acute lymphoblastic leukemia in infants. In: *Education Program Book*, Education Program Book Society of Hematology: Washington, DC, pp. 294-302.

368. Feller AC, Griesser H, Schilling CV, Wacker HH, Dallenbach F, Bartels H, Kuse R, Mak TW, Lennert K (1988). Clonal gene rearrangement patterns correlate with immunophenotype and clinical parameters in patients with angioimmunoblastic lymphadenopathy. *Am J Pathol* 133: 549-556.

369. Felman P, Bryon PA, Gentilhomme O, Ffrench M, Charrin C, Espinouse D, Viala JJ (1988). The syndrome of abnormal chromatin clumping in leucocytes: a myelodysplastic disorder with proliferative features? *Br J Haematol* 70: 49-54.

370. Felman P, Bryon PA, Gentilhomme O, Magaud JP, Manel AM, Coiffier B, Lenoir G (1985). Burkitt's lymphoma. Distinction of subgroups by morphometric analysis of the characteristics of 55 cell lines. *Anal Quant Cytol Histol* 7: 275-282.

371. Feltkamp CA, van Heerde P, Feltkamp-Vroom TM, Koudstaal J (1981). A malignant tumor arising from interdigitating cells; light microscopical, ultrastructural, immuno- and enzyme-histochemical characteristics. *Virchows Arch [Pathol Anat]* 393: 183-192.

372. Fenaux P, Beuscart R, Lai JL, Jouet JP, Bauters F (1988). Prognostic factors in adult chronic myelomonocytic leukemia: an analysis of 107 cases. *J Clin Oncol* 6: 1417-1424.

373. Fenaux P, Chomienne C, Degos L (1997). Acute promyelocytic leukemia: biology and treatment. *Semin Oncol* 24: 92-102.

374. Fenaux P, Jouet JP, Zandecki M, Lai JL, Simon M, Pollet JP, Bauters F (1987). Chronic and subacute myelomonocytic leukaemia in the adult: a report of 60 cases with special reference to prognostic factors. *Br J Haematol* 65: 101-106.

375. Fenaux P, Morel P, Lai JL (1996). Cytogenetics of myelodysplastic syndromes. *Semin Hematol* 33: 127-138.

376. Fermand JP, Brouet JC (1999). Heavy-chain diseases. *Hematol Oncol Clin North Am* 13: 1281-1294.

377. Fermand JP, Brouet JC, Danon F, Seligmann M (1989). Gamma heavy chain "disease": heterogeneity of the clinico-pathologic features. Report of 16 cases and review of the literature. *Medicine (Baltimore)* 68: 321-335.

378. Fernandez-Robles E, Vermylen C, Martiat P, Ninane J, Cornu G (1990). Familial essential thrombocythemia. *Pediatr Hematol Oncol* 7: 373-376.

379. Ferry JA, Harris NL, Picker LJ, Weinberg DS, Rosales RK, Tapia J, Richardson EP, Jr. (1988). Intravascular lymphomatosis (malignant angioendotheliomatosis). A B-cell neoplasm expressing surface homing receptors. *Mod Pathol* 1: 444-452.

380. Ferry JA, Jacobson JO, Conti D, Delmonico F, Harris NL (1989). Lymphoproliferative disorders and hematologic malignancies following organ transplantation. *Mod Pathol* 2: 583-592.

381. Ferry JA, Zukerberg LR, Harris NL (1992). Florid progressive transformation of germinal centers. A syndrome affecting young men, without early progression to nodular lymphocyte predominance Hodgkin's disease. *Am J Surg Pathol* 16: 252-258.

382. Fialkow PJ, Faguet GB, Jacobson RJ, Vaidya K, Murphy S (1981). Evidence that essential thrombocythemia is a clonal disorder with origin in a multipotent stem cell. *Blood* 58: 916-919.

383. Filipovich AH, Stone JV, Tomany SC, Ireland M, Kollman C, Pelz CJ, Casper JT, Cowan MJ, Edwards JR, Fasth A, Gale RP, Junker A, Kamani NR, Loechelt BJ, Pietryga DW, Ringden O, Vowels M, Hegland J, Williams AV, Klein JP, Sobocinski KA, Rowlings PA, Horowitz MM (2001). Impact of donor type on outcome of bone marrow transplantation for Wiskott-Aldrich syndrome: collaborative study of the International Bone Marrow Transplant Registry and the National Marrow Donor Program. *Blood* 97: 1598-1603.

384. Finn LS, Viswanatha DS, Belasco JB, Snyder H, Huebner D, Sorbara L, Raffeld M, Jaffe ES, Salhany KE (1999). Primary follicular lymphoma of the testis in childhood. *Cancer* 85: 1626-1635.

385. Fioretos T, Strombeck B, Sandberg T, Johansson B, Billstrom R, Borg A, Nilsson PG, Van den BH, Hagemeijer A, Mitelman F, Hoglund M (1999). Isochromosome 17q in blast crisis of chronic myeloid leukemia and in other hematologic malignancies is the result of clustered breakpoints in 17p11 and is not associated with coding TP53 mutations. *Blood* 94: 225-232.

386. Fisher RI, Dahlberg S, Nathwani BN, Banks PM, Miller TP, Grogan TM (1995). A clinical analysis of two indolent lymphoma entities: mantle cell lymphoma and marginal zone lymphoma (including the mucosa-associated lymphoid tissue and monocytoid B-cell subcategories): a Southwest Oncology Group study. *Blood* 85: 1075-1082.

387. Flaum MA, Schooley RT, Fauci AS, Gralnick HR (1981). A clinicopathologic correlation of the idiopathic hypereosinophilic syndrome. I. Hematologic manifestations. *Blood* 58: 1012-1020.

388. Flinn IW, Kopecky KJ, Foucar K, Head D, et al (2000). Long-term follow-up of remission duration, mortality and second malignancies in hairy cell leukemia patients treated with pentostain. *Blood* (in press).

389. Flotho C, Valcamonica S, Mach-Pascual S, Schmahl G, Corral L, Ritterbach J, Hasle H, Arico M, Biondi A, Niemeyer CM (1999). RAS mutations and clonality analysis in children with juvenile myelomonocytic leukemia (JMML). *Leukemia* 13: 32-37.

390. Foss HD, Anagnostopoulos I, Araujo I, Assaf C, Demel G, Kummer JA, Hummel M, Stein H (1996). Anaplastic large-cell lymphomas of T-cell and null-cell phenotype express cytotoxic molecules. *Blood* 88: 4005-4011.

391. Foss HD, Reusch R, Demel G, Lenz G, Anagnostopoulos I, Hummel M, Stein H (1999). Frequent expression of the B-cell-specific activator protein in Reed-Sternberg cells of classical Hodgkin's disease provides further evidence for its B-cell origin. *Blood* 94: 3108-3113.

392. Foucar K (1999). Chronic lymphoid leukemias and lymphoproliferative disorders. *Mod Pathol* 12: 141-150.

393. Foucar K, Armitage JO, Dick FR (1983). Malignant lymphoma, diffuse mixed small and large cell. A clinicopathologic study of 47 cases. *Cancer* 51: 2090-2099.

394. Fraga M, Brousset P, Schlaifer D, Payen C, Robert A, Rubie H, Huguet-Rigal F, Delsol G (1995). Bone marrow involvement in anaplastic large cell lymphoma. Immunohistochemical detection of minimal disease and its prognostic significance. *Am J Clin Pathol* 103: 82-89.

395. Franchini G (1995). Molecular mechanisms of human T-cell leukemia/lymphotropic virus type I infection. *Blood* 86: 3619-3639.

396. Franchino C, Reich C, Distenfeld A, Ubriaco A, Knowles DM (1988). A clinicopathologically distinctive primary splenic histiocytic neoplasm. Demonstration of its histiocyte derivation by immunophenotypic and molecular genetic analysis. *Am J Surg Pathol* 12: 398-404.

397. Franco V, Florena AM, Campesi G (1996). Intrasinusoidal bone marrow infiltration: a possible hallmark of splenic lymphoma. *Histopathology* 29: 571-575.

398. Francois A, Lesesve JF, Stamatoullas A, Comoz F, Lenormand B, Etienne I, Mendel I, Hemet J, Bastard C, Tilly H (1997). Hepatosplenic gamma/delta T-cell lymphoma: a report of two cases in immunocompromised patients, associated with isochromosome 7q. *Am J Surg Pathol* 21: 781-790.

399. Frangione B, Franklin EC (1973). Heavy chain diseases: clinical features and molecular significance of the disordered immunoglobulin structure. *Semin Hematol* 10: 53-64.

400. Frangione B, Franklin EC, Prelli F (1976). Mu heavy-chain disease – a defect in immunoglobulin assembly. Structural studies of the kappa chain. *Scand J Immunol* 5: 623-627.

401. Frank D, Cesarman E, Liu YF, Michler RE, Knowles DM (1995). Posttransplantation lymphoproliferative disorders frequently contain type A and not type B Epstein-Barr virus. *Blood* 85: 1396-1403.

402. Franklin EC, Kyle R, Seligmann M, Frangione B (1979). Correlation of protein structure and immunoglobulin gene organization in the light of two new deleted heavy chain disease proteins. *Mol Immunol* 16: 919-921.

403. Frassoldati A, Lamparelli T, Federico M, Annino L, Capnist G, Pagnucco G, Dini E, Resegotti L, Damasio EE, Silingardi V (1994). Hairy cell leukemia: a clinical review based on 725 cases of the Italian Cooperative Group (ICGHCL). Italian Cooperative Group for Hairy Cell Leukemia. *Leuk Lymphoma* 13: 307-316.

404. Freedman MH, Cohen A, Grunberger T, Bunin N, Luddy RE, Saunders EF, Shahidi N, Lau A, Estrov Z (1992). Central role of tumour necrosis factor, GM-CSF, and interleukin 1 in the pathogenesis of juvenile chronic myelogenous leukaemia. *Br J Haematol* 80: 40-48.

405. French DL, Laskov R, Scharff MD (1989). The role of somatic hypermutation in the generation of antibody diversity. *Science* 244: 1152-1157.

406. Frieri M, Linn N, Schweitzer M, Angadi C, Pardanani B (1990). Lymphadenopathic mastocytosis with eosinophilia and biclonal gammopathy [clinical conference]. *J Allergy Clin Immunol* 86: 126-132.

407. Frizzera G, Hanto DW, Gajl-Peczalska KJ, Rosai J, McKenna RW, Sibley RK, Holahan KP, Lindquist LL (1981). Polymorphic diffuse B-cell hyperplasias and lymphomas in renal transplant recipients. *Cancer Res* 41: 4262-4279.

408. Frizzera G, Kaneko Y, Sakurai M (1989). Angioimmunoblastic lymphadenopathy and related disorders: a retrospective look in search of definitions. *Leukemia* 3: 1-5.

409. Froberg MK, Brunning RD, Dorion P, Litz CE, Torlakovic E (1998). Demonstration of clonality in neutrophils using FISH in a case of chronic neutrophilic leukemia. *Leukemia* 12: 623-626.

410. Gahn B, Haase D, Unterhalt M, Drescher M, Schoch C, Fonatsch C, Terstappen LW, Hiddemann W, Buchner T, Bennett JM, Wormann B (1996). De novo AML with dysplastic hematopoiesis: cytogenetic and prognostic significance. *Leukemia* 10: 946-951.

411. Gaidano G, Ballerini P, Gong JZ, Inghirami G, Neri A, Newcomb EW, Magrath IT, Knowles DM, Dalla-Favera R (1991). p53 mutations in human lymphoid malignancies: association with Burkitt lymphoma and chronic lymphocytic leukemia. *Proc Natl Acad Sci U S A* 88: 5413-5417.

412. Gaidano G, Carbone A (1995). AIDS-related lymphomas: from pathogenesis to pathology. *Br J Haematol* 90: 235-243.

413. Gaidano G, Carbone A, Pastore C, Capello D, Migliazza A, Gloghini A, Roncella S, Ferrarini M, Saglio G, Dalla-Favera R (1997). Frequent mutation of the 5' noncoding region of the BCL-6 gene in acquired immunodeficiency syndrome-related non-Hodgkin's lymphomas. *Blood* 89: 3755-3762.

414. Gaidano G, Lo CF, Ye BH, Shibata D, Levine AM, Knowles DM, Dalla-Favera R (1994). Rearrangements of the BCL-6 gene in acquired immunodeficiency syndrome-associated non-Hodgkin's lymphoma: association with diffuse large-cell subtype. *Blood* 84: 397-402.

415. Gall EA, Mallory TB (1942). Malignant lymphoma: a clinico-pathologic survey of 618 cases. *Am J Pathol* 18: 381-429.

416. Gallagher CJ, Gregory WM, Jones AE, Stansfeld AG, Richards MA, Dhaliwal HS, Malpas JS, Lister TA (1986). Follicular lymphoma: prognostic factors for response and survival. *J Clin Oncol* 4: 1470-1480.

417. Gallo G, Goni F, Boctor F, Vidal R, Kumar A, Stevens FJ, Frangione B, Ghiso J (1996). Light chain cardiomyopathy. Structural analysis of the light chain tissue deposits. *Am J Pathol* 148: 1397-1406.

418. Galton DA, Goldman JM, Wiltshaw E, Catovsky D, Henry K, Goldenberg GJ (1974). Prolymphocytic leukaemia. *Br J Haematol* 27: 7-23.

419. Garand R, Duchayne E, Blanchard D, Robillard N, Kuhlein E, Fenneteau O, Salomon-Nguyen F, Grange MJ, Rousselot P, Demur C (1995). Minimally differentiated erythroleukaemia (AML M6 'variant'): a rare subset of AML distinct from AML M6. Groupe Francais d'Hematologie Cellulaire. *Br J Haematol* 90: 868-875.

420. Garand R, Goasguen J, Brizard A, Buisine J, Charpentier A, Claisse JF, Duchayne E, Lagrange M, Segonds C, Troussard X, Flandrin G (1998). Indolent course as a relatively frequent presentation in T-prolymphocytic leukaemia. Groupe Francais d'Hematologie Cellulaire. *Br J Haematol* 103: 488-494.

421. Garcia-Sanz R, Orfao A, Gonzalez M, Tabernero MD, Blade J, Moro MJ, Fernandez-Calvo J, Sanz MA, Perez-Simon JA, Rasillo A, Miguel JF (1999). Primary plasma cell leukemia: clinical, immunophenotypic, DNA ploidy, and cytogenetic characteristics. *Blood* 93: 1032-1037.

422. Gascoyne RD, Adomat SA, Krajewski S, Krajewska M, Horsman DE, Tolcher AW, O'Reilly SE, Hoskins P, Coldman AJ, Reed JC, Connors JM (1997). Prognostic significance of Bcl-2 protein expression and Bcl-2 gene rearrangement in diffuse aggressive non-Hodgkin's lymphoma. *Blood* 90: 244-251.

423. Gascoyne RD, Aoun P, Wu D, Chhanabhai M, Skinnider BF, Greiner TC, Morris SW, Connors JM, Vose JM, Viswanatha DS, Coldman A, Weisenburger DD (1999). Prognostic significance of anaplastic lymphoma kinase (ALK) protein expression in adults with anaplastic large cell lymphoma. *Blood* 93: 3913-3921.

424. Geissmann F, Ruskone-Fourmestraux A, Hermine O, Bourquelot P, Belanger C, Audouin J, Delmer A, Macintyre EA, Varet B, Brousse N (1998). Homing receptor alpha4beta7 integrin expression predicts digestive tract involvement in mantle cell lymphoma. *Am J Pathol* 153: 1701-1705.

425. Gelb AB, van de RM, Regula DP, Jr., Cornbleet JP, Kamel OW, Horoupian DS, Cleary ML, Warnke RA (1994). Epstein-Barr virus-associated natural killer-large granular lymphocyte leukemia. *Hum Pathol* 25: 953-960.

426. Gentile TC, Hadlock KG, Uner AH, Delal B, Squiers E, Crowley S, Woodman RC, Foung SK, Poiesz BJ, Loughran TP, Jr. (1998). Large granular lymphocyte leukaemia occurring after renal transplantation. *Br J Haematol* 101: 507-512.

427. Gentile TC, Uner AH, Hutchison RE, Wright J, Ben Ezra J, Russell EC, Loughran TP, Jr. (1994). CD3+, CD56+ aggressive variant of large granular lymphocyte leukemia. *Blood* 84: 2315-2321.

428. Georgescu L, Quinn GC, Schwartzman S, Paget SA (1997). Lymphoma in patients with rheumatoid arthritis: association with the disease state or methotrexate treatment. *Semin Arthritis Rheum* 26: 794-804.

429. Georgii A, Buesche G, Kreft A (1998). The histopathology of chronic myeloproliferative diseases. *Baillieres Clin Haematol* 11: 721-749.

430. Georgii A, Buhr T, Buesche G, Kreft A, Choritz H (1996). Classification and staging of Ph-negative myeloproliferative disorders by histopathology from bone marrow biopsies. *Leuk Lymphoma* 22 Suppl 1:15-29: 15-29.

431. Georgii A, Vykoupil KF, Buhr T, Choritz H, Dohler U, Kaloutsi V, Werner M (1990). Chronic myeloproliferative disorders in bone marrow biopsies. *Pathol Res Pract* 186: 3-27.

432. Germing U, Gattermann N, Minning H, Heyll A, Aul C (1998). Problems in the classification of CMML – dysplastic versus proliferative type. *Leuk Res* 22: 871-878.

433. Germing U, Gattermann N, Strupp C, Aivado M, Aul C (2000). Validation of the WHO proposals for the classification of primary myelodysplastic syndromes. *Leuk Res* (in press).

434. Ghosh SK, Abrams JT, Terunuma H, Vonderheid EC, DeFreitas E (1994). Human T-cell leukemia virus type I tax/rex DNA and RNA in cutaneous T-cell lymphoma. *Blood* 84: 2663-2671.

435. Gibson LE, Muller SA, Leiferman KM, Peters MS (1989). Follicular mucinosis: clinical and histopathologic study. *J Am Acad Dermatol* 20: 441-446.

436. Giles FJ, O'Brien SM, Keating MJ (1998). Chronic lymphocytic leukemia in (Richter's) transformation. *Semin Oncol* 25: 117-125.

437. Gilmour KC, Cranston T, Jones A, Davies EG, Goldblatt D, Thrasher A, Kinnon C, Nichols KE, Gaspar HB (2000). Diagnosis of X-linked lymphoproliferative disease by analysis of SLAM-associated protein expression. *Eur J Immunol* 30: 1691-1697.

438. Gisselbrecht C, Gaulard P, Lepage E, Coiffier B, Briere J, Haioun C, Cazals-Hatem D, Bosly A, Xerri L, Tilly H, Berger F, Bouhabdallah R, Diebold J (1998). Prognostic significance of T-cell phenotype in aggressive non-Hodgkin's lymphomas. Groupe d'Etudes des Lymphomes de l'Adulte (GELA). *Blood* 92: 76-82.

439. Gisselbrecht C, Spina M, Gabarre J, Rizzardini G, Schlaifer D, Nigra E, Bouabdallah R, Moulet I, Carbone A, Raphael M, Lepage E, Tirelli U (1999). Dose ajusted treatment in human immuno-deficiency virus related lymphoma. *Blood* 94 Suppl 1:599a: 599a.

440. Glass AG, Karnell LH, Menck HR (1997). The National Cancer Data Base report on non-Hodgkin's lymphoma. *Cancer* 80: 2311-2320.

441. Glick JH, Barnes JM, Ezdinli EZ, Berard CW, Orlow EL, Bennett JM (1981). Nodular mixed lymphoma: results of a randomized trial failing to confirm prolonged disease-free survival with COPP chemotherapy. *Blood* 58: 920-925.

442. Glick JH, McFadden E, Costello W, Ezdinli E, Berard CW, Bennett JM (1982). Nodular histiocytic lymphoma: factors influencing prognosis and implications for aggressive chemotherapy. *Cancer* 49: 840-845.

443. Goedert JJ (2000). The epidemiology of acquired immunodeficiency syndrome malignancies. *Semin Oncol* 27: 390-401.

444. Golomb HM, Rowley JD, Vardiman JW, Testa JR, Butler A (1980). "Microgranular" acute promyelocytic leukemia: a distinct clinical, ultrastructural, and cytogenetic entity. *Blood* 55: 253-259.

445. Golub TR, Barker GF, Lovett M, Gilliland DG (1994). Fusion of PDGF receptor beta to a novel ets-like gene, tel, in chronic myelomonocytic leukemia with t(5;12) chromosomal translocation. *Cell* 77: 307-316.

446. Gonzalez CL, Jaffe ES (1990). The histiocytoses: clinical presentation and differential diagnosis. *Oncology (Huntingt)* 4: 47-60.

447. Gonzalez CL, Medeiros LJ, Braziel RM, Jaffe ES (1991). T-cell lymphoma involving subcutaneous tissue. A clinicopathologic entity commonly associated with hemophagocytic syndrome. *Am J Surg Pathol* 15: 17-27.

448. Gordon MY, Goldman JM (1996). Cellular and molecular mechanisms in chronic myeloid leukaemia: biology and treatment. *Br J Haematol* 95: 10-20.

449. Goyal RK, McEvoy L, Wilson DB (1996). Hodgkin disease after renal transplantation in childhood. *J Pediatr Hematol Oncol* 18: 392-395.

450. Gravel S, Delsol G, al Saati T (1998). Single-cell analysis of the t(14;18)(q32;q21) chromosomal translocation in Hodgkin's disease demonstrates the absence of this translocation in neoplastic Hodgkin and Reed-Sternberg cells. *Blood* 91: 2866-2874.

451. Greenberg P, Cox C, LeBeau MM, Fenaux P, Morel P, Sanz G, Sanz M, Vallespi T, Hamblin T, Oscier D, Ohyashiki K, Toyama K, Aul C, Mufti G, Bennett J (1997). International scoring system for evaluating prognosis in myelodysplastic syndromes. *Blood* 89: 2079-2088.

452. Greenberger JS, Crocker AC, Vawter G, Jaffe N, Cassady JR (1981). Results of treatment of 127 patients with systemic histiocytosis (Letterer-Siwe syndrome, Schuller-Christian syndrome and multifocal eosinophilic granuloma). *Medicine (Baltimore)* 60: 311-338.

453. Greiner TC, Gascoyne RD, Anderson ME, Kingma DW, Adomat SA, Said J, Jaffe ES (1996). Nodular lymphocyte-predominant Hodgkin's disease associated with large-cell lymphoma: analysis of Ig gene rearrangements by V-J polymerase chain reaction. *Blood* 88: 657-666.

454. Greiner TC, Moynihan MJ, Chan WC, Lytle DM, Pedersen A, Anderson JR, Weisenburger DD (1996). p53 mutations in mantle cell lymphoma are associated with variant cytology and predict a poor prognosis. *Blood* 87: 4302-4310.

455. Greiner TC, Raffeld M, Lutz C, Dick F, Jaffe ES (1995). Analysis of T cell receptor-gamma gene rearrangements by denaturing gradient gel electrophoresis of GC-clamped polymerase chain reaction products. Correlation with tumor-specific sequences. *Am J Pathol* 146: 46-55.

456. Greipp PR, Leong T, Bennett JM, Gaillard JP, Klein B, Stewart JA, Oken MM, Kay NE, Van Ness B, Kyle RA (1998). Plasmablastic morphology – an independent prognostic factor with clinical and laboratory correlates: Eastern Cooperative Oncology Group (ECOG) myeloma trial E9486 report by the ECOG Myeloma Laboratory Group. *Blood* 91: 2501-2507.

457. Gretz JE, Anderson AO, Shaw S (1997). Cords, channels, corridors and conduits: critical architectural elements facilitating cell interactions in the lymph node cortex. *Immunol Rev* 156: 11-24.

458. Grever M, Kopecky K, Foucar MK, Head D, Bennett JM, Hutchison RE, Corbett WE, Cassileth PA, Habermann T, Golomb H (1995). Randomized comparison of pentostatin versus interferon alfa-2a in previously untreated patients with hairy cell leukemia: an intergroup study. *J Clin Oncol* 13: 974-982.

459. Griffin CA, Hawkins AL, Dvorak C, Henkle C, Ellingham T, Perlman EJ (1999). Recurrent involvement of 2p23 in inflammatory myofibroblastic tumors. *Cancer Res* 59: 2776-2780.

460. Griffin JD, Ritz J, Nadler LM, Schlossman SF (1981). Expression of myeloid differentiation antigens on normal and malignant myeloid cells. *J Clin Invest* 68: 932-941.

461. Grimwade D, Walker H, Oliver F, Wheatley K, Harrison C, Harrison G, Rees J, Hann I, Stevens R, Burnett A, Goldstone A (1998). The importance of diagnostic cytogenetics on outcome in AML: analysis of 1,612 patients entered into the MRC AML 10 trial. The Medical Research Council Adult and Children's Leukaemia Working Parties. *Blood* 92: 2322-2333.

462. Gritti C, Dastot H, Soulier J, Janin A, Daniel MT, Madani A, Grimber G, Briand P, Sigaux F, Stern MH (1998). Transgenic mice for MTCP1 develop T-cell prolymphocytic leukemia. *Blood* 92: 368-373.

463. Grogan TM, Durie BG, Lomen C, Spier C, Wirt DP, Nagle R, Wilson GS, Richter L, Vela E, Maxey V (1987). Delineation of a novel pre-B cell component in plasma cell myeloma: immunochemical, immunophenotypic, genotypic, cytologic, cell culture, and kinetic features. *Blood* 70: 932-942.

464. Grogan TM, Durie BG, Spier CM, Richter L, Vela E (1989). Myelomonocytic antigen positive multiple myeloma. *Blood* 73: 763-769.

465. Grogan TM, Spier CM (2001). The B cell immunoproliferative disorders, icluding multiple myeloma and amyloidosis. In: *Neoplastic Hematopathology*, Knowles DM, ed. 2nd. Lippincott Williams and Wilkins: Philadelphia, pp.

466. Gronbaek K, Straten PT, Ralfkiaer E, Ahrenkiel V, Andersen MK, Hansen NE, Zeuthen J, Hou-Jensen K, Guldberg P (1998). Somatic Fas mutations in non-Hodgkin's lymphoma: association with extranodal disease and autoimmunity. *Blood* 92: 3018-3024.

467. Grulich AE (1999). AIDS-associated non-Hodgkin's lymphoma in the era of highly active antiretroviral therapy. *J Acquir Immune Defic Syndr* 21 Suppl 1:S27-30: S27-S30.

468. Grulich AE, Wan X, Law MG, Milliken ST, Lewis CR, Garsia RJ, Gold J, Finlayson RJ, Cooper DA, Kaldor JM (2000). B-cell stimulation and prolonged immune deficiency are risk factors for non-Hodgkin's lymphoma in people with AIDS. *AIDS* 14: 133-140.

469. Gruszka-Westwood AM, Matutes E, Coignet LJ, Wotherspoon A, Catovsky D (1999). The incidence of trisomy 3 in splenic lymphoma with villous lymphocytes: a study by FISH. *Br J Haematol* 104: 600-604.

470. Guinee D, Jr., Jaffe E, Kingma D, Fishback N, Wallberg K, Krishnan J, Frizzera G, Travis W, Koss M (1994). Pulmonary lymphomatoid granulomatosis. Evidence for a proliferation of Epstein-Barr virus infected B-lymphocytes with a prominent T-cell component and vasculitis. *Am J Surg Pathol* 18: 753-764.

471. Guinee DG, Jr., Perkins SL, Travis WD, Holden JA, Tripp SR, Koss MN (1998). Proliferation and cellular phenotype in lymphomatoid granulomatosis: implications of a higher proliferation index in B cells. *Am J Surg Pathol* 22: 1093-1100.

472. Guitart J (2000). HIV-1 and an HTLV-II-associated cutaneous T-cell lymphoma. *N Engl J Med* 343: 303-304.

473. Gunz FW (1977). The epidemiology and genetics of the chronic leukaemias. *Clin Haematol* 6: 3-20.

474. Gupta R, Abdalla SH, Bain BJ (1999). Thrombocytosis with sideroblastic erythropoiesis: a mixed myeloproliferative myelodysplastic syndrome. *Leuk Lymphoma* 34: 615-619.

475. Gutierrez MI, Bhatia K, Barriga F, Diez B, Muriel FS, de Andreas ML, Epelman S, Risueno C, Magrath IT (1992). Molecular epidemiology of Burkitt's lymphoma from South America: differences in breakpoint location and Epstein-Barr virus association from tumors in other world regions. *Blood* 79: 3261-3266.

476. Haase D, Fonatsch C, Freund M, Wormann B, Bodenstein H, Bartels H, Stollmann-Gibbels B, Lengfelder E (1995). Cytogenetic findings in 179 patients with myelodysplastic syndromes. *Ann Hematol* 70: 171-187.

477. Hadzic N, Pagliuca A, Rela M, Portmann B, Jones A, Veys P, Heaton ND, Mufti GJ, Mieli-Vergani G (2000). Correction of the hyper-IgM syndrome after liver and bone marrow transplantation. *N Engl J Med* 342: 320-324.

478. Hage C, Willman CL, Favara BE, Isaacson PG (1993). Langerhans' cell histiocytosis (histiocytosis X): immunophenotype and growth fraction. *Hum Pathol* 24: 840-845.

479. Haghighi B, Smoller BR, LeBoit PE, Warnke RA, Sander CA, Kohler S (2000). Pagetoid reticulosis (Woringer-Kolopp disease): an immunophenotypic, molecular, and clinicopathologic study. *Mod Pathol* 13: 502-510.

480. Hallek M, Bergsagel PL, Anderson KC (1998). Multiple myeloma: increasing evidence for a multistep transformation process. *Blood* 91: 3-21.

481. Hamblin TJ, Davis Z, Gardiner A, Oscier DG, Stevenson FK (1999). Unmutated Ig V(H) genes are associated with a more aggressive form of chronic lymphocytic leukemia. *Blood* 94: 1848-1854.

482. Hamilton-Dutoit SJ, Raphael M, Audouin J, Diebold J, Lisse I, Pedersen C, Oksenhendler E, Marelle L, Pallesen G (1993). In situ demonstration of Epstein-Barr virus small RNAs (EBER 1) in acquired immunodeficiency syndrome-related lymphomas: correlation with tumor morphology and primary site. *Blood* 82: 619-624.

483. Hansen U, Wiese R, Knolle J (1994). [Shock and coagulation disorders in systemic mastocytosis]. *Dtsch Med Wochenschr* 119: 1231-1234.

484. Hansmann ML, Stein H, Fellbaum C, Hui PK, Parwaresch MR, Lennert K (1989). Nodular paragranuloma can transform into high-grade malignant lymphoma of B type. *Hum Pathol* 20: 1169-1175.

485. Hanson CA, Abaza M, Sheldon S, Ross CW, Schnitzer B, Stoolman LM (1993). Acute biphenotypic leukaemia: immunophenotypic and cytogenetic analysis. *Br J Haematol* 84: 49-60.

486. Hanson CA, Jaszcz W, Kersey JH, Astorga MG, Peterson BA, Gajl-Peczalska KJ, Frizzera G (1989). True histiocytic lymphoma: histopathologic, immunophenotypic and genotypic analysis. *Br J Haematol* 73: 187-198.

487. Hanson MN, Morrison VA, Peterson BA, Stieglbauer KT, Kubic VL, McCormick SR, McGlennen RC, Manivel JC, Brunning RD, Litz CE (1996). Posttransplant T-cell lymphoproliferative disorders – an aggressive, late complication of solid-organ transplantation. *Blood* 88: 3626-3633.

488. Hanto DW, Gajl-Peczalska KJ, Frizzera G, Arthur DC, Balfour HH, Jr., McClain K, Simmons RL, Najarian JS (1983). Epstein-Barr virus (EBV) induced polyclonal and monoclonal B-cell lymphoproliferative diseases occurring after renal transplantation. Clinical, pathologic, and virologic findings and implications for therapy. *Ann Surg* 198: 356-369.

489. Haque AK, Myers JL, Hudnall SD, Gelman BB, Lloyd RV, Payne D, Borucki M (1998). Pulmonary lymphomatoid granulomatosis in acquired immunodeficiency syndrome: lesions with Epstein-Barr virus infection. *Mod Pathol* 11: 347-356.

490. Harada H, Kawano MM, Huang N, Harada Y, Iwato K, Tanabe O, Tanaka H, Sakai A, Asaoku H, Kuramoto A (1993). Phenotypic difference of normal plasma cells from mature myeloma cells. *Blood* 81: 2658-2663.

491. Haralambieva E, Pulford KA, Lamant L, Pileri S, Roncador G, Gatter KC, Delsol G, Mason DY (2000). Anaplastic large-cell lymphomas of B-cell phenotype are anaplastic lymphoma kinase (ALK) negative and belong to the spectrum of diffuse large B-cell lymphomas. *Br J Haematol* 109: 584-591.

492. Harris MB, Shuster JJ, Carroll A, Look AT, Borowitz MJ, Crist WM, Nitschke R, Pullen J, Steuber CP, Land VJ (1992). Trisomy of leukemic cell chromosomes 4 and 10 identifies children with B-progenitor cell acute lymphoblastic leukemia with a very low risk of treatment failure: a Pediatric Oncology Group study. *Blood* 79: 3316-3324.

493. Harris NL, Demirjian Z (1991). Plasmacytoid T-zone cell proliferation in a patient with chronic myelomonocytic leukemia. Histologic and immunohistologic characterization. *Am J Surg Pathol* 15: 87-95.

494. Harris NL, Ferry JA, Swerdlow SH (1997). Posttransplant lymphoproliferative disorders: summary of Society for Hematopathology Workshop. *Semin Diagn Pathol* 14: 8-14.

495. Harris NL, Jaffe ES, Diebold J, Flandrin G, Muller-Hermelink HK, Vardiman J, Lister TA, Bloomfield CD (1999). World Health Organization classification of neoplastic diseases of the hematopoietic and lymphoid tissues: report of the Clinical Advisory Committee meeting-Airlie House, Virginia, November 1997. *J Clin Oncol* 17: 3835-3849.

496. Harris NL, Jaffe ES, Stein H, Banks PM, Chan JK, Cleary ML, Delsol G, Wolf-Peeters C, Falini B, Gatter KC (1994). A revised European-American classification of lymphoid neoplasms: a proposal from the International Lymphoma Study Group. *Blood* 84: 1361-1392.

497. Harris NL, Nadler LM, Bhan AK (1984). Immunohistologic characterization of two malignant lymphomas of germinal center type (centroblastic/centrocytic and centrocytic) with monoclonal antibodies. Follicular and diffuse lymphomas of small-cleaved-cell type are related but distinct entities. *Am J Pathol* 117: 262-272.

498. Harrison CN, Gale RE, Machin SJ, Linch DC (1999). A large proportion of patients with a diagnosis of essential thrombocythemia do not have a clonal disorder and may be at lower risk of thrombotic complications. *Blood* 93: 417-424.

499. Hart DN, Baker BW, Inglis MJ, Nimmo JC, Starling GC, Deacon E, Rowe M, Beard ME (1992). Epstein-Barr viral DNA in acute large granular lymphocyte (natural killer) leukemic cells. *Blood* 79: 2116-2123.

500. Hasenclever D, Diehl V (1998). A prognostic score for advanced Hodgkin's disease. International Prognostic Factors Project on Advanced Hodgkin's Disease. *N Engl J Med* 339: 1506-1514.

501. Hasle H (1994). Myelodysplastic syndromes in childhood – classification, epidemiology, and treatment. *Leuk Lymphoma* 13: 11-26.

502. Hasle H, Olesen G, Kerndrup G, Philip P, Jacobsen N (1996). Chronic neutrophil leukaemia in adolescence and young adulthood. *Br J Haematol* 94: 628-630.

503. Hastrup N, Hamilton-Dutoit S, Ralfkiaer E, Pallesen G (1991). Peripheral T-cell lymphomas: an evaluation of reproducibility of the updated Kiel classification. *Histopathology* 18: 99-105.

504. Hastrup N, Ralfkiaer E, Pallesen G (1989). Aberrant phenotypes in peripheral T cell lymphomas. *J Clin Pathol* 42: 398-402.

505. Hayhoe FG, Flemans RJ, Cowling DC (1979). Acquired lipidosis of marrow macrophages: birefringent blue crystals and Gaucher-like cells, sea-blue histiocytes, and grey-green crystals. *J Clin Pathol* 32: 420-428.

506. Head DR (1996). Revised classification of acute myeloid leukemia. *Leukemia* 10: 1826-1831.

507. Headington JT, Roth MS, Schnitzer B (1987). Regressing atypical histiocytosis: a review and critical appraisal. *Semin Diagn Pathol* 4: 28-37.

508. Heaney ML, Golde DW (1999). Myelodysplasia. *N Engl J Med* 340: 1649-1660.

509. Heerema NA, Sather HN, Sensel MG, Zhang T, Hutchinson RJ, Nachman JB, Lange BJ, Steinherz PG, Bostrom BC, Reaman GH, Gaynon PS, Uckun FM (2000). Prognostic impact of trisomies of chromosomes 10, 17, and 5 among children with acute lymphoblastic leukemia and high hyperdiploidy (>50 chromosomes). *J Clin Oncol* 18: 1876-1887.

510. Hehlmann R, Jahn M, Baumann B, Kopcke W (1988). Essential thrombocythemia. Clinical characteristics and course of 61 cases. *Cancer* 61: 2487-2496.

511. Hell K, Pringle JH, Hansmann ML, Lorenzen J, Colloby P, Lauder I, Fischer R (1993). Demonstration of light chain mRNA in Hodgkin's disease. *J Pathol* 171: 137-143.

512. Herbst H, Foss HD, Samol J, Araujo I, Klotzbach H, Krause H, Agathanggelou A, Niedobitek G, Stein H (1996). Frequent expression of interleukin-10 by Epstein-Barr virus-harboring tumor cells of Hodgkin's disease. *Blood* 87: 2918-2929.

513. Hermine O, Haioun C, Lepage E, d'Agay MF, Briere J, Lavignac C, Fillet G, Salles G, Marolleau JP, Diebold J, Reyas F, Gaulard P (1996). Prognostic significance of bcl-2 protein expression in aggressive non-Hodgkin's lymphoma. Groupe d'Etude des Lymphomes de l'Adulte (GELA). *Blood* 87: 265-272.

514. Hernandez JM, del Canizo MC, Cuneo A, Garcia JL, Gutierrez NC, Gonzalez M, Castoldi G, San Miguel JF (2000). Clinical, hematological and cytogenetic characteristics of atypical chronic myeloid leukemia. *Ann Oncol* 11: 441-444.

515. Hernandez L, Pinyol M, Hernandez S, Bea S, Pulford K, Rosenwald A, Lamant L, Falini B, Ott G, Mason DY, Delsol G, Campo E (1999). TRK-fused gene (TFG) is a new partner of ALK in anaplastic large cell lymphoma producing two structurally different TFG-ALK translocations. *Blood* 94: 3265-3268.

516. Herndier BG, Sanchez HC, Chang KL, Chen YY, Weiss LM (1993). High prevalence of Epstein-Barr virus in the Reed-Sternberg cells of HIV-associated Hodgkin's disease. *Am J Pathol* 142: 1073-1079.

517. Herzenberg AM, Lien J, Magil AB (1996). Monoclonal heavy chain (immunoglobulin G3) deposition disease: report of a case. *Am J Kidney Dis* 28: 128-131.

518. Hess JL, Bodis S, Pinkus G, Silver B, Mauch P (1994). Histopathologic grading of nodular sclerosis Hodgkin's disease. Lack of prognostic significance in 254 surgically staged patients. *Cancer* 74: 708-714.

519. Hess JL, Zutter MM, Castleberry RP, Emanuel PD (1996). Juvenile chronic myelogenous leukemia. *Am J Clin Pathol* 105: 238-248.

520. Hetet G, Dastot H, Baens M, Brizard A, Sigaux F, Grandchamp B, Stern MH (2000). Recurrent molecular deletion of the 12p13 region, centomeric to ETV6/TEL, in T-cell prolymphocytic leukemia. *Hematol J* 1: 42-47.

521. Higgins JP, Warnke RA (1999). CD30 expression is common in mediastinal large B-cell lymphoma. *Am J Clin Pathol* 112: 241-247.

522. Hill ME, MacLennan KA, Cunningham DC, Vaughan HB, Burke M, Clarke P, Di Stefano F, Anderson L, Vaughan HG, Mason D, Selby P, Linch DC (1996). Prognostic significance of BCL-2 expression and bcl-2 major breakpoint region rearrangement in diffuse large cell non-Hodgkin's lymphoma: a British National Lymphoma Investigation Study. *Blood* 88: 1046-1051.

523. Hisada M, Okayama A, Shioiri S, Spiegelman DL, Stuver SO, Mueller NE (1998). Risk factors for adult T-cell leukemia among carriers of human T-lymphotropic virus type I. *Blood* 92: 3557-3561.

524. Ho FC, Choy D, Loke SL, Kung IT, Fu KH, Liang R, Todd D, Khoo RK (1990). Polymorphic reticulosis and conventional lymphomas of the nose and upper aerodigestive tract: a clinicopathologic study of 70 cases, and immunophenotypic studies of 16 cases. *Hum Pathol* 21: 1041-1050.

525. Ho FC, Srivastava G, Loke SL, Fu KH, Leung BP, Liang R, Choy D (1990). Presence of Epstein-Barr virus DNA in nasal lymphomas of B and 'T' cell type. *Hematol Oncol* 8: 271-281.

526. Hockenbery DM, Zutter M, Hickey W, Nahm M, Korsmeyer SJ (1991). BCL2 protein is topographically restricted in tissues characterized by apoptotic cell death. *Proc Natl Acad Sci U S A* 88: 6961-6965.

527. Hodges KB, Collins RD, Greer JP, Kadin ME, Kinney MC (1999). Transformation of the small cell variant Ki-1+ lymphoma to anaplastic large cell lymphoma: pathologic and clinical features. *Am J Surg Pathol* 23: 49-58.

528. Hodgkin T (1832). On some morbid appearances of the absorbent glands and spleen. *Med Chir Soc Tr* 17: 68.

529. Hollingsworth HC, Stetler-Stevenson M, Gagneten D, Kingma DW, Raffeld M, Jaffe ES (1994). Immunodeficiency-associated malignant lymphoma. Three cases showing genotypic evidence of both T- and B-cell lineages. *Am J Surg Pathol* 18: 1092-1101.

530. Hollowood K, Stamp G, Zouvani I, Fletcher CD (1995). Extranodal follicular dendritic cell sarcoma of the gastrointestinal tract. Morphologic, immunohistochemical and ultrastructural analysis of two cases. *Am J Clin Pathol* 103: 90-97.

531. Holm LE, Blomgren H, Lowhagen T (1985). Cancer risks in patients with chronic lymphocytic thyroiditis. *N Engl J Med* 312: 601-604.

532. Horan RF, Austen KF (1991). Systemic mastocytosis: retrospective review of a decade's clinical experience at the Brigham and Women's Hospital. *J Invest Dermatol* 96: 5S-13S.

533. Horenstein MG, Nador RG, Chadburn A, Hyjek EM, Inghirami G, Knowles DM, Cesarman E (1997). Epstein-Barr virus latent gene expression in primary effusion lymphomas containing Kaposi's sarcoma-associated herpesvirus/human herpesvirus-8. *Blood* 90: 1186-1191.

534. Horning SJ, Rosenberg SA (1984). The natural history of initially untreated low-grade non-Hodgkin's lymphomas. *N Engl J Med* 311: 1471-1475.

535. Horny HP, Kaiserling E, Campbell M, Parwaresch MR, Lennert K (1989). Liver findings in generalized mastocytosis. A clinicopathologic study. *Cancer* 63: 532-538.

536. Horny HP, Kaiserling E, Handgretinger R, Ruck P, Frank D, Weber R, Jaschonek KG, Waller HD (1995). Evidence for a lymphotropic nature of circulating plasmacytoid monocytes: findings from a case of CD56+ chronic myelomonocytic leukemia. Eur J Haematol 54: 209-216.

537. Horny HP, Kaiserling E, Parwaresch MR, Lennert K (1992). Lymph node findings in generalized mastocytosis. Histopathology 21: 439-446.

538. Horny HP, Parwaresch MR, Kaiserling E, Muller K, Olbermann M, Mainzer K, Lennert K (1986). Mast cell sarcoma of the larynx. J Clin Pathol 39: 596-602.

539. Horny HP, Parwaresch MR, Lennert K (1985). Bone marrow findings in systemic mastocytosis. Hum Pathol 16: 808-814.

540. Horny HP, Ruck MT, Kaiserling E (1992). Spleen findings in generalized mastocytosis. A clinicopathologic study. Cancer 70: 459-468.

541. Horny HP, Sillaber C, Menke D, Kaiserling E, Wehrmann M, Stehberger B, Chott A, Lechner K, Lennert K, Valent P (1998). Diagnostic value of immunostaining for tryptase in patients with mastocytosis. Am J Surg Pathol 22: 1132-1140.

542. Horsman DE, Gascoyne RD, Coupland RW, Coldman AJ, Adomat SA (1995). Comparison of cytogenetic analysis, southern analysis, and polymerase chain reaction for the detection of t(14; 18) in follicular lymphoma. Am J Clin Pathol 103: 472-478.

543. Hounie H, Chittal SM, al Saati T, de Mascarel A, Sabattini E, Pileri S, Falini B, Ralfkiaer E, Le Tourneau A, Selves J (1992). Hairy cell leukemia. Diagnosis of bone marrow involvement in paraffin-embedded sections with monoclonal antibody DBA.44. Am J Clin Pathol 98: 26-33.

544. Howell WM, Leung ST, Jones DB, Nakshabendi I, Hall MA, Lanchbury JS, Ciclitira PJ, Wright DH (1995). HLA-DRB, -DQA, and -DQB polymorphism in celiac disease and enteropathy-associated T-cell lymphoma. Common features and additional risk factors for malignancy. Hum Immunol 43: 29-37.

545. Hsi ED, Picken MM, Alkan S (1998). Post-transplantation lymphoproliferative disorder of the NK-cell type: a case report and review of the literature. Mod Pathol 11: 479-484.

546. Hsu SM, Jaffe ES (1984). Leu M1 and peanut agglutinin stain the neoplastic cells of Hodgkin's disease. Am J Clin Pathol 82: 29-32.

547. Hu E, Weiss LM, Hoppe RT, Horning SJ (1985). Follicular and diffuse mixed small-cleaved and large-cell lymphoma – a clinicopathologic study. J Clin Oncol 3: 1183-1187.

548. Hu H (1987). Benzene-associated myelofibrosis. Ann Intern Med 106: 171-172.

549. Hui PK, Feller AC, Lennert K (1988). High-grade non-Hodgkin's lymphoma of B-cell type. I. Histopathology. Histopathology 12: 127-143.

550. Hummel M, Tamaru J, Kalvelage B, Stein H (1994). Mantle cell (previously centrocytic) lymphomas express VH genes with no or very little somatic mutations like the physiologic cells of the follicle mantle. Blood 84: 403-407.

551. Hurwitz CA, Raimondi SC, Head D, Krance R, Mirro J, Jr., Kalwinsky DK, Ayers GD, Behm FG (1992). Distinctive immunophenotypic features of t(8;21)(q22;q22) acute myeloblastic leukemia in children. Blood 80: 3182-3188.

552. Husby G, Blichfeldt P, Brinch L, Brandtzaeg P, Mellbye OJ, Sletten K, Stenstad T (1998). Chronic arthritis and gamma heavy chain disease: coincidence or pathogenic link? Scand J Rheumatol 27: 257-264.

553. Hussell T, Isaacson PG, Crabtree JE, Spencer J (1993). The response of cells from low-grade B-cell gastric lymphomas of mucosa-associated lymphoid tissue to Helicobacter pylori. Lancet 342: 571-574.

554. Iida S, Rao PH, Nallasivam P, Hibshoosh H, Butler M, Louie DC, Dyomin V, Ohno H, Chaganti RS, Dalla-Favera R (1996). The t(9;14)(p13;q32) chromosomal translocation associated with lymphoplasmacytoid lymphoma involves the PAX-5 gene. Blood 88: 4110-4117.

555. Iida S, Rao PH, Ueda R, Chaganti RS, Dalla-Favera R (1999). Chromosomal rearrangement of the PAX-5 locus in lymphoplasmacytic lymphoma with t(9;14)(p13;q32). Leuk Lymphoma 34: 25-33.

556. Ilowite NT, Flignar CL, Ochs HD, Brichacek B, Harada S, Haas JE, Purtilo DT, Wedgwood RJ (1986). Pulmonary angiitis with atypical lymphoreticular infiltrates in Wiskott-Aldrich syndrome: possible relationship of lymphomatoid granulomatosis and EBV infection. Clin Immunol Immunopathol 41: 479-484.

557. Imamura N, Kusunoki Y, Kawa-Ha K, Yumura K, Hara J, Oda K, Abe K, Dohy H, Inada T, Kajihara H (1990). Aggressive natural killer cell leukaemia/lymphoma: report of four cases and review of the literature. Possible existence of a new clinical entity originating from the third lineage of lymphoid cells. Br J Haematol 75: 49-59.

558. Imamura N, Kusunoki Y, Oda K, Abe K, Dohi H, Inada T, Kuramoto A, Kajihara H, Fujii H, Kawa K (1989). [Aggressive natural killer cell leukaemia/lymphoma – possible existence of a new clinical entity originating from the third lineage of lymphoid cells]. Rinsho Ketsueki 30: 193-201.

559. Inghirami G, Foitl DR, Sabichi A, Zhu BY, Knowles DM (1991). Autoantibody-associated cross-reactive idiotype-bearing human B lymphocytes: distribution and characterization, including Ig VH gene and CD5 antigen expression. Blood 78: 1503-1515.

560. Inhorn RC, Aster JC, Roach SA, Slapak CA, Soiffer R, Tantravahi R, Stone RM (1995). A syndrome of lymphoblastic lymphoma, eosinophilia, and myeloid hyperplasia/malignancy associated with t(8;13)(p11;q11): description of a distinctive clinicopathologic entity. Blood 85: 1881-1887.

561. Invernizzi R, Custodi P, de Fazio P, Bergamaschi G, Fenoglio C, Ricevuti G, Rosti V, Zambelli LM, Ascari E (1990). The syndrome of abnormal chromatin clumping in leucocytes: clinical and biological study of a case. Haematologica 75: 532-536.

562. Inwald DP, Peters MJ, Walshe D, Jones A, Davies EG, Klein NJ (2000). Absence of platelet CD40L identifies patients with X-linked hyper IgM syndrome. Clin Exp Immunol 120: 499-502.

563. Isaacson PG (1994). Gastrointestinal lymphoma. Hum Pathol 25: 1020-1029.

564. Isaacson PG, Dogan A, Price SK, Spencer J (1989). Immunoproliferative small-intestinal disease. An immunohistochemical study. Am J Surg Pathol 13: 1023-1033.

565. Isaacson PG, Matutes E, Burke M, Catovsky D (1994). The histopathology of splenic lymphoma with villous lymphocytes. Blood 84: 3828-3834.

566. Isaacson PG, Norton AJ (1994). Extranodal lymphomas. Churchill Livingstone: Edinburgh, London, Madrid, Melbourne, New York, Tokyo.

567. Isaacson PG, Norton AJ, Addis BJ (1987). The human thymus contains a novel population of B lymphocytes. Lancet 2: 1488-1491.

568. Isaacson PG, O'Connor NT, Spencer J, Bevan DH, Connolly CE, Kirkham N, Pollock DJ, Wainscoat JS, Stein H, Mason DY (1985). Malignant histiocytosis of the intestine: a T-cell lymphoma. Lancet 2: 688-691.

569. Isaacson PG, Spencer J (1987). Malignant lymphoma of mucosa-associated lymphoid tissue. Histopathology 11: 445-462.

570. Isaacson PG, Wotherspoon AC, Diss T, Pan LX (1991). Follicular colonization in B-cell lymphoma of mucosa-associated lymphoid tissue. Am J Surg Pathol 15: 819-828.

571. Ishihara S, Ohshima K, Tokura Y, Yabuta R, Imaishi H, Wakiguchi H, Kurashige T, Kishimoto H, Katayama I, Okada S, Kawa-Ha K (1997). Hypersensitivity to mosquito bites conceals clonal lymphoproliferation of Epstein-Barr viral DNA-positive natural killer cells. Jpn J Cancer Res 88: 82-87.

572. Ishihara S, Okada S, Wakiguchi H, Kurashige T, Hirai K, Kawa-Ha K (1997). Clonal lymphoproliferation following chronic active Epstein-Barr virus infection and hypersensitivity to mosquito bites. Am J Hematol 54: 276-281.

573. Isomaki HA, Hakulinen T, Joutsenlahti U (1978). Excess risk of lymphomas, leukemia and myeloma in patients with rheumatoid arthritis. J Chronic Dis 31: 691-696.

574. Jacknow G, Frizzera G, Gajl-Peczalska K, Banks PM, Arthur DC, McGlave PB, Hurd DD (1985). Extramedullary presentation of the blast crisis of chronic myelogenous leukaemia. Br J Haematol 61: 225-236.

575. Jacob J, Kelsoe G, Rajewsky K, Weiss U (1991). Intraclonal generation of antibody mutants in germinal centres. Nature 354: 389-392.

576. Jaffe ES (1995). Angioimmunoblastic T-cell lymphoma: new insights, but the clinical challenge remains. Ann Oncol 6: 631-632.

577. Jaffe ES (1995). Malignant histiocytosis and true histiocytic lymphomas. In: Surgical pathology of lymph nodes and related organs., Jaffe ES, ed. 2nd. W.B. Saunders Co.: Philadelphia, 560-593.

578. Jaffe ES (1995). Nasal and nasal-type T/NK cell lymphoma: a unique form of lymphoma associated with the Epstein-Barr virus [comment]. Histopathology 27: 581-583.

579. Jaffe ES (1995). Post-thymic T-cell lymphomas. In: Surgical Pathology of the Lymph Nodes and Related Organs (Major Problems in Pathology Series, Vol. 16) 2nd ed., W.B. Saunders Company: Philadelphia, pp. 360.

580. Jaffe ES (1996). Classification of natural killer (NK) cell and NK-like T-cell malignancies. Blood 87: 1207-1210.

581. Jaffe ES (1999). Nasal/nasal type NK/T cell lymphoma (angiocentric lymphoma) and lymphomatoid granulomatosis. In: Human Lymphoma: Clinical Implications of the REAL Classification, Mason DY, Harris NL, eds. Springer: London, pp. 32.1-32.6.

582. Jaffe ES (2001). Anaplastic large cell lymphoma: the shifting sands of diagnostic hematopathology. Mod Pathol 14: 219-228.

583. Jaffe ES, Blattner WA, Blayney DW, Bunn PA, Jr., Cossman J, Robert-Guroff M, Gallo RC (1984). The pathologic spectrum of adult T-cell leukemia/lymphoma in the United States. Human T-cell leukemia/lymphoma virus-associated lymphoid malignancies. Am J Surg Pathol 8: 263-275.

584. Jaffe ES, Chan JK, Su IJ, Frizzera G, Mori S, Feller AC, Ho FC (1996). Report of the Workshop on Nasal and Related Extranodal Angiocentric T/Natural Killer Cell Lymphomas. Definitions, differential diagnosis, and epidemiology. Am J Surg Pathol 20: 103-111.

585. Jaffe ES, Costa J, Fauci AS, Cossman J, Tsokos M (1983). Malignant lymphoma and erythrophagocytosis simulating malignant histiocytosis. Am J Med 75: 741-749.

586. Jaffe ES, Harris NL, Diebold J, Muller-Hermelink HK (1998). World Health Organization Classification of lymphomas: a work in progress. Ann Oncol 9 Suppl 5:S25-30: S25-S30.

587. Jaffe ES, Krenacs L, Kumar S, Kingma DW, Raffeld M (1999). Extranodal peripheral T-cell and NK-cell neoplasms. Am J Clin Pathol 111: S46-S55.

588. Jaffe ES, Krenacs L, Raffeld M (1997). Classification of T-cell and NK-cell neoplasms based on the REAL classification. Ann Oncol 8 Suppl 2: 17-24.

589. Jaffe ES, Puck JM, Jackson CE, Dale JK, Sneller MC, Fisher RE, Hsu AP, Lenardo MJ, Straus.S.E. (1999). Increased risk for diverse lymphomas in autoimmune lymphoproliferative syndrome (ALPS), an inherited disorder due to defective lymphocyte apoptosis. Blood 94: 597a.

590. Jaffe ES, Wilson WH (1997). Lymphomatoid granulomatosis: pathogenesis, pathology and clinical implications. *Cancer Surv* 30:233-48: 233-248.

591. Jaffe ES, Zarate-Osorno A, Medeiros LJ (1992). The interrelationship of Hodgkin's disease and non-Hodgkin's lymphomas – lessons learned from composite and sequential malignancies. *Semin Diagn Pathol* 9: 297-303.

592. James JM, Brouet JC, Orvoenfrija E, Capron F, Brechot J, Danon F, Diebold J, Rochemaure J, Zittoun R (1987). Waldenstrom's macroglobulinaemia in a bird breeder: a case history with pulmonary involvement and antibody activity of the monoclonal IgM to canary's droppings. *Clin Exp Immunol* 68: 397-401.

593. Janckila AJ, Gentile PS, Yam LT (1991). Hemopoietic inhibition in hairy cell leukemia. *Am J Hematol* 38: 30-39.

594. Jantunen R, Juvonen E, Ikkala E, Oksanen K, Anttila P, Hormila P, Jansson SE, Kekomaki R, Ruutu T (1998). Essential thrombocythemia at diagnosis: causes of diagnostic evaluation and presence of positive diagnostic findings. *Ann Hematol* 77: 101-106.

595. Jary L, Mossafa H, Fourcade C, Genet P, Pulik M, Flandrin G (1997). The 17p-syndrome: a distinct myelodysplastic syndrome entity? *Leuk Lymphoma* 25: 163-168.

596. Jensen RT (2000). Gastrointestinal abnormalities and involvement in systemic mastocytosis. *Hematol Oncol Clin North Am* 14: 579-623.

597. Jerne NK (1974). Towards a network theory of the immune system. *Ann Immunol (Paris)* 125C: 373-389.

598. Jhala DN, Medeiros LJ, Lopez-Terrada D, Jhala NC, Krishnan B, Shahab I (2000). Neutrophil-rich anaplastic large cell lymphoma of T-cell lineage. A report of two cases arising in HIV-positive patients. *Am J Clin Pathol* 114: 478-482.

599. Jones AM, Gaspar HB (2000). Immunogenetics: changing the face of immunodeficiency. *J Clin Pathol* 53: 60-65.

600. Jones D, Jorgensen JL, Shahsafaei A, Dorfman DM (1998). Characteristic proliferations of reticular and dendritic cells in angioimmunoblastic lymphoma. *Am J Surg Pathol* 22: 956-964.

601. Jones D, O'Hara C, Kraus MD, Perez-Atayde AR, Shahsafaei A, Wu L, Dorfman DM (2000). Expression pattern of T-cell-associated chemokine receptors and their chemokines correlates with specific subtypes of T-cell non-Hodgkin lymphoma. *Blood* 96: 685-690.

602. Jones SE, Fuks Z, Bull M, Kadin ME, Dorfman RF, Kaplan HS, Rosenberg SA, Kim H (1973). Non-Hodgkin's lymphomas. IV. Clinicopathologic correlation in 405 cases. *Cancer* 31: 806-823.

603. Joos S, Kupper M, Ohl S, von Bonin F, Mechtersheimer G, Bentz M, Marynen P, Moller P, Pfreundschuh M, Trumper L, Lichter P (2000). Genomic imbalances including amplification of the tyrosine kinase gene JAK2 in CD30+ Hodgkin cells. *Cancer Res* 60: 549-552.

604. Joos S, Otano-Joos MI, Ziegler S, Bruderlein S, du MS, Bentz M, Moller P, Lichter P (1996). Primary mediastinal (thymic) B-cell lymphoma is characterized by gains of chromosomal material including 9p and amplification of the REL gene. *Blood* 87: 1571-1578.

605. Jorgensen C, Legouffe MC, Perney P, Coste J, Tissot B, Segarra C, Bologna C, Bourrat L, Combe B, Blanc F, Sany J (1996). Sicca syndrome associated with hepatitis C virus infection. *Arthritis Rheum* 39: 1166-1171.

606. Joseph G, Barker RL, Yuan B, Martin A, Medeiros J, Peiper SC (1994). Post-transplantation plasma cell dyscrasias. *Cancer* 74: 1959-1964.

607. Josting A, Wolf J, Diehl V (2000). Hodgkin disease: prognostic factors and treatment strategies. *Curr Opin Oncol* 12: 403-411.

608. Jox A, Zander T, Kuppers R, Irsch J, Kanzler H, Kornacker M, Bohlen H, Diehl V, Wolf J (1999). Somatic mutations within the untranslated regions of rearranged Ig genes in a case of classical Hodgkin's disease as a potential cause for the absence of Ig in the lymphoma cells. *Blood* 93: 3964-3972.

609. Juliusson G, Merup M (1998). Cytogenetics in chronic lymphocytic leukemia. *Semin Oncol* 25: 19-26.

610. Jundt F, Anagnostopoulos I, Bommert K, Emmerich F, Muller G, Foss HD, Royer HD, Stein H, Dorken B (1999). Hodgkin/Reed-Sternberg cells induce fibroblasts to secrete eotaxin, a potent chemoattractant for T cells and eosinophils. *Blood* 94: 2065-2071.

611. Juneja SK, Imbert M, Jouault H, Scoazec JY, Sigaux F, Sultan C (1983). Haematological features of primary myelodysplastic syndromes (PMDS) at initial presentation: a study of 118 cases. *J Clin Pathol* 36: 1129-1135.

612. Juneja SK, Imbert M, Sigaux F, Jouault H, Sultan C (1983). Prevalence and distribution of ringed sideroblasts in primary myelodysplastic syndromes. *J Clin Pathol* 36: 566-569.

613. Jungnickel B, Staratschek-Jox A, auninger A, Spieker T, Wolf J, Diehl V, Hansmann ML, Rajewsky K, uppers R (2000). Clonal deleterious mutations in the IkappaBalpha gene in the malignant cells in Hodgkin's lymphoma. *J Exp Med* 191: 395-402.

614. Kadin M, Nasu K, Sako D, Said J, Vonderheid E (1985). Lymphomatoid papulosis. A cutaneous proliferation of activated helper T cells expressing Hodgkin's disease-associated antigens. *Am J Pathol* 119: 315-325.

615. Kadin ME, Agnarsson BA, Ellingsworth LR, Newcom SR (1990). Immunohistochemical evidence of a role for transforming growth factor beta in the pathogenesis of nodular sclerosing Hodgkin's disease. *Am J Pathol* 136: 1209-1214.

616. Kadin ME, Berard CW, Nanba K, Wakasa H (1983). Lymphoproliferative diseases in Japan and Western countries: Proceedings of the United States-Japan Seminar, September 6 and 7, 1982, in Seattle, Washington. *Hum Pathol* 14: 745-772.

617. Kadin ME, Liebowitz DN (1999). Cytokines and cytokine receptors in Hodgkin's disease. In: *Hodgkin's Disease*, Mauch P, Armitage JO, Diehl V, eds. Lippincott Williams & Wilkins: Philadelphia, pp. 139.

618. Kambham N, Markowitz GS, Appel GB, Kleiner MJ, Aucouturier P, D'agati VD (1999). Heavy chain deposition disease: the disease spectrum. *Am J Kidney Dis* 33: 954-962.

619. Kamel OW, Gocke CD, Kell DL, Cleary ML, Warnke RA (1995). True histiocytic lymphoma: a study of 12 cases based on current definition. *Leuk Lymphoma* 18: 81-86.

620. Kamel OW, Holly EA, van de RM, Lele C, Sah A (1999). A population based, case control study of non-Hodgkin's lymphoma in patients with rheumatoid arthritis. *J Rheumatol* 26: 1676-1680.

621. Kamel OW, van de RM, LeBrun DP, Weiss LM, Warnke RA, Dorfman RF (1994). Lymphoid neoplasms in patients with rheumatoid arthritis and dermatomyositis: frequency of Epstein-Barr virus and other features associated with immunosuppression. *Hum Pathol* 25: 638-643.

622. Kamel OW, van de RM, Weiss LM, Del Zoppo GJ, Hench PK, Robbins BA, Montgomery PG, Warnke RA, Dorfman RF (1993). Brief report: reversible lymphomas associated with Epstein-Barr virus occurring during methotrexate therapy for rheumatoid arthritis and dermatomyositis. *N Engl J Med* 328: 1317-1321.

623. Kamel OW, Weiss LM, van de RM, Colby TV, Kingma DW, Jaffe ES (1996). Hodgkin's disease and lymphoproliferations resembling Hodgkin's disease in patients receiving long-term low-dose methotrexate therapy. *Am J Surg Pathol* 20: 1279-1287.

624. Kanavaros P, Gaulard P, Charlotte F, Martin N, Ducos C, Lebezu M, Mason DY (1995). Discordant expression of immunoglobulin and its associated molecule mb-1/CD79a is frequently found in mediastinal large B cell lymphomas. *Am J Pathol* 146: 735-741.

625. Kanavaros P, Lescs MC, Briere J, Divine M, Galateau F, Joab I, Bosq J, Farcet JP, Reyes F, Gaulard P (1993). Nasal T-cell lymphoma: a clinicopathologic entity associated with peculiar phenotype and with Epstein-Barr virus. *Blood* 81: 2688-2695.

626. Kaneko Y, Maseki N, Sakurai M, Takayama S, Nanba K, Kikuchi M, Frizzera G (1988). Characteristic karyotypic pattern in T-cell lymphoproliferative disorders with reactive "angioimmunoblastic lymphadenopathy with dysproteinemia-type" features. *Blood* 72: 413-421.

627. Kant JA, Hubbard SM, Longo DL, Simon RM, DeVita VT, Jaffe ES (1986). The pathologic and clinical heterogeneity of lymphocyte-depleted Hodgkin's disease. *J Clin Oncol* 4: 284-294.

628. Kantarjian HM, Deisseroth A, Kurzrock R, Estrov Z, Talpaz M (1993). Chronic myelogenous leukemia: a concise update. *Blood* 82: 691-703.

629. Kantarjian HM, Keating MJ, Smith TL, Talpaz M, McCredie KB (1990). Proposal for a simple synthesis prognostic staging system in chronic myelogenous leukemia. *Am J Med* 88: 1-8.

630. Kantarjian HM, McLaughlin P, Fuller LM, Dixon DO, Osborne BM, Cabanillas FF (1984). Follicular large cell lymphoma: analysis and prognostic factors in 62 patients. *J Clin Oncol* 2: 811-819.

631. Kanzler H, Kuppers R, Hansmann ML, Rajewsky K (1996). Hodgkin and Reed-Sternberg cells in Hodgkin's disease represent the outgrowth of a dominant tumor clone derived from (crippled) germinal center B cells. *J Exp Med* 184: 1495-1505.

632. Kaplan MA, Ferry JA, Harris NL, Jacobson JO (1994). Clonal analysis of posttransplant lymphoproliferative disorders, using both episomal Epstein-Barr virus and immunoglobulin genes as markers. *Am J Clin Pathol* 101: 590-596.

633. Kaplan MA, Jacobson JO, Ferry JA, Harris NL (1993). T-cell lymphoma of the vulva in a renal allograft recipient with associated hemophagocytosis. *Am J Surg Pathol* 17: 842-849.

634. Kapp U, Yeh WC, Patterson B, Elia AJ, Kagi D, Ho A, Hessel A, Tipsword M, Williams A, Mirtsos C, Itie A, Moyle M, Mak TW (1999). Interleukin 13 is secreted by and stimulates the growth of Hodgkin and Reed-Sternberg cells. *J Exp Med* 189: 1939-1946.

635. Kaptain S, Zukerberg LR, Ferry JA, Harris NL (1998). BCL-1 cyclin D1+CD5+ mantle cell lymphoma. *Mod Pathol* 11: 133a.

636. Karp JE, Smith MA (1997). The molecular pathogenesis of treatment-induced (secondary) leukemias: foundations for treatment and prevention. *Semin Oncol* 24: 103-113.

637. Kassan SS, Thomas TL, Moutsopoulos HM, Hoover R, Kimberly RP, Budman DR, Costa J, Decker JL, Chused TM (1978). Increased risk of lymphoma in sicca syndrome. *Ann Intern Med* 89: 888-892.

638. Kato I, Tajima K, Suchi T, Aozasa K, Matsuzuka F, Kuma K, Tominaga S (1985). Chronic thyroiditis as a risk factor of B-cell lymphoma in the thyroid gland. *Jpn J Cancer Res* 76: 1085-1090.

639. Kato K, Ohshima K, Ishihara S, Anzai K, Suzumiya J, Kikuchi M (1998). Elevated serum soluble Fas ligand in natural killer cell proliferative disorders. *Br J Haematol* 103: 1164-1166.

640. Katzenstein AL, Carrington CB, Liebow AA (1979). Lymphomatoid granulomatosis: a clinicopathologic study of 152 cases. *Cancer* 43: 360-373.

641. Katzenstein AL, Peiper SC (1990). Detection of Epstein-Barr virus genomes in lymphomatoid granulomatosis: analysis of 29 cases by the polymerase chain reaction technique. *Mod Pathol* 3: 435-441.

642. Kawa-Ha K, Ishihara S, Ninomiya T, Yumura-Yagi K, Hara J, Murayama F, Tawa A, Hirai K (1989). CD3-negative lymphoproliferative disease of granular lymphocytes containing Epstein-Barr viral DNA. *J Clin Invest* 84: 51-55.

643. Kawaguchi H, Miyashita T, Herbst H, Niedobitek G, Asada M, Tsuchida M, Hanada R, Kinoshita A, Sakurai M, Kobayashi N, . (1993). Epstein-Barr virus-infected T lymphocytes in Epstein-Barr virus-associated hemophagocytic syndrome. *J Clin Invest* 92: 1444-1450.

644. Kawano F, Yamaguchi K, Nishimura H, Tsuda H, Takatsuki K (1985). Variation in the clinical courses of adult T-cell leukemia. *Cancer* 55: 851-856.

645. Keating MJ, Kantarjian H, O'Brien S, Koller C, Talpaz M, Schachner J, Childs CC, Freireich EJ, McCredie KB (1991). Fludarabine: a new agent with marked cytoreductive activity in untreated chronic lymphocytic leukemia. *J Clin Oncol* 9: 44-49.

646. Keller RT, Roth HP (1970). Hyperchlorhydria and hyperhistaminemia in a patient with systemic mastocytosis. *N Engl J Med* 283: 1449-1450.

647. Kern DE, Kidd PG, Moe R, Hanke D, Olerud JE (1998). Analysis of T-cell receptor gene rearrangement in lymph nodes of patients with mycosis fungoides. Prognostic implications. *Arch Dermatol* 134: 158-164.

648. Kern WF, Spier CM, Hanneman EH, Miller TP, Matzner M, Grogan TM (1992). Neural cell adhesion molecule-positive peripheral T-cell lymphoma: a rare variant with a propensity for unusual sites of involvement. *Blood* 79: 2432-2437.

649. Kersey JH (1997). Fifty years of studies of the biology and therapy of childhood leukemia. *Blood* 90: 4243-4251.

650. Khalidi HS, Brynes RK, Medeiros LJ, Chang KL, Slovak ML, Snyder DS, Arber DA (1998). The immunophenotype of blast transformation of chronic myelogenous leukemia: a high frequency of mixed lineage phenotype in "lymphoid" blasts and A comparison of morphologic, immunophenotypic, and molecular findings. *Mod Pathol* 11: 1211-1221.

651. Khouri IF, Lee MS, Romaguera J, Mirza N, Kantarjian H, Korbling M, Albitar M, Giralt S, Samuels B, Anderlini P, Rodriguez J, von Wolff B, Gajewski J, Cabanillas F, Champlin R (1999). Allogeneic hematopoietic transplantation for mantle-cell lymphoma: molecular remissions and evidence of graft-versus-malignancy. *Ann Oncol* 10: 1293-1299.

652. Khouri IF, Romaguera J, Kantarjian H, Palmer JL, Pugh WC, Korbling M, Hagemeister F, Samuels B, Rodriguez A, Giralt S, Younes A, Przepiorka D, Claxton D, Cabanillas F, Champlin R (1998). Hyper-CVAD and high-dose methotrexate/cytarabine followed by stem-cell transplantation: an active regimen for aggressive mantle-cell lymphoma. *J Clin Oncol* 16: 3803-3809.

653. Kilgore ES (1927). Polycythemia in feather dyers. *JAMA* 89: 343-344.

654. Killick S, Matutes E, Powles RL, Hamblin M, Swansbury J, Treleaven JG, Zomas A, Atra A, Catovsky D (1999). Outcome of biphenotypic acute leukemia. *Haematologica* 84: 699-706.

655. Kim YH, Hoppe RT (1999). Mycosis fungoides and the Sezary syndrome. *Semin Oncol* 26: 276-289.

656. Kingma DW, Mueller BU, Frekko K, Sorbara LR, Wood LV, Katz D, Raffeld M, Jaffe ES (1999). Low-grade monoclonal Epstein-Barr virus-associated lymphoproliferative disorder of the brain presenting as human immunodeficiency virus-associated encephalopathy in a child with acquired immunodeficiency syndrome. *Arch Pathol Lab Med* 123: 83-87.

657. Kinney MC, Collins RD, Greer JP, Whitlock JA, Sioutos N, Kadin ME (1993). A small-cell-predominant variant of primary Ki-1 (CD30)+ T-cell lymphoma. *Am J Surg Pathol* 17: 859-868.

658. Kipps TJ (1989). The CD5 B cell. *Adv Immunol* 47: 117-185.

659. Kipps TJ, Carson DA (1993). Autoantibodies in chronic lymphocytic leukemia and related systemic autoimmune diseases. *Blood* 81: 2475-2487.

660. Kirn D, Mauch P, Shaffer K, Pinkus G, Shipp MA, Kaplan WD, Tung N, Wheeler C, Beard CJ, Canellos GP (1993). Large-cell and immunoblastic lymphoma of the mediastinum: prognostic features and treatment outcome in 57 patients. *J Clin Oncol* 11: 1336-1343.

661. Kirshenbaum AS, Goff JP, Semere T, Foster B, Scott LM, Metcalfe DD (1999). Demonstration that human mast cells arise from a progenitor cell population that is CD34(+), c-kit(+), and expresses aminopeptidase N (CD13). *Blood* 94: 2333-2342.

662. Kita K, Nakase K, Miwa H, Masuya M, Nishii K, Morita N, Takakura N, Otsuji A, Shirakawa S, Ueda T (1992). Phenotypical characteristics of acute myelocytic leukemia associated with the t(8;21)(q22;q22) chromosomal abnormality: frequent expression of immature B-cell antigen CD19 together with stem cell antigen CD34. *Blood* 80: 470-477.

663. Kitano K, Ichikawa N, Mahbub B, Ueno M, Ito T, Shimodaira S, Kodaira H, Ishida F, Kobayashi H, Saito H, Okubo Y, Enokihara H, Kiyosawa K (1996). Eosinophilia associated with proliferation of CD(3+)4-(8-) alpha beta+ T cells with chromosome 16 anomalies. *Br J Haematol* 92: 315-317.

664. Kiyokawa T, Yamaguchi K, Takeya M, Takahashi K, Watanabe T, Matsumoto T, Lee SY, Takatsuki K (1987). Hypercalcemia and osteoclast proliferation in adult T-cell leukemia. *Cancer* 59: 1187-1191.

665. Klein U, Klein G, Ehlin-Henriksson B, Rajewsky K, Kuppers R (1995). Burkitt's lymphoma is a malignancy of mature B cells expressing somatically mutated V region genes. *Mol Med* 1: 495-505.

666. Klein U, Rajewsky K, Kuppers R (1998). Human immunoglobulin (Ig)M+IgD+ peripheral blood B cells expressing the CD27 cell surface antigen carry somatically mutated variable region genes: CD27 as a general marker for somatically mutated (memory) B cells. *J Exp Med* 188: 1679-1689.

667. Kluin PM, Feller A, Gaulard P, Jaffe ES, Meijer CJ, Muller-Hermelink HK, Pileri S (2001). Peripheral T/NK-cell lymphoma: a report of the IXth Workshop of the European Assocation for Haematopathology Conference report. *Histopathology* 38: 250-270.

668. Knowles DM (1999). Morphologic, immunologic and genetic features of lymphoproliferative disorders associated with immunodeficiency. In: *Human Lymphoma: Clinical Implications of the REAL Classification*, Mason DY, Harris NL, eds. Springer: London, pp.

669. Knowles DM (2001). *Neoplastic Hematopathology*. 2nd. Lippincott Williams & Wilkins: Philadelphia.

670. Knowles DM, Cesarman E, Chadburn A, Frizzera G, Chen J, Rose EA, Michler RE (1995). Correlative morphologic and molecular genetic analysis demonstrates three distinct categories of posttransplantation lymphoproliferative disorders. *Blood* 85: 552-565.

671. Knowles DM, Chamulak GA, Subar M, Burke JS, Dugan M, Wernz J, Slywotzky C, Pelicci G, Dalla-Favera R, Raphael B (1988). Lymphoid neoplasia associated with the acquired immunodeficiency syndrome (AIDS). The New York University Medical Center experience with 105 patients (1981-1986). *Ann Intern Med* 108: 744-753.

672. Knowles DM, Inghirami G, Ubriaco A, Dalla-Favera R (1989). Molecular genetic analysis of three AIDS-associated neoplasms of uncertain lineage demonstrates their B-cell derivation and the possible pathogenetic role of the Epstein-Barr virus. *Blood* 73: 792-799.

673. Knuutila S, Alitalo R, Ruutu T (1993). Power of the MAC (morphology-antibody-chromosomes) method in distinguishing reactive and clonal cells: report of a patient with acute lymphatic leukemia, eosinophilia, and t(5;14). *Genes Chromosomes Cancer* 8: 219-223.

674. Ko YH, Kim SH, Ree HJ (1998). Blastic NK-cell lymphoma expressing terminal deoxynucleotidyl transferase with Homer-Wright type pseudorosettes formation. *Histopathology* 33: 547-553.

675. Kobashi Y, Nakamura S, Sasajima Y, Koshikawa T, Yatabe Y, Kitoh K, Mori S, Ueda R, Yamabe H, Suchi T (1996). Inconsistent association of Epstein-Barr virus with CD56 (NCAM)-positive angiocentric lymphoma occuring in sites other than the upper and lower respiratory tract. *Histopathology* 28: 111-120.

676. Kobayashi Y, Uehara S, Inamori K, Shirato R, Ozawa K, Sklar J, Asano S (1996). Hemophagocytosis as a para-neoplastic syndrome in NK cell leukemia. *Int J Hematol* 64: 135-142.

677. Koeffler HP, Levine AM, Sparkes M, Sparkes RS (1980). Chronic myelocytic leukemia: eosinophils involved in the malignant clone. *Blood* 55: 1063-1065.

678. Koike T, Uesugi Y, Toba K, Narita M, Fuse I, Takahashi M, Shibata A (1995). 5q-syndrome presenting as essential thrombocythemia: myelodysplastic syndrome or chronic myeloproliferative disorders? *Leukemia* 9: 517-518.

679. Koita H, Suzumiya J, Ohshima K, Takeshita M, Kimura N, Kikuchi M, Koono M (1997). Lymphoblastic lymphoma expressing natural killer cell phenotype with involvement of the mediastinum and nasal cavity. *Am J Surg Pathol* 21: 242-248.

680. Koizumi K, Sawada K, Nishio M, Katagiri E, Fukae J, Fukada Y, Tarumi T, Notoya A, Shimizu T, Abe R, Kobayashi H, Koike T (1997). Effective high-dose chemotherapy followed by autologous peripheral blood stem cell transplantation in a patient with the aggressive form of cytophagic histiocytic panniculitis. *Bone Marrow Transplant* 20: 171-173.

681. Kojima M, Nakamura S, Itoh H, Ohno Y, Masawa N, Joshita T, Suchi T (1999). Mast cell sarcoma with tissue eosinophilia arising in the ascending colon. *Mod Pathol* 12: 739-743.

682. Kolde G, Brocker EB (1986). Multiple skin tumors of indeterminate cells in an adult. *J Am Acad Dermatol* 15: 591-597.

683. Kondo T, Kono H, Miyamoto N, Yoshida R, Toki H, Matsumoto I, Hara M, Inoue H, Inatsuki A, Funatsu T (1989). Age- and sex-specific cumulative rate and risk of ATLL for HTLV-I carriers. *Int J Cancer* 43: 1061-1064.

684. Konigsberg R, Zojer N, Ackermann J, Kromer E, Kittler H, Fritz E, Kaufmann H, Nosslinger T, Riedl L, Gisslinger H, Jager U, Simonitsch I, Heinz R, Ludwig H, Huber H, Drach J (2000). Predictive role of interphase cytogenetics for survival of patients with multiple myeloma. *J Clin Oncol* 18: 804-812.

685. Konrad RJ, Kricka LJ, Goodman DB, Goldman J, Silberstein LE (1993). Brief report: myeloma-associated paraprotein directed against the HIV-1 p24 antigen in an HIV-1-seropositive patient. *N Engl J Med* 328: 1817-1819.

686. Koss MN, Hochholzer L, Langloss JM, Wehunt WD, Lazarus AA, Nichols PW (1986). Lymphomatoid granulomatosis: a clinicopathologic study of 42 patients. *Pathology* 18: 283-288.

687. Kouides PA, Bennett JM (1996). Morphology and classification of the myelodysplastic syndromes and their pathologic variants. *Semin Hematol* 33: 95-110.

688. Kounami S, Aoyagi N, Tsuno H, Suzuki H, Kitano N, Koike M (1997). Additional chromosome abnormalities in transient abnormal myelopoiesis in Down's syndrome patients. *Acta Haematol* 98: 109-112.

689. Krafft AE, Taubenberger JK, Sheng ZM, Bijwaard KE, Abbondanzo SL, Aguilera NS, Lichy JH (1999). Enhanced sensitivity with a novel TCRgamma PCR assay for clonality studies in 569 formalin-fixed, paraffin-embedded (FFPE) cases. *Mol Diagn* 4: 119-133.

690. Krappmann D, Emmerich F, Kordes U, Scharschmidt E, Dorken B, Scheidereit C (1999). Molecular mechanisms of constitutive NF-kappaB/Rel activation in Hodgkin/Reed-Sternberg cells. *Oncogene* 18: 943-953.

691. Kraus MD, Crawford DF, Kaleem Z, Shenoy S, MacArthur CA, Longtine JA (1998). T gamma/delta hepatosplenic lymphoma in a heart transplant patient after an Epstein-Barr virus positive lymphoproliferative disorder: a case report. *Cancer* 82: 983-992.

692. Krenacs L, Himmelmann AW, Quintanilla-Martinez L, Fest T, Riva A, Wellmann A, Bagdi E, Kehrl JH, Jaffe ES, Raffeld M (1998). Transcription factor B-cell-specific activator protein (BSAP) is differentially expressed in B cells and in subsets of B-cell lymphomas. *Blood* 92: 1308-1316.

693. Krenacs L, Tiszalvicz L, Krenacs T, Boumsell L (1993). Immunohistochemical detection of CD1A antigen in formalin-fixed and paraffin-embedded tissue sections with monoclonal antibody 010. *J Pathol* 171: 99-104.

694. Krenacs L, Wellmann A, Sorbara L, Himmelmann AW, Bagdi E, Jaffe ES, Raffeld M (1997). Cytotoxic cell antigen expression in anaplastic large cell lymphomas of T- and null-cell type and Hodgkin's disease: evidence for distinct cellular origin. *Blood* 89: 980-989.

695. Kroft SH, Finn WG, Peterson LC (1995). The pathology of the chronic lymphoid leukaemias. *Blood Rev* 9: 234-250.

696. Kronland R, Grogan T, Spier C, Wirt D, Rangel C, Richter L, Durie B, Greenberg B, Miller T, Jones S (1985). Immunotopographic assessment of lymphoid and plasma cell malignancies in the bone marrow. *Hum Pathol* 16: 1247-1254.

697. Kubagawa H, Vogler LB, Capra JD, Conrad ME, Lawton AR, Cooper MD (1979). Studies on the clonal origin of multiple myeloma. Use of individually specific (idiotype) antibodies to trace the oncogenic event to its earliest point of expression in B-cell differentiation. *J Exp Med* 150: 792-807.

698. Kueck BD, Smith RE, Parkin J, Peterson LC, Hanson CA (1991). Eosinophilic leukaemia: a myeloproliferative disorder distinct from the hypereosinophilic syndrome. *Hematol Pathol* 5: 195-205.

699. Kulkarni S, Heath C, Parker S, Chase A, Iqbal S, Pocock CF, Kaeda J, Cwynarski K, Goldman JM, Cross NC (2000). Fusion of H4/D10S170 to the platelet-derived growth factor receptor beta in BCR-ABL-negative myeloproliferative disorders with a t(5;10)(q33;q21). *Cancer Res* 60: 3592-3598.

700. Kumar S, Green GA, Teruya-Feldstein J, Raffeld M, Jaffe ES (1996). Use of CD23 (BU38) on paraffin sections in the diagnosis of small lymphocytic lymphoma and mantle cell lymphoma. *Mod Pathol* 9: 925-929.

701. Kumar S, Krenacs L, Medeiros J, Elenitoba-Johnson KS, Greiner TC, Sorbara L, Kingma DW, Raffeld M, Jaffe ES (1998). Subcutaneous panniculitic T-cell lymphoma is a tumor of cytotoxic T lymphocytes. *Hum Pathol* 29: 397-403.

702. Kumar S, Krenacs L, Otsuki T, Kumar D, Harris CA, Wellmann A, Jaffe ES, Raffeld M (1996). bcl-1 rearrangement and cyclin D1 protein expression in multiple lymphomatous polyposis. *Am J Clin Pathol* 105: 737-743.

703. Kumar S, Kumar D, Kingma DW, Jaffe ES (1993). Epstein-Barr virus-associated T-cell lymphoma in a renal transplant patient. *Am J Surg Pathol* 17: 1046-1053.

704. Kummer JA, Vermeer MH, Dukers D, Meijer CJ, Willemze R (1997). Most primary cutaneous CD30-positive lymphoproliferative disorders have a CD4-positive cytotoxic T-cell phenotype. *J Invest Dermatol* 109: 636-640.

705. Kuppers R, Klein U, Hansmann ML, Rajewsky K (1999). Cellular origin of human B-cell lymphomas. *N Engl J Med* 341: 1520-1529.

706. Kushner JP, Lee GR, Wintrobe MM, Cartwright GE (1971). Idiopathic refractory sideroblastic anemia: clinical and laboratory investigation of 17 patients and review of the literature. *Medicine (Baltimore)* 50: 139-159.

707. Kvasnicka HM, Thiele J, Werden C, Zankovich R, Diehl V, Fischer R (1997). Prognostic factors in idiopathic (primary) osteomyelofibrosis. *Cancer* 80: 708-719.

708. Kwaan HC, Pierre RV, Long DL (1969). Meningeal involvement as first manifestation of acute myeloblastic transformation in chronic granulocytic leukemia. *Blood* 33: 348-352.

709. Kwong YL, Chan AC, Liang R, Chiang AK, Chim CS, Chan TK, Todd D, Ho FC (1997). CD56+ NK lymphomas: clinicopathological features and prognosis. *Br J Haematol* 97: 821-829.

710. Kwong YL, Chan AC, Liang RH (1997). Natural killer cell lymphoma/leukemia: pathology and treatment. *Hematol Oncol* 15: 71-79.

711. Kwong YL, Wong KF (1998). Association of pure red cell aplasia with T large granular lymphocyte leukaemia. *J Clin Pathol* 51: 672-675.

712. Kwong YL, Wong KF, Chan LC, Liang RH, Chan JK, Lin CK, Chan TK (1995). Large granular lymphocyte leukemia. A study of nine cases in a Chinese population. *Am J Clin Pathol* 103: 76-81.

713. Kyle RA (1978). Monoclonal gammopathy of undetermined significance. Natural history in 241 cases. *Am J Med* 64: 814-826.

714. Kyle RA (1993). "Benign" monoclonal gammopathy — after 20 to 35 years of follow-up. *Mayo Clin Proc* 68: 26-36.

715. Kyle RA, Bayrd ED (1976). Multiple myeloma: variant forms. In: *The monoclonal gammopathies, multiple myeloma and related plasma cell disorders*, Charles C. Thomas: Springfield, 141-145.

716. Kyle RA, Gertz MA (1990). Systemic amyloidosis. *Crit Rev Oncol Hematol* 10: 49-87.

717. Kyle RA, Gertz MA (1995). Primary systemic amyloidosis: clinical and laboratory features in 474 cases. *Semin Hematol* 32: 45-59.

718. Kyle RA, Greipp PR (1980). Smoldering multiple myeloma. *N Engl J Med* 302: 1347-1349.

719. Lai JL, Preudhomme C, Zandecki M, Flactif M, Vanrumbeke M, Lepelley P, Wattel E, Fenaux P (1995). Myelodysplastic syndromes and acute myeloid leukemia with 17p deletion. An entity characterized by specific dysgranulopoiesis and a high incidence of P53 mutations. *Leukemia* 9: 370-381.

720. Lai JL, Zandecki M, Mary JY, Bernardi F, Izydorczyk V, Flactif M, Morel P, Jouet JP, Bauters F, Facon T (1995). Improved cytogenetics in multiple myeloma: a study of 151 patients including 117 patients at diagnosis. *Blood* 85: 2490-2497.

721. Lai R, Arber DA, Chang KL, Wilson CS, Weiss LM (1998). Frequency of bcl-2 expression in non-Hodgkin's lymphoma: a study of 778 cases with comparison of marginal zone lymphoma and monocytoid B-cell hyperplasia. *Mod Pathol* 11: 864-869.

722. Lai R, Larratt LM, Etches W, Mortimer ST, Jewell LD, Dabbagh L, Coupland RW (2000). Hepatosplenic T-cell lymphoma of alphabeta lineage in a 16-year-old boy presenting with hemolytic anemia and thrombocytopenia. *Am J Surg Pathol* 24: 459-463.

723. Lai R, Weiss LM, Chang KL, Arber DA (1999). Frequency of CD43 expression in non-Hodgkin lymphoma. A survey of 742 cases and further characterization of rare CD43+ follicular lymphomas. *Am J Clin Pathol* 111: 488-494.

724. Lam KP, Kuhn R, Rajewsky K (1997). In vivo ablation of surface immunoglobulin on mature B cells by inducible gene targeting results in rapid cell death. *Cell* 90: 1073-1083.

725. Lamant L, Dastugue N, Pulford K, Delsol G, Mariame B (1999). A new fusion gene TPM3-ALK in anaplastic large cell lymphoma created by a (1;2)(q25;p23) translocation. *Blood* 93: 3088-3095.

726. Lamant L, Meggetto F, al Saati T, Brugieres L, de Paillerets BB, Dastugue N, Bernheim A, Rubie H, Terrier-Lacombe MJ, Robert A, Rigal F, Schlaifer D, Shiuta M, Mori S, Delsol G (1996). High incidence of the t(2;5)(p23;q35) translocation in anaplastic large cell lymphoma and its lack of detection in Hodgkin's disease. Comparison of cytogenetic analysis, reverse transcriptase-polymerase chain reaction, and P-80 immunostaining. *Blood* 87: 284-291.

727. Lambertenghi-Deliliers G, Annaloro C, Oriani A, Soligo D (1992). Myelodysplastic syndrome associated with bone marrow fibrosis. *Leuk Lymphoma* 8: 51-55.

728. Lampert I, Catovsky D, Marsh GW, Child JA, Galton DA (1980). The histopathology of prolymphocytic leukaemia with particular reference to the spleen: a comparison with chronic lymphocytic leukaemia. *Histopathology* 4: 3-19.

729. Lamy T, Loughran TP, Jr. (1999). Current concepts: large granular lymphocyte leukemia. *Blood Rev* 13: 230-240.

729a. Landis SH, Murray T, Bolden S, Wingo PA (1999). Cancer statistics, 1999. *CA Cancer J Clin* 49: 8-31.

730. Lange BJ (2000). The ultra low risk child with acute lymphoblastic leukemia. In: *Education Program Book*, Education Program Book American Society of Hematology: Washington, DC, 286-294.

731. Lardelli P, Bookman MA, Sundeen J, Longo DL, Jaffe ES (1990). Lymphocytic lymphoma of intermediate differentiation. Morphologic and immunophenotypic spectrum and clinical correlations. *Am J Surg Pathol* 14: 752-763.

732. Larson RS, Scott MA, McCurley TL, Vnencak-Jones CL (1996). Microsatellite analysis of posttransplant lymphoproliferative disorders: determination of donor/recipient origin and identification of putative lymphomagenic mechanism. *Cancer Res* 56: 4378-4381.

733. Laszewski MJ, Kemp JD, Goeken JA, Mitros FA, Platz CE, Dick FR (1990). Clonal immunoglobulin gene rearrangement in nodular lymphoid hyperplasia of the gastrointestinal tract associated with common variable immunodeficiency. *Am J Clin Pathol* 94: 338-343.

734. Laumen H, Nielsen PJ, Wirth T (2000). The BOB.1 / OBF.1 co-activator is essential for octamer-dependent transcription in B cells. *Eur J Immunol* 30: 458-469.

735. Lauritzen AF, Delsol G, Hansen NE, Horn T, Ersboll J, Hou-Jensen K, Ralfkiaer E (1994). Histiocytic sarcomas and monoblastic leukemias. A clinical, histologic, and immunophenotypical study. *Am J Clin Pathol* 102: 45-54.

736. Lauritzen AF, Hou-Jensen K, Ralfkiaer E (1993). P53 protein expression in Hodgkin's disease. *APMIS* 101: 689-694.

737. Lay JD, Tsao CJ, Chen JY, Kadin ME, Su IJ (1997). Upregulation of tumor necrosis factor-alpha gene by Epstein-Barr virus and activation of macrophages in Epstein-Barr virus-infected T cells in the pathogenesis of hemophagocytic syndrome. *J Clin Invest* 100: 1969-1979.

738. Lazzarino M, Morra E, Castello A, Inverardi D, Coci A, Pagnucco G, Magrini U, Zei G, Bernasconi C (1986). Myelofibrosis in chronic granulocytic leukaemia: clinicopathologic correlations and prognostic significance. *Br J Haematol* 64: 227-240.

739. Lazzarino M, Orlandi E, Paulli M, Strater J, Klersy C, Gianelli U, Gargantini L, Rousset MT, Gambacorta M, Marra E, Lavabre-Bertrand T, Magrini U, Manegold C, Bernasconi C, Moller P (1997). Treatment outcome and prognostic factors for primary mediastinal (thymic) B-cell lymphoma: a multicenter study of 106 patients. *J Clin Oncol* 15: 1646-1653.

740. Le Beau MM (2001). Role of cytogenetics in the diagnosis and classification of hematopoietic neoplasms. In: *Neoplastic Hematopathology*, Knowles D, ed. 2nd. Lippincott Williams & Wilkins: Philadelphia, pp. 319-418.

741. Le Beau MM, Larson RA, Bitter MA, Vardiman JW, Golomb HM, Rowley JD (1983). Association of an inversion of chromosome 16 with abnormal marrow eosinophils in acute myelomonocytic leukemia. A unique cytogenetic-clinicopathological association. *N Engl J Med* 309: 630-636.

742. Leblond V, Davi F, Charlotte F, Dorent R, Bitker MO, Sutton L, Gandjbakhch I, Binet JL, Raphael M (1998). Posttransplant lymphoproliferative disorders not associated with Epstein-Barr virus: a distinct entity? *J Clin Oncol* 16: 2052-2059.

743. LeBoit PE (1994). Granulomatous slack skin. *Dermatol Clin* 12: 375-389.

744. Legrand O, Perrot JY, Simonin G, Baudard M, Cadiou M, Blanc C, Ramond S, Viguie F, Marie JP, Zittoun R (1998). Adult biphenotypic acute leukaemia: an entity with poor prognosis which is related to unfavourable cytogenetics and P-glycoprotein over-expression. *Br J Haematol* 100: 147-155.

745. Leith CP, Kopecky KJ, Chen IM, Eijdems L, Slovak ML, McConnell TS, Head DR, Weick J, Grever MR, Appelbaum FR, Willman CL (1999). Frequency and clinical significance of the expression of the multidrug resistance proteins MDR1/P-glycoprotein, MRP1, and LRP in acute myeloid leukemia: a Southwest Oncology Group Study. *Blood* 94: 1086-1099.

746. Leith CP, Kopecky KJ, Godwin J, McConnell T, Slovak ML, Chen IM, Head DR, Appelbaum FR, Willman CL (1997). Acute myeloid leukemia in the elderly: assessment of multidrug resistance (MDR1) and cytogenetics distinguishes biologic subgroups with remarkably distinct responses to standard chemotherapy. A Southwest Oncology Group study. *Blood* 89: 3323-3329.

747. Lennert K (1978). *Malignant Lymphomas other than Hodgkin's disease*. Springer Verlag: New York.

748. Lennert K, Feller AC (1990). *Histopathologie der Non-Hodgkin Lymphome*. 2nd. Springer Verlag: Berlin.

749. Lennert K, Feller AC (1992). *Histopathology of non-Hodgkin's lymphomas*. 2nd. Springer Verlag: Berlin.

750. Lennert K, Parwaresch MR (1979). Mast cells and mast cell neoplasia: a review. *Histopathology* 3: 349-365.

751. Lennert K, Stein H, Kaiserling E (1975). Cytological and functional criteria for the classification of malignant lymphomata. *Br J Cancer* 31 SUPPL 2:29-43: 29-43.

752. Lennert K, Tamm I, Wacker HH (1991). Histopathology and immunocytochemistry of lymph node biopsies in chronic lymphocytic leukemia and immunocytoma. *Leuk Lymphoma* Supplement: 157-160.

753. Lens D, De Schouwer PJ, Hamoudi RA, Abdul-Rauf M, Farahat N, Matutes E, Crook T, Dyer MJ, Catovsky D (1997). p53 abnormalities in B-cell prolymphocytic leukemia. *Blood* 89: 2015-2023.

754. Lens D, Matutes E, Catovsky D, Coignet LJ (2000). Frequent deletions at 11q23 and 13q14 in B cell prolymphocytic leukemia (B-PLL). *Leukemia* 14: 427-430.

755. Lepretre S, Buchonnet G, Stamatoullas A, Lenain P, Duval C, d'Anjou J, Callat MP, Tilly H, Bastard C (2000). Chromosome abnormalities in peripheral T-cell lymphoma. *Cancer Genet Cytogenet* 117: 71-79.

756. Lessin SR, Vowels BR, Rook AH (1994). Retroviruses and cutaneous T-cell lymphoma. *Dermatol Clin* 12: 243-253.

757. Levine AM (1993). AIDS-related malignancies: the emerging epidemic. *J Natl Cancer Inst* 85: 1382-1397.

758. Levine AM (1996). HIV-associated Hodgkin's disease. Biologic and clinical aspects. *Hematol Oncol Clin North Am* 10: 1135-1148.

759. Levine EG, Arthur DC, Frizzera G, Peterson BA, Hurd DD, Bloomfield CD (1988). Cytogenetic abnormalities predict clinical outcome in non-Hodgkin lymphoma. *Ann Intern Med* 108: 14-20.

760. Levine PH, Blattner WA, Clark J, Tarone R, Maloney EM, Murphy EM, Gallo RC, Robert-Guroff M, Saxinger WC (1988). Geographic distribution of HTLV-I and identification of a new high-risk population. *Int J Cancer* 42: 7-12.

761. Levine PH, Kamaraju LS, Connelly RR, Berard CW, Dorfman RF, Magrath I, Easton JM (1982). The American Burkitt's Lymphoma Registry: eight years' experience. *Cancer* 49: 1016-1022.

762. Lewis EB (1963). Leukemia, multiple myeloma and anaplastic anemia in American Radiologists. *Science* 142: 1494.

763. Li JY, Gaillard F, Moreau A, Harousseau JL, Laboisse C, Milpied N, Bataille R, Avet-Loiseau H (1999). Detection of translocation t(11;14)(q13;q32) in mantle cell lymphoma by fluorescence in situ hybridization. *Am J Pathol* 154: 1449-1452.

764. Li WV, Kapadia SB, Sonmez-Alpan E, Swerdlow SH (1996). Immunohistochemical characterization of mast cell disease in paraffin sections using tryptase, CD68, myeloperoxidase, lysozyme, and CD20 antibodies. *Mod Pathol* 9: 982-988.

765. Liang R, Todd D, Chan TK, Chiu E, Lie A, Kwong YL, Choy D, Ho FC (1995). Treatment outcome and prognostic factors for primary nasal lymphoma. *J Clin Oncol* 13: 666-670.

766. Lieberman PH, Jones CR, Steinman RM, Erlandson RA, Smith J, Gee T, Huvos A, Garin-Chesa P, Filippa DA, Urmacher C, Gangi MD, Sperber M (1996). Langerhans cell (eosinophilic) granulomatosis. A clinicopathologic study encompassing 50 years. *Am J Surg Pathol* 20: 519-552.

767. Liebross RH, Ha CS, Cox JD, Weber D, Delasalle K, Alexanian R (1998). Solitary bone plasmacytoma: outcome and prognostic factors following radiotherapy. *Int J Radiat Oncol Biol Phys* 41: 1063-1067.

768. Lim MS, Straus SE, Dale JK, Fleisher TA, Stetler-Stevenson M, Strober W, Sneller MC, Puck JM, Lenardo MJ, Elenitoba-Johnson KS, Lin AY, Raffeld M, Jaffe ES (1998). Pathological findings in human autoimmune lymphoproliferative syndrome. *Am J Pathol* 153: 1541-1550.

769. Lin P, Jones D, Dorfman DM, Medeiros LJ (2000). Precursor B-cell lymphoblastic lymphoma: a predominantly extranodal tumor with low propensity for leukemic involvement. *Am J Surg Pathol* 24: 1480-1490.

770. Lindfors KK, Meyer JE, Dedrick CG, Hassell LA, Harris NL (1985). Thymic cysts in mediastinal Hodgkin disease. *Radiology* 156: 37-41.

771. Linet MS, Harlow SD, McLaughlin JK (1987). A case-control study of multiple myeloma in whites: chronic antigenic stimulation, occupation, and drug use. *Cancer Res* 47: 2978-2981.

772. Ling NR, MacLennan IC, Mason DY (1987). B-cell and plasma cell antigens: new and previously defined clusters. In: *Leukocyte Typing III: White Cell Differentiation Antigens*, McMichael AJ, Beverly PCL, Cobbold S, et al, eds. Oxford University Press: Oxford, pp. 302.

773. Lipford E, Wright JJ, Urba W, Whang-Peng J, Kirsch IR, Raffeld M, Cossman J, Longo DL, Bakhshi A, Korsmeyer SJ (1987). Refinement of lymphoma cytogenetics by the chromosome 18q21 major breakpoint region. *Blood* 70: 1816-1823.

774. Lipford EH, Smith HR, Pittaluga S, Jaffe ES, Steinberg AD, Cossman J (1987). Clonality of angioimmunoblastic lymphadenopathy and implications for its evolution to malignant lymphoma. *J Clin Invest* 79: 637-642.

775. Lipford EH, Jr., Margolick JB, Longo DL, Fauci AS, Jaffe ES (1988). Angiocentric immunoproliferative lesions: a clinicopathologic spectrum of post-thymic T-cell proliferations. *Blood* 72: 1674-1681.

776. Liso V, Troccoli G, Specchia G, Magno M (1977). Cytochemical "normal" and "abnormal" eosinophils in acute leukemias. *Am J Hematol* 2: 123-131.

777. Lister TA, Crowther D, Sutcliffe SB, Glatstein E, Canellos GP, Young RC, Rosenberg SA, Coltman CA, Tubiana M (1989). Report of a committee convened to discuss the evaluation and staging of patients with Hodgkin's disease: Cotswolds meeting. *J Clin Oncol* 7: 1630-1636.

778. Liu H, Ruskon-Fourmestraux A, Lavergne-Slove A, Ye H, Molina T, Bouhnik Y, Hamoudi RA, Diss TC, Dogan A, Megraud F, Rambaud JC, Du MQ, Isaacson PG (2001). Resistance of t(11;18) positive gastric mucosa-associated lymphoid tissue lymphoma to Helicobacter pylori eradication therapy. *Lancet* 357: 39-40.

779. Liu YJ, Zhang J, Lane PJ, Chan EY, MacLennan IC (1991). Sites of specific B cell activation in primary and secondary responses to T cell-dependent and T cell-independent antigens. *Eur J Immunol* 21: 2951-2962.

780. Lones MA, Mishalani S, Shintaku IP, Weiss LM, Nichols WS, Said JW (1995). Changes in tonsils and adenoids in children with posttransplant lymphoproliferative disorder: report of three cases with early involvement of Waldeyer's ring. *Hum Pathol* 26: 525-530.

781. Longley BJ, Metcalfe DD (2000). A proposed classification of mastocytosis incorporating molecular genetics. *Hematol Oncol Clin North Am* 14: 697-701, viii.

782. Longley BJ, Tyrrell L, Lu SZ, Ma YS, Langley K, Ding TG, Duffy T, Jacobs P, Tang LH, Modlin I (1996). Somatic c-KIT activating mutation in urticaria pigmentosa and aggressive mastocytosis: establishment of clonality in a human mast cell neoplasm. *Nat Genet* 12: 312-314.

783. Longley BJ, Jr., Metcalfe DD, Tharp M, Wang X, Tyrrell L, Lu SZ, Heitjan D, Ma Y (1999). Activating and dominant inactivating c-KIT catalytic domain mutations in distinct clinical forms of human mastocytosis. *Proc Natl Acad Sci U S A* 96: 1609-1614.

784. Longley BJ, Jr., Morganroth GS, Tyrrell L, Ding TG, Anderson DM, Williams DE, Halaban R (1993). Altered metabolism of mast-cell growth factor (c-kit ligand) in cutaneous mastocytosis. *N Engl J Med* 328: 1302-1307.

785. Longley J, Duffy TP, Kohn S (1995). The mast cell and mast cell disease. *J Am Acad Dermatol* 32: 545-561.

786. Longo DL, Young RC, Hubbard SM, Wesley M, Fisher RI, Jaffe E, Berard C, DeVita VT, Jr. (1984). Prolonged initial remission in patients with nodular mixed lymphoma. *Ann Intern Med* 100: 651-656.

787. Lopez-Guillermo A, Cid J, Salar A, Lopez A, Montalban C, Castrillo JM, Gonzalez M, Ribera JM, Brunet S, Garcia-Conde J, Fernandez dS, Bosch F, Montserrat E (1998). Peripheral T-cell lymphomas: initial features, natural history, and prognostic factors in a series of 174 patients diagnosed according to the R.E.A.L. Classification. *Ann Oncol* 9: 849-855.

788. Lorand-Metze I, Vassallo J, Souza CA (1987). Histological and cytological heterogeneity of bone marrow in Philadelphia-positive chronic myelogenous leukaemia at diagnosis. *Br J Haematol* 67: 45-49.

789. Loughran TP, Jr., Kadin ME, Starkebaum G, Abkowitz JL, Clark EA, Disteche C, Lum LG, Slichter SJ (1985). Leukemia of large granular lymphocytes: association with clonal chromosomal abnormalities and autoimmune neutropenia, thrombocytopenia, and hemolytic anemia. *Ann Intern Med* 102: 169-175.

790. Loughran TP, Jr., Starkebaum G, Aprile JA (1988). Rearrangement and expression of T-cell receptor genes in large granular lymphocyte leukemia. *Blood* 71: 822-824.

791. Louie DC, Offit K, Jaslow R, Parsa NZ, Murty VV, Schluger A, Chaganti RS (1995). p53 overexpression as a marker of poor prognosis in mantle cell lymphomas with t(11;14)(q13;q32). *Blood* 86: 2892-2899.

792. Luk IS, Shek TW, Tang VW, Ng WF (1999). Interdigitating dendritic cell tumor of the testis: a novel testicular spindle cell neoplasm. *Am J Surg Pathol* 23: 1141-1148.

793. Lukes R, Butler J, Hicks E (1966). Natural history of Hodgkin's disease as related to its pathologal picture. *Cancer* 19: 317-344.

794. Lukes RJ, Craver L, Hall T, Rappaport H, Ruben P (1966). Report of the nomenclature committee. *Cancer Res* 26: 1311.

795. Luna-Fineman S, Shannon KM, Atwater SK, Davis J, Masterson M, Ortega J, Sanders J, Steinherz P, Weinberg V, Lange BJ (1999). Myelodysplastic and myeloproliferative disorders of childhood: a study of 167 patients. *Blood* 93: 459-466.

796. Luna-Fineman S, Shannon KM, Lange BJ (1995). Childhood monosomy 7: epidemiology, biology, and mechanistic implications. *Blood* 85: 1985-1999.

797. Lydyard P, Grossi C (1998). Cells involved in the immune response. In: *Immunology*, Roitt I, Brostoff J, Male D, eds. Mosby: London, pp. 13-30.

798. Lynch JW, Jr., Linoilla I, Sausville EA, Steinberg SM, Ghosh BC, Nguyen DT, Schechter GP, Fischmann AB, Ihde DC, Stocker JL (1992). Prognostic implications of evaluation for lymph node involvement by T-cell antigen receptor gene rearrangement in mycosis fungoides. *Blood* 79: 3293-3299.

799. MacLennan IC (1994). Germinal centers. *Annu Rev Immunol* 12: 117-139.

800. MacLennan IC, Liu YJ, Oldfield S, Zhang J, Lane PJ (1990). The evolution of B-cell clones. *Curr Top Microbiol Immunol* 159:37-63: 37-63.

801. MacLennan KA, Bennett MH, Vaughan HB, Vaughan HG (1992). Diagnosis and grading of nodular sclerosing Hodgkin's disease: a study of 2190 patients. *Int Rev Exp Pathol* 33: 27-51.

802. Macon WR, Levy NB, Kurtin PJ, Salhany KE, Elkhalifa MY, Casey TT, Craig FE, Vnencak-Jones CL, Gulley ML, Park JP, Cousar JB (2001). Hepatosplenic alphabeta T-cell lymphomas: a report of 14 cases and comparison with hepatosplenic gammadelta T-cell lymphomas. *Am J Surg Pathol* 25: 285-296.

803. Magrath IT, Janus C, Edwards BK, Spiegel R, Jaffe ES, Berard CW, Miliauskas J, Morris K, Barnwell R (1984). An effective therapy for both undifferentiated (including Burkitt's) lymphomas and lymphoblastic lymphomas in children and young adults. *Blood* 63: 1102-1111.

804. Magrath IT, Sariban E (1985). Clinical features of Burkitt's lymphoma in the USA. *IARC Sci Publ* 119-127.

805. Mahmoud MS, Huang N, Nobuyoshi M, Lisukov IA, Tanaka H, Kawano MM (1996). Altered expression of Pax-5 gene in human myeloma cells. *Blood* 87: 4311-4315.

806. Maitra A, McKenna RW, Weinberg AG, et al (2001). Precursor B-cell lymphoblastic lymphoma. *in press* (in press).

807. Majlis A, Pugh WC, Rodriguez MA, Benedict WF, Cabanillas F (1997). Mantle cell lymphoma: correlation of clinical outcome and biologic features with three histologic variants. *J Clin Oncol* 15: 1664-1671.

808. Maljaei SH, Brito-Babapulle V, Hiorns LR, Catovsky D (1998). Abnormalities of chromosomes 8, 11, 14, and X in T-prolymphocytic leukemia studied by fluorescence in situ hybridization. *Cancer Genet Cytogenet* 103: 110-116.

809. Maloum K, Magnac C, Azgui Z, Cau C, Charlotte F, Binet JL, Merle-Beral H, Dighiero G (1998). VH gene expression in hairy cell leukaemia. *Br J Haematol* 101: 171-178.

810. Manaloor EJ, Neiman RS, Heilman DK, Albitar M, Casey T, Vattuone T, Kotylo P, Orazi A (2000). Immunohistochemistry can be used to subtype acute myeloid leukemia in routinely processed bone marrow biopsy specimens. Comparison with flow cytometry. *Am J Clin Pathol* 113: 814-822.

811. Mann RB, Berard CW (1983). Criteria for the cytologic subclassification of follicular lymphomas: a proposed alternative method. *Hematol Oncol* 1: 187-192.

812. Mann RB, Jaffe ES, Braylan RC, Nanba K, Frank MM, Ziegler JL, Berard CW (1976). Non-endemic Burkitts's lymphoma. A B-cell tumor related to germinal centers. *N Engl J Med* 295: 685-691.

813. Marafioti T, Hummel M, Anagnostopoulos I, Foss HD, Falini B, Delsol G, Isaacson PG, Pileri S, Stein H (1997). Origin of nodular lymphocyte-predominant Hodgkin's disease from a clonal expansion of highly mutated germinal-center B cells. *N Engl J Med* 337: 453-458.

814. Marafioti T, Hummel M, Foss HD, Laumen H, Korbjuhn P, Anagnostopoulos I, Lammert H, Demel G, Theil J, Wirth T, Stein H (2000). Hodgkin and reed-sternberg cells represent an expansion of a single clone originating from a germinal center B-cell with functional immunoglobulin gene rearrangements but defective immunoglobulin transcription. *Blood* 95: 1443-1450.

815. Marlton P, Keating M, Kantarjian H, Pierce S, O'Brien S, Freireich EJ, Estey E (1995). Cytogenetic and clinical correlates in AML patients with abnormalities of chromosome 16. *Leukemia* 9: 965-971.

816. Martiat P, Michaux JL, Rodhain J (1991). Philadelphia-negative (Ph-) chronic myeloid leukemia (CML): comparison with Ph+ CML and chronic myelomonocytic leukemia. The Groupe Francais de Cytogenetique Hematologique. *Blood* 78: 205-211.

817. Martin A, Flaman JM, Frebourg T, Davi F, El Mansouri S, Amouroux J, Raphael M (1998). Functional analysis of the p53 protein in AIDS-related non-Hodgkin's lymphomas and polymorphic lymphoproliferations. *Br J Haematol* 101: 311-317.

818. Martin AR, Weisenburger DD, Chan WC, Ruby EI, Anderson JR, Vose JM, Bierman PJ, Bast MA, Daley DT, Armitage JO (1995). Prognostic value of cellular proliferation and histologic grade in follicular lymphoma. *Blood* 85: 3671-3678.

819. Martin PL, Look AT, Schnell S, Harris MB, Pullen J, Shuster JJ, Carroll AJ, Pettenati MJ, Rao PN (1996). Comparison of fluorescence in situ hybridization, cytogenetic analysis, and DNA index analysis to detect chromosomes 4 and 10 aneuploidy in pediatric acute lymphoblastic leukemia: a Pediatric Oncology Group study. *J Pediatr Hematol Oncol* 18: 113-121.

820. Martyre MC, Romquin N, Bousse-Kerdiles MC, Chevillard S, Benyahia B, Dupriez B, Demory JL, Bauters F (1994). Transforming growth factor-beta and megakaryocytes in the pathogenesis of idiopathic myelofibrosis. *Br J Haematol* 88: 9-16.

821. Maruyama N, Ishida Y, Sato H, Koike T, Nagao K (1987). Expression of lymphocyte-associated antigens on neoplastic angioendotheliomatosis. *Appl Pathol* 5: 246-252.

822. Maschek H, Georgii A, Kaloutsi V, Werner M, Bandecar K, Kressel MG, Choritz H, Freund M, Hufnagl D (1992). Myelofibrosis in primary myelodysplastic syndromes: a retrospective study of 352 patients. *Eur J Haematol* 48: 208-214.

823. Mason DY, Bastard C, Rimokh R, Dastugue N, Huret JL, Kristoffersson U, Magaud JP, Nezelof C, Tilly H, Vannier JP (1990). CD30-positive large cell lymphomas ('Ki-1 lymphoma') are associated with a chromosomal translocation involving 5q35. *Br J Haematol* 74: 161-168.

824. Mason DY, Pulford KA, Bischof D, Kuefer MU, Butler LH, Lamant L, Delsol G, Morris SW (1998). Nucleolar localization of the nucleophosmin-anaplastic lymphoma kinase is not required for malignant transformation. *Cancer Res* 58: 1057-1062.

825. Mastovich S, Ratech H, Ware RE, Moore JO, Borowitz MJ (1994). Hepatosplenic T-cell lymphoma: an unusual case of a gamma delta T-cell lymphoma with a blast-like terminal transformation. *Hum Pathol* 25: 102-108.

826. Matano S, Nakamura S, Kobayashi K, Yoshida T, Matsuda T, Sugimoto T (1997). Deletion of the long arm of chromosome 20 in a patient with chronic neutrophilic leukemia: cytogenetic findings in chronic neutrophilic leukemia. *Am J Hematol* 54: 72-75.

827. Matano S, Nakamura S, Nakamura S, Annen Y, Hattori N, Kobayashi K, Kyoda K, Sugimoto T (1999). Monomorphic agranular natural killer cell lymphoma/leukemia with no Epstein-Barr virus association. *Acta Haematol* 101: 206-208.

828. Mateo M, Mollejo M, Villuendas R, Algara P, Sanchez-Beato M, Martinez P, Piris MA (1999). 7q31-32 allelic loss is a frequent finding in splenic marginal zone lymphoma. *Am J Pathol* 154: 1583-1589.

829. Mathew P, Tefferi A, Dewald GW, Goldberg SL, Su J, Hoagland HC, Noel P (1993). The 5q- syndrome: a single-institution study of 43 consecutive patients. *Blood* 81: 1040-1045.

830. Matolcsy A, Chadburn A, Knowles DM (1995). De novo CD5-positive and Richter's syndrome-associated diffuse large B cell lymphomas are genotypically distinct. *Am J Pathol* 147: 207-216.

831. Matolcsy A, Nador RG, Cesarman E, Knowles DM (1998). Immunoglobulin VH gene mutational analysis suggests that primary effusion lymphomas derive from different stages of B cell maturation. *Am J Pathol* 153: 1609-1614.

832. Matthews GV, Bower M, Mandalia S, Powles T, Nelson MR, Gazzard BG (2000). Changes in acquired immunodeficiency syndrome-related lymphoma since the introduction of highly active antiretroviral therapy. *Blood* 96: 2730-2734.

833. Matutes E, Brito-Babapulle V, Swansbury J, Ellis J, Morilla R, Dearden C, Sempere A, Catovsky D (1991). Clinical and laboratory features of 78 cases of T-prolymphocytic leukemia. *Blood* 78: 3269-3274.

834. Matutes E, Carrara P, Coignet L, Brito-Babapulle V, Villamor N, Wotherspoon A, Catovsky D (1999). FISH analysis for BCL-1 rearrangements and trisomy 12 helps the diagnosis of atypical B cell leukaemias. *Leukemia* 13: 1721-1726.

835. Matutes E, Crockard AD, O'Brien M, Catovsky D (1983). Ultrastructural cytochemistry of chronic T-cell leukaemias. A study with four acid hydrolases. *Histochem J* 15: 895-909.

836. Matutes E, Garcia TJ, O'Brien M, Catovsky D (1986). The morphological spectrum of T-prolymphocytic leukaemia. *Br J Haematol* 64: 111-124.

837. Matutes E, Morilla R, Farahat N, Carbonell F, Swansbury J, Dyer M, Catovsky D (1997). Definition of acute biphenotypic leukaemia. *Haematologica* 82: 64-66.

838. Matutes E, Morilla R, Owusu-Ankomah K, Houlihan A, Catovsky D (1994). The immunophenotype of splenic lymphoma with villous lymphocytes and its relevance to the differential diagnosis with other B-cell disorders. *Blood* 83: 1558-1562.

839. Matutes E, Oscier D, Garcia-Marco J, Ellis J, Copplestone A, Gillingham R, Hamblin T, Lens D, Swansbury GJ, Catovsky D (1996). Trisomy 12 defines a group of CLL with atypical morphology: correlation between cytogenetic, clinical and laboratory features in 544 patients. *Br J Haematol* 92: 382-388.

840. Matutes E, Owusu-Ankomah K, Morilla R, Garcia MJ, Houlihan A, Que TH, Catovsky D (1994). The immunological profile of B-cell disorders and proposal of a scoring system for the diagnosis of CLL. *Leukemia* 8: 1640-1645.

841. Mauch P, Armitage JO, Diehl V (1999). *Hodgkin's Disease*. Lippincott Williams & Wilkins: Philadelphia.

842. Mauri C, Torelli U, di Prisco U, Silingardi V, Artusi T, Emila G (1977). Lymphoid blastic crisis at the onset of chronic granulocytic leukemia: report of two cases. *Cancer* 40: 865-870.

843. Mazzaro C, Franzin F, Tulissi P, Pussini E, Crovatto M, Carniello GS, Efremov DG, Burrone O, Santini G, Pozzato G (1996). Regression of monoclonal B-cell expansion in patients affected by mixed cryoglobulinemia responsive to alpha-interferon therapy. *Cancer* 77: 2604-2613.

844. McCarty MJ, Vukelja SJ, Sausville EA, Perry JJ, James WD, Jaffe ES, Weiss RB (1994). Lymphomatoid papulosis associated with Ki-1-positive anaplastic large cell lymphoma. A report of two cases and a review of the literature. *Cancer* 74: 3051-3058.

845. McClain K, Jin H, Gresik V, Favara B (1994). Langerhans cell histiocytosis: lack of a viral etiology. *Am J Hematol* 47: 16-20.

846. McClain KL, Leach CT, Jenson HB, Joshi VV, Pollock BH, Hutchison RE, Murphy SB (2000). Molecular and virologic characteristics of lymphoid malignancies in children with AIDS. *J Acquir Immune Defic Syndr* 23: 152-159.

847. McClure RF, Dewald GW, Hoyer JD, Hanson CA (1999). Isolated isochromosome 17q: a distinct type of mixed myeloproliferative disorder/myelodysplastic syndrome with an aggressive clinical course. *Br J Haematol* 106: 445-454.

848. McDonnell TJ, Deane N, Platt FM, Nunez G, Jaeger U, McKearn JP, Korsmeyer SJ (1989). bcl-2-immunoglobulin transgenic mice demonstrate extended B cell survival and follicular lymphoproliferation. *Cell* 57: 79-88.

849. McIntyre KJ, Hoagland HC, Silverstein MN, Petitt RM (1991). Essential thrombocythemia in young adults. *Mayo Clin Proc* 66: 149-154.

850. McKenna RW, Parkin J, Brunning RD (1979). Morphologic and ultrastructural characteristics of T-cell acute lymphoblastic leukemia. *Cancer* 44: 1290-1297.

851. McKenna RW, Parkin J, Kersey JH, Gajl-Peczalska KJ, Peterson L, Brunning RD (1977). Chronic lymphoproliferative disorder with unusual clinical, morphologic, ultrastructural and membrane surface marker characteristics. *Am J Med* 62: 588-596.

852. McLaughlin P, Fuller LM, Velasquez WS, Butler JJ, Hagemeister FB, Sullivan-Halley JA, Dixon DO (1987). Stage III follicular lymphoma: durable remissions with a combined chemotherapy-radiotherapy regimen. *J Clin Oncol* 5: 867-874.

853. McNiff JM, Cooper D, Howe G, Crotty PL, Tallini G, Crouch J, Eisen RN (1996). Lymphomatoid granulomatosis of the skin and lung. An angiocentric T-cell-rich B-cell lymphoproliferative disorder. *Arch Dermatol* 132: 1464-1470.

854. Medeiros LJ, Lardelli P, Stetler-Stevenson M, Longo DL, Jaffe ES (1991). Genotypic analysis of diffuse, mixed cell lymphomas. Comparison with morphologic and immunophenotypic findings. *Am J Clin Pathol* 95: 547-555.

855. Medeiros LJ, Peiper SC, Elwood L, Yano T, Raffeld M, Jaffe ES (1991). Angiocentric immunoproliferative lesions: a molecular analysis of eight cases. *Hum Pathol* 22: 1150-1157.

856. Meeker TC, Hardy D, Willman C, Hogan T, Abrams J (1990). Activation of the interleukin-3 gene by chromosome translocation in acute lymphocytic leukemia with eosinophilia. *Blood* 76: 285-289.

857. Melnick A, Licht JD (1999). Deconstructing a disease: RARalpha, its fusion partners, and their roles in the pathogenesis of acute promyelocytic leukemia. *Blood* 93: 3167-3215.

858. Melnyk A, Rodriguez A, Pugh WC, Cabannillas F (1997). Evaluation of the Revised European-American Lymphoma classification confirms the clinical relevance of immunophenotype in 560 cases of aggressive non-Hodgkin's lymphoma. *Blood* 89: 4514-4520.

859. Melo JV (1996). The diversity of BCR-ABL fusion proteins and their relationship to leukemia phenotype. *Blood* 88: 2375-2384.

860. Melo JV, Catovsky D, Galton DA (1986). The relationship between chronic lymphocytic leukaemia and prolymphocytic leukaemia. I. Clinical and laboratory features of 300 patients and characterization of an intermediate group. *Br J Haematol* 63: 377-387.

861. Melo JV, Catovsky D, Gregory WM, Galton DA (1987). The relationship between chronic lymphocytic leukaemia and prolymphocytic leukaemia. IV. Analysis of survival and prognostic features. *Br J Haematol* 65: 23-29.

862. Melo JV, Hegde U, Parreira A, Thompson I, Lampert IA, Catovsky D (1987). Splenic B cell lymphoma with circulating villous lymphocytes: differential diagnosis of B cell leukaemias with large spleens. *J Clin Pathol* 40: 642-651.

863. Melo JV, Myint H, Galton DA, Goldman JM (1994). P190BCR-ABL chronic myeloid leukaemia: the missing link with chronic myelomonocytic leukaemia? *Leukemia* 8: 208-211.

864. Menke DM, Griesser H, Moder KG, Tefferi A, Luthra HS, Cohen MD, Colon-Otero G, Lloyd RV (2000). Lymphomas in patients with connective tissue disease. Comparison of p53 protein expression and latent EBV infection in patients immunosuppressed and not immunosuppressed with methotrexate. *Am J Clin Pathol* 113: 212-218.

865. Mercieca J, Matutes E, Dearden C, MacLennan K, Catovsky D (1994). The role of pentostatin in the treatment of T-cell malignancies: analysis of response rate in 145 patients according to disease subtype. *J Clin Oncol* 12: 2588-2593.

866. Mercieca J, Matutes E, Moskovic E, MacLennan K, Matthey F, Costello C, Behrens J, Basu S, Roath S, Fairhead S (1992). Massive abdominal lymphadenopathy in hairy cell leukaemia: a report of 12 cases. *Br J Haematol* 82: 547-554.

867. Mesa RA, Silverstein MN, Jacobsen SJ, Wollan PC, Tefferi A (1999). Population-based incidence and survival figures in essential thrombocythemia and agnogenic myeloid metaplasia: an Olmsted County Study, 1976-1995. *Am J Hematol* 61: 10-15.

868. Messinezy M, Westwood NB, Woodcock SP, Strong RM, Pearson TC (1995). Low serum erythropoietin – a strong diagnostic criterion of primary polycythaemia even at normal haemoglobin levels. *Clin Lab Haematol* 17: 217-220.

869. Metcalfe DD (1991). The liver, spleen, and lymph nodes in mastocytosis. *J Invest Dermatol* 96: 45S-46S.

870. Metter GE, Nathwani BN, Burke JS, Winberg CD, Mann RB, Barcos M, Kjeldsberg CR, Whitcomb CC, Dixon DO, Miller TP (1985). Morphological subclassification of follicular lymphoma: variability of diagnoses among hematopathologists, a collaborative study between the Repository Center and Pathology Panel for Lymphoma Clinical Studies. *J Clin Oncol* 3: 25-38.

871. Meytes D, Katz D, Ramot B (1976). Preleukemia and leukemia in polycythemia vera. *Blood* 47: 237-241.

872. Michaux JL, Martiat P (1993). Chronic myelomonocytic leukaemia (CMML) – a myelodysplastic or myeloproliferative syndrome? *Leuk Lymphoma* 9: 35-41.

873. Michels SD, McKenna RW, Arthur DC, Brunning RD (1985). Therapy-related acute myeloid leukemia and myelodysplastic syndrome: a clinical and morphologic study of 65 cases. *Blood* 65: 1364-1372.

874. Miettinen M, Fletcher CD, Lasota J (1993). True histiocytic lymphoma of small intestine. Analysis of two S-100 protein-positive cases with features of interdigitating reticulum cell sarcoma. *Am J Clin Pathol* 100: 285-292.

875. Miettinen M, Franssila KO, Saxen E (1983). Hodgkin's disease, lymphocytic predominance nodular. Increased risk for subsequent non-Hodgkin's lymphomas. *Cancer* 51: 2293-2300.

876. Miles DK, Freedman MH, Stephens K, Pallavicini M, Sievers EL, Weaver M, Grunberger T, Thompson P, Shannon KM (1996). Patterns of hematopoietic lineage involvement in children with neurofibromatosis type 1 and malignant myeloid disorders. *Blood* 88: 4314-4320.

877. Miller RL, Purvis JD, III, Weick JK (1989). Familial polycythemia vera. *Cleve Clin J Med* 56: 813-818.

878. Miller TP, Grogan TM, Dahlberg S, Spier CM, Braziel RM, Banks PM, Foucar K, Kjeldsberg CR, Levy N, Nathwani BN (1994). Prognostic significance of the Ki-67-associated proliferative antigen in aggressive non-Hodgkin's lymphomas: a prospective Southwest Oncology Group trial. *Blood* 83: 1460-1466.

879. Miralles GD, O'Fallon JR, Talley NJ (1992). Plasma-cell dyscrasia with polyneuropathy. The spectrum of POEMS syndrome. *N Engl J Med* 327: 1919-1923.

880. Miranda RN, Esparza AR, Sambandam S, Medeiros LJ (1994). Systemic mast cell disease presenting with peripheral blood eosinophilia. *Hum Pathol* 25: 727-730.

881. Mitelman F (1993). The cytogenetic scenario of chronic myeloid leukemia. *Leuk Lymphoma* 11 Suppl 1:11-5: 11-15.

882. Mitelman F, Levan G, Nilsson PG, Brandt L (1976). Non-random karyotypic evolution in chronic myeloid leukemia. *Int J Cancer* 18: 24-30.

883. Mittal K, Neri A, Feiner H, Schinella R, Alfonso F (1990). Lymphomatoid granulomatosis in the acquired immunodeficiency syndrome. Evidence of Epstein-Barr virus infection and B-cell clonal selection without myc rearrangement. *Cancer* 65: 1345-1349.

884. Modan B (1965). An epidemiological study of polycythemia vera. *Blood* 26: 657-667.

885. Molina A, Lombard C, Donlon T, Bangs CD, Dorfman RF (1990). Immunohistochemical and cytogenetic studies indicate that malignant angioendotheliomatosis is a primary intravascular (angiotropic) lymphoma. *Cancer* 66: 474-479.

886. Mollejo M, Menarguez J, Lloret E, Sanchez A, Campo E, Algara P, Cristobal E, Sanchez E, Piris MA (1995). Splenic marginal zone lymphoma: a distinctive type of low-grade B-cell lymphoma. A clinicopathological study of 13 cases. *Am J Surg Pathol* 19: 1146-1157.

887. Moller P, Herrmann B, Moldenhauer G, Momburg F (1987). Defective expression of MHC class I antigens is frequent in B-cell lymphomas of high-grade malignancy. *Int J Cancer* 40: 32-39.

888. Moller P, Lammler B, Eberlein-Gonska M, Feichter GE, Hofmann WJ, Schmitteckert H, Otto HF (1986). Primary mediastinal clear cell lymphoma of B-cell type. *Virchows Arch A Pathol Anat Histopathol* 409: 79-92.

889. Moller P, Moldenhauer G, Momburg F, Lammler B, Eberlein-Gonska M, Kiesel S, Dorken B (1987). Mediastinal lymphoma of clear cell type is a tumor corresponding to terminal steps of B cell differentiation. *Blood* 69: 1087-1095.

890. Momose H, Jaffe ES, Shin SS, Chen YY, Weiss LM (1992). Chronic lymphocytic leukemia/small lymphocytic lymphoma with Reed-Sternberg-like cells and possible transformation to Hodgkin's disease. Mediation by Epstein-Barr virus. *Am J Surg Pathol* 16: 859-867.

891. Monda L, Warnke R, Rosai J (1986). A primary lymph node malignancy with features suggestive of dendritic reticulum cell differentiation. A report of 4 cases. *Am J Pathol* 122: 562-572.

892. Monsalve MV, Helgason A, Devine DV (1999). Languages, geography and HLA haplotypes in native American and Asian populations. *Proc R Soc Lond B Biol Sci* 266: 2209-2216.

893. Montesinos-Rongen M, Roers A, Kuppers R, Rajewsky K, Hansmann ML (1999). Mutation of the p53 gene is not a typical feature of Hodgkin and Reed-Sternberg cells in Hodgkin's disease. *Blood* 94: 1755-1760.

894. Montserrat E, Villamor N, Reverter JC, Brugues RM, Tassies D, Bosch F, Aguilar JL, Vives-Corrons JL, Rozman M, Rozma C (1996). Bone marrow assessment in B-cell chronic lymphocytic leukaemia: aspirate or biopsy? A comparative study in 258 patients. *Br J Haematol* 93: 111-116.

895. Moreau EJ, Matutes E, A'Hern RP, Morilla AM, Morilla RM, Owusu-Ankomah KA, Seon BK, Catovsky D (1997). Improvement of the chronic lymphocytic leukemia scoring system with the monoclonal antibody SN8 (CD79b). *Am J Clin Pathol* 108: 378-382.

896. Mori N, Yatabe Y, Oka K, Kinoshita T, Kobayashi T, Ono T, Asai J (1996). Expression of perforin in nasal lymphoma. Additional evidence of its natural killer cell derivation. *Am J Pathol* 149: 699-705.

897. Morris SW, Kirstein MN, Valentine MB, Dittmer KG, Shapiro DN, Saltman DL, Look AT (1994). Fusion of a kinase gene, ALK, to a nucleolar protein gene, NPM, in non-Hodgkin's lymphoma. *Science* 263: 1281-1284.

898. Morrison AM, Jager U, Chott A, Schebesta M, Haas OA, Busslinger M (1998). Deregulated PAX-5 transcription from a translocated IgH promoter in marginal zone lymphoma. *Blood* 92: 3865-3878.

899. Mrozek K, Heinonen K, de la CA, Bloomfield CD (1997). Clinical significance of cytogenetics in acute myeloid leukemia. *Semin Oncol* 24: 17-31.

900. Muehleck SD, McKenna RW, Arthur DC, Parkin JL, Brunning RD (1984). Transformation of chronic myelogenous leukemia: clinical, morphologic, and cytogenetic features. *Am J Clin Pathol* 82: 1-14.

901. Mueller NC, Grufferman (1999). The epidemiology of Hodgkin's disease. In: *Hodgkin's Disease*, Mauch P, Armitage JO, Diehl V, eds. Lippincott Williams & Wilkins: Philadelphia, 61.

902. Mukai HY, Kojima H, Suzukawa K, Hori M, Komeno T, Hasegawa Y, Ninomiya H, Mori N, Nagasawa T (1999). High-dose chemotherapy with peripheral blood stem cell rescue in blastoid natural killer cell lymphoma. *Leuk Lymphoma* 32: 583-588.

903. Mullaney BP, Ng VL, Herndier BG, McGrath MS, Pallavicini MG (2000). Comparative genomic analyses of primary effusion lymphoma. *Arch Pathol Lab Med* 124: 824-826.

904. Mulligan SP, Matutes E, Dearden C, Catovsky D (1991). Splenic lymphoma with villous lymphocytes: natural history and response to therapy in 50 cases. *Br J Haematol* 78: 206-209.

905. Munn SE, McGregor JM, Jones A, Amlot P, Rustin MH, Russell JR, Whittaker S (1996). Clinical and pathological heterogeneity in cutaneous gamma-delta T-cell lymphoma: a report of three cases and a review of the literature. *Br J Dermatol* 135: 976-981.

906. Murphy S (1992). Polycythemia vera. *Dis Mon* 38: 153-212.

907. Murphy S (1999). Diagnostic criteria and prognosis in polycythemia vera and essential thrombocythemia. *Semin Hematol* 36: 9-13.

908. Murphy S, Iland H, Rosenthal D, Laszlo J (1986). Essential thrombocythemia: an interim report from the Polycythemia Vera Study Group. *Semin Hematol* 23: 177-182.

909. Murphy S, Peterson P, Iland H, Laszlo J (1997). Experience of the Polycythemia Vera Study Group with essential thrombocythemia: a final report on diagnostic criteria, survival, and leukemic transition by treatment. *Semin Hematol* 34: 29-39.

910. Murphy SB (1978). Childhood non-Hodgkin's lymphoma. *N Engl J Med* 299: 1446-1448.

911. Murphy SB, Hustu HO (1980). A randomized trial of combined modality therapy of childhood non-Hodgkin's lymphoma. *Cancer* 45: 630-637.

912. Murray A, Cuevas EC, Jones DB, Wright DH (1995). Study of the immunohistochemistry and T cell clonality of enteropathy-associated T cell lymphoma. *Am J Pathol* 146: 509-519.

913. Muschen M, Rajewsky K, Brauninger A, Baur AS, Oudejans JJ, Roers A, Hansmann ML, Kuppers R (2000). Rare occurrence of classical Hodgkin's disease as a T cell lymphoma. *J Exp Med* 191: 387-394.

914. Nador RG, Cesarman E, Chadburn A, Dawson DB, Ansari MQ, Sald J, Knowles DM (1996). Primary effusion lymphoma: a distinct clinicopathologic entity associated with the Kaposi's sarcoma-associated herpes virus. *Blood* 88: 645-656.

915. Nador RG, Chadburn A, Cesarman E, Said JW, Knowles DM (1997). AIDS-related polymorphic lymphoproliferative disorders. *J Acquir Immune Defic Syndr Hum Retrovirol* 14: 45a.

916. Nagata H, Worobec AS, Oh CK, Chowdhury BA, Tannenbaum S, Suzuki Y, Metcalfe DD (1995). Identification of a point mutation in the catalytic domain of the protooncogene c-kit in peripheral blood mononuclear cells of patients who have mastocytosis with an associated hematologic disorder. *Proc Natl Acad Sci U S A* 92: 10560-10564.

917. Nair C, Chopra H, Shinde S, Barbhaya S, Kumar A, Dhond S, Yejamanam B, Sapre R, Chougule A, Advani S (1995). Immunophenotype and ultrastructural studies in blast crisis of chronic myeloid leukemia. *Leuk Lymphoma* 19: 309-313.

918. Najean Y, Arrago JP, Rain JD, Dresch C (1984). The 'spent' phase of polycythaemia vera: hypersplenism in the absence of myelofibrosis. *Br J Haematol* 56: 163-170.

919. Najean Y, Deschamps A, Dresch C, Daniel MT, Rain JD, Arrago JP (1988). Acute leukemia and myelodysplasia in polycythaemia vera. A clinical study with long-term follow-up. *Cancer* 61: 89-95.

920. Najean Y, Mugnier P, Dresch C, Rain JD (1987). Polycythaemia vera in young people: an analysis of 58 cases diagnosed before 40 years. *Br J Haematol* 67: 285-291.

921. Najean Y, Rain JD (1997). The very long-term evolution of polycythemia vera: an analysis of 318 patients initially treated by phlebotomy or 32P between 1969 and 1981. *Semin Hematol* 34: 6-16.

922. Nakamura S, Aoyagi K, Furuse M, Suekane H, Matsumoto T, Yao T, Sakai Y, Fuchigami T, Yamamoto I, Tsuneyoshi M, Fujishima M (1998). B-cell monoclonality precedes the development of gastric MALT lymphoma in Helicobacter pylori-associated chronic gastritis. *Am J Pathol* 152: 1271-1279.

923. Nakamura S, Hara K, Suchi T, Ito M, Ikeda H, Nagahama M, Nakayama A, Nakagawa A, Kaneshima H, Asai J (1988). Interdigitating cell sarcoma. A morphologic, immunohistologic, and enzyme-histochemical study. *Cancer* 61: 562-568.

924. Nakamura S, Katoh E, Koshikawa T, Yatabe Y, Nagasaka T, Ishida H, Tokoro Y, Koike K, Kagami Y, Ogura M, Kojima M, Nara Y, Mizoguchi Y, Hara K, Kurita S, Seto M, Suchi T (1997). Clinicopathologic study of nasal T/NK-cell lymphoma among the Japanese. *Pathol Int* 47: 38-53.

925. Nakamura S, Koshikawa T, Kitoh K, Nakayama A, Yamakawa M, Imai Y, Ishii K, Fujita M, Suchi T (1994). Interdigitating cell sarcoma: a morphologic and immunologic study of lymph node lesions in four cases. *Pathol Int* 44: 374-386.

926. Nakamura S, Koshikawa T, Yatabe Y, Suchi T (1998). Lymphoblastic lymphoma expressing CD56 and TdT. *Am J Surg Pathol* 22: 135-137.

927. Nakamura S, Shiota M, Nakagawa A, Yatabe Y, Kojima M, Motoori T, Suzuki R, Kagami Y, Ogura M, Morishima Y, Mizoguchi Y, Okamoto M, Seto M, Koshikawa T, Mori S, Suchi T (1997). Anaplastic large cell lymphoma: a distinct molecular pathologic entity: a reappraisal with special reference to p80(NPM/ALK) expression. *Am J Surg Pathol* 21: 1420-1432.

928. Nakamura S, Suchi T (1991). A clinicopathologic study of node-based, low-grade, peripheral T-cell lymphoma. Angioimmunoblastic lymphoma, T-zone lymphoma, and lymphoepithelioid lymphoma. *Cancer* 67: 2566-2578.

929. Nakamura S, Suchi T, Koshikawa T, Kitoh K, Koike K, Komatsu H, Iida S, Kagami Y, Ogura M, Katoh E (1995). Clinicopathologic study of CD56 (NCAM)-positive angiocentric lymphoma occurring in sites other than the upper and lower respiratory tract. *Am J Surg Pathol* 19: 284-296.

930. Nakamura S, Yao T, Aoyagi K, Iida M, Fujishima M, Tsuneyoshi M (1997). Helicobacter pylori and primary gastric lymphoma. A histopathologic and immunohistochemical analysis of 237 patients. *Cancer* 79: 3-11.

931. Nalesnik MA, Jaffe R, Starzl TE, Demetris AJ, Porter K, Burnham JA, Makowka L, Ho M, Locker J (1988). The pathology of posttransplant lymphoproliferative disorders occurring in the setting of cyclosporine A-prednisone immunosuppression. *Am J Pathol* 133: 173-192.

932. Nalesnik MA, Randhawa P, Demetris AJ, Casavilla A, Fung JJ, Locker J (1993). Lymphoma resembling Hodgkin disease after posttransplant lymphoproliferative disorder in a liver transplant recipient. *Cancer* 72: 2568-2573.

933. Nathwani BN, Anderson JR, Armitage JO, Cavalli F, Diebold J, Drachenberg MR, Harris NL, MacLennan KA, Muller-Hermelink HK, Ullrich FA, Weisenburger DD (1999). Clinical significance of follicular lymphoma with monocytoid B cells. Non-Hodgkin's Lymphoma Classification Project. *Hum Pathol* 30: 263-268.

934. Nathwani BN, Anderson JR, Armitage JO, Cavalli F, Diebold J, Drachenberg MR, Harris NL, MacLennan KA, Muller-Hermelink HK, Ullrich FA, Weisenburger DD (1999). Marginal zone B-cell lymphoma: A clinical comparison of nodal and mucosa-associated lymphoid tissue types. Non-Hodgkin's Lymphoma Classification Project. *J Clin Oncol* 17: 2486-2492.

935. Nathwani BN, Metter GE, Miller TP, Burke JS, Mann RB, Barcos M, Kjeldsberg CR, Dixon DO, Winberg CD, Whitcomb CC (1986). What should be the morphologic criteria for the subdivision of follicular lymphomas? *Blood* 68: 837-845.

936. Natkunam Y, Rouse RV (2000). Utility of paraffin section immunohistochemistry for C-KIT (CD117) in the differential diagnosis of systemic mast cell disease involving the bone marrow. *Am J Surg Pathol* 24: 81-91.

937. Natkunam Y, Warnke RA, Zehnder JL, Cornbleet PJ (1999). Aggressive natural killer-like T-cell malignancy with leukemic presentation following solid organ transplantation. *Am J Clin Pathol* 111: 663-671.

938. Navas IC, Ortiz-Romero PL, Villuendas R, Martinez P, Garcia C, Gomez E, Rodriguez JL, Garcia D, Vanaclocha F, Iglesias L, Piris MA, Algara P (2000). p16(INK4a) gene alterations are frequent in lesions of mycosis fungoides. *Am J Pathol* 156: 1565-1572.

939. Navid F, Mosijczuk AD, Head DR, Borowitz MJ, Carroll AJ, Brandt JM, Link MP, Rozans MK, Thomas GA, Schwenn MR, Shields DJ, Vietti TJ, Pullen DJ (1999). Acute lymphoblastic leukemia with the (8;14)(q24;q32) translocation and FAB L3 morphology associated with a B-precursor immunophenotype: the Pediatric Oncology Group experience. *Leukemia* 13: 135-141.

940. Neiman RS, Rosen PJ, Lukes RJ (1973). Lymphocyte-depletion Hodgkin's disease. A clinicopathological entity. *N Engl J Med* 288: 751-755.

941. Nelson BP, Nalesnik MA, Bahler DW, Locker J, Fung JJ, Swerdlow SH (2000). Epstein-Barr virus-negative post-transplant lymphoproliferative disorders: a distinct entity? *Am J Surg Pathol* 24: 375-385.

942. Neri A, Barriga F, Knowles DM, Magrath IT, Dalla-Favera R (1988). Different regions of the immunoglobulin heavy-chain locus are involved in chromosomal translocations in distinct pathogenetic forms of Burkitt lymphoma. *Proc Natl Acad Sci U S A* 85: 2748-2752.

943. Neubauer A, Thiede C, Morgner A, Alpen B, Ritter M, Neubauer B, Wundisch T, Ehninger G, Stolte M, Bayerdorffer E (1997). Cure of Helicobacter pylori infection and duration of remission of low-grade gastric mucosa-associated lymphoid tissue lymphoma. *J Natl Cancer Inst* 89: 1350-1355.

944. Neumann MP, Frizzera G (1986). The coexistence of Langerhans' cell granulomatosis and malignant lymphoma may take different forms: report of seven cases with a review of the literature. *Hum Pathol* 17: 1060-1065.

945. Neuwirtova R, Mocikova K, Musilova J, Jelinek J, Havlicek F, Michalova K, Adamkov M (1996). Mixed myelodysplastic and myeloproliferative syndromes. *Leuk Res* 20: 717-726.

946. Nezelof C, Basset F (1998). Langerhans cell histiocytosis research. Past, present, and future. *Hematol Oncol Clin North Am* 12: 385-406.

947. Ng CS, Lo ST, Chan JK (1999). Peripheral T and putative natural killer cell lymphomas commonly coexpress CD95 and CD95 ligand. *Hum Pathol* 30: 48-53.

948. Ng CS, Lo ST, Chan JK, Chan WC (1997). CD56+ putative natural killer cell lymphomas: production of cytolytic effectors and related proteins mediating tumor cell apoptosis? *Hum Pathol* 28: 1276-1282.

949. Nguyen DT, Diamond LW, Hansmann ML, Hell K, Fischer R (1994). Follicular dendritic cell sarcoma. Identification by monoclonal antibodies in paraffin sections. *Appl Immunohistochem* 2: 60-64.

950. Nichols CR, Roth BJ, Heerema N, Griep J, Tricot G (1990). Hematologic neoplasia associated with primary mediastinal germ-cell tumors. *N Engl J Med* 322: 1425-1429.

951. Nicholson HS, Egeler RM, Nesbit ME (1998). The epidemiology of Langerhans cell histiocytosis. *Hematol Oncol Clin North Am* 12: 379-384.

952. Niemeyer CM, Arico M, Basso G, Biondi A, Cantu RA, Creutzig U, Haas O, Harbott J, Hasle H, Kerndrup G, Locatelli F, Mann G, Stollmann-Gibbels B, Veer-Korthof ET, van Wering E, Zimmermann M (1997). Chronic myelomonocytic leukemia in childhood: a retrospective analysis of 110 cases. European Working Group on Myelodysplastic Syndromes in Childhood (EWOG-MDS). *Blood* 89: 3534-3543.

953. Niemeyer CM, Fenu S, Hasle H, Mann G, Stary J, van Wering E (1998). Responce: Differentiating juvenile myelomonocytic leukemia from infectious disease. *Blood* 91: 365-366.

954. Nizze H, Cogliatti SB, von Schilling C, Feller AC, Lennert K (1991). Monocytoid B-cell lymphoma: morphological variants and relationship to low-grade B-cell lymphoma of the mucosa-associated lymphoid tissue. *Histopathology* 18: 403-414.

955. Norrby A, Ridell B, Swolin B, Westin J (1982). Rearrangement of chromosome no. 3 in a case of preleukemia with thrombocytosis. *Cancer Genet Cytogenet* 5: 257-263.

956. Norton AJ, Matthews J, Pappa V, Shamash J, Love S, Rohatiner AZ, Lister TA (1995). Mantle cell lymphoma: natural history defined in a serially biopsied population over a 20-year period. *Ann Oncol* 6: 249-256.

957. Nowell P, Finan J, Glover D, Guerry D (1981). Cytogenetic evidence for the clonal nature of Richter's syndrome. *Blood* 58: 183-186.

958. Nowell PC, Hungerford DA (1960). A minutre chromosome in human chronic granulocytic leukemia. *Science* 132: 1497-1500.

959. Nunez G, London L, Hockenbery D, Alexander M, McKearn JP, Korsmeyer SJ (1990). Deregulated Bcl-2 gene expression selectively prolongs survival of growth factor-deprived hemopoietic cell lines. *J Immunol* 144: 3602-3610.

960. O'Briain DS, Kennedy MJ, Daly PA, O'Brien AA, Tanner WA, Rogers P, Lawlor E (1989). Multiple lymphomatous polyposis of the gastrointestinal tract. A clinicopathologically distinctive form of non-Hodgkin's lymphoma of B-cell centrocytic type. *Am J Surg Pathol* 13: 691-699.

961. O'Connor NT, Crick JA, Wainscoat JS, Gatter KC, Stein H, Falini B, Mason DY (1986). Evidence for monoclonal T lymphocyte proliferation in angioimmunoblastic lymphadenopathy. *J Clin Pathol* 39: 1229-1232.

962. O'Shea JJ, Jaffe ES, Lane HC, MacDermott RP, Fauci AS (1987). Peripheral T cell lymphoma presenting as hypereosinophilia with vasculitis. Clinical, pathologic, and immunologic features. *Am J Med* 82: 539-545.

963. Offit K, Lo CF, Louie DC, Parsa NZ, Leung D, Portlock C, Ye BH, Lista F, Filippa DA, Rosenbaum A (1994). Rearrangement of the bcl-6 gene as a prognostic marker in diffuse large-cell lymphoma. *N Engl J Med* 331: 74-80.

964. Offit K, Parsa NZ, Gaidano G, Filippa DA, Louie D, Pan D, Jhanwar SC, Dalla-Favera R, Chaganti RS (1993). 6q deletions define distinct clinico-pathologic subsets of non-Hodgkin's lymphoma. *Blood* 82: 2157-2162.

965. Ohno T, Smir BN, Weisenburger DD, Gascoyne RD, Hinrichs SD, Chan WC (1998). Origin of the Hodgkin/Reed-Sternberg cells in chronic lymphocytic leukemia with "Hodgkin's transformation". *Blood* 91: 1757-1761.

966. Ohno T, Stribley JA, Wu G, Hinrichs SH, Weisenburger DD, Chan WC (1997). Clonality in nodular lymphocyte-predominant Hodgkin's disease. *N Engl J Med* 337: 459-465.

967. Ohno Y, Amakawa R, Fukuhara S, Huang CR, Kamesaki H, Amano H, Imanaka T, Takahashi Y, Arita Y, Uchiyama T (1989). Acute transformation of chronic large granular lymphocyte leukemia associated with additional chromosome abnormality. *Cancer* 64: 63-67.

968. Ohshima K, Kikuchi M, Mizuno S, Akashi K, Moriyama K, Yoneda S, Takeshita M, Shibata T (1995). Hepatosinusoidal leukaemia/lymphoma consisting of Epstein-Barr virus-containing natural killer cell leukaemia/lymphoma and T-cell lymphoma; mimicking malignant histiocytosis. *Hematol Oncol* 13: 83-97.

969. Ohshima K, Mukai Y, Shiraki H, Suzumiya J, Tashiro K, Kikuchi M (1997). Clonal integration and expression of human T-cell lymphotropic virus type I in carriers detected by polymerase chain reaction and inverse PCR. *Am J Hematol* 54: 306-312.

970. Ohshima K, Suzumiya J, Kato A, Tashiro K, Kikuchi M (1997). Clonal HTLV-I-infected CD4+ T-lymphocytes and non-clonal non-HTLV-I-infected giant cells in incipient ATLL with Hodgkin-like histologic features. *Int J Cancer* 72: 592-598.

971. Ohshima K, Suzumiya J, Sato K, Kanda M, Simazaki T, Kawasaki C, Haraoka S, Kikuchi M (1999). Survival of patients with HTLV-I-associated lymph node lesions. *J Pathol* 189: 539-545.

972. Ohshima K, Suzumiya J, Sato K, Kanda M, Sugihara M, Haraoka S, Takeshita M, Kikuchi M (1998). Nodal T-cell lymphoma in an HTLV-I-endemic area: proviral HTLV-I DNA, histological classification and clinical evaluation. *Br J Haematol* 101: 703-711.

973. Ohshima K, Suzumiya J, Shimazaki K, Kato A, Tanaka T, Kanda M, Kikuchi M (1997). Nasal T/NK cell lymphomas commonly express perforin and Fas ligand: important mediators of tissue damage. *Histopathology* 31: 444-450.

974. Okuda T, Fisher R, Downing JR (1996). Molecular diagnostics in pediatric acute lymphoblastic leukemia. *Mol Diagn* 1: 139-151.

975. Okuda T, Sakamoto S, Deguchi T, Misawa S, Kashima K, Yoshihara T, Ikushima S, Hibi S, Imashuku S (1991). Hemophagocytic syndrome associated with aggressive natural killer cell leukemia. *Am J Hematol* 38: 321-323.

976. Okun DB, Tanaka KR (1978). Leukocyte alkaline phosphatase. *Am J Hematol* 4: 293-299.

977. Opelz G, Henderson R (1993). Incidence of non-Hodgkin lymphoma in kidney and heart transplant recipients. *Lancet* 342: 1514-1516.

978. Orfao A, Chillon MC, Bortoluci AM, Lopez-Berges MC, Garcia-Sanz R, Gonzalez M, Tabernero MD, Garcia-Marcos MA, Rasillo AI, Hernandez-Rivas J, San Miguel JF (1999). The flow cytometric pattern of CD34, CD15 and CD13 expression in acute myeloblastic leukemia is highly characteristic of the presence of PML-RARalpha gene rearrangements. *Haematologica* 84: 405-412.

979. Orfao A, Escribano L, Villarrubia J, Velasco JL, Cervero C, Ciudad J, Navarro JL, San Miguel JF (1996). Flow cytometric analysis of mast cells from normal and pathological human bone marrow samples: identification and enumeration. *Am J Pathol* 149: 1493-1499.

980. Orlandi E, Castelli G, Brusamolino E, Canevari A, Morra E, Lazzarino M, Bernasconi C (1989). Hemorrhagic and thrombotic complications in polycythemia vera. A clinical study. *Haematologica* 74: 45-49.

981. Osborne BM, Butler JJ, Gresik MV (1992). Progressive transformation of germinal centers: comparison of 23 pediatric patients to the adult population. *Mod Pathol* 5: 135-140.

982. Osborne BM, Mackay B (1994). True histiocytic lymphoma with multiple skin nodules. *Ultrastruct Pathol* 18: 241-246.

983. Oscier DG, Thompsett A, Zhu D, Stevenson FK (1997). Differential rates of somatic hypermutation in V(H) genes among subsets of chronic lymphocytic leukemia defined by chromosomal abnormalities. *Blood* 89: 4153-4160.

984. Oshimi K (1996). Lymphoproliferative disorders of natural killer cells. *Int J Hematol* 63: 279-290.

985. Oshimi K, Yamada O, Kaneko T, Nishinarita S, Iizuka Y, Urabe A, Inamori T, Asano S, Takahashi S, Hattori M (1993). Laboratory findings and clinical courses of 33 patients with granular lymphocyte-proliferative disorders. *Leukemia* 7: 782-788.

986. Otsuki T, Kumar S, Ensoli B, Kingma DW, Yano T, Stetler-Stevenson M, Jaffe ES, Raffeld M (1996). Detection of HHV-8/KSHV DNA sequences in AIDS-associated extranodal lymphoid malignancies. *Leukemia* 10: 1358-1362.

987. Ott G, Kalla J, Hanke A, Muller JG, Rosenwald A, Katzenberger T, Kretschmar R, Kreipe H, Muller-Hermelink HK (1998). The cytomorphological spectrum of mantle cell lymphoma is reflected by distinct biological features. *Leuk Lymphoma* 32: 55-63.

988. Ott G, Kalla J, Ott MM, Schryen B, Katzenberger T, Muller JG, Muller-Hermelink HK (1997). Blastoid variants of mantle cell lymphoma: frequent bcl-1 rearrangements at the major translocation cluster region and tetraploid chromosome clones. *Blood* 89: 1421-1429.

989. Ott G, Katzenberger T, Greiner A, Kalla J, Rosenwald A, Heinrich U, Ott MM, Muller-Hermelink HK (1997). The t(11;18)(q21;q21) chromosome translocation is a frequent and specific aberration in low-grade but not high-grade malignant non-Hodgkin's lymphomas of the mucosa-associated lymphoid tissue (MALT-) type. *Cancer Res* 57: 3944-3948.

990. Ottensmeier CH, Thompsett AR, Zhu D, Wilkins BS, Sweetenham JW, Stevenson FK (1998). Analysis of VH genes in follicular and diffuse lymphoma shows ongoing somatic mutation and multiple isotype transcripts in early disease with changes during disease progression. *Blood* 91: 4292-4299.

991. Padeh S, Sharon N, Schiby G, Rechavi G, Passwell JH (1997). Hodgkin's lymphoma in systemic onset juvenile rheumatoid arthritis after treatment with low dose methotrexate. *J Rheumatol* 24: 2035-2037.

992. Pagliuca A, Layton DM, Manoharan A, Gordon S, Green PJ, Mufti GJ (1989). Myelofibrosis in primary myelodysplastic syndromes: a clinico-morphological study of 10 cases. *Br J Haematol* 71: 499-504.

993. Pallesen G, Myhre-Jensen O (1987). Immunophenotypic analysis of neoplastic cells in follicular dendritic cell sarcoma. *Leukemia* 1: 549-557.

994. Pancake BA, Wassef EH, Zucker-Franklin D (1996). Demonstration of antibodies to human T-cell lymphotropic virus-I tax in patients with the cutaneous T-cell lymphoma, mycosis fungoides, who are seronegative for antibodies to the structural proteins of the virus. *Blood* 88: 3004-3009.

995. Pancake BA, Zucker-Franklin D, Coutavas EE (1995). The cutaneous T cell lymphoma, mycosis fungoides, is a human T cell lymphotropic virus-associated disease. A study of 50 patients. *J Clin Invest* 95: 547-554.

996. Pandolfi F, Loughran TP, Jr., Starkebaum G, Chisesi T, Barbui T, Chan WC, Brouet JC, De Rossi G, McKenna RW, Salsano F (1990). Clinical course and prognosis of the lymphoproliferative disease of granular lymphocytes. A multicenter study. *Cancer* 65: 341-348.

997. Pane F, Frigeri F, Camera A, Sindona M, Brighel F, Martinelli V, Luciano L, Selleri C, Del Vecchio N, Rotoli B, Salvatore F (1996). Complete phenotypic and genotypic lineage switch in a Philadelphia chromosome-positive acute lymphoblastic leukemia. *Leukemia* 10: 741-745.

998. Pane F, Frigeri F, Sindona M, Luciano L, Ferrara F, Cimino R, Meloni G, Saglio G, Salvatore F, Rotoli B (1996). Neutrophilic-chronic myeloid leukemia: a distinct disease with a specific molecular marker (BCR/ABL with C3/A2 junction). *Blood* 88: 2410-2414.

999. Paquette RL, Landaw EM, Pierre RV, Kahan J, Lubbert M, Lazcano O, Isaac G, McCormick F, Koeffler HP (1993). N-ras mutations are associated with poor prognosis and increased risk of leukemia in myelodysplastic syndrome. *Blood* 82: 590-599.

999a. Parkin DM, Pisani P, Ferlay J (1999). Global cancer statistics. *CA Cancer J Clin* 49: 33-64.

1000. Parkin JL, Arthur DC, Abramson CS, McKenna RW, Kersey JH, Heideman RL, Brunning RD (1982). Acute leukemia associated with the t(4;11) chromosome rearrangement: ultrastructural and immunologic characteristics. *Blood* 60: 1321-1331.

1001. Parreira L, Tavares dC, Hibbin JA, Marsh JC, Marcus RE, Babapulle VB, Spry CJ, Goldman JM, Catovsky D (1986). Chromosome and cell culture studies in eosinophilic leukaemia. *Br J Haematol* 62: 659-669.

1002. Parwaresch MR, Horny HP, Lennert K (1985). Tissue mast cells in health and disease. *Pathol Res Pract* 179: 439-461.

1003. Pasqualucci L, Migliazza A, Fracchiolla N, William C, Neri A, Baldini L, Chaganti RS, Klein U, Kuppers R, Rajewsky K, Dalla-Favera R (1998). BCL-6 mutations in normal germinal center B cells: evidence of somatic hypermutation acting outside Ig loci. *Proc Natl Acad Sci U S A* 95: 11816-11821.

1004. Passmore SJ, Hann IM, Stiller CA, Ramani P, Swansbury GJ, Gibbons B, Reeves BR, Chessells JM (1995). Pediatric myelodysplasia: a study of 68 children and a new prognostic scoring system. *Blood* 85: 1742-1750.

1005. Pastore C, Gaidano G, Ghia P, Fassone L, Cilia AM, Gloghini A, Capello D, Buonaiuto D, Gonella S, Roncella S, Carbone A, Saglio G (1998). Patterns of cytokine expression in AIDS-related non-Hodgkin's lymphoma. *Br J Haematol* 103: 143-149.

1006. Patakfalvi A, Csete B, Horvath T (1969). Familial myelofibrosis. *Haematologia* 3: 217-224.

1007. Patsouris E, Engelhard M, Zwingers T, Lennert K (1993). Lymphoepithelioid cell lymphoma (Lennert's lymphoma): clinical features derived from analysis of 108 cases. *Br J Haematol* 84: 346-348.

1008. Patte C, Leverger G, Perel Y, Rubie H, Otten J, Nelken B, et al (1990). Up-dated results of the LMB86 protocol of the French Society of Pediatric Oncology for B-cell non-Hodgkin's lymphoma with CNS involvement B-ALL. *Med Pediatr Oncol* 18: 397.

1009. Patte C, Philip T, Rodary C, Zucker JM, Behrendt H, Gentet JC, Lamagnere JP, Otten J, Dufillot D, Pein F (1991). High survival rate in advanced-stage B-cell lymphomas and leukemias without CNS involvement with a short intensive poly-chemotherapy: results from the French Pediatric Oncology Society of a randomized trial of 216 children. *J Clin Oncol* 9: 123-132.

1010. Paul C, Le Tourneau A, Cayuela JM, Devidas A, Robert C, Molinie V, Dubertret L (1997). Epstein-Barr virus-associated lymphoproliferative disease during methotrexate therapy for psoriasis. *Arch Dermatol* 133: 867-871.

1011. Paulli M, Berti E, Rosso R, Boveri E, Kindl S, Klersy C, Lazzarino M, Borroni G, Menestrina F, Santucci M (1995). CD30/Ki-1-positive lymphoproliferative disorders of the skin – clinicopathologic correlation and statistical analysis of 86 cases: a multicentric study from the European Organization for Research and Treatment of Cancer Cutaneous Lymphoma Project Group. *J Clin Oncol* 13: 1343-1354.

1012. Paulli M, Strater J, Gianelli U, Rousset MT, Gambacorta M, Orlandi E, Klersy C, Lavabre-Bertrand T, Morra E, Manegold C, Lazzarino M, Magrini U, Moller P (1999). Mediastinal B-cell lymphoma: a study of its histomorphologic spectrum based on 109 cases. *Hum Pathol* 30: 178-187.

1013. Pawson R, Dyer MJ, Barge R, Matutes E, Thornton PD, Emmett E, Kluin-Nelemans JC, Fibbe WE, Willemze R, Catovsky D (1997). Treatment of T-cell prolymphocytic leukemia with human CD52 antibody. *J Clin Oncol* 15: 2667-2672.

1014. Pawson R, Matutes E, Brito-Babapulle V, Maljaie H, Hedges M, Mercieca J, Dyer M, Catovsky D (1997). Sezary cell leukaemia: a distinct T cell disorder or a variant form of T prolymphocytic leukaemia? *Leukemia* 11: 1009-1013.

1015. Pearson TC (1991). Primary thrombocythaemia: diagnosis and management. *Br J Haematol* 78: 145-148.

1016. Pedersen-Bjergaard J, Philip P, Larsen SO, Andersson M, Daugaard G, Ersboll J, Hansen SW, Hou-Jensen K, Nielsen D, Sigsgaard TC (1993). Therapy-related myelodysplasia and acute myeloid leukemia. Cytogenetic characteristics of 115 consecutive cases and risk in seven cohorts of patients treated intensively for malignant diseases in the Copenhagen series. *Leukemia* 7: 1975-1986.

1017. Pekarsky Y, Hallas C, Isobe M, Russo G, Croce CM (1999). Abnormalities at 14q32.1 in T cell malignancies involve two oncogenes. *Proc Natl Acad Sci U S A* 96: 2949-2951.

1018. Pelicci PG, Knowles DM, Arlin ZA, Wieczorek R, Luciw P, Dina D, Basilico C, Dalla-Favera R (1986). Multiple monoclonal B cell expansions and c-myc oncogene rearrangements in acquired immune deficiency syndrome-related lymphoproliferative disorders. Implications for lymphomagenesis. *J Exp Med* 164: 2049-2060.

1019. Pelicci PG, Knowles DM, Magrath I, Dalla-Favera R (1986). Chromosomal breakpoints and structural alterations of the c-myc locus differ in endemic and sporadic forms of Burkitt lymphoma. *Proc Natl Acad Sci U S A* 83: 2984-2988.

1020. Peng HZ, Du MQ, Koulis A, Aiello A, Dogan A, Pan LX, Isaacson PG (1999). Nonimmunoglobulin gene hypermutation in germinal center B cells. *Blood* 93: 2167-2172.

1021. Penn I (1991). The changing pattern of posttransplant malignancies. *Transplant Proc* 23: 1101-1103.

1022. Perentesis J, Ramsey NKC, Brunning RD, et al (1983). Biphenotypic leukemia: immunologic and morphologic evidence for a common lymphoid-myeloid progenitor in man. *J Ped* 101: 63-67.

1023. Perez-Ordonez B, Erlandson RA, Rosai J (1996). Follicular dendritic cell tumor: report of 13 additional cases of a distinctive entity. *Am J Surg Pathol* 20: 944-955.

1024. Perez-Ordonez B, Rosai J (1998). Follicular dendritic cell tumor: review of the entity. *Semin Diagn Pathol* 15: 144-154.

1025. Perniciaro C, Winkelmann RK, Daoud MS, Su WP (1995). Malignant angioendotheliomatosis is an angiotropic intravascular lymphoma. Immunohistochemical, ultrastructural, and molecular genetics studies. *Am J Dermatopathol* 17: 242-248.

1026. Perrone T, Frizzera G, Rosai J (1986). Mediastinal diffuse large-cell lymphoma with sclerosis. A clinicopathologic study of 60 cases. *Am J Surg Pathol* 10: 176-191.

1027. Perry DA, Bast MA, Armitage JO, Weisenburger DD (1990). Diffuse intermediate lymphocytic lymphoma. A clinicopathologic study and comparison with small lymphocytic lymphoma and diffuse small cleaved cell lymphoma. *Cancer* 66: 1995-2000.

1028. Peters AM, Kohfink B, Martin H, Griesinger F, Wormann B, Gahr M, Roesler J (1999). Defective apoptosis due to a point mutation in the death domain of CD95 associated with autoimmune lymphoproliferative syndrome, T-cell lymphoma, and Hodgkin's disease. *Exp Hematol* 27: 868-874.

1029. Peterson LC, Brown BA, Crosson JT, Mladenovic J (1986). Application of the immunoperoxidase technic to bone marrow trephine biopsies in the classification of patients with monoclonal gammopathies. *Am J Clin Pathol* 85: 688-693.

1030. Peterson LC, Parkin JL, Arthur DC, Brunning RD (1991). Acute basophilic leukemia. A clinical, morphologic, and cytogenetic study of eight cases. *Am J Clin Pathol* 96: 160-170.

1031. Petrella T, Dalac S, Maynadie M, Mugneret F, Thomine E, Courville P, Joly P, Lenormand B, Arnould L, Wechsler J, Bagot M, Rieux C, Bosq J, Avril MF, Bernheim A, Molina T, Devidas A, Delfau-Larue MH, Gaulard P, Lambert D (1999). CD4+ CD56+ cutaneous neoplasms: a distinct hematological entity? Groupe Francais d'Etude des Lymphomes Cutanes (GFELC). *Am J Surg Pathol* 23: 137-146.

1032. Petrella T, Delfau-Larue MH, Caillot D, Morcillo JL, Casasnovas O, Portier H, Gaulard P, Farcet JP, Arnould L (1996). Nasopharyngeal lymphomas: further evidence for a natural killer cell origin. *Hum Pathol* 27: 827-833.

1033. Pettit CK, Zukerberg LR, Gray MH, Ferry JA, Rosenberg AE, Harmon DC, Harris NL (1990). Primary lymphoma of bone. A B-cell neoplasm with a high frequency of multilobated cells. *Am J Surg Pathol* 14: 329-334.

1034. Picker LJ, Weiss LM, Medeiros LJ, Wood GS, Warnke RA (1987). Immunophenotypic criteria for the diagnosis of non-Hodgkin's lymphoma. *Am J Pathol* 128: 181-201.

1035. Pileri SA, Grogan TM, Harris NL, Banks P, Campo E, Chan JK, Dalla-Favera R, Delsol G, De Wolf PC, Falini B, Gascoyne RD, Gaulard P, Isaacson PG, Jaffe E, Kluin P, Knowles DM, Mason DY, Mori S, Muller-Hermelink HK, Piris MA, Ralfkiaer E, Stein H, Su IJ, Warnke RA, Weiss LM (2001). Tumors of histiocytes and accessory dendritic cells. An immunohistochemical approach to classification from the International Lymphoma Study Group based on 61 cases. *Histopathology* (in press).

1036. Pileri SA, Pulford K, Mori S, Mason DY, Sabattini E, Roncador G, Piccioli M, Ceccarelli C, Piccaluga PP, Santini D, Leone O, Stein H, Falini B (1997). Frequent expression of the NPM-ALK chimeric fusion protein in anaplastic large-cell lymphoma, lympho-histiocytic type. *Am J Pathol* 150: 1207-1211.

1037. Pilozzi E, Muller-Hermelink HK, Falini B, Wolf-Peeters C, Fidler C, Gatter K, Wainscoat J (1999). Gene rearrangements in T-cell lymphoblastic lymphoma. *J Pathol* 188: 267-270.

1038. Pinkel D (1998). Differentiating juvenile myelomonocytic leukemia from infectious disease. *Blood* 91: 365-367.

1039. Pinkus GS, O'Hara CJ, Said JW (1990). Peripheral/post-thymic T-cell lymphomas: a spectrum of disease. Clinical, pathologic, and immunologic features of 78 cases. *Cancer* 65: 971-998.

1040. Pinkus GS, Said JW (1985). Hodgkin's disease, lymphocyte predominance type, nodular – a distinct entity? Unique staining profile for L&H variants of Reed-Sternberg cells defined by monoclonal antibodies to leukocyte common antigen, granulocyte-specific antigen, and B-cell-specific antigen. *Am J Pathol* 118: 1-6.

1041. Pinkus GS, Said JW (1988). Hodgkin's disease, lymphocyte predominance type, nodular – further evidence for a B cell derivation. L & H variants of Reed-Sternberg cells express L26, a pan B cell marker. *Am J Pathol* 133: 211-217.

1042. Pinto A, Hutchison RE, Grant LH, Trevenen CL, Berard CW (1990). Follicular lymphomas in pediatric patients. *Mod Pathol* 3: 308-313.

1043. Pinyol M, Cobo F, Bea S, Jares P, Nayach I, Fernandez PL, Montserrat E, Cardesa A, Campo E (1998). p16(INK4a) gene inactivation by deletions, mutations, and hypermethylation is associated with transformed and aggressive variants of non-Hodgkin's lymphomas. *Blood* 91: 2977-2984.

1044. Piris M, Brown DC, Gatter KC, Mason DY (1990). CD30 expression in non-Hodgkin's lymphoma. *Histopathology* 17: 211-218.

1045. Piro LD, Carrera CJ, Carson DA, Beutler E (1990). Lasting remissions in hairy-cell leukemia induced by a single infusion of 2-chlorodeoxyadenosine. *N Engl J Med* 322: 1117-1121.

1046. Pittaluga S, Ayoubi TA, Wlodarska I, Stul M, Cassiman JJ, Mecucci C, Van den BH, Van De Ven WJ, Wolf-Peeters C (1996). BCL-6 expression in reactive lymphoid tissue and in B-cell non-Hodgkin's lymphomas. *J Pathol* 179: 145-150.

1047. Pittaluga S, Tierens A, Pinyol M, Campo E, Delabie J, Wolf-Peeters C (1998). Blastic variant of mantle cell lymphoma shows a heterogenous pattern of somatic mutations of the rearranged immunoglobulin heavy chain variable genes. *Br J Haematol* 102: 1301-1306.

1048. Pittaluga S, Verhoef G, Criel A, Maes A, Nuyts J, Boogaerts M, De Wolf PC (1996). Prognostic significance of bone marrow trephine and peripheral blood smears in 55 patients with mantle cell lymphoma. *Leuk Lymphoma* 21: 115-125.

1049. Pittaluga S, Wiodarska I, Pulford K, Campo E, Morris SW, Van den BH, Wolf-Peeters C (1997). The monoclonal antibody ALK1 identifies a distinct morphological subtype of anaplastic large cell lymphoma associated with 2p23/ALK rearrangements. *Am J Pathol* 151: 343-351.

1050. Ponzoni M, Arrigoni G, Gould VE, Del Curto B, Maggioni M, Scapinello A, Paolino S, Cassisa A, Patriarca C (2000). Lack of CD 29 (beta1 integrin) and CD 54 (ICAM-1) adhesion molecules in intravascular lymphomatosis. *Hum Pathol* 31: 220-226.

1051. Poppema S (1980). The diversity of the immunohistological staining pattern of Sternberg-Reed cells. *J Histochem Cytochem* 28: 788-791.

1052. Porter SR, Diz DP, Kumar N, Stock C, Barrett AW, Scully C (1999). Oral plasmablastic lymphoma in previously undiagnosed HIV disease. *Oral Surg Oral Med Oral Pathol Oral Radiol Endod* 87: 730-734.

1053. Potter M, Boyce CR (1962). Induction of plasma cell neoplasms in strain BALB/C mice with mineral oil and mineral oil adjuvants. *Nature* 193: 1086-1087.

1054. Pozzato G, Mazzaro C, Crovatto M, Modolo ML, Ceselli S, Mazzi G, Sulfaro S, Franzin F, Tulissi P, Moretti M (1994). Low-grade malignant lymphoma, hepatitis C virus infection, and mixed cryoglobulinemia. *Blood* 84: 3047-3053.

1055. Prchal JT (2001). Pathogenetic mechanisms of polycythemia vera and congenital polycythemic disorders. *Semin Hematol* 38: 10-20.

1056. Preud'Homme JL, Aucouturier P, Touchard G, Striker L, Khamlichi AA, Rocca A, Denoroy L, Cogne M (1994). Monoclonal immunoglobulin deposition disease (Randall type). Relationship with structural abnormalities of immunoglobulin chains. *Kidney Int* 46: 965-972.

1057. Preudhomme C, Dervite I, Wattel E, Vanrumbeke M, Flactif M, Lai JL, Hecquet B, Coppin MC, Nelken B, Gosselin B (1995). Clinical significance of p53 mutations in newly diagnosed Burkitt's lymphoma and acute lymphoblastic leukemia: a report of 48 cases. *J Clin Oncol* 13: 812-820.

1058. Prevot S, Hamilton-Dutoit S, Audouin J, Walter P, Pallesen G, Diebold J (1992). Analysis of African Burkitt's and high-grade B cell non-Burkitt's lymphoma for Epstein-Barr virus genomes using in situ hybridization. *Br J Haematol* 80: 27-32.

1059. Price SK (1990). Immunoproliferative small intestinal disease: a study of 13 cases with alpha heavy-chain disease. *Histopathology* 17: 7-17.

1060. Pui CH, Campana D, Crist WM (1995). Toward a clinically useful classification of the acute leukemias. *Leukemia* 9: 2154-2157.

1061. Pui CH, Relling MV, Rivera GK, Hancock ML, Raimondi SC, Heslop HE, Santana VM, Ribeiro RC, Sandlund JT, Mahmoud HH (1995). Epipodophyllotoxin-related acute myeloid leukemia: a study of 35 cases. *Leukemia* 9: 1990-1996.

1062. Pulford K, Lamant L, Morris SW, Butler LH, Wood KM, Stroud D, Delsol G, Mason DY (1997). Detection of anaplastic lymphoma kinase (ALK) and nucleolar protein nucleophosmin (NPM)-ALK proteins in normal and neoplastic cells with the monoclonal antibody ALK1. *Blood* 89: 1394-1404.

1063. Pulford KA, Rigney EM, Micklem KJ, Jones M, Stross WP, Gatter KC, Mason DY (1989). KP1: a new monoclonal antibody that detects a monocyte/macrophage associated antigen in routinely processed tissue sections. *J Clin Pathol* 42: 414-421.

1064. Pulford KA, Sipos A, Cordell JL, Stross WP, Mason DY (1990). Distribution of the CD68 macrophage/myeloid associated antigen. *Int Immunol* 2: 973-980.

1065. Purtilo DT, Strobach RS, Okano M, Davis JR (1992). Epstein-Barr virus-associated lymphoproliferative disorders. *Lab Invest* 67: 5-23.

1066. Qin Y, Greiner A, Trunk MJ, Schmausser B, Ott MM, Muller-Hermelink HK (1995). Somatic hypermutation in low-grade mucosa-associated lymphoid tissue-type B-cell lymphoma. *Blood* 86: 3528-3534.

1067. Quesnel B, Kantarjian H, Bjergaard JP, Brault P, Estey E, Lai JL, Tilly H, Stoppa AM, Archimbaud E, Harousseau JL (1993). Therapy-related acute myeloid leukemia with t(8;21), inv(16), and t(8;16): a report on 25 cases and review of the literature. *J Clin Oncol* 11: 2370-2379.

1068. Quintanilla-Martinez L, Fend F, Moguel LR, Spilove L, Beaty MW, Kingma DW, Raffeld M, Jaffe ES (1999). Peripheral T-cell lymphoma with Reed-Sternberg-like cells of B-cell phenotype and genotype associated with Epstein-Barr virus infection. *Am J Surg Pathol* 23: 1233-1240.

1069. Quintanilla-Martinez L, Franklin JL, Guerrero I, Krenacs L, Naresh KN, Rama-Rao C, Bhatia K, Raffeld M, Magrath IT (1999). Histological and immunophenotypic profile of nasal NK/T cell lymphomas from Peru: high prevalence of p53 overexpression. *Hum Pathol* 30: 849-855.

1070. Quintanilla-Martinez L, Kumar S, Fend F, Reyes E, Teruya-Feldstein J, Kingma DW, Sorbara L, Raffeld M, Straus SE, Jaffe ES (2000). Fulminant EBV(+) T-cell lymphoproliferative disorder following acute/chronic EBV infection: a distinct clinicopathologic syndrome. *Blood* 96: 443-451.

1071. Quintanilla-Martinez L, Lome-Maldonado C, Ott G, Gschwendtner A, Gredler E, Angeles-Angeles A, Reyes E, Fend F (1998). Primary intestinal non-Hodgkin's lymphoma and Epstein-Barr virus: high frequency of EBV-infection in T-cell lymphomas of Mexican origin. *Leuk Lymphoma* 30: 111-121.

1072. Rabbani GR, Phyliky RL, Tefferi A (1999). A long-term study of patients with chronic natural killer cell lymphocytosis. *Br J Haematol* 106: 960-966.

1073. Radaszkiewicz T, Dragosics B, Bauer P (1992). Gastrointestinal malignant lymphomas of the mucosa-associated lymphoid tissue: factors relevant to prognosis. *Gastroenterology* 102: 1628-1638.

1074. Rai KR, Sawitsky A, Cronkite EP, Chanana AD, Levy RN, Pasternack BS (1975). Clinical staging of chronic lymphocytic leukemia. *Blood* 46: 219-234.

1075. Raimondi SC (1993). Current status of cytogenetic research in childhood acute lymphoblastic leukemia. *Blood* 81: 2237-2251.

1076. Raimondi SC, Chang MN, Ravindranath Y, Behm FG, Gresik MV, Steuber CP, Weinstein HJ, Carroll AJ (1999). Chromosomal abnormalities in 478 children with acute myeloid leukemia: clinical characteristics and treatment outcome in a cooperative pediatric oncology group study-POG 8821. *Blood* 94: 3707-3716.

1077. Raimondi SC, Pui CH, Hancock ML, Behm FG, Filatov L, Rivera GK (1996). Heterogeneity of hyperdiploid (51-67) childhood acute lymphoblastic leukemia. *Leukemia* 10: 213-224.

1078. Rajkumar SV, Greipp PR (1999). Prognostic factors in multiple myeloma. *Hematol Oncol Clin North Am* 13: 1295-314, xi.

1079. Ralfkiaer E (1991). Immunohistological markers for the diagnosis of cutaneous lymphomas. *Semin Diagn Pathol* 8: 62-72.

1080. Ralfkiaer E, Delsol G, O'Connor NT, Brandtzaeg P, Brousset P, Vejlsgaard GL, Mason DY (1990). Malignant lymphomas of true histiocytic origin. A clinical, histological, immunophenotypic and genotypic study. *J Pathol* 160: 9-17.

1081. Ralfkiaer E, Stein H, Wantzin GL, Thomsen K, Ralfkiaer N, Mason DY (1985). Lymphomatoid papulosis. Characterization of skin infiltrates by monoclonal antibodies. *Am J Clin Pathol* 84: 587-593.

1082. Rambaldi A, Pelicci PG, Allavena P, Knowles DM, Rossini S, Bassan R, Barbui T, Dalla-Favera R, Mantovani A (1985). T cell receptor beta chain gene rearrangements in lymphoproliferative disorders of large granular lymphocytes/natural killer cells. *J Exp Med* 162: 2156-2162.

1083. Ramot B SNBJ (0 AD). Malabsorption syndrome in lymphoma of the small intestine. A study of 13 cases. *Isr J Med Sci* 1221-1226.

1084. Ramsay AD, Smith WJ, Isaacson PG (1988). T-cell-rich B-cell lymphoma. *Am J Surg Pathol* 12: 433-443.

1085. Randall RE, Williamson WC, Mullinax F, Tung MY, Still WJ (1976). Manifestations of systemic light chain deposition. *Am J Med* 60: 293-299.

1086. Randi ML, Putti MC, Fabris F, Sainati L, Zanesco L, Girolami A (2000). Features of essential thrombocythaemia in childhood: a study of five children. *Br J Haematol* 108: 86-89.

1087. Raphael M, Gentilhomme O, Tulliez M, Byron PA, Diebold J (1991). Histopathologic features of high-grade non-Hodgkin's lymphomas in acquired immunodeficiency syndrome. The French Study Group of Pathology for Human Immunodeficiency Virus-Associated Tumors. *Arch Pathol Lab Med* 115: 15-20.

1088. Raphael MM, Audouin J, Lamine M, Delecluse HJ, Vuillaume M, Lenoir GM, Gisselbrecht C, Lennert K, Diebold J (1994). Immunophenotypic and genotypic analysis of acquired immunodeficiency syndrome-related non-Hodgkin's lymphomas. Correlation with histologic features in 36 cases. French Study Group of Pathology for HIV-Associated Tumors. *Am J Clin Pathol* 101: 773-782.

1089. Rappaport H (1966). *Tumors of the Hematopoietic system. Atlas of Tumor Pathology.* AFIP: Washington, DC.

1090. Rappaport H, Winter W, Hicks E (1956). Follicular lymphoma. A re-evaluation of its position in the scheme of malignant lymphoma, based on a survey of 253 cases. *Cancer* 9: 792-821.

1091. Reardon DA, Hanson CA, Roth MS, Castle VP (1994). Lineage switch in Philadelphia chromosome-positive acute lymphoblastic leukemia. *Cancer* 73: 1526-1532.

1092. Redner RL, Rush EA, Faas S, Rudert WA, Corey SJ (1996). The t(5;17) variant of acute promyelocytic leukemia expresses a nucleophosmin-retinoic acid receptor fusion. *Blood* 87: 882-886.

1093. Ree HJ, Kadin ME, Kikuchi M, Ko YH, Go JH, Suzumiya J, Kim DS (1998). Angioimmunoblastic lymphoma (AILD-type T-cell lymphoma) with hyperplastic germinal centers. *Am J Surg Pathol* 22: 643-655.

1094. Rege-Cambrin G, Mecucci C, Tricot G, Michaux JL, Louwagie A, Van Hove W, Francart H, Van den BH (1987). A chromosomal profile of polycythemia vera. *Cancer Genet Cytogenet* 25: 233-245.

1095. Rege K, Swansburg GJ, Atra AA, et al (2000). Influence of age, secondary karyotype abnormalities CD19 status and extramedullary leukemia on survival. *in press* (in press).

1096. Reilly JT, Snowden JA, Spearing RL, Fitzgerald PM, Jones N, Watmore A, Potter A (1997). Cytogenetic abnormalities and their prognostic significance in idiopathic myelofibrosis: a study of 106 cases. *Br J Haematol* 98: 96-102.

1097. Reisman RP, Greco MA (1984). Virus-associated hemophagocytic syndrome due to Epstein-Barr virus. *Hum Pathol* 15: 290-293.

1098. Remstein ED, James CD, Kurtin PJ (2000). Incidence and subtype specificity of API2-MALT1 fusion translocations in extranodal, nodal, and splenic marginal zone lymphomas. *Am J Pathol* 156: 1183-1188.

1099. Requena L (1992). Erythrodermic mastocytosis. *Cutis* 49: 189-192.

1100. Richter M (1928). Generalized reticular cell sarcoma of lymph nodes associated with lymphocytic leukemia. *Am J Pathol* 4: 285-292.

1101. Ridell B, Carneskog J, Wedel H, Vilen L, Hogh D, I, Mellqvist UH, Brywe N, Wadenvik H, Kutti J (2000). Incidence of chronic myeloproliferative disorders in the city of Goteborg, Sweden 1983-1992. *Eur J Haematol* 65: 267-271.

1102. Ridley RC, Xiao H, Hata H, Woodliff J, Epstein J, Sanderson RD (1993). Expression of syndecan regulates human myeloma plasma cell adhesion to type I collagen. *Blood* 81: 767-774.

1103. Ries LAG, Kosary CL, Hankey BF, et al (1999). *SEER Cancer Statistics Review, 1973-1996.* National Cancer Institute: Bethesda, MD.

1104. Rijlaarsdam JU, Toonstra J, Meijer OW, Noordijk EM, Willemze R (1996). Treatment of primary cutaneous B-cell lymphomas of follicle center cell origin: a clinical follow-up study of 55 patients treated with radiotherapy or polychemotherapy. *J Clin Oncol* 14: 549-555.

1105. Rimsza LM, Campbell K, Dalton WS, Salmon S, Willcox G, Grogan TM (1999). The major vault protein (MVP), a new multidrug resistance associated protein, is frequently expressed in multiple myeloma. *Leuk Lymphoma* 34: 315-324.

1106. Rimsza LM, Larson RS, Winter SS, Foucar K, Chong YY, Garner KW, Leith CP (2000). Benign hematogone-rich lymphoid proliferations can be distinguished from B-lineage acute lymphoblastic leukemia by integration of morphology, immunophenotype, adhesion molecule expression, and architectural features. *Am J Clin Pathol* 114: 66-75.

1107. Risdall RJ, Dehner LP, Duray P, Kobrinsky N, Robison L, Nesbit ME, Jr. (1983). Histiocytosis X (Langerhans' cell histiocytosis): Prognostic role of histopathology. *Arch Pathol Lab Med* 107: 59-63.

1108. Risdall RJ, McKenna RW, Nesbit ME, Krivit W, Balfour HH, Simmons RL, Brunning RD (1979). Virus-associated hemophagocytic syndrome: a benign histiocytic proliferation distinct from malignant histiocytosis. *Cancer* 44: 993-1002.

1109. Roitt I (1997). *Roitt's Essential Immunology.* Blackwell Science: London.

1110. Rosati S, Mick R, Xu F, Stonys E, Le Beau MM, Larson R, Vardiman JW (1996). Refractory cytopenia with multilineage dysplasia: further characterization of an 'unclassifiable' myelodysplastic syndrome. *Leukemia* 10: 20-26.

1111. Rosenberg CL, Wong E, Petty EM, Bale AE, Tsujimoto Y, Harris NL, Arnold A (1991). PRAD1, a candidate BCL1 oncogene: mapping and expression in centrocytic lymphoma. *Proc Natl Acad Sci U S A* 88: 9638-9642.

1112. Rosenwald A, Ott G, Pulford K, Katzenberger T, Kuhl J, Kalla J, Ott MM, Mason DY, Muller-Hermelink HK (1999). t(1;2)(q21;p23) and t(2;3)(p23;q35) in anaplastic large cell lymphoma. *Blood* 94: 362-364.

1113. Ross CW, Schnitzer B, Sheldon S, Braun DK, Hanson CA (1994). Gamma/delta T-cell posttransplantation lymphoproliferative disorder primarily in the spleen. *Am J Clin Pathol* 102: 310-315.

1114. Rossi G, Donisi A, Casari S, Re A, Cadeo G, Carosi G (1999). The International Prognostic Index can be used as a guide to treatment decisions regarding patients with human immunodeficiency virus-related systemic non-Hodgkin lymphoma. *Cancer* 86: 2391-2397.

1115. Rottem M, Okada T, Goff JP, Metcalfe DD (1994). Mast cells cultured from the peripheral blood of normal donors and patients with mastocytosis originate from a CD34+/Fc epsilon RI- cell population. *Blood* 84: 2489-2496.

1116. Rousselet MC, Francois S, Croue A, Maigre M, Saint-Andre JP, Ifrah N (1994). A lymph node interdigitating reticulum cell sarcoma. *Arch Pathol Lab Med* 118: 183-188.

1117. Rowe M, Rowe DT, Gregory CD, Young LS, Farrell PJ, Rupani H, Rickinson AB (1987). Differences in B cell growth phenotype reflect novel patterns of Epstein-Barr virus latent gene expression in Burkitt's lymphoma cells. *EMBO J* 6: 2743-2751.

1118. Rowley JD (1973). Letter: A new consistent chromosomal abnormality in chronic myelogenous leukaemia identified by quinacrine fluorescence and Giemsa staining. *Nature* 243: 290-293.

1119. Rowley JD (1988). Chromosome studies in the non-Hodgkin's lymphomas: the role of the 14;18 translocation. *J Clin Oncol* 6: 919-925.

1120. Rowlings PA, Curtis RE, Passweg JR, Deeg HJ, Socie G, Travis LB, Kingma DW, Jaffe ES, Sobocinski KA, Horowitz MM (1999). Increased incidence of Hodgkin's disease after allogeneic bone marrow transplantation. *J Clin Oncol* 17: 3122-3127.

1121. Rozman C, Montserrat E (1995). Chronic lymphocytic leukemia. *N Engl J Med* 333: 1052-1057.

1122. Rubin D, Hudnall SD, Aisenberg A, Jacobson JO, Harris NL (1994). Richter's transformation of chronic lymphocytic leukemia with Hodgkin's-like cells is associated with Epstein-Barr virus infection. *Mod Pathol* 7: 91-98.

1123. Ruco LP, Gearing AJ, Pigott R, Pomponi D, Burgio VL, Cafolla A, Baiocchini A, Baroni CD (1991). Expression of ICAM-1, VCAM-1 and ELAM-1 in angiofollicular lymph node hyperplasia (Castleman's disease): evidence for dysplasia of follicular dendritic reticulum cells. *Histopathology* 19: 523-528.

1123a. Rudiger T, Jaffe ES, Delsol G, Dewolf-Peeters C, Gascoyne RD, Georgii A, Harris NL, Kadin ME, MacLennan KA, Poppema S, Stein H, Weiss LE, Muller-Hermelink HK (1998). Workshop report on Hodgkin's disease and related diseases ('grey zone' lymphoma). *Ann Oncol* 9 Suppl 5: S31-S38.

1124. Rupoli S, Da Lio L, Sisti S, Campanati G, Salvi A, Brianzoni MF, D'Amico S, Cinciripini A, Leoni P (1994). Primary myelofibrosis: a detailed statistical analysis of the clinicopathological variables influencing survival. *Ann Hematol* 68: 205-212.

1125. Ruskone-Fourmestraux A, Delmer A, Lavergne A, Molina T, Brousse N, Audouin J, Rambaud JC (1997). Multiple lymphomatous polyposis of the gastrointestinal tract: prospective clinicopathologic study of 31 cases. Groupe D'etude des Lymphomes Digestifs. *Gastroenterology* 112: 7-16.

1126. Russell-Jones R, Whittaker S (1999). T-cell receptor gene analysis in the diagnosis of Sezary syndrome. *J Am Acad Dermatol* 41: 254-259.

1127. Saglio G, Pane F, Gottardi E, Frigeri F, Buonaiuto MR, Guerrasio A, de Micheli D, Parziale A, Fornaci MN, Martinelli G, Salvatore F (1996). Consistent amounts of acute leukemia-associated P190BCR/ABL transcripts are expressed by chronic myelogenous leukemia patients at diagnosis. *Blood* 87: 1075-1080.

1128. Said JW, Rettig MR, Heppner K, Vescio RA, Schiller G, Ma HJ, Belson D, Savage A, Shintaku IP, Koeffler HP, Asou H, Pinkus G, Pinkus J, Schrage M, Green E, Berenson JR (1997). Localization of Kaposi's sarcoma-associated herpesvirus in bone marrow biopsy samples from patients with multiple myeloma. *Blood* 90: 4278-4282.

1129. Said W, Chien K, Takeuchi S, Tasaka T, Asou H, Cho SK, de Vos S, Cesarman E, Knowles DM, Koeffler HP (1996). Kaposi's sarcoma-associated herpesvirus (KSHV or HHV8) in primary effusion lymphoma: ultrastructural demonstration of herpesvirus in lymphoma cells. *Blood* 87: 4937-4943.

1130. Saikia T, Advani S, Dasgupta A, Ramakrishnan G, Nair C, Gladstone B, Kumar MS, Badrinath Y, Dhond S (1988). Characterisation of blast cells during blastic phase of chronic myeloid leukaemia by immunophenotyping – experience in 60 patients. *Leuk Res* 12: 499-506.

1131. Sainati L, Matutes E, Mulligan S, de Oliveira MP, Rani S, Lampert IA, Catovsky D (1990). A variant form of hairy cell leukemia resistant to alpha-interferon: clinical and phenotypic characteristics of 17 patients. *Blood* 76: 157-162.

1132. Sainty D, Liso V, Cantu-Rajnoldi A, Head D, Mozziconacci MJ, Arnoulet C, Benattar L, Fenu S, Mancini M, Duchayne E, Mahon FX, Gutierrez N, Birg F, Biondi A, Grimwade D, Lafage-Pochitaloff M, Hagemeijer A, Flandrin G (2000). A new morphologic classification system for acute promyelocytic leukemia distinguishes cases with underlying PLZF/RARA gene rearrangements. Group Francais de Cytogenetique Hematologique, UK Cancer Cytogenetics Group and BIOMED 1 European Coomunity-Concerted Acion "Molecular Cytogenetic Diagnosis in Haematological Malignancies. *Blood* 96: 1287-1296.

1133. Salar A, Fernandez dS, Romagosa V, Domingo-Claros A, Gonzalez-Barca E, Pera J, Climent J, Granena A (1998). Diffuse large B-cell lymphoma: is morphologic subdivision useful in clinical management? *Eur J Haematol* 60: 202-208.

1134. Salhany KE, Macon WR, Choi JK, Elenitsas R, Lessin SR, Felgar RE, Wilson DM, Przybylski GK, Lister J, Wasik MA, Swerdlow SH (1998). Subcutaneous panniculitis-like T-cell lymphoma: clinicopathologic, immunophenotypic, and genotypic analysis of alpha/beta and gamma/delta subtypes. *Am J Surg Pathol* 22: 881-893.

1135. Salloum E, Cooper DL, Howe G, Lacy J, Tallini G, Crouch J, Schultz M, Murren J (1996). Spontaneous regression of lymphoproliferative disorders in patients treated with methotrexate for rheumatoid arthritis and other rheumatic diseases. *J Clin Oncol* 14: 1943-1949.

1136. Salmon SE, Cassady JR (1988). Plasma cell neoplasms. In: *Cancer, Principles and Practice of Oncology*, DeVita VT, Hellman S, Rosenberg S, eds. J.B.Lippincott: Philadelphia, pp. 1854.

1137. Salmon SE, Seligmann M (1974). B-cell neoplasia in man. *Lancet* 2: 1230-1233.

1138. Samoszuk M, Nansen L (1990). Detection of interleukin-5 messenger RNA in Reed-Sternberg cells of Hodgkin's disease with eosinophilia. *Blood* 75: 13-16.

1139. Sander CA, Jaffe ES, Gebhardt FC, Yano T, Medeiros LJ (1992). Mediastinal lymphoblastic lymphoma with an immature B-cell immunophenotype. *Am J Surg Pathol* 16: 300-305.

1140. Sander CA, Medeiros LJ, Weiss LM, Yano T, Sneller MC, Jaffe ES (1992). Lymphoproliferative lesions in patients with common variable immunodeficiency syndrome. *Am J Surg Pathol* 16: 1170-1182.

1141. Sander CA, Yano T, Clark HM, Harris C, Longo DL, Jaffe ES, Raffeld M (1993). p53 mutation is associated with progression in follicular lymphomas. *Blood* 82: 1994-2004.

1142. Sanderson CJ (1992). Interleukin-5, eosinophils, and disease. *Blood* 79: 3101-3109.

1143. Sandler DP, Ross JA (1997). Epidemiology of acute leukemia in children and adults. *Semin Oncol* 24: 3-16.

1144. Sansonno D, De Vita S, Cornacchiulo V, Carbone A, Boiocchi M, Dammacco F (1996). Detection and distribution of hepatitis C virus-related proteins in lymph nodes of patients with type II mixed cryoglobulinemia and neoplastic or non-neoplastic lymphoproliferation. *Blood* 88: 4638-4645.

1145. Sarris A, Jhanwar S, Cabanillas F (1999). Cytogenetics of Hodgkin's disease. In: *Hodgkin's Disease*, Mauch P, Armitage JO, Diehl V, eds. Lippincott Williams & Wilkins: Philadelphia, pp. 195.

1146. Savage DG, Szydlo RM, Chase A, Apperley JF, Goldman JM (1997). Bone marrow transplantation for chronic myeloid leukaemia: the effects of differing criteria for defining chronic phase on probabilities of survival and relapse. *Br J Haematol* 99: 30-35.

1147. Savage DG, Szydlo RM, Goldman JM (1997). Clinical features at diagnosis in 430 patients with chronic myeloid leukaemia seen at a referral centre over a 16-year period. *Br J Haematol* 96: 111-116.

1148. Saven A, Burian C, Koziol JA, Piro LD (1998). Long-term follow-up of patients with hairy cell leukemia after cladribine treatment. *Blood* 92: 1918-1926.

1149. Savilo E, Campo E, Mollejo M, Pinyol M, Piris MA, Zukerberg LR, Yang WI, Koelliker DD, Nguyen PL, Harris NL (1998). Absence of cyclin D1 protein expression in splenic marginal zone lymphoma. *Mod Pathol* 11: 601-606.

1150. Sawyer JR, Waldron JA, Jagannath S, Barlogie B (1995). Cytogenetic findings in 200 patients with multiple myeloma. *Cancer Genet Cytogenet* 82: 41-49.

1151. Scarisbrick JJ, Woolford AJ, Russell-Jones R, Whittaker SJ (2000). Loss of heterozygosity on 10q and microsatellite instability in advanced stages of primary cutaneous T-cell lymphoma and possible association with homozygous deletion of PTEN. *Blood* 95: 2937-2942.

1152. Schaffner C, Idler I, Stilgenbauer S, Dohner H, Lichter P (2000). Mantle cell lymphoma is characterized by inactivation of the ATM gene. *Proc Natl Acad Sci U S A* 97: 2773-2778.

1153. Schaffner C, Stilgenbauer S, Rappold GA, Dohner H, Lichter P (1999). Somatic ATM mutations indicate a pathogenic role of ATM in B-cell chronic lymphocytic leukemia. *Blood* 94: 748-753.

1154. Scheck O, Horny HP, Ruck P, Schmelzle R, Kaiserling E (1987). Solitary mastocytoma of the eyelid. A case report with special reference to the immunocytology of human tissue mast cells, and a review of the literature. *Virchows Arch A Pathol Anat Histopathol* 412: 31-36.

1155. Scheffer E, Meijer CJ, van Vloten WA (1980). Dermatopathic lymphadenopathy and lymph node involvement in mycosis fungoides. *Cancer* 45: 137-148.

1156. Schlegelberger B, Himmler A, Godde E, Grote W, Feller AC, Lennert K (1994). Cytogenetic findings in peripheral T-cell lymphomas as a basis for distinguishing low-grade and high-grade lymphomas. *Blood* 83: 505-511.

1157. Schlegelberger B, Weber-Matthiesen K, Himmler A, Bartels H, Sonnen R, Kuse R, Feller AC, Grote W (1994). Cytogenetic findings and results of combined immunophenotyping and karyotyping in Hodgkin's disease. *Leukemia* 8: 72-80.

1158. Schlegelberger B, Zhang Y, Weber-Matthiesen K, Grote W (1994). Detection of aberrant clones in nearly all cases of angioimmunoblastic lymphadenopathy with dysproteinemia-type T-cell lymphoma by combined interphase and metaphase cytogenetics. *Blood* 84: 2640-2648.

1159. Schmid C, Pan L, Diss T, Isaacson PG (1991). Expression of B-cell antigens by Hodgkin's and Reed-Sternberg cells. *Am J Pathol* 139: 701-707.

1160. Schmid C, Sargent C, Isaacson PG (1991). L and H cells of nodular lymphocyte predominant Hodgkin's disease show immunoglobulin light-chain restriction. *Am J Pathol* 139: 1281-1289.

1161. Schmitz LL, McClure JS, Litz CE, Dayton V, Weisdorf DJ, Parkin JL, Brunning RD (1994). Morphologic and quantitative changes in blood and marrow cells following growth factor therapy. *Am J Clin Pathol* 101: 67-75.

1162. Schoch C, Haase D, Haferlach T, Gudat H, Buchner T, Freund M, Link H, Lengfelder E, Wandt H, Sauerland MC, Loffler H, Fonatsch C (1996). Fifty-one patients with acute myeloid leukemia and translocation t(8;21)(q22;q22): an additional deletion in 9q is an adverse prognostic factor. *Leukemia* 10: 1288-1295.

1163. Schooley RT, Flaum MA, Gralnick HR, Fauci AS (1981). A clinicopathologic correlation of the idiopathic hypereosinophilic syndrome. II. Clinical manifestations. *Blood* 58: 1021-1026.

1164. Schwarting R, Stein H, Wang CY (1985). The monoclonal antibodies alpha S-HCL 1 (alpha Leu-14) and alpha S-HCL 3 (alpha Leu-M5) allow the diagnosis of hairy cell leukemia. *Blood* 65: 974-983.

1165. Schwartz LB, Sakai K, Bradford TR, Ren S, Zweiman B, Worobec AS, Metcalfe DD (1995). The alpha form of human tryptase is the predominant type present in blood at baseline in normal subjects and is elevated in those with systemic mastocytosis. *J Clin Invest* 96: 2702-2710.

1166. Scott AA, Head DR, Kopecky KJ, Appelbaum FR, Theil KS, Grever MR, Chen IM, Whittaker MH, Griffith BB, Licht JD (1994). HLA-DR-, CD33+, CD56+, CD16-myeloid/natural killer cell acute leukemia: a previously unrecognized form of acute leukemia potentially misdiagnosed as French-American-British acute myeloid leukemia-M3. *Blood* 84: 244-255.

1167. Scott RB, Robb-Smith AHT (1939). Histiocytic medullary reticulosis. *Lancet* 2: 194.

1168. Secker-Walker LM, Mehta A, Bain B (1995). Abnormalities of 3q21 and 3q26 in myeloid malignancy: a United Kingdom Cancer Cytogenetic Group study. *Br J Haematol* 91: 490-501.

1169. Secker-Walker LM, Moorman AV, Bain BJ, Mehta AB (1998). Secondary acute leukemia and myelodysplastic syndrome with 11q23 abnormalities. EU Concerted Action 11q23 Workshop. *Leukemia* 12: 840-844.

1170. Seitz V, Hummel M, Marafioti T, Anagnostopoulos I, Assaf C, Stein H (2000). Detection of clonal T-cell receptor gamma-chain gene rearrangements in Reed-Sternberg cells of classic Hodgkin disease. *Blood* 95: 3020-3024.

1171. Sekhar M, Prentice HG, Popat U, Anderson D, Janmohammed R, Roberts I, Britt RP (1996). Idiopathic myelofibrosis in children. *Br J Haematol* 93: 394-397.

1172. Seligmann M (1975). Immunohistochemical, clinical and pathological features of alpha-heavy chain disease. *Arch Intern Med* 135: 78-82.

1173. Seligmann M, Mihaesco E, Preud'Homme JL, Danon F, Brouet JC (1979). Heavy chain diseases: current findings and concepts. *Immunol Rev* 48: 145-167.

1174. Seligmann M, Sassy C, Chevalier A (1973). A human IgG myeloma protein with anti-2 macroglobulin antibody activity. *J Immunol* 110: 85-90.

1175. Selves J, Meggetto F, Brousset P, Voigt JJ, Pradere B, Grasset D, Icart J, Mariame B, Knecht H, Delsol G (1996). Inflammatory pseudotumor of the liver. Evidence for follicular dendritic reticulum cell proliferation associated with clonal Epstein-Barr virus. *Am J Surg Pathol* 20: 747-753.

1176. Semenzato G, Zambello R, Starkebaum G, Oshimi K, Loughran TP, Jr. (1997). The lymphoproliferative disease of granular lymphocytes: updated criteria for diagnosis. *Blood* 89: 256-260.

1177. Sepp N, Schuler G, Romani N, Geissler D, Gattringer C, Burg G, Bartram CR, Fritsch P (1990). "Intravascular lymphomatosis" (angioendotheliomatosis): evidence for a T-cell origin in two cases. *Hum Pathol* 21: 1051-1058.

1178. Serpell LC, Sunde M, Blake CC (1997). The molecular basis of amyloidosis. *Cell Mol Life Sci* 53: 871-887.

1179. Sessarego M, Defferrari R, Dejana AM, Rebuttato AM, Fugazza G, Salvidio E, Ajmar F (1989). Cytogenetic analysis in essential thrombocythemia at diagnosis and at transformation. A 12-year study. *Cancer Genet Cytogenet* 43: 57-65.

1180. Shannon KM, O'Connell P, Martin GA, Paderanga D, Olson K, Dinndorf P, McCormick F (1994). Loss of the normal NF1 allele from the bone marrow of children with type 1 neurofibromatosis and malignant myeloid disorders. *N Engl J Med* 330: 597-601.

1181. Shapiro RS, McClain K, Frizzera G, Gajl-Peczalska KJ, Kersey JH, Blazar BR, Arthur DC, Patton DF, Greenberg JS, Burke B (1988). Epstein-Barr virus associated B cell lymphoproliferative disorders following bone marrow transplantation. *Blood* 71: 1234-1243.

1182. Sheibani K, Burke JS, Swartz WG, Nademanee A, Winberg CD (1988). Monocytoid B-cell lymphoma. Clinicopathologic study of 21 cases of a unique type of low-grade lymphoma. *Cancer* 62: 1531-1538.

1183. Shepherd PC, Ganesan TS, Galton DA (1987). Haematological classification of the chronic myeloid leukaemias. *Baillieres Clin Haematol* 1: 887-906.

1184. Shibata K, Shimamoto Y, Suga K, Sano M, Matsuzaki M, Yamaguchi M (1994). Essential thrombocythemia terminating in acute leukemia with minimal myeloid differentiation — a brief review of recent literature. *Acta Haematol* 91: 84-88.

1185. Shimodaira S, Ishida F, Kobayashi H, Mahbub B, Kawa-Ha K, Kitano K (1995). The detection of clonal proliferation in granular lymphocyte-proliferative disorders of natural killer cell lineage. *Br J Haematol* 90: 578-584.

1186. Shimoyama M (1991). Diagnostic criteria and classification of clinical subtypes of adult T-cell leukaemia-lymphoma. A report from the Lymphoma Study Group (1984-87). *Br J Haematol* 79: 428-437.

1187. Shiong YS, Lian JD, Lin CY, Shu KH, Lu YS, Chou G (1992). Epstein-Barr virus-associated T-cell lymphoma of the maxillary sinus in a renal transplant recipient. *Transplant Proc* 24: 1929-1931.

1188. Shiota M, Nakamura S, Ichinohasama R, Abe M, Akagi T, Takeshita M, Mori N, Fujimoto J, Miyauchi J, Mikata A (1995). Anaplastic large cell lymphomas expressing the novel chimeric protein p80NPM/ALK: a distinct clinicopathologic entity. *Blood* 86: 1954-1960.

1189. Shiramizu B, Barriga F, Neequaye J, Jafri A, Dalla-Favera R, Neri A, Guttierez M, Levine P, Magrath I (1991). Patterns of chromosomal breakpoint locations in Burkitt's lymphoma: relevance to geography and Epstein-Barr virus association. *Blood* 77: 1516-1526.

1190. Shukralla N, Finiewicz K, Roulston D, et al (1997). Is atypical chronic myeloid leukemia a high white count myelodysplastic disorder? *Mod Pathol* 10: 134a.

1191. Sibilia J, Liote F, Mariette X (1998). Lymphoproliferative disorders in rheumatoid arthritis patients on low-dose methotrexate. *Rev Rhum Engl Ed* 65: 267-273.

1192. Side LE, Emanuel PD, Taylor B, Franklin J, Thompson P, Castleberry RP, Shannon KM (1998). Mutations of the NF1 gene in children with juvenile myelomonocytic leukemia without clinical evidence of neurofibromatosis, type 1. *Blood* 92: 267-272.

1193. Siebert JD, Ambinder RF, Napoli VM, Quintanilla-Martinez L, Banks PM, Gulley ML (1995). Human immunodeficiency virus-associated Hodgkin's disease contains latent, not replicative, Epstein-Barr virus. *Hum Pathol* 26: 1191-1195.

1194. Siegert W, Nerl C, Agthe A, Engelhard M, Brittinger G, Tiemann M, Lennert K, Huhn D (1995). Angioimmunoblastic lymphadenopathy (AILD)-type T-cell lymphoma: prognostic impact of clinical observations and laboratory findings at presentation. The Kiel Lymphoma Study Group. *Ann Oncol* 6: 659-664.

1195. Siena S, Sammarelli G, Grimoldi MG, Schiavo R, Nozza A, Roncalli M, Mecucci C, Santoro A, Carlo-Stella C (1999). New reciprocal translocation t(5;10)(q33;q22) associated with atypical chronic myeloid leukemia. *Haematologica* 84: 369-372.

1196. Silverstein MN, Lanier AP (1971). Polycythemia vera, 1935-1969: an epidemiologic survey in Rochester, Minnesota. *Mayo Clin Proc* 46: 751-753.

1197. Simon HU, Plotz SG, Dummer R, Blaser K (1999). Abnormal clones of T cells producing interleukin-5 in idiopathic eosinophilia. *N Engl J Med* 341: 1112-1120.

1198. Siu LL, Wong KF, Chan JK, Kwong YL (1999). Comparative genomic hybridization analysis of natural killer cell lymphoma/leukemia. Recognition of consistent patterns of genetic alterations. *Am J Pathol* 155: 1419-1425.

1199. Skinnider BF, Elia AJ, Gascoyne RD, Trumper LH, von Bonin F, Kapp U, Patterson B, Snow BE, Mak TW (2001). Interleukin 13 and interleukin 13 receptor are frequently expressed by hodgkin and reed-sternberg cells of hodgkin lymphoma. *Blood* 97: 250-255.

1200. Slovak ML, Kopecky KJ, Cassileth PA, Harrington DH, Theil KS, Mohamed A, Paietta E, Willman CL, Head DR, Rowe JM, Forman SJ, Appelbaum FR (2000). Karyotypic analysis predicts outcome of preremission and postremission therapy in adult acute myeloid leukemia: a southwest oncology Group/Eastern cooperative oncology group study. *Blood* 96: 4075-4083.

1201. Smith JL, Hodges E, Quin CT, McCarthy KP, Wright DH (2000). Frequent T and B cell oligoclones in histologically and immunophenotypically characterized angioimmunoblastic lymphadenopathy. *Am J Pathol* 156: 661-669.

1202. Smith MA, Reis LA, Gurnew JG, et al (1995). *Cancer incidence and survival among children and adolescents: United States SEER program 1975-1995.* NIH Pub 99-4649. National Cancer Institute, SEER Program: Bethesda, MD.

1203. Sneller MC, Wang J, Dale JK, Strober W, Middelton LA, Choi Y, Fleisher TA, Lim MS, Jaffe ES, Puck JM, Lenardo MJ, Straus SE (1997). Clincial, immunologic, and genetic features of an autoimmune lymphoproliferative syndrome associated with abnormal lymphocyte apoptosis. *Blood* 89: 1341-1348.

1204. Sokal JE, Baccarani M, Russo D, Tura S (1988). Staging and prognosis in chronic myelogenous leukemia. *Semin Hematol* 25: 49-61.

1205. Solal-Celigny P, Desaint B, Herrera A, Chastang C, Amar M, Vroclans M, Brousse N, Mancilla F, Renoux M, Bernard JF (1984). Chronic myelomonocytic leukemia according to FAB classification: analysis of 35 cases. *Blood* 63: 634-638.

1206. Soler J, Bordes R, Ortuno F, Montagud M, Martorell J, Pons C, Nomdedeu J, Lopez-Lopez JJ, Prat J, Rutllant M (1994). Aggressive natural killer cell leukaemia/lymphoma in two patients with lethal midline granuloma. *Br J Haematol* 86: 659-662.

1207. Sood R, Stewart CC, Aplan PD, Murai H, Ward P, Barcos M, Baer MR (1998). Neutropenia associated with T-cell large granular lymphocyte leukemia: long-term response to cyclosporine therapy despite persistence of abnormal cells. *Blood* 91: 3372-3378.

1208. Sordillo PP, Epremian B, Koziner B, Lacher M, Lieberman P (1982). Lymphomatoid granulomatosis: an analysis of clinical and immunologic characteristics. *Cancer* 49: 2070-2076.

1209. Soria C, Orradre JL, Garcia-Almagro D, Martinez B, Algara P, Piris MA (1992). True histiocytic lymphoma (monocytic sarcoma). *Am J Dermatopathol* 14: 511-517.

1210. Sorour A, Brito-Babapulle V, Smedley D, Yuille M, Catovsky D (2000). Unusual breakpoint distribution of 8p abnormalities in T-prolymphocytic leukaemia: A study with Yacs mapping to 8p11-12. *Cancer Genet Cytogenet* (in press).

1211. Soter NA (2000). Mastocytosis and the skin. *Hematol Oncol Clin North Am* 14: 537-55, vi.

1212. Soussain C, Patte C, Ostronoff M, Delmer A, Rigal-Huguet F, Cambier N, Leprise PY, Francois S, Cony-Makhoul P, Harousseau JL (1995). Small noncleaved cell lymphoma and leukemia in adults. A retrospective study of 65 adults treated with the LMB pediatric protocols. *Blood* 85: 664-674.

1213. Specht L, Hasenclever D (1999). Prognostic factors of Hodgkin's disease. In: *Hodgkin's Disease*, Mauch P, Armitage JO, Diehl V, eds. Lippincott Williams & Wilkins: Philadelphia, pp. 295.

1214. Spencer J, Cerf-Bensussan N, Jarry A, Brousse N, Guy-Grand D, Krajewski AS, Isaacson PG (1988). Enteropathy-associated T cell lymphoma (malignant histiocytosis of the intestine) is recognized by a monoclonal antibody (HML-1) that defines a membrane molecule on human mucosal lymphocytes. *Am J Pathol* 132: 1-5.

1215. Spencer J, Finn T, Pulford KA, Mason DY, Isaacson PG (1985). The human gut contains a novel population of B lymphocytes which resemble marginal zone cells. *Clin Exp Immunol* 62: 607-612.

1216. Sperr WR, Walchshofer S, Horny HP, Fodinger M, Simonitsch I, Fritsche-Polanz R, Schwarzinger I, Tschachler E, Sillaber C, Hagen W, Geissler K, Chott A, Lechner K, Valent P (1998). Systemic mastocytosis associated with acute myeloid leukaemia: report of two cases and detection of the c-kit mutation Asp-816 to Val. *Br J Haematol* 103: 740-749.

1217. Spiers AS, Bain BJ, Turner JE (1977). The peripheral blood in chronic granulocytic leukaemia. Study of 50 untreated Philadelphia-positive cases. *Scand J Haematol* 18: 25-38.

1218. Spina D, Leoncini L, Megha T, Gallorini M, Disanto A, Tosi P, Abinya O, Nyong'O A, Pileri S, Kraft R, Laissue JA, Cottier H (1997). Cellular kinetic and phenotypic heterogeneity in and among Burkitt's and Burkitt-like lymphomas. *J Pathol* 182: 145-150.

1219. Spina M, Vaccher E, Nasti G, Tirelli U (2000). Human immunodeficiency virus-associated Hodgkin's disease. *Semin Oncol* 27: 480-488.

1220. Spiro IJ, Yandell DW, Li C, Saini S, Ferry J, Powelson J, Katkov WN, Cosimi AB (1993). Brief report: lymphoma of donor origin occurring in the porta hepatis of a transplanted liver. *N Engl J Med* 329: 27-29.

1221. Spits H, Blom B, Jaleco AC, Weijer K, Verschuren MC, van Dongen JJ, Heemskerk MH, Res PC (1998). Early stages in the development of human T, natural killer and thymic dendritic cells. *Immunol Rev* 165: 75-86.

1222. Spry CJ, Davies J, Tai PC, Olsen EG, Oakley CM, Goodwin JF (1983). Clinical features of fifteen patients with the hypereosinophilic syndrome. *Q J Med* 52: 1-22.

1223. Standen GR, Jasani B, Wagstaff M, Wardrop CA (1990). Chronic neutrophilic leukemia and multiple myeloma. An association with lambda light chain expression. *Cancer* 66: 162-166.

1224. Standen GR, Steers FJ, Jones L (1993). Clonality of chronic neutrophilic leukaemia associated with myeloma: analysis using the X-linked probe M27 beta. *J Clin Pathol* 46: 297-298.

1225. Stanley M, McKenna RW, Ellinger G, Brunning RD (1985). Classification of 358 cases of Acute Myeloid Leukemia by FAB criteria: analysis of clinical and morphologic findings in chronic and acute leukemias in adults. Martin Nijhoff Publishers: Boston.

1226. Stark B, Resnitzky P, Jeison M, Luria D, Blau O, Avigad S, Shaft D, Kodman Y, Gobuzov R, Ash S (1995). A distinct subtype of M4/M5 acute myeloblastic leukemia (AML) associated with t(8:16)(p11:p13), in a patient with the variant t(8:19)(p11:q13) – case report and review of the literature. *Leuk Res* 19: 367-379.

1227. Starzl TE, Nalesnik MA, Porter KA, Ho M, Iwatsuki S, Griffith BP, Rosenthal JT, Hakala TR, Shaw BW, Jr., Hardesty RL (1984). Reversibility of lymphomas and lymphoproliferative lesions developing under cyclosporin-steroid therapy. *Lancet* 1: 583-587.

1228. Stein H, Diehl V, Marafioti T, Jox A, Wolf J, Hummel M (1999). The nature of Reed-Sternberg cells, lymphocytic and histiocytic cells and their molecular biology in Hodgkin's disease. In: *Hodgkin's Disease*, Mauch P, Armitage JO, Diehl V, eds. Lippincott Williams & Wilkins: Philadelphia, 121.

1229. Stein H, Foss HD, Durkop H, Marafioti T, Delsol G, Pulford K, Pileri S, Falini B (2000). CD30(+) anaplastic large cell lymphoma: a review of its histopathologic, genetic, and clinical features. *Blood* 96: 3681-3695.

1230. Stein H, Gerdes J, Kirchner H, Schaadt M, Diehl V (1981). Hodgkin and Sternberg-Reed cell antigen(s) detected by an antiserum to a cell line (L428) derived from Hodgkin's disease. *Int J Cancer* 28: 425-429.

1231. Stein H, Hansmann ML, Lennert K, Brandtzaeg P, Gatter KC, Mason DY (1986). Reed-Sternberg and Hodgkin cells in lymphocyte-predominant Hodgkin's disease of nodular subtype contain J chain. *Am J Clin Pathol* 86: 292-297.

1232. Stein H, Lennert K, Feller AC, Mason DY (1984). Immunohistological analysis of human lymphoma: correlation of histological and immunological categories. *Adv Cancer Res* 42:67-147: 67-147.

1233. Stein H, Marafioti T, Foss HD, Laumen H, Hummel M, Anagnostopoulos I, Wirth T, Demel G, Falini B (2001). Down-regulation of BOB.1/OBF.1 and Oct2 in classical Hodgkin disease but not in lymphocyte predominant Hodgkin disease correlates with immunoglobulin transcription. *Blood* 97: 496-501.

1234. Stein H, Mason DY, Gerdes J, O'Connor N, Wainscoat J, Pallesen G, Gatter K, Falini B, Delsol G, Lemke H (1985). The expression of the Hodgkin's disease associated antigen Ki-1 in reactive and neoplastic lymphoid tissue: evidence that Reed-Sternberg cells and histiocytic malignancies are derived from activated lymphoid cells. *Blood* 66: 848-858.

1235. Stein H, Uchanska-Ziegler B, Gerdes J, Ziegler A, Wernet P (1982). Hodgkin and Sternberg-Reed cells contain antigens specific to late cells of granulopoiesis. *Int J Cancer* 29: 283-290.

1236. Stern MH, Soulier J, Rosenzwajg M, Nakahara K, Canki-Klain N, Aurias A, Sigaux F, Kirsch IR (1993). MTCP-1: a novel gene on the human chromosome Xq28 translocated to the T cell receptor alpha/delta locus in mature T cell proliferations. *Oncogene* 8: 2475-2483.

1237. Stilgenbauer S, Schaffner C, Litterst A, Liebisch P, Gilad S, Bar-Shira A, James MR, Lichter P, Dohner H (1997). Biallelic mutations in the ATM gene in T-prolymphocytic leukemia. *Nat Med* 3: 1155-1159.

1238. Stilgenbauer S, Winkler D, Ott G, Schaffner C, Leupolt E, Bentz M, Moller P, Muller-Hermelink HK, James M, Lichter P, Dohner H (1999). Molecular characterization of 11q deletions points to a pathogenic role of the ATM gene in mantle cell lymphoma. *Blood* 94: 3262-3264.

1239. Storniolo AM, Moloney WC, Rosenthal DS, Cox C, Bennett JM (1990). Chronic myelomonocytic leukemia. *Leukemia* 4: 766-770.

1240. Straus DJ, Huang J, Testa MA, Levine AM, Kaplan LD (1998). Prognostic factors in the treatment of human immunodeficiency virus-associated non-Hodgkin's lymphoma: analysis of AIDS Clinical Trials Group protocol 142 – low-dose versus standard-dose m-BACOD plus granulocyte-macrophage colony-stimulating factor. National Institute of Allergy and Infectious Diseases. *J Clin Oncol* 16: 3601-3606.

1241. Strazzabosco M, Corneo B, Iemmolo RM, Menin C, Gerunda G, Bonaldi L, Merenda R, Neri D, Poletti A, Montagna M, Del Mistro A, Faccioli AM, D'Andrea E (1997). Epstein-Barr virus-associated post-transplant lympho-proliferative disease of donor origin in liver transplant recipients. *J Hepatol* 26: 926-934.

1242. Streeter RR, Presant CA, Reinhard E (1977). Prognostic significance of thrombocytosis in idiopathic sideroblastic anemia. *Blood* 50: 427-432.

1243. Strickler JG, Meneses MF, Habermann TM, Ilstrup DM, Earle JD, McDonald TJ, Chang KL, Weiss LM (1994). Polymorphic reticulosis: a reappraisal. *Hum Pathol* 25: 659-665.

1244. Suchi T, Lennert K, Tu LY, Kikuchi M, Sato E, Stansfeld AG, Feller AC (1987). Histopathology and immunohistochemistry of peripheral T cell lymphomas: a proposal for their classification. *J Clin Pathol* 40: 995-1015.

1245. Suda T, Miura Y, Mizoguchi H, Ijima H, Eguchi M, Kaku H, Ide C (1982). Characterization of hemopoietic precursor cells in juvenile-type chronic myelocytic leukemia. *Leuk Res* 6: 43-53.

1246. Sugimoto K, Hirano N, Toyoshima H, Chiba S, Mano H, Takaku F, Yazaki Y, Hirai H (1993). Mutations of the p53 gene in myelodysplastic syndrome (MDS) and MDS-derived leukemia. *Blood* 81: 3022-3026.

1247. Sulak LE, Clare CN, Morale BA, Hansen KL, Montiel MM (1990). Biphenotypic acute leukemia in adults. *Am J Clin Pathol* 94: 54-58.

1248. Sultan C, Sigaux F, Imbert M, Reyes F (1981). Acute myelodysplasia with myelofibrosis: a report of eight cases. *Br J Haematol* 49: 11-16.

1249. Suster S, Rosai J (1989). Intranodal hemorrhagic spindle-cell tumor with "amianthoid" fibers. Report of six cases of a distinctive mesenchymal neoplasm of the inguinal region that simulates Kaposi's sarcoma. *Am J Surg Pathol* 13: 347-357.

1250. Suzuki R, Yamamoto K, Seto M, Kagami Y, Ogura M, Yatabe Y, Suchi T, Kodera Y, Morishima Y, Takahashi T, Saito H, Ueda R, Nakamura S (1997). CD7+ and CD56+ myeloid/natural killer cell precursor acute leukemia: a distinct hematolymphoid disease entity. *Blood* 90: 2417-2428.

1251. Suzumiya J, Takeshita M, Kimura N, Morioka E, Sakai T, Hisano S, Okumura M, Kikuchi M (1993). Sinonasal malignant lymphoma of natural killer cell phenotype associated with diffuse pancreatic involvement. *Leuk Lymphoma* 10: 231-236.

1252. Swerdlow SH, Habeshaw JA, Murray LJ, Dhaliwal HS, Lister TA, Stansfeld AG (1983). Centrocytic lymphoma: a distinct clinicopathologic and immunologic entity. A multiparameter study of 18 cases at diagnosis and relapse. *Am J Pathol* 113: 181-197.

1253. Swerdlow SH, Yang WI, Zukerberg LR, Harris NL, Arnold A, Williams ME (1995). Expression of cyclin D1 protein in centrocytic/mantle cell lymphomas with and without rearrangement of the BCL1/cyclin D1 gene. *Hum Pathol* 26: 999-1004.

1254. Swerdlow SH, Zukerberg LR, Yang WI, Harris NL, Williams ME (1996). The morphologic spectrum of non-Hodgkin's lymphomas with BCL1/cyclin D1 gene rearrangements. *Am J Surg Pathol* 20: 627-640.

1255. Swolin B, Weinfeld A, Westin J (1988). A prospective long-term cytogenetic study in polycythemia vera in relation to treatment and clinical course. *Blood* 72: 386-395.

1256. Symmons DP (1985). Neoplasms of the immune system in rheumatoid arthritis. *Am J Med* 78: 22-28.

1257. Taillan B, Garnier G, Castanet J, Ferrari E, Pesce A, Dujardin P (1993). Lymphoma developing in a patient with rheumatoid arthritis taking methotrexate. *Clin Rheumatol* 12: 93-94.

1258. Tajima K, Hinuma Y (1992). Epidemiology of HTLV-I/II in Japan and the world. In: *Advances in Adult T-Cell Leukemia and HTLV-I Research (Gann Monograph on Cancer Research)*, Takatsuki K, Hinuma Y, Yoshida M, eds. Japan Scientific Societies Press: Tokyo, pp. 129-149.

1259. Takeshita M, Akamatsu M, Ohshima K, Kobari S, Kikuchi M, Suzumiya J, Uike N, Okamura T (1995). CD30 (Ki-1) expression in adult T-cell leukaemia/lymphoma is associated with distinctive immunohistological and clinical characteristics. *Histopathology* 26: 539-546.

1260. Talal N, Sokoloff L, Barth WF (1967). Extrasalivary lymphoid abnormalities in Sjogren's syndrome (reticulum cell sarcoma, "pseudolymphoma," macroglobulinemia). *Am J Med* 43: 50-65.

1261. Tallman MS, Andersen JW, Schiffer CA, Appelbaum FR, Feusner JH, Ogden A, Shepherd L, Willman C, Bloomfield CD, Rowe JM, Wiernik PH (1997). All-trans-retinoic acid in acute promyelocytic leukemia. *N Engl J Med* 337: 1021-1028.

1262. Tallman MS, Peterson LC, Hakimian D, Gillis S, Polliack A (1999). Treatment of hairy-cell leukemia: current views. *Semin Hematol* 36: 155-163.

1263. Tamaru J, Hummel M, Marafioti T, Kalvelage B, Leoncini L, Minacci C, Tosi P, Wright D, Stein H (1995). Burkitt's lymphomas express VH genes with a moderate number of antigen-selected somatic mutations. *Am J Pathol* 147: 1398-1407.

1264. Tamura H, Ogata K, Mori S, An E, Tajika K, Sugisaki Y, Dan K (1998). Lymphoblastic lymphoma of natural killer cell origin, presenting as pancreatic tumour. *Histopathology* 32: 508-511.

1265. Tanaka M, Suda T, Haze K, Nakamura N, Sato K, Kimura F, Motoyoshi K, Mizuki M, Tagawa S, Ohga S, Hatake K, Drummond AH, Nagata S (1996). Fas ligand in human serum. *Nat Med* 2: 317-322.

1266. Tangye SG, Phillips JH, Lanier LL, Nichols KE (2000). Functional requirement for SAP in 2B4-mediated activation of human natural killer cells as revealed by the X-linked lymphoproliferative syndrome. *J Immunol* 165: 2932-2936.

1267. Taniere P, Thivolet-Bejui F, Vitrey D, Isaac S, Loire R, Cordier JF, Berger F (1998). Lymphomatoid granulomatosis – a report on four cases: evidence for B phenotype of the tumoral cells. *Eur Respir J* 12: 102-106.

1268. Tao J, Valderrama E (1999). Epstein-Barr virus-associated polymorphic B-cell lymphoproliferative disorders in the lungs of children with AIDS: a report of two cases. *Am J Surg Pathol* 23: 560-566.

1269. Tao Q, Robertson KD, Manns A, Hildesheim A, Ambinder RF (1998). Epstein-Barr virus (EBV) in endemic Burkitt's lymphoma: molecular analysis of primary tumor tissue. *Blood* 91: 1373-1381.

1270. Taylor AM, Metcalfe JA, Thick J, Mak YF (1996). Leukemia and lymphoma in ataxia telangiectasia. *Blood* 87: 423-438.

1271. Tefferi A (2000). Myelofibrosis with myeloid metaplasia. *N Engl J Med* 342: 1255-1265.

1272. Tefferi A, Hoagland HC, Therneau TM, Pierre RV (1989). Chronic myelomonocytic leukemia: natural history and prognostic determinants. *Mayo Clin Proc* 64: 1246-1254.

1273. Tefferi A, Li CY, Witzig TE, Dhodapkar MV, Okuno SH, Phyliky RL (1994). Chronic natural killer cell lymphocytosis: a descriptive clinical study. *Blood* 84: 2721-2725.

1274. Teruya-Feldstein J, Jaffe ES, Burd PR, Kanegane H, Kingma DW, Wilson WH, Longo DL, Tosato G (1997). The role of Mig, the monokine induced by interferon-gamma, and IP-10, the interferon-gamma-inducible protein-10, in tissue necrosis and vascular damage associated with Epstein-Barr virus-positive lymphoproliferative disease. *Blood* 90: 4099-4105.

1275. Teruya-Feldstein J, Jaffe ES, Burd PR, Kingma DW, Setsuda JE, Tosato G (1999). Differential chemokine expression in tissues involved by Hodgkin's disease: direct correlation of eotaxin expression and tissue eosinophilia. *Blood* 93: 2463-2470.

1276. Teruya-Feldstein J, Setsuda J, Yao X, Kingma DW, Straus S, Tosato G, Jaffe ES (1999). MIP-1alpha expression in tissues from patients with hemophagocytic syndrome. *Lab Invest* 79: 1583-1590.

1277. Teruya-Feldstein J, Temeck BK, Sloas MM, Kingma DW, Raffeld M, Pass HI, Mueller B, Jaffe ES (1995). Pulmonary malignant lymphoma of mucosa-associated lymphoid tissue (MALT) arising in a pediatric HIV-positive patient. *Am J Surg Pathol* 19: 357-363.

1278. Teruya-Feldstein J, Zauber P, Setsuda JE, Berman EL, Sorbara L, Raffeld M, Tosato G, Jaffe ES (1998). Expression of human herpesvirus-8 oncogene and cytokine homologues in an HIV-seronegative patient with multicentric Castleman's disease and primary effusion lymphoma. *Lab Invest* 78: 1637-1642.

1279. Tew JG, Wu J, Qin D, Helm S, Burton GF, Szakal AK (1997). Follicular dendritic cells and presentation of antigen and costimulatory signals to B cells. *Immunol Rev* 156: 39-52.

1280. Thangavelu M, Finn WG, Yelavarthi KK, Roenigk HH, Jr., Samuelson E, Peterson L, Kuzel TM, Rosen ST (1997). Recurring structural chromosome abnormalities in peripheral blood lymphocytes of patients with mycosis fungoides/Sezary syndrome. *Blood* 89: 3371-3377.

1281. Theaker JM, Gatter KC, Esiri MM, Easterbrook P (1986). Neoplastic angioendotheliosis – further evidence supporting a lymphoid origin. *Histopathology* 10: 1261-1270.

1282. Theil J, Laumen H, Marafioti T, Hummel M, Lenz G, Wirth T, Stein H (2001). Defective octamer dependent transcription is responsible for silenced immunoglobulin transcription in Reed-Sternberg cells (in press).

1283. Thieblemont C, Bastion Y, Berger F, Rieux C, Salles G, Dumontet C, Felman P, Coiffier B (1997). Mucosa-associated lymphoid tissue gastrointestinal and nongastrointestinal lymphoma behavior: analysis of 108 patients. *J Clin Oncol* 15: 1624-1630.

1284. Thieblemont C, Berger F, Dumontet C, Moullet I, Bouafia F, Felman P, Salles G, Coiffier B (2000). Mucosa-associated lymphoid tissue lymphoma is a disseminated disease in one third of 158 patients analyzed. *Blood* 95: 802-806.

1285. Thiele J, Bennewitz FG, Bertsch HP, Falk S, Fischer R, Stutte HJ (1993). Splenic haematopoiesis in primary (idiopathic) osteomyelofibrosis: immunohistochemical and morphometric evaluation of proliferative activity of erytro- and endoreduplicative capacity of megakaryopoiesis (PCNA- and Ki-67 staining). *Virchows Arch B Cell Pathol Incl Mol Pathol* 64: 281-286.

1286. Thiele J, Hoeppner B, Zankovich R, Fischer R (1989). Histomorphometry of bone marrow biopsies in primary osteomyelofibrosis/-sclerosis (agnogenic myeloid metaplasia) – correlations between clinical and morphological features. *Virchows Arch A Pathol Anat Histopathol* 415: 191-202.

1287. Thiele J, Kvasnicka HM, Boeltken B, Zankovich R, Diehl V, Fischer R (1999). Initial (prefibrotic) stages of idiopathic (primary) myelofibrosis (IMF) – a clinicopathological study. *Leukemia* 13: 1741-1748.

1288. Thiele J, Kvasnicka HM, Diehl V, Fischer R, Michiels J (1999). Clinicopathological diagnosis and differential criteria of thrombocythemias in various myeloproliferative disorders by histopathology, histochemistry and immunostaining from bone marrow biopsies. *Leuk Lymphoma* 33: 207-218.

1289. Thiele J, Kvasnicka HM, Fischer R (1999). Histochemistry and morphometry on bone marrow biopsies in chronic myeloproliferative disorders – aids to diagnosis and classification. *Ann Hematol* 78: 495-506.

1290. Thiele J, Kvasnicka HM, Schmitt-Graeff A, Zirbes TK, Birnbaum F, Kressmann C, Melguizo-Grahmann M, Frackenpohl H, Sprungmann C, Leder LD, Diehl V, Zankovich R, Schaefer HE, Niederle N, Fischer R (2000). Bone marrow features and clinical findings in chronic myeloid leukemia – a comparative, multicenter, immunohistological and morphometric study on 614 patients. *Leuk Lymphoma* 36: 295-308.

1291. Thiele J, Kvasnicka HM, Werden C, Zankovich R, Diehl V, Fischer R (1996). Idiopathic primary osteo-myelofibrosis: a clinico-pathological study on 208 patients with special emphasis on evolution of disease features, differentiation from essential thrombocythemia and variables of prognostic impact. *Leuk Lymphoma* 22: 303-317.

1292. Thiele J, Kvasnicka HM, Zirbes TK, Flucke U, Niederle N, Leder LD, Diehl V, Fischer R (1998). Impact of clinical and morphological variables in classification and regression tree-based survival (CART) analysis of CML with special emphasis on dynamic features. *Eur J Haematol* 60: 35-46.

1293. Thiele J, Schneider G, Hoeppner B, Wienhold S, Zankovich R, Fischer R (1988). Histomorphometry of bone marrow biopsies in chronic myeloproliferative disorders with associated thrombocytosis – features of significance for the diagnosis of primary (essential) thrombocythaemia. *Virchows Arch A Pathol Anat Histopathol* 413: 407-417.

1294. Thiele J, Zankovich R, Steinberg T, Fischer R, Diehl V (1989). Agnogenic myeloid metaplasia (AMM) – correlation of bone marrow lesions with laboratory data: a longitudinal clinicopathological study on 114 patients. *Hematol Oncol* 7: 327-343.

1295. Thiele J, Zirbes TK, Kvasnicka HM, Fischer R (1999). Focal lymphoid aggregates (nodules) in bone marrow biopsies: differentiation between benign hyperplasia and malignant lymphoma – a practical guideline. *J Clin Pathol* 52: 294-300.

1296. Thomason RW, Craig FE, Banks PM, Sears DL, Myerson GE, Gulley ML (1996). Epstein-Barr virus and lymphoproliferation in methotrexate-treated rheumatoid arthritis. *Mod Pathol* 9: 261-266.

1297. Tilly H, Rossi A, Stamatoullas A, Lenormand B, Bigorgne C, Kunlin A, Monconduit M, Bastard C (1994). Prognostic value of chromosomal abnormalities in follicular lymphoma. *Blood* 84: 1043-1049.

1298. Tinguely M, Vonlanthen R, Muller E, Dommann-Scherrer CC, Schneider J, Laissue JA, Borisch B (1998). Hodgkin's disease-like lymphoproliferative disorders in patients with different underlying immunodeficiency states. *Mod Pathol* 11: 307-312.

1299. Tirelli U, Errante D, Dolcetti R, Gloghini A, Serraino D, Vaccher E, Franceschi S, Boiocchi M, Carbone A (1995). Hodgkin's disease and human immunodeficiency virus infection: clinicopathologic and virologic features of 114 patients from the Italian Cooperative Group on AIDS and Tumors. *J Clin Oncol* 13: 1758-1767.

1300. Tolksdorf G, Stein H, Lennert K (1980). Morphological and immunological definition of a malignant lymphoma derived from germinal-centre cells with cleaved nuclei (centrocytes). *Br J Cancer* 41: 168-182.

1301. Tomita Y, Ohsawa M, Qiu K, Hashimoto M, Yang WI, Kim GE, Aozasa K (1997). Epstein-Barr virus in lymphoproliferative diseases in the sino-nasal region: close association with CD56+ immunophenotype and polymorphic-reticulosis morphology. *Int J Cancer* 70: 9-13.

1302. Topar G, Staudacher C, Geisen F, Gabl C, Fend F, Herold M, Greil R, Fritsch P, Sepp N (1998). Urticaria pigmentosa: a clinical, hematopathologic, and serologic study of 30 adults. *Am J Clin Pathol* 109: 279-285.

1303. Toro JR, Beaty M, Sorbara L, Turner ML, White J, Kingma DW, Raffeld M, Jaffe ES (2000). gamma delta T-cell lymphoma of the skin: a clinical, microscopic, and molecular study. *Arch Dermatol* 136: 1024-1032.

1304. Touhy EA (1920). A case of splenomegaly with polymorphonuclear neutrophil hyperleukocytosis. *Am J Med Sci* 160: 18-25.

1305. Touriol C, Greenland C, Lamant L, Pulford K, Bernard F, Rousset T, Mason DY, Delsol G (2000). Further demonstration of the diversity of chromosomal changes involving 2p23 in ALK-positive lymphoma: 2 cases expressing ALK kinase fused to CLTCL (clathrin chain polypeptide-like). *Blood* 95: 3204-3207.

1306. Toyama K, Ohyashiki K, Yoshida Y, Abe T, Asano S, Hirai H, Hirashima K, Hotta T, Kuramoto A, Kuriya S (1993). Clinical implications of chromosomal abnormalities in 401 patients with myelodysplastic syndromes: a multicentric study in Japan. *Leukemia* 7: 499-508.

1307. Travis WD, Li CY (1988). Pathology of the lymph node and spleen in systemic mast cell disease. *Mod Pathol* 1: 4-14.

1308. Travis WD, Li CY, Bergstralh EJ, Yam LT, Swee RG (1988). Systemic mast cell disease. Analysis of 58 cases and literature review. *Medicine (Baltimore)* 67: 345-368.

1309. Travis WD, Li CY, Hoagland HC, Travis LB, Banks PM (1986). Mast cell leukemia: report of a case and review of the literature. *Mayo Clin Proc* 61: 957-966.

1310. Travis WD, Li CY, Yam LT, Bergstralh EJ, Swee RG (1988). Significance of systemic mast cell disease with associated hematologic disorders. *Cancer* 62: 965-972.

1311. Trinei M, Lanfrancone L, Campo E, Pulford K, Mason DY, Pelicci PG, Falini B (2000). A new variant anaplastic lymphoma kinase (ALK)-fusion protein (ATIC-ALK) in a case of ALK-positive anaplastic large cell lymphoma. *Cancer Res* 60: 793-798.

1312. Tsang P, Cesarman E, Chadburn A, Liu YF, Knowles DM (1996). Molecular characterization of primary mediastinal B cell lymphoma. *Am J Pathol* 148: 2017-2025.

1313. Tsang WY, Chan JK, Ng CS, Pau MY (1996). Utility of a paraffin section-reactive CD56 antibody (123C3) for characterization and diagnosis of lymphomas. *Am J Surg Pathol* 20: 202-210.

1314. Tsukasaki K, Tsushima H, Yamamura M, Hata T, Murata K, Maeda T, Atogami S, Sohda H, Momita S, Ideda S, Katamine S, Yamada Y, Kamihira S, Tomonaga M (1997). Integration patterns of HTLV-I provirus in relation to the clinical course of ATL: frequent clonal change at crisis from indolent disease. *Blood* 89: 948-956.

1315. Tursz T, Flandrin G, Brouet JC, Seligmann M (1974). [Coexistence of a myeloma and a granulocytic leukemia in the absence of any treatment. Study of 4 cases]. *Nouv Rev Fr Hematol* 14: 693-704.

1316. Uccini S, Monardo F, Stoppacciaro A, Gradilone A, Agliano AM, Faggioni A, Manzari V, Vago L, Costanzi G, Ruco LP, . (1990). High frequency of Epstein-Barr virus genome detection in Hodgkin's disease of HIV-positive patients. *Int J Cancer* 46: 581-585.

1317. Utz GL, Swerdlow SH (1993). Distinction of follicular hyperplasia from follicular lymphoma in B5-fixed tissues: comparison of MT2 and bcl-2 antibodies. *Hum Pathol* 24: 1155-1158.

1318. Vaandrager JW, Schuuring E, Zwikstra E, De Boer CJ, Kleiverda KK, Van Krieken JH, Kluin-Nelemans HC, van Ommen GJ, Raap AK, Kluin PM (1996). Direct visualization of dispersed 11q13 chromosomal translocations in mantle cell lymphoma by multicolor DNA fiber fluorescence in situ hybridization. *Blood* 88: 1177-1182.

1319. Valent P (1995). 1995 Mack-Forster Award Lecture. Review. Mast cell differentiation antigens: expression in normal and malignant cells and use for diagnostic purposes. *Eur J Clin Invest* 25: 715-720.

1320. Valent P (1996). Biology, classification and treatment of human mastocytosis. *Wien Klin Wochenschr* 108: 385-397.

1321. Valent P, Ashman LK, Hinterberger W, Eckersberger F, Majdic O, Lechner K, Bettelheim P (1989). Mast cell typing: demonstration of a distinct hematopoietic cell type and evidence for immunophenotypic relationship to mononuclear phagocytes. *Blood* 73: 1778-1785.

1322. Valent P, Horny HP, Escribano L, Longley BJ, Li CY, Schwartz LB, Marone G, Nunez R, Akin C, Sotlar K, Sperr WR, Wolff K, Brunning RD, Parwaresch MR, Austen KF, Lennert K, Metcalfe DD, Vardiman JW, Bennett JM (2001). Diagnostic criteria and classification of mastocytosis: a consensus proposal. *Leuk Res* 25.

1323. Valla D, Casadevall N, Huisse MG, Tulliez M, Grange JD, Muller O, Binda T, Varet B, Rueff B, Benhamou JP (1988). Etiology of portal vein thrombosis in adults. A prospective evaluation of primary myeloproliferative disorders. *Gastroenterology* 94: 1063-1069.

1324. van Baarlen J, Schuurman HJ, van Unnik JA (1988). Multilobated non-Hodgkin's lymphoma. A clinicopathologic entity. *Cancer* 61: 1371-1376.

1325. Van Camp B, Durie BG, Spier C, De Waele M, Van R, I, Vela E, Frutiger Y, Richter L, Grogan TM (1990). Plasma cells in multiple myeloma express a natural killer cell-associated antigen: CD56 (NKH-1; Leu-19). *Blood* 76: 377-382.

1326. van den Oord JJ, Wolf-Peeters C, Desmet VJ (1986). The marginal zone in the human reactive lymph node. *Am J Clin Pathol* 86: 475-479.

1327. van den Oord JJ, Wolf-Peeters C, Desmet VJ (1989). Marginal zone lymphocytes in the lymph node. *Hum Pathol* 20: 1225-1227.

1328. van den BA, Visser L, Poppema S (1999). High expression of the CC chemokine TARC in Reed-Sternberg cells. A possible explanation for the characteristic T-cell infiltratein Hodgkin's lymphoma. *Am J Pathol* 154: 1685-1691.

1329. van Doorn R, Van Haselen CW, Voorst Vader PC, Geerts ML, Heule F, de Rie M, Steijlen PM, Dekker SK, van Vloten WA, Willemze R (2000). Mycosis fungoides: disease evolution and prognosis of 309 Dutch patients. *Arch Dermatol* 136: 504-510.

1330. van Gorp J, Doornewaard H, Verdonck LF, Klopping C, Vos PF, van den Tweel JG (1994). Posttransplant T-cell lymphoma. Report of three cases and a review of the literature. Cancer 73: 3064-3072.

1331. van Gorp J, Weiping L, Jacobse K, Liu YH, Li FY, De Weger RA, Li G (1994). Epstein-Barr virus in nasal T-cell lymphomas (polymorphic reticulosis/midline malignant reticulosis) in western China. J Pathol 173: 81-87.

1332. Van Krieken JH, von Schilling C, Kluin PM, Lennert K (1989). Splenic marginal zone lymphocytes and related cells in the lymph node: a morphologic and immunohistochemical study. Hum Pathol 20: 320-325.

1333. van Spronsen DJ, Vrints LW, Hofstra G, Crommelin MA, Coebergh JW, Breed WP (1997). Disappearance of prognostic significance of histopathological grading of nodular sclerosing Hodgkin's disease for unselected patients, 1972-92. Br J Haematol 96: 322-327.

1334. Vandenberghe E, Wolf-Peeters C, van den OJ, Wlodarska I, Delabie J, Stul M, Thomas J, Michaux JL, Mecucci C, Cassiman JJ (1991). Translocation (11;14): a cytogenetic anomaly associated with B-cell lymphomas of non-follicle centre cell lineage. J Pathol 163: 13-18.

1335. Vasef MA, Medeiros LJ, Yospur LS, Sun NC, McCourty A, Brynes RK (1997). Cyclin D1 protein in multiple myeloma and plasmacytoma: an immunohistochemical study using fixed, paraffin-embedded tissue sections. Mod Pathol 10: 927-932.

1336. Vasef MA, Zaatari GS, Chan WC, Sun NC, Weiss LM, Brynes RK (1995). Dendritic cell tumors associated with low-grade B-cell malignancies. Report of three cases. Am J Clin Pathol 104: 696-701.

1337. Vassallo R, Ryu JH, Colby TV, Hartman T, Limper AH (2000). Pulmonary Langerhans'-cell histiocytosis. N Engl J Med 342: 1969-1978.

1338. Velders GA, Kluin-Nelemans JC, De Boer CJ, Hermans J, Noordijk EM, Schuuring E, Kramer MH, Van Dijk WA, Rahder JB, Kluin PM, Van Krieken JH (1996). Mantle cell lymphoma: a population-based clinical study. J Clin Oncol 14: 1269-1274.

1339. Venditti A, Del Poeta G, Stasi R, Masi M, Bruno A, Buccisano F, Cox C, Coppetelli U, Aronica G, Simone MD (1994). Minimally differentiated acute myeloid leukaemia (AML-M0): cytochemical, immunophenotypic and cytogenetic analysis of 19 cases. Br J Haematol 88: 784-793.

1340. Verbov JL, Borrie PF (1971). Diffuse cutaneous mastocytosis. Br J Dermatol 84: 190-191.

1341. Verfaillie CM (1998). Biology of chronic myelogenous leukemia. Hematol Oncol Clin North Am 12: 1-29.

1342. Vergier B, Beylot-Barry M, Pulford K, Michel P, Bosq J, de Muret A, Beylot C, Delaunay MM, Avril MF, Dalac S, Bodemer C, Joly P, Groppi A, de Mascarel A, Bagot M, Mason DY, Wechsler J, Merlio JP (1998). Statistical evaluation of diagnostic and prognostic features of CD30+ cutaneous lymphoproliferative disorders: a clinicopathologic study of 65 cases. Am J Surg Pathol 22: 1192-1202.

1343. Vergier B, de Muret A, Beylot-Barry M, Vaillant L, Ekouevi D, Chene G, Carlotti A, Franck N, Dechelotte P, Souteyrand P, Courville P, Joly P, Delaunay M, Bagot M, Grange F, Fraitag S, Bosq J, Petrella T, Durlach A, de Mascarel A, Merlio JP, Wechsler J (2000). Transformation of mycosis fungoides: clinicopathological and prognostic features of 45 cases. French Study Group of Cutaneious Lymphomas. Blood 95: 2212-2218.

1344. Vermeer MH, Geelen FA, Kummer JA, Meijer CJ, Willemze R (1999). Expression of cytotoxic proteins by neoplastic T cells in mycosis fungoides increases with progression from plaque stage to tumor stage disease. Am J Pathol 154: 1203-1210.

1345. Vidal AU, Gessain A, Yoshida M, Mahieux R, Nishioka K, Tekaia F, Rosen L, De The G (1994). Molecular epidemiology of HTLV type I in Japan: evidence for two distinct ancestral lineages with a particular geographical distribution. AIDS Res Hum Retroviruses 10: 1557-1566.

1346. Vie H, Chevalier S, Garand R, Moisan JP, Praloran V, Devilder MC, Moreau JF, Soulillou JP (1989). Clonal expansion of lymphocytes bearing the gamma delta T-cell receptor in a patient with large granular lymphocyte disorder. Blood 74: 285-290.

1347. Virgilio L, Lazzeri C, Bichi R, Nibu K, Narducci MG, Russo G, Rothstein JL, Croce CM (1998). Deregulated expression of TCL1 causes T cell leukemia in mice. Proc Natl Acad Sci U S A 95: 3885-3889.

1348. Virgilio L, Narducci MG, Isobe M, Billips LG, Cooper MD, Croce CM, Russo G (1994). Identification of the TCL1 gene involved in T-cell malignancies. Proc Natl Acad Sci U S A 91: 12530-12534.

1349. Visani G, Finelli C, Castelli U, Petti MC, Ricci P, Vianelli N, Gianni L, Zuffa E, Aloe Spiriti MA, Latagliata R (1990). Myelofibrosis with myeloid metaplasia: clinical and haematological parameters predicting survival in a series of 133 patients. Br J Haema-tol 75: 4-9.

1350. Vorechovsky I, Luo L, Dyer MJ, Catovsky D, Amlot PL, Yaxley JC, Foroni L, Hammarstrom L, Webster AD, Yuille MA (1997). Clustering of missense mutations in the ataxia-telangiectasia gene in a sporadic T-cell leukaemia. Nat Genet 17: 96-99.

1351. Vose JM, Bierman PJ, Lynch JC, Weisenburger DD, Kessinger A, Chan WC, Greiner TC, Armitage JO (1998). Effect of follicularity on autologous transplantation for large-cell non-Hodgkin's lymphoma. J Clin Oncol 16: 844-849.

1352. Waggott W, Delsol G, Jarret RF, Mason DY, Gatter KC, Boultwood J, Wainscoat JS (1997). NPM-ALK gene fusion and Hodgkin's disease. Blood 90: 1712-1713.

1353. Wagner SD, Martinelli V, Luzzatto L (1994). Similar patterns of V kappa gene usage but different degrees of somatic mutation in hairy cell leukemia, prolymphocytic leukemia, Waldenstrom's macroglobulinemia, and myeloma. Blood 83: 3647-3653.

1354. Wahner-Roedler DL, Kyle RA (1992). Mu-heavy chain disease: presentation as a benign monoclonal gammapathy. Am J Hematol 40: 56-60.

1355. Wahner-Roedler DL, Kyle RA (1998). Heavy chain disease. In: Myeloma, Biology and Management, Malpas JA, Bergsagel DE, Kyle RA, Anderson KC, eds. 2nd. Oxford University Press: New York, 604-638.

1356. Walts AE, Shintaku IP, Said JW (1990). Diagnosis of malignant lymphoma in effusions from patients with AIDS by gene rearrangement. Am J Clin Pathol 94: 170-175.

1357. Wang CC, Tien HF, Lin MT, Su IJ, Wang CH, Chuang SM, Shen MC, Liu CH (1995). Consistent presence of isochromosome 7q in hepatosplenic T gamma/delta lymphoma: a new cytogenetic-clinicopathologic entity. Genes Chromosomes Cancer 12: 161-164.

1358. Wano Y, Hattori T, Matsuoka M, Takatsuki K, Chua AO, Gubler U, Greene WC (1987). Interleukin 1 gene expression in adult T cell leukemia. J Clin Invest 80: 911-916.

1359. Ward HP, Block MH (1971). The natural history of agnogenic myeloid metaplasia (AMM) and a critical evaluation of its relationship with the myeloproliferative syndrome. Medicine (Baltimore) 50: 357-420.

1360. Warnke RA, Kim H, Fuks Z, Dorfman RF (1977). The coexistence of nodular and diffuse patterns in nodular non-Hodgkin's lymphomas: significance and clinicopathologic correlation. Cancer 40: 1229-1233.

1361. Warnke RA, Weiss LM, Chan JKC, Cleary ML, Dorfman RF (1995). Tumors of the lymph nodes and spleen. In: Atlas of tumor pathology, Atlas of tumor pathology Armed Forces Institute of Pathology: Washington, D.C.pp.

1362. Washington LT, Ansari MQ, Picker LJ, et al (1999). Immunophenotypic analysis of B-cell precursors (BCP) in 661 bone marrow (BM) specimens by 4 color floc cytometry. Mod Pathol 12: 148A.

1363. Webb TA, Li CY, Yam LT (1982). Systemic mast cell disease: a clinical and hematopathologic study of 26 cases. Cancer 49: 927-938.

1364. Weinreb M, Day PJ, Niggli F, Green EK, Nyong'o AO, Othieno-Abinya NA, Riyat MS, Raafat F, Mann JR (1996). The consistent association between Epstein-Barr virus and Hodgkin's disease in children in Kenya. Blood 87: 3828-3836.

1365. Weinreb M, Day PJ, Niggli F, Powell JE, Raafat F, Hesseling PB, Schneider JW, Hartley PS, Tzortzatou-Stathopoulou F, Khalek ER, Mangoud A, El Safy UR, Madanat F, Al Sheyyab M, Mpofu C, Revesz T, Rafii R, Tiedemann K, Waters KD, Barrantes JC, Nyongo A, Riyat MS, Mann JR (1996). The role of Epstein-Barr virus in Hodgkin's disease from different geographical areas. Arch Dis Child 74: 27-31.

1366. Weisenburger DD, Anderson J, Armitage J, et al (1998). Grading of follicular lymphoma: diagnostic accuracy, reproducibility, and clinical relevance. Mod Pathol 11: 142a.

1367. Weiss LM, Berry GJ, Dorfman RF, Banks P, Kaiserling E, Curtis J, Rosai J, Warnke RA (1990). Spindle cell neoplasms of lymph nodes of probable reticulum cell lineage. True reticulum cell sarcoma? Am J Surg Pathol 14: 405-414.

1368. Weiss LM, Jaffe ES, Liu XF, Chen YY, Shibata D, Medeiros LJ (1992). Detection and localization of Epstein-Barr viral genomes in angioimmunoblastic lymphadenopathy and angioimmunoblastic lymphadenopathy-like lymphoma. Blood 79: 1789-1795.

1369. Weiss LM, Strickler JG, Dorfman RF, Horning SJ, Warnke RA, Sklar J (1986). Clonal T-cell populations in angioimmunoblastic lymphadenopathy and angioimmunoblastic lymphadenopathy-like lymphoma. Am J Pathol 122: 392-397.

1370. Weiss LM, Warnke RA, Sklar J, Cleary ML (1987). Molecular analysis of the t(14;18) chromosomal translocation in malignant lymphomas. N Engl J Med 317: 1185-1189.

1371. Weiss LM, Wood GS, Trela M, Warnke RA, Sklar J (1986). Clonal T-cell populations in lymphomatoid papulosis. Evidence of a lymphoproliferative origin for a clinically benign disease. N Engl J Med 315: 475-479.

1372. Weiss SW, Gnepp DR, Bratthauer GL (1989). Palisaded myofibroblastoma. A benign mesenchymal tumor of lymph node. Am J Surg Pathol 13: 341-346.

1373. Weissmann DJ, Ferry JA, Harris NL, Louis DN, Delmonico F, Spiro I (1995). Posttransplantation lymphoproliferative disorders in solid organ recipients are predominantly aggressive tumors of host origin. Am J Clin Pathol 103: 748-755.

1374. Weitzman S, Greenberg ML, Thorner P (1991). Treatment of non-Hodgkin's lymphoma in childhood. In: Neoplastic diseases of blood, PH Wiernik, GP Canellos, RA Kyle, Schiffer CA. 1 vol. 2nd ed. Churchill Livingstone: New York, pp. 753-768.

1375. Weller PF, Bubley GJ (1994). The idiopathic hypereosinophilic syndrome. Blood 83: 2759-2779.

1376. Wellmann A, Otsuki T, Vogelbruch M, Clark HM, Jaffe ES, Raffeld M (1995). Analysis of the t(2;5)(p23;q35) translocation by reverse transcription-polymerase chain reaction in CD30+ anaplastic large-cell lymphomas, in other non-Hodgkin's lymphomas of T-cell phenotype, and in Hodgkin's disease. Blood 86: 2321-2328.

1377. Wellmann A, Thieblemont C, Pittaluga S, Sakai A, Jaffe ES, Siebert P, Raffeld M (2000). Detection of differentially expressed genes in lymphomas using cDNA arrays: identification of clusterin as a new diagnostic marker for anaplastic large-cell lymphomas. Blood 96: 398-404.

1378. Wendum D, Sebban C, Gaulard P, Coiffier B, Tilly H, Cazals D, Boehn A, Casasnovas RO, Bouabdallah R, Jaubert J, Ferrant A, Diebold J, de Mascarel A, Gisselbrecht C (1997). Follicular large-cell lymphoma treated with intensive chemotherapy: an analysis of 89 cases included in the LNH87 trial and comparison with the outcome of diffuse large B-cell lymphoma. Groupe d'Etude des Lymphomes de l'Adulte. *J Clin Oncol* 15: 1654-1663.

1379. Werner M, Kaloutsi V, Kausche F, Buhr T, Georgii A (1993). Evidence from molecular genetic and cytogenetic analyses that bone marrow histopathology is reliable in the diagnosis of chronic myeloproliferative disorders. *Virchows Arch B Cell Pathol Incl Mol Pathol* 63: 199-204.

1380. Westbrook CA (1992). The role of molecular techniques in the clinical management of leukemia. Lessons from the Philadelphia chromosome. *Cancer* 70: 1695-1700.

1381. Westhoff DD, Samaha RJ, Barnes A, Jr. (1975). Arsenic intoxication as a cause of megaloblastic anemia. *Blood* 45: 241-246.

1382. Whang-Peng J, Bunn P, Knutsen T, Schechter GP, Gazdar AF, Matthews MJ, Minna JD (1979). Cytogenetic abnormalities in patients with cutaneous T-cell lymphomas. *Cancer Treat Rep* 63: 575-580.

1383. Whittaker S, Smith N, Jones RR, Luzzatto L (1991). Analysis of beta, gamma, and delta T-cell receptor genes in lymphomatoid papulosis: cellular basis of two distinct histologic subsets. *J Invest Dermatol* 96: 786-791.

1384. Wickert RS, Weisenburger DD, Tierens A, Greiner TC, Chan WC (1995). Clonal relationship between lymphocytic predominance Hodgkin's disease and concurrent or subsequent large-cell lymphoma of B lineage. *Blood* 86: 2312-2320.

1385. Wilks S (1856). Cases of lardaceous disease and some allied affections, with remarks. *Guy's Hosp Rep* 17: 103.

1386. Wilks S (1856). Enlargement of the lymphatic glands and spleen (or, Hodgkin's disease) with remarks. *Guy's Hosp Rep* 11: 56.

1387. Willemze R, Kerl H, Sterry W, Berti E, Cerroni L, Chimenti S, Diaz-Perez JL, Geerts ML, Goos M, Knobler R, Ralfkiaer E, Santucci M, Smith N, Wechsler J, van Vloten WA, Meijer CJ (1997). EORTC classification for primary cutaneous lymphomas: a proposal from the Cutaneous Lymphoma Study Group of the European Organization for Research and Treatment of Cancer. *Blood* 90: 354-371.

1388. Willemze R, Ruiter DJ, Scheffer E, van Vloten WA (1980). Diffuse cutaneous mastocytosis with multiple cutaneous mastocytomas. Report of a case with clinical, histopathological and ultrastructural aspects. *Br J Dermatol* 102: 601-607.

1389. Williams ME, Swerdlow SH, Rosenberg CL, Arnold A (1993). Chromosome 11 translocation breakpoints at the PRAD1/ cyclin D1 gene locus in centrocytic lymphoma. *Leukemia* 7: 241-245.

1390. Williams ME, Westermann CD, Swerdlow SH (1990). Genotypic characterization of centrocytic lymphoma: frequent rearrangement of the chromosome 11 bcl-1 locus. *Blood* 76: 1387-1391.

1391. Williams ME, Whitefield M, Swerdlow SH (1997). Analysis of the cyclin-dependent kinase inhibitors p18 and p19 in mantle-cell lymphoma and chronic lymphocytic leukemia. *Ann Oncol* 8 Suppl 2:71-3: 71-73.

1392. Williams ME, Woytowitz D, Finkelstein SD, Swerdlow SH (1995). MTS1/MTS2 (p15/p16) deletions and p53 mutations in mantle-cell (centrocytic) lymphoma. *Blood* 86: 747a.

1393. Williamson PJ, Kruger AR, Reynolds PJ, Hamblin TJ, Oscier DG (1994). Establishing the incidence of myelodysplastic syndrome. *Br J Haematol* 87: 743-745.

1394. Willman CL (1998). Molecular genetic features of myelodysplastic syndromes (MDS). *Leukemia* 12 Suppl 1:S2-6: S2-S6.

1395. Willman CL, Busque L, Griffith BB, Favara BE, McClain KL, Duncan MH, Gilliland DG (1994). Langerhans'-cell histiocytosis (histiocytosis X) – a clonal proliferative disease. *N Engl J Med* 331: 154-160.

1396. Wilson MS, Weiss LM, Gatter KC, Mason DY, Dorfman RF, Warnke RA (1990). Malignant histiocytosis. A reassessment of cases previously reported in 1975 based on paraffin section immunophenotyping studies. *Cancer* 66: 530-536.

1397. Wilson WH, Kingma DW, Raffeld M, Wittes RE, Jaffe ES (1996). Association of lymphomatoid granulomatosis with Epstein-Barr viral infection of B lymphocytes and response to interferon-alpha 2b. *Blood* 87: 4531-4537.

1398. Wilson WH, Teruya-Feldstein J, Fest T, Harris C, Steinberg SM, Jaffe ES, Raffeld M (1997). Relationship of p53, bcl-2, and tumor proliferation to clinical drug resistance in non-Hodgkin's lymphomas. *Blood* 89: 601-609.

1399. Wlodarska I, Mecucci C, Marynen P, Guo C, Franckx D, La Starza R, Aventin A, Bosly A, Martelli MF, Cassiman JJ (1995). TEL gene is involved in myelodysplastic syndromes with either the typical t(5;12)(q33;p13) translocation or its variant t(10;12)(q24;p13). *Blood* 85: 2848-2852.

1400. Wlodarska I, Wolf-Peeters C, Falini B, Verhoef G, Morris SW, Hagemeijer A, Van den BH (1998). The cryptic inv(2)(p23q35) defines a new molecular genetic subtype of ALK-positive anaplastic large-cell lymphoma. *Blood* 92: 2688-2695.

1401. Wolf BC, Banks PM, Mann RB, Neiman RS (1988). Splenic hematopoiesis in polycythemia vera. A morphologic and immunohistologic study. *Am J Clin Pathol* 89: 69-75.

1402. Wolf BC, Brady K, O'Murchadha MT, Neiman RS (1990). An evaluation of immunohistochemical stains for immunoglobulin light chains in bone marrow biopsies in benign and malignant plasma cell proliferations. *Am J Clin Pathol* 94: 742-746.

1403. Wolf BC, Kumar A, Vera JC, Neiman RS (1986). Bone marrow morphology and immunology in systemic amyloidosis. *Am J Clin Pathol* 86: 84-88.

1404. Wolf BC, Neiman RS (1985). Myelofibrosis with myeloid metaplasia: pathophysiologic implications of the correlation between bone marrow changes and progression of splenomegaly. *Blood* 65: 803-809.

1405. Wolf BC, Neiman RS (1989). Essential thrombocythemia. In: *Disorders of the spleen*, Disorders of the spleen. W.B. Saunders Company: Philadelphia, pp. 173-174.

1406. Wong KF, Chan JK, Ng CS, Lee KC, Tsang WY, Cheung MM (1992). CD56 (NKH1)-positive hematolymphoid malignancies: an aggressive neoplasm featuring frequent cutaneous/mucosal involvement, cytoplasmic azurophilic granules, and angiocentricity. *Hum Pathol* 23: 798-804.

1407. Wong KF, Zhang YM, Chan JK (1999). Cytogenetic abnormalities in natural killer cell lymphoma/leukaemia – is there a consistent pattern? *Leuk Lymphoma* 34: 241-250.

1408. Wood C, Wood GS, Deneau DG, Oseroff A, Beckstead JH, Malin J (1984). Malignant histiocytosis X. Report of a rapidly fatal case in an elderly man. *Cancer* 54: 347-352.

1409. Wood GS, Hardman DL, Boni R, Dummer R, Kim YH, Smoller BR, Takeshita M, Kikuchi M, Burg G (1996). Lack of the t(2;5) or other mutations resulting in expression of anaplastic lymphoma kinase catalytic domain in CD30+ primary cutaneous lymphoproliferative disorders and Hodgkin's disease. *Blood* 88: 1765-1770.

1410. Wood GS, Hu CH, Beckstead JH, Turner RR, Winkelmann RK (1985). The indeterminate cell proliferative disorder: report of a case manifesting as an unusual cutaneous histiocytosis. *J Dermatol Surg Oncol* 11: 1111-1119.

1411. Woodlock TJ, Seshi B, Sham RL, Cyran EM, Bennett JM (1994). Use of cell surface antigen phenotype in guiding therapeutic decisions in chronic myelomonocytic leukemia. *Leuk Res* 18: 173-181.

1412. Worobec AS (2000). Treatment of systemic mast cell disorders. *Hematol Oncol Clin North Am* 14: 659-87, vii.

1413. Worobec AS, Semere T, Nagata H, Metcalfe DD (1998). Clinical correlates of the presence of the Asp816Val c-kit mutation in the peripheral blood mononuclear cells of patients with mastocytosis. *Cancer* 83: 2120-2129.

1414. Worsley A, Oscier DG, Stevens J, Darlow S, Figes A, Mufti GJ, Hamblin TJ (1988). Prognostic features of chronic myelomonocytic leukaemia: a modified Bournemouth score gives the best prediction of survival. *Br J Haematol* 68: 17-21.

1415. Wotherspoon AC, Doglioni C, Diss TC, Pan L, Moschini A, de Boni M, Isaacson PG (1993). Regression of primary low-grade B-cell gastric lymphoma of mucosa-associated lymphoid tissue type after eradication of Helicobacter pylori. *Lancet* 342: 575-577.

1416. Wotherspoon AC, Finn TM, Isaacson PG (1995). Trisomy 3 in low-grade B-cell lymphomas of mucosa-associated lymphoid tissue. *Blood* 85: 2000-2004.

1417. Wotherspoon AC, Ortiz-Hidalgo C, Falzon MR, Isaacson PG (1991). Helicobacter pylori-associated gastritis and primary B-cell gastric lymphoma. *Lancet* 338: 1175-1176.

1418. Wright D, McKeever P, Carter R (1997). Childhood non-Hodgkin lymphomas in the United Kingdom: findings from the UK Children's Cancer Study Group. *J Clin Pathol* 50: 128-134.

1419. Wright DH (1971). Burkitt's lymphoma: a review of the pathology, immunology and possible aetiological factors. Pathology annual. In: *SC Sommers*, Pathology annual., ed. Appleton-Century-Crofts: New York, pp. 337-363.

1420. Wright DH (1997). Enteropathy associated T cell lymphoma. *Cancer Surv* 30:249-61: 249-261.

1421. Wright DH (1997). What is Burkitt's lymphoma? *J Pathol* 182: 125-127.

1422. Wrotnowski U, Mills SE, Cooper PH (1985). Malignant angioendotheliomatosis. An angiotropic lymphoma? *Am J Clin Pathol* 83: 244-248.

1423. Wu CD, Wickert RS, Williamson JE, Sun NC, Brynes RK, Chan WC (1999). Using fluorescence-based human androgen receptor gene assay to analyze the clonality of microdissected dendritic cell tumors. *Am J Clin Pathol* 111: 105-110.

1424. Wu TT, Swerdlow SH, Locker J, Bahler D, Randhawa P, Yunis EJ, Dickman PS, Nalesnik MA (1996). Recurrent Epstein-Barr virus-associated lesions in organ transplant recipients. *Hum Pathol* 27: 157-164.

1425. Xiao S, Nalabolu SR, Aster JC, Ma J, Abruzzo L, Jaffe ES, Stone R, Weissman SM, Hudson TJ, Fletcher JA (1998). FGFR1 is fused with a novel zinc-finger gene, ZNF198, in the t(8;13) leukemia/lymphoma syndrome. *Nat Genet* 18: 84-87.

1426. Yam LT, Yam CF, Li CY (1980). Eosinophilia in systemic mastocytosis. *Am J Clin Pathol* 73: 48-54.

1427. Yamaguchi K (1994). Human T-lymphotropic virus type I in Japan. *Lancet* 343: 213-216.

1428. Yamaguchi K, Nishimura H, Kohrogi H, Jono M, Miyamoto Y, Takatsuki K (1983). A proposal for smoldering adult T-cell leukemia: a clinicopathologic study of five cases. *Blood* 62: 758-766.

1429. Yamamura M, Yamada Y, Momita S, Kamihira S, Tomonaga M (1998). Circulating interleukin-6 levels are elevated in adult T-cell leukaemia/lymphoma patients and correlate with adverse clinical features and survival. *Br J Haematol* 100: 129-134.

1430. Yanagisawa K, Ohminami H, Sato M, Takada K, Hasegawa H, Yasukawa M, Fujita S (1998). Neoplastic involvement of granulocytic lineage, not granulocytic-monocytic, monocytic, or erythrocytic lineage, in a patient with chronic neutrophilic leukemia. *Am J Hematol* 57: 221-224.

1431. Yang WI, Zukerberg LR, Motokura T, Arnold A, Harris NL (1994). Cyclin D1 (Bcl-1, PRAD1) protein expression in low-grade B-cell lymphomas and reactive hyperplasia. *Am J Pathol* 145: 86-96.

1432. Yano T, Sander CA, Clark HM, Dolezal MV, Jaffe ES, Raffeld M (1993). Clustered mutations in the second exon of the MYC gene in sporadic Burkitt's lymphoma. *Oncogene* 8: 2741-2748.

1433. You W, Weisbrot IM (1979). Chronic neutrophilic leukemia. Report of two cases and review of the literature. *Am J Clin Pathol* 72: 233-242.

1434. Young JL, Jr., Percy CL, Asire AJ, Berg JW, Cusano MM, Gloeckler LA, Horm JW, Lourie WI, Jr., Pollack ES, Shambaugh EM (1981). Cancer incidence and mortality in the United States, 1973-77. *Natl Cancer Inst Monogr* 1-187.

1435. Yu RC, Chu AC (1995). Lack of T-cell receptor gene rearrangements in cells involved in Langerhans cell histiocytosis. *Cancer* 75: 1162-1166.

1436. Yu RC, Chu C, Buluwela L, Chu AC (1994). Clonal proliferation of Langerhans cells in Langerhans cell histiocytosis. *Lancet* 343: 767-768.

1437. Yunis JJ, Mayer MG, Arnesen MA, Aeppli DP, Oken MM, Frizzera G (1989). bcl-2 and other genomic alterations in the prognosis of large-cell lymphoma. *N Engl J Med* 320: 1047-1054.

1438. Zhu D, Oscier DG, Stevenson FK (1995). Splenic lymphoma with villous lymphocytes involves B cells with extensively mutated Ig heavy chain variable region genes. *Blood* 85: 1603-1607.

1439. Ziegler JL, Beckstead JA, Volberding PA, Abrams DI, Levine AM, Lukes RJ, Gill PS, Burkes RL, Meyer PR, Metroka CE (1984). Non-Hodgkin's lymphoma in 90 homosexual men. Relation to generalized lymphadenopathy and the acquired immunodeficiency syndrome. *N Engl J Med* 311: 565-570.

1440. Ziegler JL, Bluming AZ, Morrow RH, Fass L, Carbone PP (1970). Central nervous system involvement in Burkitt's lymphoma. *Blood* 36: 718-728.

1441. Zipursky A, Brown EJ, Christensen H, Doyle J (1999). Transient myeloproliferative disorder (transient leukemia) and hematologic manifestations of Down syndrome. *Clin Lab Med* 19: 157-67, vii.

1442. Zipursky A, Thorner P, De Harven E, Christensen H, Doyle J (1994). Myelodysplasia and acute megakaryoblastic leukemia in Down's syndrome. *Leuk Res* 18: 163-171.

1443. Zittoun R, Rea D, Ngoc LH, Ramond S (1994). Chronic neutrophilic leukemia. A study of four cases. *Ann Hematol* 68: 55-60.

1444. Zoldan MC, Inghirami G, Masuda Y, Vandekerckhove F, Raphael B, Amorosi E, Hymes K, Frizzera G (1996). Large-cell variants of mantle cell lymphoma: cytologic characteristics and p53 anomalies may predict poor outcome. *Br J Haematol* 93: 475-486.

1445. Zouali M, Fine JM, Eyquem A (1984). Anti-DNA autoantibody activity and idiotypic relationships of human monoclonal proteins. Eur J Immunol 14: 1085-1089.

1446. Zucca E, Stein H, Coiffier B (1994). European Lymphoma Task Force (ELTF): Report of the workshop on Mantle Cell Lymphoma (MCL). Ann Oncol 5: 507-511.

1447. Zuckerman E, Zuckerman T, Levine AM, Douer D, Gutekunst K, Mizokami M, Qian DG, Velankar M, Nathwani BN, Fong TL (1997). Hepatitis C virus infection in patients with B-cell non-Hodgkin lymphoma. Ann Intern Med 127: 423-428.

1448. Zukerberg LR, Collins AB, Ferry JA, Harris NL (1991). Coexpression of CD15 and CD20 by Reed-Sternberg cells in Hodgkin's disease. Am J Pathol 139: 475-483.

1449. Zukerberg LR, Medeiros LJ, Ferry JA, Harris NL (1993). Diffuse low-grade B-cell lymphomas. Four clinically distinct subtypes defined by a combination of morphologic and immunophenotypic features. Am J Clin Pathol 100: 373-385.

1450. Zukerberg LR, Yang WI, Arnold A, Harris NL (1995). Cyclin D1 expression in non-Hodgkin's lymphomas. Detection by immunohistochemistry. Am J Clin Pathol 103: 756-760.

1451. Zutter MM, Martin PJ, Sale GE, Shulman HM, Fisher L, Thomas ED, Durnam DM (1988). Epstein-Barr virus lymphoproliferation after bone marrow transplantation. Blood 72: 520-529.

Subject index

Common variable immunodeficiency (CVID), 257-259
Convoluted T cell lymphoma, 115
Crow-Fukase syndrome, 154
Cutaneous CD4, 214
Cutaneous follicular lymphoma, 165
Cutaneous mastocytosis (CM), 293, 294, 296, 297, 301
CVID, see Common variable immunodeficiency
CYCLIN D1, 124, 129, 136, 148, 160, 169, 173
cyt-mu, 113

D

DBA.44, 139, 140
DEK/CAN, 94
del (13q), 34, 38
del (20q), 28, 34, 38, 67
del(11q), 89
del(12p), 54, 89, 113
del(20q), 54, 66, 68, 70, 71, 89
del(5q), 64, 66, 67, 70, 71, 73, 77, 89
del(7q), 70, 71, 77, 89
Dendritic cell sarcoma, 275, 284-288
Dendritic cell sarcoma, not otherwise specified, 289
Dermatopathic lymphadenopathy, 217, 219
DIC, see Disseminated intravascular coagulation
Diffuse centroblastic/centrocytic lymphoma, 167
Diffuse cutaneous mastocytosis, 293, 297
Diffuse large B-cell lymphoma (DLCBCL), 121, 125, 128, 134, 159, 160, 164-167, 171-177, 179, 185, 187, 243, 258, 260-267, 269-271
Diffuse large B-cell lymphoma with expression of full-length ALK, 174
Diffuse large cell (immunoblastic) lymphoma, 134
Disseminated intravascular coagulation (DIC), 84, 86, 117
DLCBCL, see Diffuse large B-cell lymphoma
Down syndrome, 101
Drosophila trithorax gene, 87
Duncan syndrome, 257, 258
Dutcher bodies, 133
Dyserythropoiesis, 50, 53, 54, 65, 68, 69, 71, 88, 90, 101
Dysgranulopoiesis, 21, 36, 50, 53, 65, 71, 88
Dysmegakaryopoiesis, 88
Dysmyelopoietic syndromes, 63

E

EBER, 180, 233, 262, 269, 286
EBNA-1, 248
EBNA-2, 248
EBV, see Epstein-Barr virus
Elastophagocytosis, 220
EMA, 174, 222, 230, 232, 233, 242, 246, 263
EMH, see Extramedullary haematopoiesis
Enteropathy-type T-cell lymphoma, 208, 211
Epstein-Barr virus (EBV), 56, 122, 145, 171, 173-175, 179-182, 184-187, 189, 199, 200, 202, 204, 205, 207, 208, 210, 214, 215, 225, 226, 229, 233, 234, 237, 239, 257-262, 264-271, 277, 281, 286

Erythremic myelosis (pure erythroid), 97
Erythroderma, 195, 216, 219
Erythroleukaemia, 90, 97-99
Erythrophagocytosis, 94, 95, 97, 231
Essential thrombocythaemia (ET), 17, 19, 39-44, 48, 59
ET, see Essential thrombocythaemia
Ewing's/PNET, 105
Extracutaneous mastocytoma, 300
Extramedullary haematopoiesis (EMH), 17, 32, 34-36, 38, 39, 41
Extramedullary monocytic sarcoma, 86, 96
Extramedullary myeloid tumour, 105
Extramedullary plasmacytoma, 149, 268
Extranodal NK/T-cell lymphoma, 185, 198, 199, 205-208, 214
Extranodal NK/T-cell lymphoma, nasal type, 185, 199, 204
Extraosseous (extramedullary) plasmacytoma, 149

F

5q- syndrome, 59, 61, 66, 73
Faggot cells, 84
Fanconi anaemia, 64
Fas, 197, 198, 199, 207
Fatal infectious mononucleosis (FIM), 257-259
Fibroblastic reticular cells (FRC), 276
FIM, see Fatal infectious mononucleosis
FL, see Follicular lymphoma
Flame cells, 146
Follicle centre lymphoma, 125, 162, 167
Follicle centre cells (FCC), FCC, 162, 168, 171
Follicular centre cells, 168
Follicular dendritic cell sarcoma, 285-287
Follicular dendritic cell tumour, 286
Follicular dendritic cell tumours, 277
Follicular dendritic cell (FDC), 123, 160, 164, 165, 169, 225, 226, 243, 252, 276, 285-288
Follicular lymphoma (FL), 119, 121, 124-126, 133, 136, 159, 160, 162-167, 171, 173, 184, 191, 270, 271
Follicular mucinosis, 220
Franklin disease, 154

G

Gamma delta T-cell lymphomas, 210
Gamma delta T cells, 192, 194, 207, 210, 211, 268, 269
Gamma heavy chain disease, 134, 154
Gaucher-like cells, 146
Glycophorin A, 78, 98, 99, 104
Granulocytic sarcoma, 81, 105
Granulomatous slack skin, 220
Granzyme B, 194, 197, 203, 207, 213, 222, 233
Graft vs Host disease (GVHD), 121, 264

H

H. pylori, see Helicobacter pylori
HCL, see Hairy cell leukaemia

HCDD, see Heavy chain deposition disease
Helicobacter pylori, 119, 122, 126, 157-160
Highly active antiretroviral therapy (HAART), 260
Haematopoiesis, 13, 17, 32, 34, 37, 41, 47, 63, 66, 105, 116, 143, 149
Haematopoietic stem cell, 67, 84, 87, 89, 90, 92
Haemoglobin A, 23, 78, 98, 99, 104
Haemorrhagic thrombocythaemia, 39
Hairy cell leukaemia (HCL), 121, 125, 136, 138-140, 275, 295
Hand mirror cells, 112
Hand-Schüller-Christian disease, 280
Hashimoto thyroiditis, 122, 157-159, 161
Heavy chain diseases, 154
Heavy chain deposition disease (HCDD), 150, 152, 153
HECA-452, 222
Helper T cells, 192
Hemophagocytosis, 94
Hepatitis C virus, 122, 133
Hepatosplenic T-cell lymphoma, 194, 210
Hepatosplenomegaly, 13, 27, 38, 56, 99, 130, 154, 155, 168, 195, 199, 200, 201, 210, 212, 225, 278, 284
HES, see Hypereosinophilic syndrome
HHV8, 122, 145, 179, 180, 255, 260, 262
Histiocytic and dendritic cell neoplasms, 273, 275
Histiocytic sarcoma, 275, 278, 279
Histiocytosis X, see Langerhans cell histiocytosis
HIV, see Human immunodeficiency virus
HL, see Hodgkin lymphoma
HLA-DR, 23, 84, 92, 94, 99, 100, 102, 106, 114, 207, 279, 281, 287
Hodgkin cells, 186, 244, 245
Hodgkin disease, 130, 239
Hodgkin lymphoma (HL), 13, 30, 128, 176, 186, 194, 220, 223, 229, 230, 232, 237, 239, 240, 243-250, 252, 253, 258-261, 268, 270, 271, 280
Hodgkin's paragranuloma, 240
Hodgkin's sarcoma, 253
Hodgkin and Reed-Sternberg cell (HRS), 239, 242-250, 252, 253
HRX, see MLL
HTLV-1, 189, 191, 195, 200, 201, 203, 216, 217, 219
Human immunodeficiency virus (HIV), 121, 122, 145, 171, 173, 179-182, 185, 244, 250, 253, 255, 260-263, 268, 281
Human immunodeficiency virus (HIV)-related lymphoma, 260, 262, 263
Hybrid acute leukaemia, 106
Hyper IgM syndrome, 257, 258, 259
Hypereosinophilic syndrome (HES), 29, 30, 31, 294
Hyperleukocytosis, 93
Hypocellular acute leukaemia, 91
Hypocellular acute myeloid leukaemia, 78

I

Idiopathic myelofibrosis, 35, 100
Idiopathic thrombocytosis, 39
IGV, 123, 124

Myeloproliferative disease, undifferentiated 42
Myelodysplastic/myeloproliferative disorder, 52, 58, 88
Myelodysplastic/myeloproliferative disorder, unclassifiable (MDS/MPD-U), 58, 59
Myeloid sarcoma, 104, 105, 116
Myelomatosis, 142
Myeloperoxidase (MPO), 23, 30, 79, 82-84, 86, 87, 92-96, 98-102, 104-106, 112, 114, 117, 215, 279, 281, 285, 287, 300
Myelosclerosis with myeloid metaplasia, 35
MYH11, 84

N

Nasal and nasal-type NK/T-cell lymphoma, 191, 194, 204, 205, 207, 211
NBS, see Nijmegen breakage syndrome
N-CAM, 207
Neuroblastoma, 100, 105, 114, 117
Neurofibromatosis type 1, 47, 55-57
Neurofibromatosis type-1, 47
Neutropenia, 49, 64, 71, 72, 91-93, 106, 111, 197-200
NHL, see Non-Hodgkin lymphoma
Nijmegen breakage syndrome (NBS), 257, 258
NK-cell neoplasms, 189, 191, 194, 204
NLPHL, see Nodular lymphocyte predominant Hodgkin lymphoma
Nodular lymphocyte predominant Hodgkin lymphoma (NLPHL), 171, 172, 239, 240, 242, 243, 247, 250, 252, 259
Nodular sclerosis Hodgkin lymphoma (NSHL), 176, 239, 244, 245, 248-250, 253, 261
Non-Hodgkin lymphoma of the lymphoblastic type, 105
Non-Hodgkin lymphoma (NHL), 13, 96, 119, 121, 127, 162, 168, 171, 191, 212, 215, 216, 225, 229, 230, 239, 247, 252, 253, 260-262, 280
Non-secretory myeloma, 143
Normoblastemia, 97
NPM, 85, 86, 174, 222, 232-235
NPM-ALK, 174, 232-235
NSHL, see Nodular sclerosis Hodgkin lymphoma
Nuclear matrix associated gene (NuMA), 85
Nucleophosmin, 85, 233, 234
NuMa, see Nuclear matrix associated gene

O

Oct2, 243, 246, 247
Oligoblastic leukaemia, 63
Organomegaly, 17, 38, 43, 102, 144
Osteosclerosis, 34, 42, 300
Osteosclerotic myeloma, 154

P

p15, 166
p16, 166, 169, 218
p24, 145, 248

p53, 128, 129, 132, 148, 170, 173, 248, 263; see also TP53
P. carini, see Pneumocystis carinii
Pagetoid reticulosis, 211, 220
Pancytopenia, 70, 88, 89, 103, 138, 177, 212, 258, 277, 278, 281
Panmyelosis, 33, 38, 90, 100, 103
Parafollicular lymphoma, see Marginal zone B-cell lymphoma
PAS, 88, 98, 100, 101, 102, 112, 133
Pautrier microabcesses, 217
Pautrier-like microabscesses, 202
PAX-5, 134, 148
PCL, 144
P-component, 151, 152
PDGFbR, 47, 54
PEL, see Primary effusion lymphoma
Perforin, 194, 197, 207, 210, 213, 222, 233
Peripheral lymphadenopathy, 130, 131, 135, 155, 161, 210, 225, 240, 244
Peripheral T-cell lymphoma, 191, 198, 207, 225, 227, 229, 231, 247, 259, 262, 268, 270
Peripheral T-cell lymphoma, unspecified, 191, 207, 227, 231, 268
Peripheral T-cell neoplasm, 200, 225, 227
Philadelphia (Ph) chromosome, 15, 18, 20, 23, 25, 27-29, 31, 34, 38, 41-44, 47, 49, 53, 54, 57-59, 100, 102, 103, 107, 265, 266, 269
PID, see Primary immune disorders
Plasma cell leukaemia, 142, 144, 146, 147, 154
Plasma cell myeloma, 121, 124-126, 134, 142-152, 154, 155, 172, 174, 267
Plasma cell neoplasm, 124, 130, 134, 142, 149, 150-154, 194
Plasma cell-related amyloid (AL), 151
Plasmacytic hyperplasia, 265, 268, 269
Plasmacytoma, 142, 147-150, 154, 268
Platelet peroxidase (PPO) reaction, 100
Platelets, 17, 18, 36, 38-41, 50, 58, 68, 71, 99, 100, 103, 132
PLZF, see Promyelocyte leukaemia zinc finger
PLZF/RARa, 86
PML, 84-86
PML/RARa, 85, 86
Pneumocystis carinii, 201, 203
POEMS syndrome, 154
Polycythaemia rubra vera, 32
Polycythaemia vera (PV), 17, 18, 19, 32-34, 42-44
Polycythaemia vera (PV), "spent" phase and post-polycythaemic myelofibrosis and myeloid metaplasia (PPMM), 34
Polymorphic PTLD, 266, 269
Polymorphic reticulosis, 204, 207
Popcorn cell, 240, 246
Post-polycythaemic myelofibrosis and myeloid metaplasia (PPMM), 34
Post-transplant lymphoproliferative disease (PTLD), 255, 258, 262, 264-266, 268, 269
Post-transplant lymphoproliferative disease, monomorphic 266
PPMM, see Post-polycythaemic myelofibrosis and myeloid metaplasia
PRAD1, 169
Precursor B ALL/lymphoma, 113
Precursor B lymphoblastic leukaemia, 31, 109, 111
Precursor B lymphoblastic lymphoma, 111, 114

Precursor B lymphoblastic neoplasm, 111
Precursor B-lymphoblast, 114
Precursor B-lymphoblastic leukaemia / lymphoma, 184
Precursor NK-cell lymphoblastic lymphoma/ leukaemia, 214
Precursor T lymphoblast, 117
Precursor T lymphoblastic leukaemia, 115
precursor T lymphoblastic leukaemia/ lymphoma, 31
Precursor T lymphoblastic lymphoma, 115
Precursor T-ALL, 115
Precursor T-lymphoblastic leukaemia / lymphoma, 215
Precursor T-lymphoblastic lymphoma/ leukaemia, 259
Preleukaemic syndromes, 63
Primary amyloidosis, 151
Primary cutaneous CD30-positive T-cell lymphoproliferative disorders, 221, 224
Primary cutaneous anaplastic large cell lymphoma (C-ALCL), 221-224
Primary cutaneous anaplastic large cell lymphoma, lymphomatoid papulosis, 221-224
Primary cutaneous anaplastic large cell lymphoma, borderline lesions, 221, 224
Primary effusion lymphoma (PEL), 122, 125, 179, 260, 262, 263
Primary immune disorders (PID), 257-259
Primary myelofibrosis, 35
Primary thrombocytosis, 39
Progressively transformed germinal centres, (PTGC), 240
Prolymphocytic leukaemia, 96, 140, 168, 195, 259
Promyelocytic leukaemia zinc finger, 85
Pseudo Chediak-Higashi granules, 65, 71, 81
Pseudo Pelger-Huet, 65, 66, 70, 71, 81, 86, 88, 93
Pseudofollicles, 127, 128, 131, 133, 168, 169
Pseudo-Gaucher cells, 21
PTEN, 218
PTGC, see Progressively transformed germinal centres
PTLD, see Post-transplant lymphoproliferative disease
Pure erythroid leukaemia, 91, 97, 98, 99, 100
Pure sideroblastic anaemia, 69
Psoralen/UVA therapy (PUVA), 223
PV, see Polycythaemia vera

R

RA, see Refractory anaemia
RAEB, see Refractory anaemia with excess blasts
Randall disease, 152
RARa, 84-86
RARS, see Refractory anaemia with ringed sideroblasts
RAS, 18, 25, 47, 52, 57, 263, 269
RCMD, see Refractory cytopenia with multilineage dysplasia
RCMD-RS, see Refractory cytopenia with multilineage dysplasia with ringed sideroblasts

WORLD HEALTH ORGANIZATION CLASSIFICATION OF TUMOURS

Third edition of the Blue Books Series, combining histological and genetic typing of human neoplasms

The new series *World Health Organization Classification of Tumours,* published by the International Agency for Research on Cancer (IARC), Lyon/France, provides standardized guidelines on the histological and genetic typing of human tumours.

Each title of the new Blue Book series is the outcome of a collaborative effort by a multidisciplinary, international working group of experts. Diagnostic criteria, pathological features and associated genetic alterations are described in a strictly disease-oriented manner. Profiles of all recognized neoplasms and their variants include new ICD-O codes, incidence, age and sex distribution, location, clinical signs and symptoms, pathology, genetics and predictive factors. The books contain more than 500 colour photographs, MRIs, CT scans, charts and an up-to-date reference list.

Authoritative and concise, the series provides an international standard for pathologists, oncologists and geneticists. It will serve as an indispensable guide for the design of trials monitoring response to therapy and clinical outcome. IARC plans to publish two to three books per year, with completion of the series due in 2004.

WHO Blue Books on the web:
http://www.iarc.fr/WHO-bluebooks

Pathology & Genetics of Tumours of the Nervous System

Edited by P. Kleihues & W.K. Cavenee
Includes new disease entities and inherited tumour syndromes.
314 pages, 600 colour photographs, MRIs, CTs and charts.

Lyon 2000 · ISBN 92 832 2409 4 · US$ 75.00

Pathology & Genetics of Tumours of the Digestive System

Edited by S.R. Hamilton & L.A. Aaltonen
Includes neoplasms of the gastrointestinal tract, liver, biliary system and exocrine pancreas.
320 pages, 700 colour photographs, MRIs, CTs and charts.
Lyon 2000 · ISBN 92 832 2410 8 · US$ 75.00

Pathology & Genetics of Tumours of the Breast and Female Genital Organs

Edited by F.A. Tavassoli, R.H. Young and M.R. Stratton
Includes a comprehensive classification of interest to pathologists, gynaecologists and basic scientists.
Ca. 300 pages, 600 coloured photographs, MRIs, CTs and charts.
ISBN 92 8322412 4 · US$ 75.00
Publication date: Spring 2002

Future volumes will cover tumours of bone and soft tissues, skin, kidney and genitourinary, endocrine organs, head and neck, and the lower respiratory tract, mediastinum and thymus.

IARC*Press* · Lyon · Washington